Management and Leadership for Nurse Administrators

Fourth Edition

Edited by

Linda Roussel, RN, DSN
Associate Professor
University of South Alabama
College of Nursing
Mobile, Alabama

with

Russell C. Swansburg, RN, PhD
Consultant in Nursing and Hospital Administration
San Antonio, Texas

and

Richard J. Swansburg, RN, BSN, MSCIS
Systems Software Specialist II
University of South Alabama
Mobile, Alabama

JONES AND BARTLETT PUBLISHERS
Sudbury, Massachusetts
BOSTON TORONTO LONDON SINGAPORE

World Headquarters
Jones and Bartlett Publishers
40 Tall Pine Drive
Sudbury, MA 01776
978-443-5000
info@jbpub.com
www.jbpub.com

Jones and Bartlett Publishers
Canada
6339 Ormindale Way
Mississauga, ON L5V 1J2
Canada

Jones and Bartlett Publishers
International
Barb House, Barb Mews
London W6 7PA
United Kingdom

Jones and Bartlett's books and products are available through most bookstores and online booksellers. To contact Jones and Bartlett Publishers directly, call 800-832-0034, fax 978-443-8000, or visit our website www.jbpub.com.

Substantial discounts on bulk quantities of Jones and Bartlett's publications are available to corporations, professional associations, and other qualified organizations. For details and specific discount information, contact the special sales department at Jones and Bartlett via the above contact information or send an email to specialsales@jbpub.com.

ISBN-13: 978-0-7637-3486-2
ISBN-10: 0-7637-3486-1

Production Credits
Acquisitions Editor: Kevin Sullivan
Production Director: Amy Rose
Associate Editor: Amy Sibley
Associate Production Editor: Carolyn Rogers
Marketing Manager: Emily Ekle
Manufacturing Buyer: Amy Bacus
Composition: Graphic World
Cover Design: Timothy Dziewit
Text Design: Nova Graphic Services, Inc.
Printing and Binding: Bradford & Bigelow
Cover Printing: Bradford & Bigelow

Library of Congress Cataloging-in-Publication Data
Management and leadership for nurse administrators / [edited by] Linda Roussel with Russell C. Swansburg, and Richard J. Swansburg.— 4th ed.
p. ; cm.
Rev. ed. of: Introduction to management and leadership for nurse managers / Russell C. Swansburg, Richard J. Swansburg. c2002.
Includes bibliographical references and index.
ISBN 0-7637-3486-1 (pbk. : alk. paper)
1. Nursing services—Administration. 2. Nurse administrators. 3. Leadership. I. Roussel, Linda. II. Swansburg, Richard J. III. Swansburg, Russell C. Introduction to management and leadership for nurse managers.
[DNLM: 1. Nursing, Supervisory. 2. Administrative Personnel. 3. Nurse Administrators. WY 105 M2655 2006]
RT89.S885 2006
362.17'3'068—dc22
2005019368

6048

Printed in the United States of America
10 09 08 07 06 10 9 8 7 6 5 4 3 2

To Russell and Laurel Clark Swansburg:
Thank you for this opportunity and your
mentorship throughout my career.

Contents

Chapter 3: Ethical Principles for the Nurse Administrator

Chapter 4: The Components of Change: Creativity and Innovation, Critical Thinking, and Planned Change

Chapter 5: Decision Making and Problem Solving: Communication Practices and Skills

Chapter 9: The Planning Process

Chapter 10: Staffing and Scheduling

Chapter 13: eNursing

Chapter 14: Health Policy, Legal, and Regulatory Issues

Chapter 17: Quality Management

Chapter 18: Performance Appraisal

Chapter 19: The Nurse Manager of Staff Development

Preface

> Management exists for the sake of the institution's results. It has to start with the intended results and has to organize the resources of the institution to attain these results. It is the organ to make the institution, whether business, church, university, hospital, or a battered women's shelter, capable of producing results outside of itself.
>
> P. F. Drucker[1]

This book is organized around the *Scope and Standards for Nurse Administrators* with the overall conceptualization of the four major management functions: planning, organizing, directing or leading, and controlling or evaluating. It is designed for management development of professional nurses in the 21st century. *Management and Leadership for Nurse Administrators, Fourth Edition*, is suitable for an introductory course in nursing administration in graduate programs. This book can also be used in upper-level baccalaureate programs in which students complete a basic course in management essentials before their senior year. This text is also designed for staff development of nurse managers in the service setting. The theory and principles of *Management and Leadership for Nurse Administrators, Fourth Edition*, apply to the entire spectrum of health care institutions and settings.

Management and Leadership for Nurse Administrators, Fourth Edition, provides theoretical and practical knowledge that will aid professional nurses in meeting the demands of constantly changing patient care services. Because the demand for nurses in some specialties and geographic areas exceeds supply, it is essential that management processes provide the environment for high morale, motivation, and productivity. Financial considerations have increasingly dominated the health care industry, making the job of managing costly human and material resources ever more important.

Health care institutions have been restructured, demassed, and decentralized along with other business and industrial institutions. This book has been revised to provide the best management concepts and theory of management available from the fields of generic management as well as nursing management sources.

Chapters have been updated and streamlined. Chapters on ethical issues for nurse administrators and emotional intelligence for professional nursing administrative practice have been added to this new edition.

The current shortages of students in generic nursing programs and graduate nurses in practice require application of sound management principles to recruit and retain nurses in these areas.

NOTE

1. Drucker, P. (1999). Management Challenges for the 21st Century. New York: HarperCollins.

Contributors

Chapter 2: Emotionally Intelligent Leadership in Nursing and Health Care Organizations
Susan H. Taft, RN, MSN, PhD
Kent State University
Kent, OH

Chapter 4: The Components of Change: Creativity and Innovation, Critical Thinking, and Planned Change
Elizabeth Simms, RN, MSN
Nurse Manager
Medical Center of Louisiana in New Orleans
New Orleans, LA

Chapter 6: Organizational Structure and Analysis
Denise Danna, RN, DNS, CNAA, CHE
Nurse Executive
Memorial Tenet Hospital
New Orleans, LA

Chapter 8: Human Resource Development: Managing a Culturally Diverse Work Force
Susan Jacob, RN, MSN
Ochsner Medical Center
New Orleans, LA

Chapter 9: The Planning Process
Elizabeth Simms, RN, MSN
Nurse Manager
Medical Center of Louisiana in New Orleans
New Orleans, LA

Chapter 10: Staffing and Scheduling
Elizabeth Simms, RN, MSN
Nurse Manager
Medical Center of Louisiana in New Orleans
New Orleans, LA

Chapter 11: Principles of Budgeting
Denise Danna, RN, DNS, CNAA, CHE
Nurse Executive
Memorial Tenet Hospital
New Orleans, LA

Chapter 13: eNursing
Richard J. Swansburg, RN, BSN, MSCIS
Systems Software Specialist II
University of South Alabama
Mobile, AL

Chapter 14: Health Policy, Legal, and Regulatory Issues
Mary-Eliese Merrill, RN, MSN
Director, Mental Health Service Line
Veterans Administration Memorial Hospital
New Orleans, LA

Chapter 17: Quality Management
Beverly Blain Wright, RNC, CAN, CPHQ
Quality Management Project Coordinator
University of South Alabama Medical Center
Mobile, AL

Chapter 19: The Nurse Manager of Staff Development
Lynn P. Norman, RN, MSN
Assistant Professor
School of Nursing
Auburn University at Montgomery
Montgomery, AL

CHAPTER 1

Conceptualization of Nursing Administration: Theory and Concepts

Linda Roussel, RN, DSN

It is only with the heart that one can see rightly; what is essential is invisible to the eye.

Antoine de Saint-Exupéry

LEARNING OBJECTIVES AND ACTIVITIES

- Identify the scope and standards for nurse administrators as a framework for practice.
- Define the terms *executive, manager, managing, management*, and *nursing management*.
- Identify five essential management practices that promote patient safety.
- Differentiate among concepts, principles, and theory.
- Describe critical theory.
- Discuss general systems theory.
- Illustrate selected principles of nursing management.
- Describe roles for nurse managers and nurse executives, differentiating among levels.
- Distinguish between two cognitive styles: intuitive thinking and rational thinking. Give examples of each.
- Discuss the use of nursing theory in managing a clinical practice.
- Discuss the responsibility of the nurse administrator for managing a clinical discipline.

CONCEPTS: Scope of practice, standards of practice for nurse administrators, management theory, nursing management theory, critical theory, general systems theory, nursing management, management principles, management development, nursing management roles, role development, cognitive styles, intuitive thinking, rational thinking, management levels, modalities of nursing.

NURSE MANAGER BEHAVIORS: Applies traditional and postmodern management theory to organizational operations. Assesses the impact of various influences from ethnic, political, social, financial, economic, and ethical issues perspectives. Networks with state, regional, national, and global peers to share ideas and conduct mutual problem solving. Demonstrates a commitment to lifelong learning and ongoing professional development through such activities as certification and participation in professional organizations.

NURSE EXECUTIVE BEHAVIORS: Examines the possibility of developing application of a nursing management theory by creating a business plan that incorporates a pilot study. Works with representatives of the professional nursing staff to develop and test the pilot study. Leads initiatives in innovative programs and new implementation alternatives. Pursues continuing education, certification, professional development, and networking. Seeks experiences to advance one's skills and knowledge base in areas of responsibilities, including the art and science of nursing, changes in health care systems, application of emerging technologies, and administrative practices.

Introduction

Providing a framework for nursing administrative practice necessitates a conceptualization of the various functions, roles, and responsibilities of a nurse administrator. Changes in the landscape of health care—such as new technology, increased diversity in the workplace, greater accountability for practice, and a new spiritual focus on the mind and body connection—require creativity and innovative leadership and management models. A roadmap, with its definitive lines of direction, is not enough. A more appropriate analogy is that of using a compass to find true north in this new age of nursing practice and health care delivery systems. Productivity and cost concerns remain important; however, there is an equal if not greater focus on safety, quality relationships, and healing environments.

Sound nursing and management theories, along with evidence-based management practices, equip the nurse administrator with the tools to foster a culture of collaborative decision making and positive patient and staff outcomes. Core competencies identified by the Institute of Medicine in its work on educating health care professionals further underscore the work that needs to be done:[1]

1. Provide patient-centered care,
2. Work in interdisciplinary teams,
3. Employ evidence-based practice,
4. Apply quality improvement, and
5. Utilize informatics.

The core competencies apply to all health care professionals and emphasize greater integration of disciplines and creating a culture specifically focused on improving safety outcomes in health care. Transformational leadership and evidence-based management are necessary components of redesigning our current health care system.

Scope and Standards for Nurse Administrators: Framework for Practice

In a joint position statement on nursing administration education, The American Association of Colleges of Nursing and the American Organization of Nurse Executives outline core abilities necessary for nurses in administrative roles. These include the abilities to use management skills that enhance collaborative relationships and team-based learning to advocate for patients and community partners, to embrace change and innovation, to manage resources effectively, to negotiate and resolve conflict, and to communicate effectively using information technology. Content for specialty education in nursing administration includes such concepts and constructs as strategic management, policy development, financial management/cost analysis, leadership, organizational development and business planning, and interdisciplinary relationships. Being mentored by expert executive nurses, engaging in research, and enacting evidence-based management (such as the tracking of effectiveness of care, cost of care, and patient outcomes) are also critical to the education of nurse administrators. *Scope and Standards for Nurse Administrators* provides a conceptual model for educating and developing nurses in the professional practice of administrative nursing and health care. This document serves as a framework for this book, which focuses on the levels of nursing administration practice, the standards of practice, and the standards of professional performance for nurse administrators. Consideration of the scope and standards, the role of certification, magnet recognition, and best practice will also be included from this frame of reference.[2] Management and leadership theory serves to further reinforce the concepts required for nursing administrative practice. Such concepts are essential to managing a clinical practice discipline.

The Nurse Administrator

The nurse administrator has been described as a "registered nurse whose primary responsibility is the management of health care delivery services and who represents nursing service."[3] Nurse administrators can be found in a wide variety of settings, with entrepreneurial opportunities available throughout the health care arena. In addition to hospitals, home health care and skilled care, nurse administrators can also serve in such settings as assisted living, community health services, residential care, and adult day care. In these settings, the nurse administrator must be adequately prepared to face challenges in diverse fields such as information management, evidence-based care and management, legal and regulatory oversight, and ethical practices.

Level of Nursing Administrative Practice

The American Nurses Association (ANA) conceptually divides nursing administration practice into two levels: nurse executive and nurse manager, each with a particular focus that makes a unique contribution to the management of health care systems. The nurse executive's scope includes overall management of nursing practice, nursing education and professional development, nursing research, nursing administration, and nursing services. "The nurse executive holds the accountability to manage within the context of the organization as a whole, and to transform organizational values into daily operations yielding an efficient, effective, and caring organization."[4] Particular functions of the nurse executive include leadership, development, implementation, and evaluation of protocols, programs, and services that are evidence-based and congruent with professional standards.

Nurse managers are responsible to a nurse executive and have more defined areas of nursing service. Advocating and allocating for available resources to facilitate effective, efficient, safe, and compassionate care based on standards of practice are the cornerstone roles of the nurse manager. A nurse manager performs these management functions to deliver health care to patients. Nurse managers or administrators work at all levels to put into practice the concepts, principles, and theories of nursing management. They manage the organizational environment to provide a climate optimal to the provision of nursing care by clinical nurses and ancillary staff.

Management knowledge is universal; so is nursing management knowledge. It uses a systematic body of knowledge that includes concepts, principles, and theories applicable to all nursing management situations. A nurse manager who has applied this knowledge successfully in one situation can be expected to do so in new situations. Nursing management occurs at unit and executive levels. At the executive level, it is frequently termed administration; however, the theories, principles, and concepts remain the same.

With decentralization and participatory management, the supervisor, or middle management, level has been largely eliminated. Nurse managers of clinical units are being educated in management theory and skills at the master's level. Clinical nurses are being educated in management skills that empower them to take action in managing groups of employees as well as clients and families. Clinical nurse managers perform more of the coordinating duties among units, departments, and services. "Nurse managers are accountable for the environment in which clinical nursing is practiced."[5] Both the nurse executive and nurse manager use the Standards of Practice and Standards of Professional Performance as priorities for nurse administrative practice.

The standards of practice (as framework for this edition) include the following:[6]

Standard 1: Assessment
Considers data collection systems and processes. Analyzes workflow in relation to effectiveness and efficiency of assessment processes. Evaluates assessment practices.

Standard 2: Problems/Diagnosis
Considers the identification and procurement of adequate resources for decision analysis. Promotes interdisciplinary collaboration. Promotes an organizational climate that supports the validation of problems and formulation of a diagnosis of the organization's environment, culture, and values that direct and support care delivery.

Standard 3: Identification of Outcomes
Considers the interdisciplinary identification of outcomes and the development and utilization of databases that include nursing measures. Promotes continuous improvement of outcome-related clinical guidelines that foster continuity of care.

Standard 4: Planning
Considers development, maintenance, and evaluation of organizational systems that facilitate planning for care delivery. Creativity and innovation that promote organizational processes for desired patient-defined and cost-effective outcomes are also included in this standard. Collaborates and advocates for staff involvement in all levels of organizational planning and decision making.

Standard 5: Implementation
Considers the appropriate personnel to implement the design and improvement of systems and processes that assure interventions. Considers the efficient documentation of interventions and patient responses.

Standard 6: Evaluation
Considers support of participative decision making. Develops policies, procedures, and guidelines based on research findings and institutional measurement of quality outcomes. Evaluation includes the integration of clinical, human resource, and financial data to adequately plan nursing and patient care.

Standards of professional performance such as quality of care and administrative practice, performance appraisal, professional knowledge, professional environment, ethics, collaboration, research, and resource utilization are also integrated in the framework of this edition. These standards are weaved within the chapters and provide continuity of processes and systems of nursing administration.

Magnet Recognition Program and *Scope and Standards for Nurse Administrators*

The American Nurses Credentialing Center (ANCC) provides guidelines for the Magnet Recognition Program. This program's purpose is to recognize health care organizations that have demonstrated the very best in nursing care and professional nursing practice. Such programs have been recognized for having the best practices in nursing, and they also serve to attract and retain quality employees. A key objective of the program is to promote positive patient outcomes. This program also offers a vehicle for communicating best practices and strategies among nursing systems. "Magnet designation helps consumers locate health care organizations that have a proven level of nursing care."[7] Quality indicators and standards of nursing practice as identified by the ANA's *Scope and Standards for Nurse Administrators* are cornerstone to the Magnet Recognition Program. Qualitative and quantitative factors in nursing are also included in the appraisal process. Certification of nurse administrators is also endorsed through the Magnet Recognition Program.

Qualifications of Nurse Administrators

Attaining the license, education, and experience required for levels of nursing administrative practice is paramount to success in the role as well as to the organizational responsibilities accepted. The nurse manager and nurse executive must hold an active registered nurse license and meet the requirements in the state in which they practice. The nurse executive should hold a bachelor's degree and master's degree (or higher) with a major in nursing. The doctoral degree in a relevant field is considered important and is a nationally recognized certification in nursing administration.

In the nurse manager's role, preparation should be a minimum of a bachelor's degree with a major in nursing. A master's degree with a focus in nursing is recommended along with nationally recognized certification in nursing administration with an appropriate specialty. "The experience backgrounds of professional nurses who serve as nurse administrators must include clinical and administrative practice, which enables these registered nurses to consistently fulfill the responsibilities inherent in their respective administrative roles."[8]

Certification of Nursing Administration

The ANCC offers two levels for Nursing Administration, including an advanced level. Both certification examinations include the following domains: organization and structure, economics, human resources, ethics, and legal and regulatory issues. The domain of organization and structure accounts for the highest percentage of questions for the advanced level. For the nurse manager level, the domain of human resources ranks highest. Both certification examinations include 175 questions with 150 questions scored. Review and resource materials for certification are available and can provide continuing education units for the certification examination.

Using management theory as an underlying framework, support the work of the nurse administrator through the *Scope and Standards for Nurse Administrators*.

Management: Premodern, Modern, and Postmodern Eras

Consideration of premodern, modern and postmodern eras provides a broader perspective on management. The premodern era includes the concepts of work as craft, apprenticeship, journeyman artisan, fraternal organization of professions, and tradition. The modern management era considers pyramids, hierarchy, systems of money, materials, manpower, inspection, distribution, and production in specialized cells that minimize interaction. The postmodern era includes networks, network stakeholders, and team planning.

Mary Parker Follett is credited with being the "mother of modern management." Taylor, Fayol, and Weber have had considerable influence on modern management and are called the "fathers of modern management." Scientific management (efficiency) provided information on standards, time/motion studies, task analysis, job simplification, and productivity incentives.

Modern management theory evolved from the work of Henri Fayol, who identified the activities or functions of the administrator as planning, organizing, coordinating, and controlling.[9] His work has been called "process management." Fayol defined management in these words:

> To manage is to forecast and plan, to organize, to command, to coordinate, and to control. To foresee and provide means [of] examining the future and drawing up the plan of action. To organize means building up the dual structure, material and human, of the undertaking. To command means binding together, unifying and harmonizing all activity and effort. To control means seeing that everything occurs in conformity with established rule and expressed demand.[10]

Although some persons believed these were technical functions that could be learned only on the job, Fayol believed that they could be taught in an educational setting if a theory of administration could be formulated.[11] He also stated that the need for managerial ability increases in relative importance as an individual advances in the chain of command.

Fayol listed the principles of management as follows:[12]

1. Division of work
2. Authority
3. Discipline
4. Unity of command
5. Unity of direction
6. Subordination of individual interests to the general interests
7. Remuneration
8. Centralization
9. Scalar chain (line of authority)
10. Order
11. Equity
12. Stability or tenure of personnel
13. Initiative
14. Esprit de corps

Urwick, a theorist in the development of the science and the art of management, believed that administrative skill was a practical art that improved with practice and required intense study and thinking. According to Urwick, the administrator must master intellectual principles, reinforcing the process through general reflection on actual problems. From his work, Urwick concluded that there are three principles of administration. He described the first principle as investigation and stated that all scientific procedure is based on investigation of the facts. The second principle is appropriateness, which underlines forecasting, enters into the process with organization, and takes effect in coordination. Exercising the third principle, planning, the administrator looks ahead and organizes resources to meet future needs. Planning enters into the process with command and is effected in control.[13]

Human relations management and behavioral science and management are also integrated into the modern management paradigm. The Hawthorne studies validated the influence of working conditions on employee efficiency and productivity. Labor and management relationships, communication, and democratization of the workplace are key aspects of human relations management. Maslow, Hertberg, MacGregor, Argyris, and Likert have been instrumental in developing behavioral science management theory. Additionally, Blake, Mouton, Fiedler, Hersey, and Blanchard are also noted for their work in this aspect of the modern era. Building on the work of human relations management, the behaviorists paid particular attention to leadership, participative management, personal motivation and hygiene factors, and hierarchy of workers' needs. During the modern management era, there was noted stability in the work force, limited diversity in the workplace, and a better educated work force.

Throughout management literature, the original functions of planning, organizing, directing (command and coordination), and controlling as defined by Fayol, Urwick, and others have been accepted as the principal functions of managers. While linear structures, bureaucracy, rationality, and control define the modern area, the postmodern era considers a new universe of pattern, purpose, and process. Postmodern organizations are described as loosely coupled, fluid, organic, and "adhocratic." Organic, continuum-based, and living systems are inherent to this era. Wilson and Porter-O'Grady contrast linear integration with meta-integration, which focuses on long-term service orientation, systems design, and population/person-driven, continuum-based and outcome-driven systems. According to the authors, the postmodern manager's role is accountability-based, resource-oriented, and service-driven. The term *service-driven* highlights the manager's role as facilitator, integrator, and coordinator.

Peter Drucker first applied the term postmodern to organization in 1957, identifying a shift from the Cartesian universe of mechanical cause and effect (subject/object duality) to this new order of pattern, purpose, and process. Knowledge workers were also included in this discussion with greater emphasis on providing management processes and systems that supported decision making at the point of service by those knowledgeable about the processes. Evidence-based management is viewed as critical to transforming work environments and providing safe and quality care.[14]

Evidence-based management has particular significance in health care, as the work environment experiences greater turbulence, chaos, and instability than do those of other disciplines. Dated and untested management practices are no longer useful and may be detrimental to providing safe care. In *Keeping Patients Safe, Transforming the Work Environment*, the Committee on the Work Environment for Nurses underscores the importance of sound, evidence-based management practices. Using an evidence-based frame of reference, managers, like their clinical counterparts, are accountable for searching for, appraising, and applying empirical evidence from management research in their practices. Additionally, thoughtful reflection, decision making, and actions by managers should be systematically recorded and evaluated in ways that further add to the evidence base of effective management practice. The committee identified five essential management practices.[15] These five practices have not been consistently applied, adding further evidence to their importance in today's health care environment.

1. Balancing the tension between efficiency and effectiveness
   Best practices in this domain include putting redundancy into work design, which has proven effective in the air traffic control industry. Consideration of production efficiency, balance and alignment of organizational goals, accountability processes, rewards, incentives, and compensation are aspects of this practice, which can improve patient outcomes.
2. Creating and sustaining trust
   Trust and honest, open communication are critical to successful organizational change. When there is openness and trust, individuals are more willing to make contributions to the organization without immediate payoffs. Trust in an organization's leaders and management practices has been linked to positive business outcomes such as increased productivity and greater profitability, whereas distrust has been linked to increased absenteeism, turnover, and risk aversion.
3. Actively managing the process of change
   This management practice is related to human resource management and includes practices such as ongoing communication; training; designing mechanisms for feedback, measurement, and redesign; sustained attention; and worker involvement. The concept of investment in change as being good for the organization and individual is illuminated in this practice.
4. Involving workers in work design and workflow decision making
   Hierarchically structured and highly controlled organizations lack the flexibility to respond to situations that are highly variable and associated with

reduced safety. The concepts of shared governance, nursing empowerment, control over nursing practice, and clinical autonomy have been noted to improve patient outcomes as well as worker satisfaction. The key element in this practice is nurses' control over their practice. This influences care of the individual patient as well as organizational policies and practices carried out within nursing units, the effects of the health care organization as a whole on nursing care, and the control of resources in care provision. Magnet hospitals support these aspects of nurses' involvement. Studies reveal that both autonomy and control over nursing practice are consistent magnet characteristics. Additionally, nurses' autonomy and control over practice are positively related to trust in management.[16]

5. Creating a learning organization
   Learning organizations constantly manage the learning process and consider all sources of knowledge, the use of systematic experimentation to generate new knowledge within the organization, and the quick and efficient transfer of knowledge within the organization. Understanding the existing knowledge culture within the organization is important to the work of creating a learning organization with enough time to think, learn, and train. Incentives and reward systems must be aligned and must facilitate knowledge management practices in the creation of a learning environment.[17]

These five essential management practices in nurses' work environment and health care at large are inconsistent at best and create barriers to positive patient outcomes. An understanding of management theory and practices provides a foundation for best practice.

Managing means accomplishing the goals of the group through effective and efficient use of resources. Specifically, project management is considered a core competency for nurses and managers. Some organizations have adopted project management as their main management approach (management-by-project); other organizations superimpose project management on their current organizational structure and management practices. The manager creates and maintains an internal environment in an enterprise in which individuals work together as a group. Managing is the art of doing, and management is the body of organized knowledge underlying the art. In modern management, staffing is frequently separated from the planning function, directing is labeled *leading*, and *controlling* is used interchangeably with *evaluating*. The ANA's standards for nursing administration are based on these principles, which support the science of nursing administration.[18]

Theory, Concepts, and Principles

The knowledge base of management science includes theory, which in turn includes concepts, methods, and principles. The principles are related and can be observed and verified to some degree when they are translated into the art or practice of management. Concepts are thoughts, ideas, and general notions about a class of objects that form a basis for action or discussion. Concepts tend to be true but are not always true. Principles are fundamental truths, laws, or doctrines on which other notions are based. Principles provide guidance to concepts and to thought or action in a situation.[19] In nursing management research, Urwick's investigation of facts underlies part of the theory of the field.

White explores a viewpoint on nursing theories in which she addresses prescriptive theories. She notes that their use as practice guidelines must be broad enough to provide a wide range of practice situations but not so broad as to be meaningless. A theory of decision making might be more beneficial in practice than a theory of nursing. If nursing is going to base its theory on laws, nurses will need to validate principles through research—a difficult task, as theorists in the social sciences have discovered. It is not easy to reduce human behavior to laws. Nurses deal with human behavior in all roles but particularly in nursing management. Nurses believe that for nursing to be a real profession, it should have a scientific and theoretical base. Nursing is thus a practice profession based on the physical and social sciences.[20]

Nurse managers learn to merge the disciplines of human relations, labor relations, personnel management, and industrial engineering into a unified force for effective management. Many nurse managers would add the theory of nursing to this list. A successful synthesis of these disciplines can promote employee commitment, increased productivity, enhanced competency, good labor relations, and competitiveness in health care. The work force is poorly managed when these goals are not achieved.

Contradictions exist in management theory because of a lack of agreement about sets of ideas and concepts among and within disciplines.[21] Two common approaches are described in the following sections.

Critical Theory Versus Critical Thinking

Steffy and Grimes note that a strict natural science approach to social science is naive, because subjective or qualitative analysis is important to quantitative research. This holds true for management and consequently for nursing management. Health care organizational models are not objective and value-free. Steffy and Grimes suggest using a critical theory approach to organizational science, rather than a phenomenological or hermeneutic approach.

A phenomenological approach uses second-order constructs, or "interpretations of interpretations." This approach requires researchers to become participants in the organization and to suspend all judgments and preconceived ideas about possible meanings. The nurse manager interprets the meaning of nursing management experiences or observations and arrives at a nursing management theory from the aggregate of meanings.

Hermeneutics is the art of textual interpretation. In this approach, the nurse manager as researcher views herself or himself as a historically produced entity and recognizes personal biases in doing research. He or she considers the specific context and historic dimensions of data collected and reflects on the relationship between theory and history.[22]

Critical theory is an empirical philosophy of social institutions. Decision makers, such as nurse managers, translate theories into practice. Theories in use are behavioral technologies that include organizational development, management by objectives or results, strategic planning, planned change, performance appraisal, and other practice-oriented activities performed by managers. Critical theory aims to do the following:

1. critique the ideology of scientism, the institutionalized form of reasoning that accepts the idea that the meaning of knowledge is defined by what the sciences do and thus can be adequately explicated through analysis of scientific procedures, and
2. develop an organizational science capable of changing organizational processes.

These aims are compatible with a theory of nursing management. Nurses are using science to legitimize the practice of clinical nursing and nursing management.[23]

Critical theory is a contemporary school of thought that strenuously criticizes oppressive established values and instructions. "In a more moderate form, critical theory maintains the necessity of examining the hidden assumptions that undergird thinking."[24]

General Systems Theory

General systems theory is an organic approach to the study of the general relationships of the empirical universe of an organization and human thought. The theory comes from the field of biology and poses an analogy between an organism and a social organization. Boulding describes nine levels of a general systems theory,[25] which are given here with nursing management applications:

1. A static structure: the framework. Nursing is a discipline with an aggregate population of registered nurses educated at several levels (including those with hospital diplomas and those with degrees from associate through doctoral levels), licensed practical nurses, and unlicensed assistive personnel (e.g., aides, orderlies, attendants, nursing assistants, and clerks). This population functions within a dynamic and flattening structure that may change frequently. Superior/subordinate relationships are giving way to decentralized, participatory, and transformational management at the practice level. Flat organizations usually have a top administrator, first-line managers, and practitioners. These nursing persons usually function in an environment in which the focus of attention is the client. One approach to a framework in nursing is that nursing persons apply the nursing process in giving care to patients. Many similarities exist between the nursing process and nursing management. (See Exhibit 1-1.)
2. A moving level of necessary predetermined motions: the clockwork. Nurse managers process the knowledge and skills of management—planning, organizing, leading, and evaluating—to produce nursing care. The function of nursing management is the use of personnel, supplies, equipment, clinical knowledge, and skills to give nursing care to clients within varying environments. The nurse manager may also have other ancillary personnel to manage, such as therapists, housekeepers, and social workers, adding to the complexity of providing overall quality services for client care. One such environment is the hospital physical plant. Nursing planning (NP) + nursing organizing (NO) + nursing leading (NL) + nursing evaluating (NE) = nursing management (NM): NP + NO + NL + NE = NM. To this we may add that nursing management (NM) + nursing practice (NPR) = nursing care of clients (NCC), or NM + NP = NCC. The move is toward equilibrium of all forces that go into the nursing management equation.
3. A control mechanism: the thermostat. In nursing administration, this thermostat could be the top administrator or any first-line manager. This person maintains a management information system that transmits and interprets information and communication to and from employees. Production of nursing care of satisfactory quality and quantity depends on the manager maintaining an environment satisfactory to employees.

EXHIBIT 1-1
An Open System

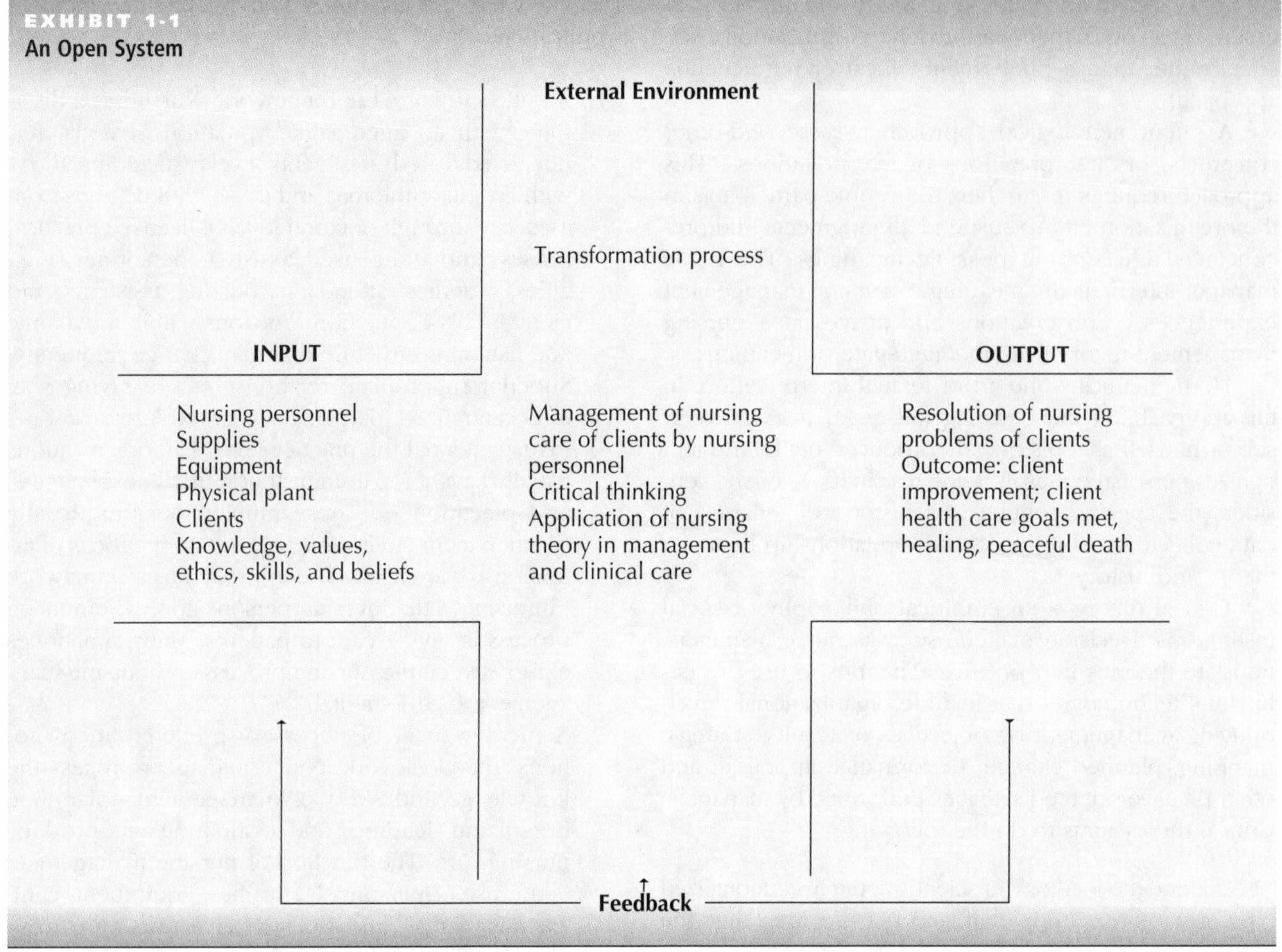

4. An open system or self-maintaining structure: the cell. Nursing management will survive and maintain the nursing organization by being open to new ideas, new management techniques, and the input of human and material resources to produce the nursing care needed by clients. An open system will reproduce itself by keeping up to date and by developing replacements. Keep up to date by adding nursing education (NDU): NM + NP + NE = NCC.
5. The genetic–societal level. There is a division of labor even within nursing management, but especially among nursing personnel who produce the nursing care of patients. Further integrating multi-skill-level personnel into the mix offers more comprehensive complimentary care in meeting clients' health care needs. The raw materials—that is, the human and material resources—are input. These resources are processed as put through by a group of nursing personnel with varying knowledge and skills using a theory-based nursing care delivery system. The output is resolution of the nursing needs and problems of clients, with their improvement, accomplishment of health care goals, and healing, or their succumbing to a peaceful death.
6. The "animal" level. This level has increased mobility, teleological (designing or purposeful) behavior, and self-awareness. Some evidence indicates that nursing management is reaching this level. As nurse managers learn the knowledge and skills of the business and industrial world, they adapt these skills to the management of health care services. This gives nursing management and nursing practice a more scientific basis, the end result of which may be that nurses will be able to demonstrate empirically and theoretically that what they do affects client outcomes.
7. The "human" level. The nurse manager develops an increased awareness and knows that he or she can process the knowledge and skills of management to produce specific results.
8. The level of social organization. Nurse managers at this level distinguish themselves from other groups of managers. Nurse managers operate within com-

plex roles; their functions are made effective by communication, relationships, and other interpersonal processes.

9. Transcendental systems. At this level nurse managers ask questions for which there are as yet no answers. Theoretical models of nursing management extend to level 4 (the cell), the level of application of most other models. Empirical knowledge is deficient at nearly all levels. Descriptive models are needed to catalogue events in nursing. The movement toward decentralization and participatory and service-line management, while still a very simple system, is growing each year as nurse scientists develop and apply new nursing administration models and theories of nursing. General systems theory is the skeleton of a science. Adding nursing research (NR) gives: NM + NP + NE + NR = NCC.

Disciplines and sciences have bodies of knowledge that grow with meaningful information. The empirical universe provides general phenomena relevant to many different disciplines; these phenomena can be built into theoretical models, including one for nursing management. Nursing as a discipline has varied populations (phenomena) that interact dynamically among themselves. These include professional nurses, technical nurses, practical nurses, and unlicensed assistive nursing personnel, as well as professional nursing teachers, researchers, and managers. Individuals within the discipline interact with the environment (another phenomenon). Through knowledge and experience they grow. The media for growth are information, interpersonal processing, relationships, and communication, which are themselves phenomena.[26]

With the emerging changes in health care systems, nurse leaders will need to accelerate changes in nursing organizations. The goal may be nursing modules centered on closely related operations, such as differentiated practice delivery models matched with intensity of care or specialized services. Standardization and flexibility can be melded to develop systems based on a requirement for a theory of nursing practice as a foundation for all modules, but with different theories being used in different modules chosen by professional clinical nurses.[27]

Full realization of systems theory is as far in the future for nursing as it is for manufacturing. Nursing is a "head, heart, and hands" discipline. Nursing management and practice tie the parts of the health care system together. Transformational nurse leaders will be fully knowledgeable about the work being done by their constituents because they will be coaches, mentors, and facilitators. Followers of the systems concept will also have to implement the integration of people, materials, machines, and time.[28]

Nursing-Theory-Based Conceptual Models of Administration: Self-Care Nursing

Sarah E. Allison established Orem's theory as the basis for nursing practice at the Mississippi Methodist Rehabilitation Hospital and Center in the mid to late 1970s. Allison, McLaughlin, and Walker state that a theory-based nursing systems design for a population of patients does the following:

- Describes the nursing characteristics of the patient population to be served
- Uses these characteristics to predict the types of client problems for which nursing is needed
- Identifies appropriate nursing technologies
- Determines the types and number of nursing personnel needed
- Organizes nursing personnel for effective performance
- Defines outcomes or results based on nursing theory[29]

Examination of a theory-based nursing system will be evident in the following:

- Mission, philosophy, and objectives statements
- Documentation tools or forms of data that provide a nursing database
- Standards of care and practice
- Staff education and development
- Quality assurance outcomes audits
- Patient acuity systems
- Position descriptions and performance evaluation
- Policies and procedures
- Career development programs that attract and retain the best nurses by motivating and clarifying the role of the nurse
- Support given by nursing administration commitment[30]

A conceptual model for nursing administrative practice will assist in solving problems associated with change.

"The new assumption on which management, both as a discipline and as a practice, will increasingly have to base itself is that the scope of management is not legal. It has to be operational. It has to embrace the entire process. It has to be focused on results and performance across the entire economic chain."[31]

Another systems-perspective model of nursing is that of Scalzi and Anderson. It comprises three elements: the nursing domain, the management domain, and the interval where the two domains interact—that is, systems concerns.[32]

Who Needs Nursing Management?

All types of health care organizations need nursing management, including nursing homes, hospitals, assisted living facilities, residential care programs, home health care agencies, ambulatory care centers, student infirmaries, and many others. Even the nurse working with one client and family needs management knowledge and skills to help people work together to accomplish a common goal. A primary nurse working with several clients must prioritize care, with the goal of assisting them to improved health, healing, or, sometimes, a peaceful death.[33]

All of the major functions of nursing management operate independently and interdependently.

General Principles

The following are some major principles of nursing management, which are discussed in more detail in subsequent chapters.

- Planning is a major function of nursing management and is primary to all other management activities or functions.
- Effective use of time is essential to effective nursing management, which takes place in the present while preparing for future performance, growth, and change.
- Decision making is a primary element of nursing management at every level.
- Nurse managers manage a clinical practice discipline in which professional nurses are primarily knowledge workers, applying their knowledge to gathering data, making nursing diagnoses and nursing prescriptions, supervising the implementation of the nursing care plan by skilled workers, and evaluating and adjusting that plan.
- Social goals are formulated by nurse managers and achieved by clinical nurses.
- Organizing is the second major function of nursing management.
- Change is a major element in nursing management.
- Organizational cultures should be managed to reflect values and beliefs, with managers in nursing having a common purpose of making productive the values, aspirations, and traditions of employees who are individuals as well as members of communities and of society.
- Directing or leading is the third major function of nursing management; it includes empowering employees, improving quality, and leading to excellence of production.
- Motivation is a basic element of the directing function of nursing management. Satisfactory performance results from job satisfaction, quality of work life, and organizational commitment, conditions that require nurse managers to motivate nurse employees.
- Effective communication and management are major elements of nursing management that result in fewer misunderstandings and give employees a common vision, common understanding, and unity of direction and effort.
- Staff development is an important element of the directing function of nursing management and serves to maintain the competency of all practicing nurses.
- Controlling or evaluating is the fourth major function of nursing management and includes the processes of evaluating the given directives and how well the adopted plan was carried out, establishing principles and standards, comparing performance with standards, evaluating patterns, and correcting deficiencies.

Management Development

Management development is big business. In the new health care environment, a variety of innovative agencies and programs are being developed. These entities serve to meet the ever-changing population and face increasing financial constraints. These organizations are no less complex than are hospitals, and they require cost controls and increased productivity to thrive. Unless nurses are educated to manage in these new environments, they will lose out to other professions or will manage poorly and be unhappy and unsuccessful.[34]

To prepare clinical nurses for beginning management roles, the Mount Sinai Medical Center of Greater Miami designed a voluntary two-day "taking charge" course. Goals included greater competence, confidence, and continuity; preparation for problem solving; job satisfaction; and a positive leadership experience. A guidebook was prepared for use during the learning experience and for reference. Topics covered included communication, leadership styles, time management, managing stress, staffing, assignments, rounds, reports, ordering supplies, unit operations, position description, policies, patient care assessment, quality assurance, conflict management, and counseling. A posttest and three-month followup showed the course to be successful. The clinical nurses were more effective, showing improved self-concept, self-esteem, and assertiveness. Both the nurses' morale and the organizational climate improved.[35]

Management development of nurses at Mount Sinai is taken seriously. Recognizing that nurse managers have "onstage" (on the scene) and "backstage" (behind the scene) roles to perform, one management program focused on communication skills required for onstage management, in which different "hats" are worn for each role: negotiator, counselor, director, delegator, collaborator, and controller. The nurse manager is a hands-on person.

The communication course consists of one 2-hour session each week for 10 weeks. It covers topics such as communication style, nonverbal communication, listening, conflict management, verbal messages, rumors, committees, team building, and communication climate. The course helps prepare the nurse manager to respond to multiple issues from multiple sources. Backstage, it provides the nurse manager with the ability to communicate with other executives in the business world. These nurse managers should also be well-versed in management theories, with knowledge of economics, finance, and accounting. They should be assertive, proactive, and collegial.[36]

A system for developing nurse administrators has been published by Fralic and O'Connor, who make frequent reference to the works of Katz and of Charns and Schaefer. Katz classifies management skills into three categories:

1. Conceptual skills, which are innate abilities, or thinking skills.
2. Technical skills, which include methods, processes, procedures, and techniques.
3. Human skills, which relate to leadership ability and intergroup relations.

In nursing, technical skills are divided into nursing management technology and nursing practice technology. Fralic and O'Connor relate the conceptual, human, and technical skills to three management levels, with the chief nurse executive needing the highest level of conceptual competence and the nurse manager needing the highest level of nursing practice technology. The necessary staff development is evident in the role requirements.[37]

Leadership training is a huge industry. Content of leadership training includes feedback, personnel growth, skill building, and conceptual awareness. Values-based leadership is the goal of training, with values shared by leaders and constituents. Investing in training and technology will improve efficiencies.[38]

Spicer indicates that scientific management knowledge is at the base of the nurse manager's role, including knowledge of a role model and the ability to conceptualize the role. Preparation for management and support during the transition are needed for the change from clinical nurse to nurse manager. The role model would demonstrate the relationships between politics and strategy and between power and influence.[39]

Preparation of nurse managers includes many things:

- Knowledge of legal labor practices and institutional policy in managing employees
- Preparation for continuing education and staff development, including principles of adult education; a needs survey; and preparation, presentation, and evaluation of programs
- Knowledge of financial matters, including budget, management of cost and revenue centers, financing of health care, and productivity

Nurse managers use performance appraisal as a continuum directed toward results. Preparation of nurse managers assists them in becoming self-directed.[40]

In the new management culture nurses will survive and prosper by updating skills. Entrepreneurial managers invest in their employees with adequate pay, fiscal quality in the workplace, and training.[41]

Roles and Nursing Management

Role Development

The nurse manager draws from the best and most applicable theories of management to create an individual management style and performance. This requires knowledge and the skills to use it. The nurse manager continues to acquire and use management knowledge to solve managerial problems, which require a contingency approach because no single approach works for all situations. The nurse manager acts with the assumption that clinical nurses and other health care providers want to be competent and that with managerial support they will be motivated to achieve competence and greater levels of productivity. With achievement of competence and productivity goals, higher goals are set. Clinical nurses will seek out the organization that fits their needs.[42]

Adding to the nurse manager's ever-expanding role is the need to increase knowledge of and sensitivity to other health care individuals providing clinical services. These services are integrated into the client's overall experience of health care, of which nursing is a critical component.

McClure points out that nurse managers manage a clinical discipline performed by professional nurses. Because most nurses are women, conflicts may arise between their professional and personal lives. The nurse manager devises strategies to deal with these conflicts. Some blue-collar nurses lack knowledge of nursing research and do not read to keep up to date; they want nurse managers to do everything. White-collar nurses often want to be treated differently; they want job enrichment, with primary nursing duties and professional autonomy, and they want to be organized like the medical staff, with staff appointments and peer review. The nurse manager manages these two groups differently.[43]

Freund surveyed chief executive officers (CEOs) and directors of nursing (DONs) of 250 university-affiliated hospitals. The sample evaluated the effectiveness of DONs on the basis of the following categories:

- General management/health/nursing knowledge, including finance, accounting, computer literacy, nursing, health care field, and productivity.
- Human management skills, including communication, interaction with people, sensitivity, and humor.
- Total view of the organization (theory and behavior), with nurses as part of the management team and nursing's interests blended with those of the entire organization.
- Support by CEOs. DONs did not think that CEOs viewed this as important.
- Medical staff relations. Smooth and peaceful nursing/medical staff relationships were important to CEOs, whereas DONs desired a collegial relationship.
- Flexibility, negotiation, and compromise. CEOs cited flexibility as an important skill in the effectiveness of DONs, whereas DONs cited negotiation and compromise.
- Political savvy. DONs thought that the political nature of their positions required political savvy, whereas CEOs did not view this as crucial for DONs.
- Knowledge of advanced clinical practice. Neither CEOs nor DONs viewed this as crucial to the effectiveness of DONs.

Of the DONs, 73.1% had graduate degrees: 60.2% had Master of Science in Nursing degrees, 8.2% had Master of Business Administration or Master of Hospital Administration degrees, and 4.7% had doctoral or Doctor of Nursing Services degrees. Of the CEOs, 92% had graduate degrees (81.6% master's and 10.4% doctorate). Management experience averaged 19 years for CEOs and 13 years for DONs. All DONs began in clinical practice.[44]

Analysis of the concept of intuition by Rew details the attributes of intuition:[45]

1. **"Knowledge of a fact or truth, as a whole;**
2. **Immediate possession of knowledge; and**
3. **Knowledge independent of the linear reasoning process."**

Management Levels

Nurse managers perform at several levels in the health care organization. These include first-line patient care management at the unit level, middle management at the department level, and top management at the executive level. In some organizations decentralization has displaced the middle management level and redistributed department-level functions to staff functions under a matrix or another organizational structure. The middle management role is often reconsidered in work redesign effort, particularly as leadership moves further away from the clinical care. The roles of managers are developmental, building on knowledge and skills as the scope of the nurse manager's role increases in breadth and depth. Middle nurse manager roles are frequently eliminated, and clinical nurses become empowered through management education.

First-Line Nurse Managers

The following are some of the knowledge and skills needed by nurses in first-line management roles:

- Financial management knowledge and skills to prepare and defend a budget for expenses of unit personnel, supplies, and capital equipment and for revenues to meet expenses. The ability to manage scarce and expensive resources for performance.
- The ability to match moral and ethical choices with respect to human needs, moral principles for behavior, and individual feelings in making decisions.
- Recognition of and advocacy for patients' rights.
- Active and assertive effort to share power within the organization, including shared power for nursing's practitioners. This includes nursing autonomy, which is threatened by authoritarian management. In turn, practicing nurses are involved in solving managerial problems.
- The ability to communicate and to promote effective communication and interpersonal relationships among nursing staff and others; presentation skills.
- Knowledge of internal factors related to purpose, tasks, people, technology, and structure.
- Knowledge of external factors related to economy, political pressures, legal aspects, sociocultural characteristics, and technology.
- The ability to study situations and use management concepts and techniques, analyze the situations correctly, make diagnoses of problems, and tie the processes together to arrive at decisions.
- The ability to provide for staff development.
- The ability to provide a climate in which nurses clearly perceive that they are pursuing meaningful and worthwhile goals through their individual efforts.
- Knowledge of organizational culture and its impact on productivity and problem solving.
- Ability to effect change through an orderly process.
- Commitment to maintain self-development by reading and attending workshops and other educational programs.

- Knowledge of how to empower clinical nurses through committee assignments, quality circles, primary nursing, and even assigning titles.[46] At Mount Sinai Medical Center of Greater Miami, head nurses are department heads who write goals and objectives, prepare and manage the unit budget, and prepare plans. They are encouraged to be organized and unified, to network, and to be community leaders in the health care field, including working with legislators.[47]
- Knowledge of recruitment and retention strategies to promote and retain valued nursing and health care personnel.

To these could be added staffing and scheduling; management reports; hiring; performance appraisal; job productivity and satisfaction; constructive discipline dealing with stress and conflict; personnel management; diversity and awareness of culture, values, norms, and ways of doing things.[48] Although these skills and this knowledge may be obtained through staff development, master's level management preparation is essential.

In no way are these lists complete. They are a beginning, however, and will be built on in succeeding chapters.

The Nurse Executive

Executive nurse managers increase their knowledge and skills by building on what they learned as lower-level managers. Executive nurse managers should be able to do the following:

- Apply financial management principles to costing and pricing nursing care and convey this knowledge to the nurses providing care.
- Coordinate the division budget.
- Empower lower-level nurse managers.
- Undertake corporate self-analysis of what nursing can do (skills, capabilities, weaknesses, the work of nursing) and its assumptions about itself, its environment, and its beliefs and convey results to employees.
- Specify, weigh, interrelate, and simultaneously accomplish multiple goals.
- Abandon obsolete principles of standardization, centralization, specialization, and concentration.
- Decentralize and share authority and power through participatory management and transformational leadership, shared governance, professional nursing models, employee involvement, and programs on the quality of work life.
- Establish a matrix organization using task forces and project teams with project leaders.
- Set the stage for clinical nursing practice. This does not necessarily require that the nurse executive be clinically competent.
- Promote application of a theory of nursing within a nursing care delivery system.
- Advise nursing educators on content of nursing administration programs.
- Set depth and breadth of nursing research programs.
- Anticipate the future of health care and of nursing.
- Manage strategic planning.
- Serve as mentor, role model, and preceptor to lower-level managers, graduate students, and others.
- Recognize and use authority and the potential for power.

Research data indicate that executive nurses prepared at the doctoral level need courses in ethical and accountable decision making, including missions and goals, policies, human resources, financial and material resources, databases, and communication management. These courses would be organized into organizational structure and governance, resources, and information management.[49]

With major changes in business practices, lessons learned from Japan offer meaningful strategies to American business, including the business of health care. For example, the Japanese have found that less variety is best when it comes to cutting costs and saving time. Consensus decision making does not always work. With the help of high-tech information systems, lone decisions based on multiple data sources and data points may be the best decisions.[50] The understanding of theories, roles and responsibilities, and evidence-based management provides the foundational work for the nurse administrator to manage a clinical practice.

Managing a Clinical Practice

Nursing is a clinical practice discipline. Professional nurses want autonomy and control of their practice. They want to apply their nursing knowledge and skills without interference from nurse managers, physicians, or persons in other disciplines. The effective nurse manager trusts the professional nurse to apply knowledge and skills correctly in caring for a group of patients. In turn, the clinical nurse trusts the nurse manager to coordinate supplies, equipment, and support systems with personnel in other departments. Clinical nurses trust a human relations management in which they participate rather than one in which they have rules and regulations imposed on them. They use the body of nursing knowledge (theory) gained in nursing school and maintained through continuing education and staff development to practice nursing as they determine it should be practiced. In doing so, they adhere to management policies regarding such issues as documentation or quality improvement, because these requirements are also part of clinical nursing practice.

Use of Nursing Theory

In developing nursing as a scientific discipline, nursing educators and researchers have developed theoretical frameworks for the clinical practice of nursing that are used by clinical nurses as models for testing and validating applications of nursing knowledge and skills. The results are added to the body of knowledge commonly called the theory of nursing. Theory gives practicing nurses a professional identity. It is based on scientific inquiry: nursing research. Each result of nursing research adds tested facts to nursing theory that can be learned by nursing students and active practitioners.

Models and Examples

Models are frequently used in the development of nursing theory. A model usually communicates in graphic format an abstract entity, structure, or process that cannot be observed directly. Models depict behavioral processes that cannot be observed directly except as indirect behaviors of those engaged in the process. They order, clarify, and systematize selected components of the phenomena they serve to depict. Because nursing theories have not been applied widely, theories are frequently described as models.[51]

Orem's and Kinlein's Theories

Dickson and Lee-Villasenor report testing of Orem's self-care nursing theory as modified by Kinlein. As independent generalist nurses, they did their research in a private nursing practice setting. They used grounded theory methodology to systematically obtain and analyze data from clients.

In performing a content analysis, Dickson and Lee-Villasenor classified events as expressions of need, self-care assets, self-care demands, and self-care measures. They catalogued events by numbers of expressions of need (a perception of self, an action taken, a want, a wish, or a question) and by perception of self according to mind/body combinations. Events were also catalogued according to evidence of patterns of self-care actions that contributed positively to the client's state of health and number of self-care assets: action, motivation, knowledge, and potential.[52] Orem's general theory of nursing is frequently used as a frame of reference.[53]

Roy's Theory

Roy advocates adaptation level theory to nursing intervention. She notes that a person adapts to the environment through four modes: physiologic needs and processes, self-concept (beliefs and feelings about oneself), role mastery (behavior among people who occupy different positions within society), and interdependence (giving and receiving nurturance).[54] Just as the individual patient adapts to changes in the environment, so does the nursing worker.

According to Roy, the goal of nursing is to assist the patient to adapt to illness so as to be able to respond to other stimuli. The patient is assessed for positive or negative behavior in the four adaptive modes. Once the assessment is made at the necessary (first or second) level, intervention is established by a nursing care plan of goals and approaches. The approach is selected to match the goal.[55] According to Mastal and Hammond, Roy's views are "that the developing body of nursing knowledge now contains verifiable theories and general laws related to: (1) persons as holistic beings, and (2) the role of nursing in promoting the person's maximum potential health and harmonious interaction with the environment."[56]

Frederickson illustrates application of the Roy adaptation model to the nursing diagnosis of anxiety. He describes or defines anxiety from the nursing perspective as exhibited by "poor nutritional status, reduction in usual physical activity, and lowered self-esteem, in addition to concern for job security." The nurse diagnoses the symptoms of anxiety through assessment of the four modes and then designs and implements intervention that promotes client adaptation.[57]

Evaluation criteria for empirical testing of nursing theory were developed by Silva and expanded by others. Theory testing includes processes of verifying whether what was purported or experienced is true or solves problems in one's discipline or practice. Silva and Sorrell define nursing theory as "a tentative body of diverse but purposeful, creative, and logically interrelated perspectives that help nurses to redefine nursing and to understand, explain, raise questions about, and seek clarification of nursing phenomena in their research and practice."[58] They list three alternative approaches of testing to verify nursing theory:

1. Through critical reasoning.
2. Through description of personal experiences.
3. Through application to nursing practice. (This concept has been applied at the National Hospital for Orthopedics and Rehabilitation, Arlington, Virginia, where the Roy adaptation model has been implemented throughout the hospital.)

Newman's Theory

Engle tested Margaret Newman's conceptual framework of health in a sample of older women. She indicates that Newman uses Rogers's concept of the life process and the relationship of the individual within the environment. In this model, aging is considered a natural process, the person's individual state being a fusion of health and disease. Movement is a correlation of health measured by a basic time factor and tempo.[59] Engle defines tempo as the characteristic rate of performing a task. Time is the second correlation of health. Tempo and time occur in a succession of events, rhythmic patterns of temperatures and movement, and patterns within the environment. Time perception and tempo are hypothesized to be altered by age and illness. Self-assessment and physical assessment of health have been shown to correlate. Self-assessment of health is altered by one's ability to perform everyday activities, by one's age self-concept, and by movement and time.[60]

In her study, Engle measured personal tempo, time perception, and self-assessment of health by using the Cantril ladder in 114 women age 60 or older. She found no age effect for time perception in this study, nor did Newman and Tompkins in similar studies, nor did they find any age effect for personal tempo.[61]

According to Engle, a significant relationship existed between time perception and personal tempo that could have implications for the patient and the clinical nurse. The patient or nurse with a physical or mental condition that alters personal tempo may have an altered perception of time. This could be true in older nurses in whom physical and mental states are more often altered. Further research in this area is needed.

Levine's Theory

Levine writes that nursing practice has mirrored prevailing theories of health and disease. Nursing creates an environment for healing that includes cleanliness, safety, and physical and emotional comfort, and nursing enhances the reparative process. Nursing was disease-oriented when diseases, rather than patients, were the focus of treatment. As nurses became concerned with the multiple factors impacting the course of disease, they developed the total-patient-care concept.[62]

People respond to illness in individual ways. Nursing intervention should match the individual response, which is identified from observation and data analysis. Assessment reveals unique needs requiring unique nursing measures. Nursing supports repair and maintenance of a person's integrated self-homeostasis and equilibrium. Equilibrium is maintained by adaptation. The nurse intervenes to support successful adaptation to achieve a therapeutic or supportive role.[63]

Johnson's Theory

Johnson incorporated the nursing process (assessment, diagnosis planning, intervention, and evaluation) into a general systems model. Rawls applied this model to care of a patient for the purpose of testing, evaluating, and determining its utility for predicting the effect of nursing care on a patient. Rawls indicates that the model has disadvantages but is a tool that can be used "to accurately predict the results of nursing interventions prior to care, formulate standards of care, and most importantly, administer truly holistic empathic nursing care."[64]

Derdiarian sampled 223 cancer patients to verify the relationship among the eight subsystems of Johnson's behavioral system model. These eight subsystems (achievement, affiliative, aggressive/protective, dependence, eliminative, ingestive, sexual, and restorative) function through behavior to meet a person's demands. Illness disrupts and changes behavior sustained in the subsystems, resulting in negative effects on the behavioral systems. Changes in one subsystem initiate changes in others. Findings of this research indicated "fairly large, statistically significant ($P < .001$) direct relationships between the aggressive/protective subsystems and each of the other subsystems." The research presents a model for continued research of Johnson's behavioral system model with "implications for comprehensive assessment, early intervention, prevention of patients' potential problems, and ultimately for efficient care."[65]

Peplau's Theory

Peplau's theory defines nursing as a "significant, therapeutic, interpersonal process."[66] Peplau's theory involves such concepts as communication techniques, assessment, definition of problems and goals, direction, and role clarification.

Peplau states that four components make up the main elements of the nurse/patient relationship: nurse, patient, professional expertise, and client need. The nurse/patient relationship has three phases: the orientation phase, the working phase, and the resolution phase. During encounters with patients, the nurse observes, interprets what he or she observes, and then decides what needs to be done.

Interpersonal relations uses the theoretical constructs of concepts, processes, and patterns:

- A concept is a small, circumscribed set of behaviors pertaining to a particular phenomenon such as conflict.
- A process is more complicated, more comprehensive, and longer lasting.
- A pattern is made up of separate acts that may have variations but share a common theme, aim, or intention.

Interpersonal theory is especially useful in psychiatric nursing and is useful in relation to psychosocial problems and nurse/patient relationships in all clinical areas of nursing. The joint effort of the nurse/patient relationship "includes identification of the presenting problems, understanding the problems and their variation in pattern, and appreciating, applying, and testing remedial measures in order to produce beneficial outcomes for patients."[67]

Orlando's Theory

Orlando's theory of nursing develops three basic concepts:

1. Professional nursing has as its function the identification and meeting of patient's immediate needs for help.
2. Professional nursing has as its intended outcome or product both verbal and nonverbal improvement in the patient's behavior.
3. Regardless of its form, the patient's presenting or initial behavior may be a plea for help.

Schmieding applied Orlando's theory to solving problems in managing the behavior of clinical nurses. She recommends that the work of one theorist be used as the practice model within a given organization. This application of Orlando's model has helped nurses apply common concepts and a framework for nursing. The model could be adapted if the nursing staff synthesized the concepts of several theories.[68]

Other Theories

Wiens presents Meyer's model of patient autonomy in care as a theoretical framework for nursing. With laws for advance directives and increased emphasis on patient's rights, the right to patient self-determination has greater implications for care providers. Historically, patients have been perceived by providers to be dependent and compliant. Autonomy competency includes a repertory of skills or abilities that contribute to an individual's life plan of value, emotional ties, and personal ideals:

- Self-reference: a person recognizes his or her response to life situations.
- Self-direction: a person expresses himself or herself in ways considered fitting and worthy of self.
- Self-definition: a person knows and acts as his or her true self.
- Self-discovery: a person examines his or her socialization for self-understanding and future self-control.
- Self-portrait or self-concept.

Patients need to be encouraged to be autonomous and to ask questions and make decisions about their care. Illness decreases the patient's autonomy competency. Nurses will have to change their nurse/patient relationships to accommodate autonomy competency in patients.

Frequently, as patients become increasingly autonomy-competent, they are viewed as noncompliant troublemakers. Informed consent requires decision making and truth telling. In the case of truth telling, providers need to be kind and caring.[69]

Sociotechnical systems theory views an organization as an open and living system interacting with the environment. The components of this system are social, technological, physical and work-setting-related. The system produces products or services. Employers participate in designing and redesigning work and jobs to achieve a high-quality work life. More studies are needed to test the assumption that the work environment is important to care delivery.[70]

Modalities of Nursing Practice

Several modalities or methods of nursing practice have evolved during the past 50 years. These include functional nursing, team nursing, primary nursing, case method, and joint practice. All are practiced in various forms in health care institutions in the United States, and all may be practiced with case management and managed care.

Functional Nursing

Functional nursing is the oldest nursing practice modality. It can best be described as a task-oriented method in which a particular nursing function is assigned to each staff member. One registered nurse is responsible for administering medications, one for providing treatments, and one for managing intravenous administration; one licensed nurse is assigned admissions and discharges, and another gives bed baths; a nurse's aide makes beds and passes meal trays. No nurse is responsible for total care of any patient. This method divides the tasks to be done, with each person being responsible to the nurse manager, who coordinates and oversees the care. It is efficient and the best system for a nursing staff confronted with a large patient load and a shortage of professional nurses:

The advantage of functional nursing is that it accomplishes the most work in the shortest amount of time. Its disadvantages include the following:

- It fragments nursing care.
- It decreases the nurse's accountability and responsibility.
- It makes the nurse/client relationship difficult to establish, if such a relationship is ever achieved.
- It gives professional nursing low status in terms of responsibility for patient care.

Functional nursing was largely a development of the World War II era, when large numbers of nurses entered military service and ancillary personnel were trained to staff many nursing functions in hospitals. It is still used in many institutions.

Team Nursing

Team nursing developed in the early 1950s when various nursing leaders decided that a team approach could unify the different categories of nursing workers. Under the leadership of a professional nurse, a group of nurses work together to fulfill the full functions of professional nurses. Patients are assigned to a team consisting of a reg-

EXHIBIT 1-2

Team Nursing Organization

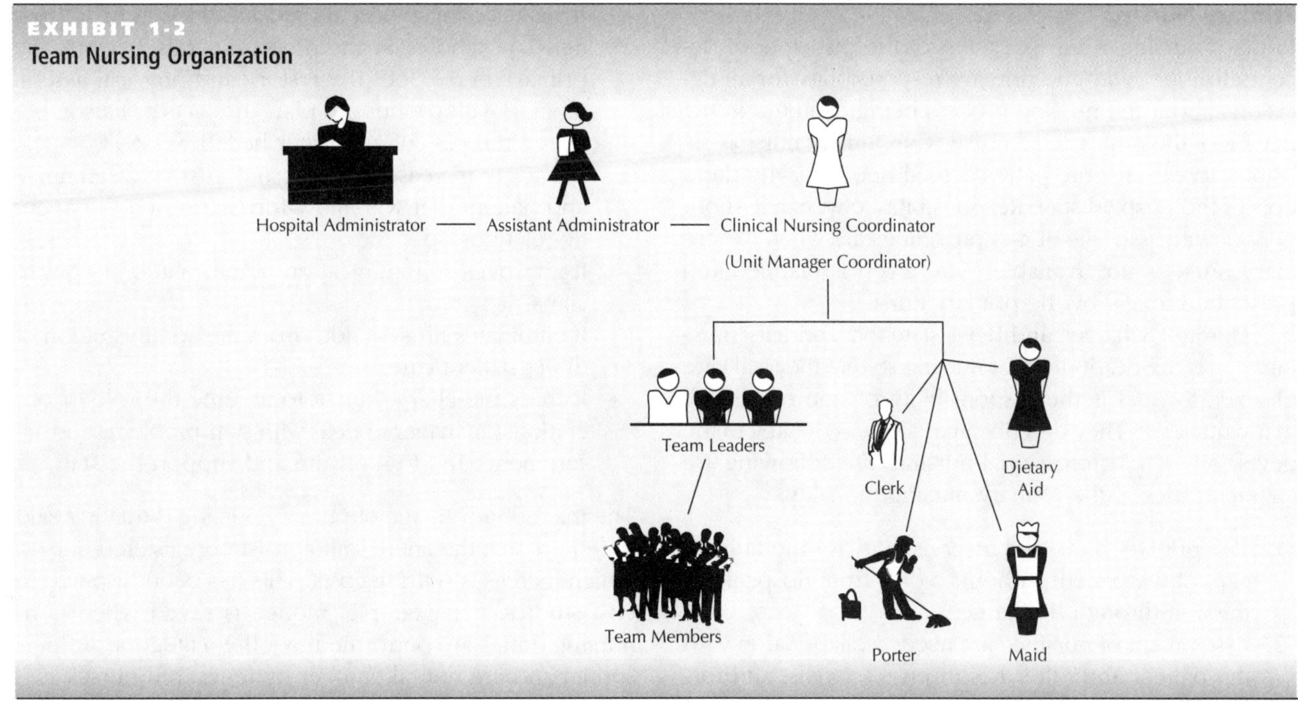

istered nurse as a team leader and other staff—RNs, LPNs, and aides—as team members. The team leader is responsible for coordinating the total care of a block of patients and is the leadership figure.

The intent of team nursing is to provide patient-centered care. The patient's nursing care needs are identified and met through nursing diagnosis and prescription. Ward clerks and unit managers perform the nonnursing functions of the unit. The process requires planning with the objective of taking nursing personnel to the bedside so that they can focus on the nursing care of patients. Implementing team nursing requires study of the literature on the team plan, development of a philosophy of team nursing, planning for appropriate utilization of all categories of nursing workers, and planning for team conferences, nursing care plans, and development of team leadership. Exhibit 1-2 depicts schema for a team nursing organization, with team members performing different but coordinated roles in self-managed work teams.

The following is a summary of the team plan:

> The team plan gives priorities to the development of leadership potential, leadership in the practice of nursing that is creative and that encourages improvement of communications among team members, patients, and leaders. It prioritizes emphasis on democratic leadership, the nurturing of cooperative effort, and free expression of ideas of all team members. It emphasizes motivation of people to grow to the self-approved or maximum level of performance. Through the team plan the contributions of all team members to improving patient care are recognized. The team plan emphasizes the strengthening of team members' weaknesses.
>
> Patient-centered care employs effective supervision and recognizes that personnel are the media by which the objectives are met in a cooperative effort between team leaders and team members. Through supervision, the team leader identifies nursing care goals, identifies team members' needs, focuses on fulfilling goals and needs, motivates team members to grow as workers and citizens, and guides team members to help set and meet high standards of patient care and job performance. All of these goals support the priorities of practicing nursing.[71]

The advantages of team nursing are as follows:

- It involves all team members in planning patients' nursing care through team conferences and written nursing care plans.
- It provides the best care at the lowest cost, according to some advocates.

Disadvantages of team nursing include the following:

- It can lead to fragmentation of care if the concept is not implemented totally.
- It can be difficult to find time for team conferences and care plans.
- It allows the registered nurse who is the team leader to have the only significant responsibility and authority.

The disadvantages of team nursing can be overcome by educating competent team leaders in the principles of nursing team leadership.

Primary Nursing

Primary nursing is an extension of the principle of decentralization, with the primary responsibility for all decisions about the nursing process being centered in the person of the professional nurse. The primary nurse is assigned to care for the patient's total needs for the duration of the hospital stay. Responsibility covers a 24-hour period, with associate nurses providing care when the primary nurse is not available. Care given is planned and prescribed totally by the primary nurse.

Marram, Schlegel, and Bevis state that "primary nursing . . . is the distribution of nursing so that the total care of an individual is the responsibility of one nurse, not many nurses."[72] They describe autonomy as the key to the development of professional nursing. The following are characteristics of the primary nursing modality:

1. The primary nurse has responsibility for the nursing care of the patient 24 hours a day, from hospital admission through discharge.
2. Assessment of nursing care needs, collaboration with the patient and other health professionals, and formulation of the plan of care are all responsibilities of the primary nurse.
3. Execution of the nursing care plan is delegated by the primary nurse to a secondary nurse during other shifts.
4. The primary nurse consults with nurse managers.
5. Authority, accountability, and autonomy rest with the primary nurse.[73]

Fagin states that research studies on primary nursing showed that it reduced hospital stays and complications of renal transplant patients at the University of Michigan Medical Center in Ann Arbor, where the savings were $51,000 in one year for the entire center. Primary nursing at Evanston (Illinois) Hospital near Chicago resulted in fewer nursing hours and less salary expense per patient during a 5-year period. Nurses aides had 27% unoccupied time per day, whereas registered nurses had 8% unoccupied time at Rush Presbyterian in Chicago. Turnover was also decreased in the operating room, with an increased registered nurse-to-operating room technician ratio. Other studies indicate that primary nursing saves money; increases job satisfaction, group adhesion, and patient satisfaction; and decreases costs of overtime, sick time, and compensatory time.[74]

The following are advantages of primary nursing:

- It provides for increased autonomy on the part of the nurse, thus increasing motivation, responsibility, and accountability.
- It ensures more continuity of care, as the primary nurse gives or directs care throughout hospitalization.
- It makes available increased knowledge of the patient's psychosocial and physical needs, because the primary nurse does the history and physical assessment, develops the care plan, and acts as liaison between the patient and other health workers.
- It leads to increased rapport and trust between nurse and patient that will allow formation of a therapeutic relationship.
- It improves communication of information to physicians.
- It eliminates nurses' aides from the administration of direct patient care.
- It frees the charge nurse to assume the role of operational manager to deal with staff problems and assignments and to motivate and support the staff.

The main disadvantage of primary nursing is that it is said to require that the entire staff consist of registered nurses, which increases staffing costs. This has been disputed in cost studies. For example, money is saved when non-nursing duties are performed by other categories of personnel and are not taken over by registered nurses.[75]

Primary nursing is sometimes modified to employ nurse extenders as technical assistants to registered nurses. The registered nurses assess the patients, develop care plans, and direct others. These are responsibilities that only the professional nurses are licensed to do, and they cannot be delegated. Modifications of team nursing and primary nursing to merge the advantages of each will result in more efficient and effective outcomes.

Case Method

The case method of nursing provides for a registered nurse-to-client ratio of 1:1 and constant care for a specified period of time. Examples are private duty, intensive care, and community health nurses. This method is similar to that of primary nursing, except that relief nurses on other shifts are not associate registered nurses.

Joint Practice

Joint practice is more than a modality. It entails nurses and physicians collaborating as colleagues to provide patient care. Nurses and physicians work together to define their roles within the joint practice setting, and their goals are reciprocal and complementary rather than mutually exclusive. They may use mutually agreed upon protocols to manage care within a primary setting.[76]

The primary nursing modality is preferred for joint practice, or collaborative practice. There must be an adequate number of professional nurses who are freed from nonnursing tasks. Decision making is decentralized, and in-service education and certification are used to upgrade the nurse's scope of practice. Compensation is increased to match increased responsibility and accountability.

Physicians are required to accept responsibility for their part in joint collaborative practice. Administration includes joint practice nurses on every committee within the hospital. It takes as long as a year to establish truly functional relationships, because both physicians and nurses have to modify their behaviors.

The following elements are needed to establish successful joint practice in a hospital setting:

1. A committee of physicians and nurses with equal representation and equal voice in establishing the objectives and ground rules of operation.
2. An integrated patient record system.
3. Primary nursing and case management.
4. Collaborative practice with honest communication and encouragement of clinical decision making by nurses.
5. Joint education of physicians and nurses.
6. Joint nurse/physician evaluation of patient care.
7. Trust.

Results of a joint practice demonstration project at four hospitals concluded the following:

- Patients receive better nursing care and are highly satisfied with their care.
- Physician/nurse communications are better, and there is increased mutual respect and trust between nurses and physicians.
- Both physicians' and nurses' job satisfaction is increased.[77]

Joint practice has developed rapidly in managed care organizations. This has led to issues and changes in licensure, clinical autonomy, prescriptive authority, and third-party insurance payments.[78] Nurse practitioners emerge from joint practice as a group of highly educated and competent providers of patient care.[79]

Case Management

Case management is more than a modality of nursing. It has been described as all of the following: clinical system that focuses on the accountability of an identified individual or group for conditioning care for a patient or a group of patients across a continuum of care; insuring and facilitating the achievement of quality and clinical and cost outcomes; negotiating, procuring, and coordinating services and resources needed by the patient or family; intervening at busy points (and/or when significant variance occurs) for individual patients; addressing and resolving patterns in aggregate variances that have a negative quality/cost impact; and creating opportunities and systems to enhance outcomes.[80]

Simply stated, case management is a process of coordinating services, and the case manager is the person who does the coordinating.[81]

The Center for Case Management's model of case management was designed as a clinical one. The model's underlying assumption was that caregivers of each discipline needed to have management skills, better patient care management tools, and more responsible administrative support to create quality clinical outcomes within a new cost-conscious milieu. The organizational structure is flat, with attending-level physician and "selected primary care nurses expanded into case managers to produce the integration of processes, aided by critical paths."[82] Critical paths have been integrated into CareMaps®. The CareMap® is used as the nursing care plan and for documentation.

A collaborative team approach is used when integration of care occurs across geographic care units such as the emergency room, the coronary care unit, the step down unit, and the ambulatory clinic. Primary nurses from these units who have undergone formal orientation join the team.[83]

Personnel at the Center for Case Management believe that 100% of patients need their care managed by a CareMap®. The CareMaps® provide the documented standards for specific patient populations and disease states. With this infrastructure of care delivery, only 20% believe that patients need a case manager in addition to a CareMap® system.[84]

In the restructuring of nursing care, Zander places increased emphasis on accountability.

Quality improvement is an integral part of the case management system. Quality management is operationalized by the use of critical paths, CareMaps®, and case management, all of which provide the tools for accomplishing the nursing process.[85] CareMaps® present problems by defining quality as a product.[86] When interventions and goals are recorded that are different from those planned, they are termed variances. A variance indicates deviations from a norm or standard. Variance indicates intervention that works or does not work. Variances alter discharge dates, expected costs, and expected outcomes.

Variances show how the CareMap® and reality differ both positively and negatively. Variance that shows negative outcomes requires action to improve quality. Variance data are collected, totaled, analyzed, and reported; they then result in decisions that revise CareMaps® critical paths, procedures, and other elements of the Plan-Do-Check-Act (PDCA) cycle.[87] Because CareMaps® can be used to document nursing care, are outcome-based, and have been found to be effective and efficient, nurses may want to use a computerized version for documentation.

Other Models of Case Management

University of Kentucky Hospital Model

The University of Kentucky Hospital model of case management uses a problem solving process. Case managers are master's-prepared nurses to whom cases are referred by quality-monitoring groups. Case managers verify problems, design strategies to fix them, and evaluate outcomes.

The priority in this model is efficient movement through the health care system. Case managers consult with finance personnel, administrators, and health care providers; they collaborate with physicians, primary nurses, and other health care providers; and they establish therapeutic relationships with patients and families. A case management advisory board meeting takes place quarterly. Members perform prospective or retrospective surveys for clinical problems. Case managers follow up with diagnoses and procedure codes specific to the cases with verified problems. Sample problems of outcomes include poor continuity in patient's care, inadequate discharge planning, inadequate patient teaching, extended preoperative and postoperative stays, and poor nutritional status of patients.

Among the results were the following:

- Reduced glucose levels in diabetic, adult open-heart surgery patients (which resulted in a savings of $11,585 in room charges during a six-month period).
- Decreased arterial blood gas charges in cardiovascular patients.
- Intensive care newborn patients home 218 days earlier than comparable patients during the previous year (a savings of $82,731 for Medicaid patients alone).

Management will pay for performance when hiring case managers in the future.[88]

Carondelet/St. Mary's Hospital and Health Center Model

Another model of case management is the Carondelet/St. Mary's Hospital and Health Center in Tucson, Arizona. In this model, nurse case managers work in partnership with high-risk individuals in the hospital (30%) and in the community (70%). Reports of applications of this model of nursing case management indicate that it results in financial savings and liability defenses. It is case management in which the nurse manages and coordinates the entire spectrum of a patient's care in all settings, hospital and community. Effective case management wins the confidence of all team members, including social workers and physicians. Nursing case management supports the highest use of clinical nursing skills. Rogers, Riordan, and Swindle report that case management reduced total admissions, mean admissions per patient, mean length of stay per patient, and net reimbursement. The authors recommend mandating Bachelor of Science in Nursing qualifications for case managers, as well as five years of clinical experience. They worked out comparable arrangements with social workers.[89]

Lyon summarizes case management models as including such hospital-based models as the Center for Case Management model, the discharge planner and arbitration model, the geriatric clinical nurse specialist model, and models such as the Arizona model that stretch across the health care continuum. Community case management models include the Denver and Indianapolis models. Lyon calls case management in hospitals managed care, as it does not make maximum use of community health services.[90]

Other Factors Related to Case Management

Bower reported that case managers at Hennepin County Medical Center in Minneapolis were responsible for the following:[91]

1. Over $1 million in direct cost savings.
2. Readmission rates for patients having major bowel procedures reduced from 67% to 26%.
3. Readmission rates for patients with cerebrovascular disorders (except transitory ischemic attacks) reduced from 43% to 31%.
4. Compliance with antibiotic protocols in patients having hip and femur procedures increased from 38% to 89%.

Nurses have been at the forefront of case management as it relates to moving patients through the hospital efficiently. There may be conflicts between nurse case managers and other providers within the community. Professional nurses should become educated about case management programs, interagency groups, use of interdisciplinary teams, and legal issues and should keep respect for clients' wishes and rights continually in mind.[92]

Strong indicates that clinical nurse specialists have the expert clinical and management skills to enhance planning, clinical decision making, and evaluation of resource use. The case management system has been applied to promote cost-effective, long-term wellness in migrant children by addressing cultural, nutritional, and dental care needs and by using available resources. This has also been done with homeless families. Case management identifies the clients' needs and makes and implements plans to meet those needs efficiently and effectively. Case management may be performed by a group practice of primary nurses.[93]

Discussing clients with learning disabilities, Thomas describes case management applied to clients in their local communities as managing a team of field workers who assess clients' needs and make action plans with them.[94] These plans address assessment, action planning, package development, and financial management. Case managers draw up contracts for clients' services.

These packages include an estimate of hours required for one month's care and residential versus home care costs, and they break down costs into those for such workers as community care assistant, respite care home outreach worker, physiotherapist, and occupational therapist, and for transportation. Contracts involving groups of clients may obtain discounts. Third-party payers usually approve contracts.

Thomas states that caseworkers are frequently social workers, and case management may develop into a new autonomous profession.

Dowling states that nursing case management makes the patient's nurse the central decision hub for the entire spectrum of patient care requirements and services.[95] He calls this matrix management. The common results of nursing case management fall into five primary areas:

1. Early, or appropriate, patient discharges.
2. Expected, or standardized, clinical outcomes.
3. Promotion of collaborative practice, coordinated patient care, and true continuity of care.
4. Promotion of nurses' professional development and job satisfaction.
5. Use of appropriate, or reduced, resources.

The model is the critical path forecasting physician intervention, diagnostic testing, ancillary department patient care, support department input, and supply and equipment requirements. The individual critical path is a communication tool for all care given. It is a production schedule. The critical path provides the hospital material manager with a dynamic distribution of patient care supplies and equipment needed in advance of any requests. Hospital information supplements provide the information needed for supplies and equipment planning to be case specific. Just-in-time programs can provide patient-specific supplies for multiple supply-retention locations on a nursing unit.

Research indicates that using the critical path technique for assessing the postoperative recovery of coronary artery bypass graph patients prevents complications, reduces lengths of stay, and reduces hospital costs. Nursing interventions such as use of inspirometers, resumption of activity, and patient education support this finding. Critical paths may be used by nurses to identify appropriate nursing interventions and their costs.[96]

Case management is outcome-based and supports evidence-based practices. The Medical Center of Central Georgia in Macon used outcome-based nursing practice. Researchers studied a population of stable cardiovascular patients receiving specialty infusions. By treating these patients on the telemetry unit rather than in the coronary care unit, the center realized cost avoidance of $46,121.83 in one year. Patient classification systems estimate caregiver time and caregiver costs. The weighted salary of caregivers was $14.34/hr in the coronary care unit and $10.00/hr in the telemetry unit. Cost per patient day was $102.45 versus $49.23, for a cost avoidance of $53.22 per patient day.[97]

Zander states that the complete results of case management must include length of stay statistics, readmission rates, and some tally of patient satisfaction.[98]

Bower catalogues the reasons for implementing case management:[99]

1. A client/family focus on the full spectrum of needs.
2. Outcome orientation to care.
3. Coordination of care by team collaboration.
4. Cost management through facilitation through the health care system.
5. Response to insurers and payers.
6. A merger of clinical and financial interests, systems, and outcomes.
7. Inclusion for marketing strategies.

Patient Outcomes

Outcomes and their relation to productivity are a major concern in human relations management. At the University of Iowa College of Nursing, nurse researchers and practitioners have developed the Nursing Outcomes Classification (NOC). At the College of Nursing, the NOC has been integrated with the Nursing Diagnoses Classification, the Nursing Interventions Classification, and the Nursing Management Minimum Data Set.[100] Patient outcomes are the outcomes resulting from care of patients by nurses or an interdisciplinary care team. Patient outcomes include those related to patient satisfaction and health status, nosocomial infection control, and risk events and adverse outcomes. Activities related to patient outcomes are directed toward improving organizational performance continually over time.[101]

Summary

Scope and Standards for Nurse Administrators provides a conceptualization for practice. Levels of nursing administration further delineate the roles of nurse manager and nurse executive.

A theory of nursing management evolves from a general theory of management that governs effective use of human and material resources. The four major functions of management are planning, organizing, directing (or leading), and controlling (or evaluating). All management activities—cognitive, affective, and psychomotor—fall within one or more of these major functions, which operate simultaneously.

Nursing management focuses on human behavior. Nurse managers with knowledge and skills in human behavior manage professional nurses and nonprofessional assistive nursing workers to achieve the highest level of productivity of patient care services. To do this, nurse managers must become competent leaders to stimulate motivation through relationships and interpersonal processes and communication with the work force.

The primary role of the nurse manager is that of managing a clinical practice discipline. To accomplish this requires numerous competencies supported by a theory of nursing management.

Nurse managers work with staff consisting of clinical practitioners. Educated in nursing management, they can assist these practitioners in their work according to the models of such theorists as Orem, Kinlein, Roy, Newman, Levine, Johnson, Peplau, and Orlando.

Several modalities of nursing have evolved over the past 50 years. Functional nursing, the oldest nursing practice modality, is a method in which each staff member is assigned a particular nursing function, such as administering medications, admitting and discharging patients, and making beds and serving meals. Later, team nursing became the modality of choice for many hospital nursing services. Under the leadership of a professional nurse, a group of nurses work together to provide patient care. Team nursing rests on theoretical knowledge related to philosophy, planning, leadership, interpersonal relationships, and nursing process.

Since the 1970s, the modality of total patient care through primary nursing has evolved. With primary nursing, the total care of a patient and a case load is the responsibility of one primary nurse. Joint or collaborative practice by a physician/nurse team has developed as a modality of nursing in a few hospitals. A more recent development is case management, a method of practicing nursing that incorporates any modality and in which the knowledgeable nurse becomes the case manager, making or facilitating all clinical nursing decisions about a case load of patients during an entire episode of illness.

As new technologies of patient treatment develop and the health care delivery system evolves around managed care, nurses will need avenues to pursue the ensuing ethical dilemmas. Nursing practice is further complicated by the need for multicultural assessments as part of the nursing process and its outcomes.

APPLICATION EXERCISES

EXERCISE 1-1

Define nursing management as it relates to your job. If you are a student, observe the work of a nurse manager and define management in terms of your observations.

EXERCISE 1-2

Describe a belief you have about nursing management in the organization in which you work or are doing clinical practice. Discuss your belief with your peers in clinical practice or students and with your nurse manager or instructor.

Summarize the conclusions. Is your belief valid? Totally? Partly? Not at all? Validity can be established by comparing your conclusions with viewpoints found in publications or by obtaining agreement from practicing nurse managers. You will codify selected theory of nursing management.

EXERCISE 1-3

Translate the management of time into nursing management theory with examples such as: "A nurse who practices good management will know how to use time effectively." The example may be one that applies to you as manager or to the observed behavior of another nurse manager. Keep a log for a day, making entries at 15-minute intervals on a separate sheet of paper. Use the following format.

TIME	ACTIVITY	DELAYS AND BOTTLENECKS

Analyze your log. How much of your day was productive? How much was unproductive? What can be done to increase productive time? Using the following format, make a management plan to make better use of your time.

Management Plan

Goal:

ACTIONS	TARGET DATES	ASSIGNED TO	ACCOMPLISHMENTS

Based on your observations from this exercise, write a theory statement that describes management as the effective use of time.

EXERCISE 1-4

The following functions originate from a theory of the institution or organization and the division of nursing:

Plans for accomplishing objectives are made.
Strategies for accomplishing objectives are formulated.
Activities are organized by priority.
Work is assigned.
Managerial jobs are designed.
An organizational structure evolves.

Describe how each of these activities is evident in your place of practice as a student or a practicing professional nurse.

EXERCISE 1-5

Write a short theory of nursing management based on information presented in this chapter. Remember that a theory of nursing management is an accumulation of concepts, methods, and principles that can be or have been observed and verified to some degree and translated into the art or practice of nursing management.

EXERCISE 1-6

Examine the periodicals listed for the last 12-month period:

The Journal of Nursing Administration
Nursing Administration Quarterly
Nursing Management
Nursing Research

Note the following:

- The number of articles on nursing theory versus nursing management theory.
- Theories of nursing that could be incorporated into a theory of nursing management. Did the research indicate that the theory fulfilled its claim? Explain.
- According to these periodicals, what theory of nursing management is being used in the organization in which you are gaining clinical experience as a student or in which you are employed?
- According to these periodicals, what theory of nursing management could be used in the organization in which you are gaining clinical experience as a student or in which you are employed? Consider the value the research has for meeting the goals of the organization, the division of nursing, and the nursing unit.
- Make a management plan for putting the research results into practice.

EXERCISE 1-7

Use your student group or form an ad hoc committee of nurses to plan for needed implementation of nursing theory in a nursing unit. Make a management plan using the following format. To help make a decision, access the Internet and find applications of theories of Orem, Roy, Margaret Newman, Levine, Johnson, Peplau, and Orlando.

MANAGEMENT PLAN

PROBLEM:

OBJECTIVE:

ACTIONS	TARGET DATES	ASSIGNED TO	ACCOMPLISHMENTS

EXERCISE 1-8 Evaluate case management as practiced in the agency in which you are employed or to which you are assigned as a student. Do this by gathering and analyzing data that do the following:

1. Describe the model of case management being used.
2. Identify the standards used to trigger the case management process.
3. Trace the continuum of case management from patient's entry through discharge.
4. Measure the achievement of stated outcomes.
5. Relate the nursing modality to case management.

NOTES

1. Greiner, A. C. & Knebel, E. (Eds.). (2003). *Health professions education: A bridge to quality*. Washington, DC: The National Academies Press.
2. American Nurses Association (ANA). (2004). *Scope and standards for nurse administrators* (2nd ed.). Washington, DC: Author.
3. Ibid., p. 9.
4. Ibid., p. 5.
5. Ibid., p. 7.
6. Ibid.
7. American Nurses Association Credentialing Center. (2004). *Certification for nurse administration*. Washington, DC: Author.
8. ANA, 2004, p. 10.
9. Fayol, H. (1949). *General and industrial management* (C. Storrs, Trans.). London: Pitman & Sons, p. 3.
10. Ibid., pp. 5–6.
11. Hodgetts, R. M. (1990). Management: Theory, process, and practice (5th ed.). Orlando, FL: Harcourt Brace, p. 38.
12. Fayol, 1949, pp. 8–9.
13. Ibid., pp. 19–20.
14. Page, A. (Ed.). (2004). *Keeping patients safe: Transforming the work environment of nurses*. Washington, DC: The National Academies Press.
15. Ibid., pp. 112–125.
16. Ibid., p. 122.
17. Ibid., p. 125.
18. ANA, 2004.
19. Megginson, L. C., Mosley, D. C., & Pietri, P.H., Jr. (1996). *Management: Leadership in action* (5th ed.). New York: Harper & Row, pp. 15–20.
20. White, V. (1984). Nursing theory: A viewpoint. *Journal of Nursing Administration*, 6, 15.
21. Skinner, W. (1982). Big hat, no cattle: Managing human resources, part I. *Journal of Nursing Administration*, pp. 27–29.
22. Steffy, B. D. & Grimes, A. J. (1986). A critical theory of organizational science. *Academy of Management Review*, 322–336.
23. Ibid.
24. McKenzie, L. (1992). Critical thinking in health care supervision. *Health Care Supervisor*, 2.
25. Boulding, K. E. (1956). General systems theory: The skeleton of science. *Management Science*, 197–208.
26. Ibid.
27. Drucker, P. F. (1990). The emerging theory of manufacturing. *Harvard Business Review*, 94–100.
28. Ibid.
29. Allison, S. E., McLaughlin, K., & Walker, D. (1991). Nursing theory: A tool to put nursing back into nursing administration. *Nursing Administration Quarterly*, 72–78.
30. Ibid.
31. Drucker, 1999, p. 34.
32. Anderson, R. (1989). A theory development role for nurse administrators, *Journal of Nursing Administration*, 23–29.
33. Henderson, V. (1966). *The nature of nursing*. New York: Macmillan, p. 15.
34. Gleeson, S., Nestor, D. W., & Riddell, A. J. (1983). Helping nurses through the management threshold. *Nursing Administration Quarterly*, 11–16.
35. Taylor, B. A. & DeSimone, A. Taking the first steps to becoming a nurse manager. *Nursing Administration Quarterly*, 17–22.
36. Reeves, D. M. & Underly, N. (1983). Nurse managers and Mickey Mouse marketing. *Nursing Administration Quarterly*, 22–27.
37. Fralic, M. F. & O'Connor, A. (1983a). A management system for nurse administrators, part I. *Journal of Nursing Administration*, 9–13; Fralic, M. F. & O'Connor, A. (1983b). A management progression system for nurse administrators, part 2. *Journal of Nursing Administration*, 32–33; Fralic, M. F. & O'Connor, A. (1983c). A management progression system for nurse administrators, part 3. *Journal of Nursing Administration*, 7–12.
38. Huey, J. (1994). The leadership industry. *Fortune*, 54–56; Perry, N. J. (1994). How to mine human resources. *Fortune*, 96.
39. Spicer, J. G. (1983). Dispelling illusions with management development. *Nursing Administration Quarterly*, 46–49.
40. Ibid.
41. Osborne, D. & Gaebler, T. (1992). *Reinventing government*. New York: Plume, pp. 275–276.
42. McClure, M. L. (1984a). Managing the professional nurse, part I: The organizational theories. *Journal of Nursing Administration*, 15–21; McClure, M. L. (1984b). Managing the professional nurse, part II: Applying management theory to the challenges. *Journal of Nursing Administration*, 11–17.
43. Ibid.
44. Freund, C. M. (1985). Director of nursing effectiveness: DON and CEO perspectives and implications for education. *Journal of Nursing Administration*, 25–30.
45. Rew, L. (1986). Intuition: Concept analysis of a group phenomenon. *Advances in Nursing Science*, 21–28.
46. O'Leary, J. (1984). Do nurse administrators' values conflict with the economic trend? *Nursing Administration Quarterly*, 1–9; McClure, 1984a; Maidique, M. A. (1983). Point of view: The new management thinkers. *California Management Review*, 151–160; Poulin, M. A. (1984a). Future directions for nursing administration. *Journal of Nursing Administration*, 37–41; Fralic & O'Connor, 1983a; Gentleman, C. (1983). G. Power at the unit level. *Nursing Administration Quarterly*, 27–31; Poulin, M. A. (1984b). The nurse executive role: A structural and functional analysis. *Journal of Nursing Administration*, 9–14.
47. Gentleman, 1983.
48. Mathews, J. J. (1988). Designing a first line manager development program using organization-appropriate strategies. *The Journal of Continuing Education in the Health Professions*, *8*(3), 181–188.

49. Princeton, J. C. (1993). Education for executive nurse administrators: A databased curricular model for doctoral (PhD) programs. *Journal of Nursing Education*, 59–63.
50. Henkoff, R. (1995). New management secrets from Japan. *Fortune*, 135–146.
51. Bush, H. A. (1979). Models for nursing. *Advances in Nursing Science*, 13–21.
52. Dickson, G. L. & Lee-Villasenor, H. (1982). Nursing theory and practice: A self-care approach. *Advances in Nursing Science*, 29–40.
53. Jaarsma, T., Halfens, R., Senten, M., Abu Saad, H. H., & Dracup, K. (1998). Developing a supportive-educative program for patients with advanced heart failure within Orem's general theory of nursing. *Nursing Science Quarterly*, 79–85.
54. Roy, C. (1971). Adaptation: A basis for nursing practice. *Nursing Outlook*, 254–257; Frederickson, K. (1993). Using a nursing model to manage symptoms: Anxiety and the Roy Adaptation Model. *Holistic Nursing Practice*, 36–43.
55. Ibid.
56. Mastal, M. F. & Hammond, H. (1980). Analysis and expansion of the Roy Adaptation Model: A contribution to holistic nursing. *Advances in Nursing Science*, 71–81.
57. Frederickson, 1993.
58. Silva, M. C. & Sorrell, J. M. (1992). Testing a nursing theory: Critique and philosophical expansion. *Advances in Nursing Science*, 12–23.
59. Engle, V. F. (1984). Newman's conceptual framework and the measurement of older adults' health. *Advances in Nursing Science*, 24–36.
60. Ibid.
61. Ibid.
62. Levine, M. E. (1966). Adaptation and assessment: A rationale for nursing intervention. *American Journal of Nursing*, 2450–2453.
63. Ibid.
64. Rawls, A. C. (1980). Evaluation of the Johnson Behavioral System Model in clinical practice. *Image*, 12–16.
65. Derdiarian, A. K. (1990). The relationships among the subsystems of Johnson's Behavioral System Model. *Image*, 219–225.
66. Thompson, L. (1986). Peplau's theory: An application to short-term individual therapy. *Journal of Psychosocial Nursing*, 26–31.
67. Peplau, H. E. (1992). Interpersonal relations: A theoretical framework for application in nursing practice. *Nursing Science Quarterly*, 13–18; Schafer, P. (1999). Working with Dave: Application of Peplau's Interpersonal Nursing Theory in the correctional environment. *Journal of Psychosocial Nursing and Mental Health Services*, 18–24.
68. Schmieding, N. J. (1984). Putting Orlando's theory into practice. *American Journal of Nursing*, 759–761; Orlando, I. J. (1972). *The discipline and teaching of nursing process: An evaluative study*. New York: G. P. Putnam's Sons; Orlando, I. J. (1961). *The dynamic nurse/patient relationship: Function, process, principles*. New York: G. P. Putnam's Sons.
69. Wiens, A. G. (1993). Patient autonomy in care: A theoretical framework for nursing. *Journal of Professional Nursing*, 95–103.
70. Happ, M. B. (1993). Sociotechnical systems theory. *Journal of Nursing Administration*, 47–54.
71. Newcomb, D. P. & Swansburg, R. C. (1971). *The team plan: A manual for nursing service administrators* (2nd ed.). New York: Putnam, p. 56.
72. Marram, G. D., Schlegel, M. W. & Bevis, E. O. (1974). *Primary nursing: A model for individualized care*. Saint Louis: Mosby, p. 1.
73. Ibid., 16–17.
74. Fagin, C. M. (1982). The economic value of nursing research. *American Journal of Nursing*, 1844–1849.
75. Lyon, J. C. (1993). *Models of nursing care delivery and case management: Clarification of terms. Nursing Economic*, 163–169.
76. The National Joint Practice Commission. (1981). *Guidelines for establishing joint or collaborative practice in hospitals*. Chicago, IL: Neely Printing.
77. Ibid.
78. Koch, L. W., Puzaki, S. H., & Campbell, J. D. (1992). The first 20 years of nurse practitioner literature: An evolution of joint practice issues. *Nurse Practitioner*, 62–66, 68, 71.
79. Herman, J. & Ziel, S. (1999). Collaborative practice agreements for advanced practice nurses: What you should know. *AACN Clinical Issues*, 337–342.
80. Center for Case Management. Toward a fully-integrated CareMap® and case management system. (1983). *The New Definition*, 1.
81. Center for Case Management. Part 1: Rationale for care-provider organizations. (1994). *The New Definition*, 1.
82. Ibid.
83. Ibid.
84. Ibid.
85. Center for Case Management. Quantifying, managing, and improving quality, part I: How CareMaps® link CQI to the patient. (1992). *The New Definition*, 1.
86. Ibid.
87. Center for Case Management. Quantifying, managing and improving quality, part III: Using variance concurrently. (1992). *The New Definition*, 1–2.
88. Brockopp, D. Y., Porter, M., Kinnaird, S., & Silberman, S. (1992). Fiscal and clinical evaluation of patient care. *Journal of Nursing Administration*, 23–27.
89. Rogers, M., Riordan, J., & Swindle, D. (1991). Community-based nursing case management pays off. *Nursing Management*, 30–34.
90. Lyon, 1993.
91. Bower, K. (1992). *Case management by nurses* (2nd ed.). Washington, DC: American Nurses Publishing, 33–34.
92. Williams, R. (1992). Nurse case management: Working with the community. *Nursing Management*, 33–34.
93. Strong, A. G. (1992). Case management and the CNS. *Clinical Nurse Specialist*, 64.
94. Thomas, J. (1992, July 15). Package Deals. *Nursing Times*, pp. 48–49.
95. Dowling, G. F. (1991). Case management nursing: Indications for material management. *Hospital Material Management Quarterly*, 26–32.
96. Strong & Sneed, 1991.
97. Servais, S. H. (1991). Nursing resource applications through outcome based nursing practice. *Nursing Economic*, 171–174, 179.
98. Zander, K., & McGill, R. (1994). Critical and anticipated recovery paths: Only the beginning. *Nurse Manager, 25*(8), 34–37, 40.
99. Bower, 1992, 7–8.
100. The University of Iowa College of Nursing. (2000). *CHAOS*. Iowa City, IA: University of Iowa Press.
101. Titler, M. G. & McCloskey, J. M. (Eds.). (1999). On the scene: University of Iowa hospitals and clinics: Outcomes management. *Nursing Administration Quarterly*, 31–65.

REFERENCES

American Academy of Nursing. (1977). *Primary care by nurses: Sphere of responsibility and accountability*. Kansas City, MO: Author.

American Nurses Association. (1994). *Nursing: A social policy statement*. Washington, DC: Author.

Bower, K. A. & Somerville, J. G. (1988). Managed care and case management outcome based practice: Creating the environment, Program presented at the Sheraton Grand Hotel, Tampa, Florida, February 15–16, 1988.

Bradshaw, M. J. (1999). Clinical pathways: A tool to evaluate clinical learning. *Journal of the Society of Pediatric Nurses*, 37–40.

Burr, J. A. & Chapman, T. (1998). Some reflections on cultural and social considerations in mental health nursing. *Journal of Psychiatric Mental Health Nursing*, 431–437.

Carr, J. M. (1998). Vigilance as a caring expression and Leininger's theory of cultural care diversity and universality. *Nursing Science Quarterly*, 74–78.

Carse, J. (1994). Diversity in the World's Religions. *National Forum*, 26–27.

Chase, M. (1992, May 21). Cancer doctors aim to improve chemotherapy. *The Wall Street Journal*, p. A88.

Chinn, P. L. & Jacobs, M. K. (1987). *Theory and nursing: A systematic approach*. St. Louis: Mosby.

Ciske, K. I. (1978). Response to Zander's "Primary nursing won't work . . . Unless the head nurse lets it." *Journal of Nursing Administration*, 26, 43, 50.

Cortes, C. E. (1994). Limits to pluribus, limits to unum. *National Forum*, 6–8.

Dickoff, J., James, P., & Wiedenbach, E. (1968a). Theory in a practice discipline, part I. Practice oriented theory. *Nursing Research*, 415–435.

Dickoff, J., James, P., & Wiedenbach, E. (1968b). Theory in a practice discipline, part II. Practice oriented research. *Nursing Research*, 545–554.

Dixon, E. L. (1999). Community health nursing practice and the Roy Adaptation Model. *Public Health Nursing*, 290–300.

Donaldson, T. (1992). Individual rights and multinational corporate responsibilities. *National Forum*, 7–9.

Etzioni, A. (1992). Too many rights, too few responsibilities. *National Forum*, 4–6.

Fadden, T. C. & Seiser, G. K. (1984). Nursing diagnosis: A matter of form. *American Journal of Nursing*, 470–472.

Felton, G. (1975). Increasing the quality of nursing care by introducing the concept of primary nursing: A model project. *Nursing Research*, 27–32.

Flaherty, M. (1998). Letting go: Facing the sensitive subject of DNR orders. *HealthWeek*, 20.

Flanagan, J. (1998). Achieving partnership: The contribution of nursing education to the production of a flexible workforce. *Journal of Nursing Management*, 135–136.

Freed, P. E., & Drake, V. K. (1999). Mandatory reporting of abuse: Practical, moral, and legal issues for psychiatric home healthcare nurses. *Issues in Mental Health Nursing*, 423–436.

Garcia, M. A., Bruce, D., Niemeyer, J., & Robbins, J. (1993). Collaborative practice: A shared success. *Nursing Management*, 72–74, 78.

Goodman, D. (1997). Application of the critical pathway and integrated case teaching method to nursing orientation. *Journal of Continuing Education in Nursing*, 205–210.

Goodman, E. (2000, April 21). Health system relies on lying. *San Antonio Express-News*.

Goodpaster, K. E., & Atkinson, G. (1992). Stakeholders, individual rights, and the common good. *National Forum*, 14–17.

Hellinghausen, M. A. (2000). Closing the gap: Program aims to add more minorities to healthcare professions. *HealthWeek*, 27.

Henry, B., Arndt, C., DiVincenti, M., & Mariner-Tomey, A. (Eds.). (1989). *Dimensions of nursing administration: Theory, research, education, practice*. Boston: Blackwell.

Hoffman, W. M., & Petry, E.S., Jr. (1992). Abusing business ethics. *National Forum*, 10–13.

Jonsdottir, H. (1999). Outcomes of implementing primary nursing in the care of people with chronic lung diseases: The nurses' experience. *Journal of Nursing Management*, 235–242.

Koleszar, A. J. (1990). The great debate. *CWRU*, 16–20.

Kols, A. J., Sherman, J. E., & Piotrow, P. T. (1999). Ethical foundations of client-centered care in family planning. *Journal of Women's Health*, 303–312.

Koziol-McLain, J. & Maeve, M. K. (1993). Nursing theory in perspective. *Nursing Outlook*, 79–81.

Leininger, M. (1988). Leininger's theory of nursing: Culture care diversity and universality. *Nursing Science Quarterly*, *1*(4), 152–160.

Leininger, M. (1993). Culture care theory: The comparative global theory to advance human care theory and practice. In D. A. Gaut (Ed.), *A global agenda for caring* (pp. 3–18). New York: National League for Nursing.

Leininger, M. (1994). Quality of life from a transcultural nursing perspective. *Nursing Science Quarterly*, *7*(1), 22–28.

Leininger, M. (1995). *Transcultural nursing: Concepts, theories, research & practices* (2nd ed.). New York: McGraw-Hill.

McLaughlin, C. (1994). Thinking about diversity. *National Forum*, 16–18.

Moffic, H. S. & Kinzie, J.D. (1996). The history of cross cultural psychiatric services. *Community Mental Health Journal*, 581–592.

Moore, J. (1992, April 29). Senator says mental hospital abuses not limited to Texas. *San Antonio Light*, p. D6.

Morgan, L. (1999). Faith meets health. *HealthWeek*, 15.

Murphy, W. J. (1999). Ethical perspectives in neuroscience nursing practice. *Nursing Clinics of North America*, 621–635.

Nelson-Marten, P., Hecomovich, K., & Pangle, M. Caring theory: A framework for advanced nursing practice. *Advanced Practice Nursing Quarterly*, 70–77.

Newman, M. A. (1984). Nursing diagnosis: Looking at the whole. *American Journal of Nursing*, 1496–1499.

Nightingale, Florence. (1959). *Notes on nursing*. Philadelphia: J. B. Lippincott.

Norman-Culp, S. (1993, May 23). No mercy for dying man, wife says. *San Antonio Express-News*, p. 3F.

Parker, R. S. (1990). Measuring nurses' moral judgments. *Image*, 213–218.

Parse, R. R. (1999). Nursing science: The transformation of practice. *Journal of Advanced Nursing*, 1383–1387.

Paul, N. (1992). For the record: Information on individuals. *National Forum*, 34–38.

Redman, B. K., & Fry, S. T. (1998). Ethical conflicts reported by certified registered rehabilitation nurses. *Rehabilitation Nursing*, 179–184.

Rogers, M. (1970). *An introduction to the theoretical basis of nursing*. Philadelphia: F. A. Davis.

Rogers, M., Riordan, J., & Swindle, D. (1991). Community-based nursing case management pays off. *Nursing Management*, 30–34.

Rothrock, J. C. (1984). Nursing diagnosis in the days of Florence Nightingale. *AORN Journal*, 189–190.

Roy, S. C. (1976). *Introduction to nursing: An adaptation model*. Englewood Cliffs, NJ: Prentice Hall.

Saliba, D., Kington, R., Buchanan, J., Bell, R., Wang, M., Lee, M. et al. (2000). Appropriateness of the decision to transfer nursing facility residents to the hospital. *Journal of the American Geriatric Society*, 154–163.

Shaw-Taylor, Y. & Benesch, B. (1998). Workforce diversity and cultural competence in healthcare. *Journal of Cultural Diversity*, 147–148.

Shukla, R. K. (1981). Structure vs people in primary nursing: An inquiry. *Nursing Research*, 236–241.

Simpson, R. D. & Anderson, W.W. (1992). Science education and the common good. *National Forum*, 30–33.

Smith, H. L. (1992). Genetic technologies: Can we do responsibly everything we can do technically? *National Forum*, 26–29.

Smith, L. S. (1988). Concept analysis: Cultural competence. *Journal of Cultural Diversity*, 4–10.

Strong, A. G. & Sneed, N.V. (1991). Clinical evaluation of a critical path for coronary artery bypass surgery patients. *Progress in Cardiovascular Nursing*, 29–37.

Swansburg, R. C. (1968). *Team nursing: A programmed learning experience* (4 vols.). New York: G. P. Putnam's Sons.

Swansburg, R. C. (1976). *Management of patient care services*. St. Louis: Mosby.

Swansburg, R. C. & Swansburg, P. W. (1984). Strategic career planning and development for nurses. Rockville, MD: Aspen Publishers.

Thomas, J. (1992, July 15). Package deals. *Nursing Times*, 48–49.

Thomas, L. H. (1992). Qualified nurse and nursing auxiliary perceptions of their work environment in primary, team, and functional nursing wards. *Journal of Advanced Nursing*, 373–382.

Thomas, N. M. & Newsome, G. G. (1992). Factors affecting the use of nursing diagnosis. *Nursing Outlook*, 182–186.

Thorns, A. R. & Ellershaw, J. E. (1999). A survey of nursing and medical staff views on the use of cardiopulmonary resuscitation in the hospice. *Palliative Medicine*, 225–232.

Tritsch, J. M. (1998). Application of King's theory of goal attainment and the Carondelet St. Mary's Case Management Model. *Nursing Science Quarterly*, 69–73.

VanLeit, B. (1995). Using the case method to develop reasoning skills in problem-based learning. *American Journal of Occupational Therapy*, 349–353.

Wagner, L., Henry, B., Giovinco, G., and Blanks C. (1988). Suggestions for graduate education in nursing administration. *Journal of Nursing Education*, 210–218.

Williams, R. (1992). Nurse case management: Working with the community. *Nursing Management*, 33–34.

Williams, R. (1999). Cultural safety—What does it mean for our work practice? *Australia New Zealand Journal of Public Health*, 213–214.

Wong, F. K. (1998). The nurse manager as a professional/managerial class: A case study. *Journal of Nursing Management*, 343–350.

Yamashita, M. (1998). Newman's theory of health as expanding consciousness: Research on family caregiving in mental illness in Japan. *Nursing Science Quarterly*, 110–115.

Yoder, M. E. (1984). Nursing diagnosis: Application during perioperative practice. *AORN Journal*, 183–188.

Zander, K. S. (1977). Primary nursing won't work . . . unless the head nurse lets it. *Journal of Nursing Administration*, 19–23.

CHAPTER 2

Emotionally Intelligent Leadership in Nursing and Health Care Organizations

Susan H. Taft, RN, MSN, PhD

LEARNING OBJECTIVES AND ACTIVITIES

- Define emotional intelligence (EI).
- Distinguish between emotional intelligence and emotional competencies (EC).
- Name the four EI clusters.
- Identify the 18 emotional competencies discussed in the EI clusters.
- Identify factors that may enhance or diminish one's innate EI and learned ECs.
- Describe the five core competencies and why they are considered crucial.
- Discuss why nursing settings are intensely emotional.
- Discuss the emotional competencies that may be most important to practicing nurses.
- Identify the EI strengths and weaknesses of the nurses in these case studies: Exhibits 2-2, 2-3, and 2-6.
- Describe how to develop emotional competencies.
- Examine the characteristics of "best" and "worst" bosses you have known.
- Identify areas of research—from nursing and other disciplines—that support emotional competencies as predictors of leadership success.
- Describe how middle- and executive-level nurse leaders might use emotional competencies in different situations.
- Discuss how emotionally intelligent nurse leaders might improve nursing work environments.
- Identify the desirable characteristics and capabilities of middle- and executive-level nurse leaders and how to select for these qualities.

CONCEPTS: Emotional intelligence, emotional competency, socioemotional leadership, effective and ineffective leaders, self-awareness, self-assessment, self-confidence, self-control, trust and trustworthiness, adaptability, achievement drive, initiative, optimism, empathy, influence, organizational politics, service orientation, developing others, inspirational leadership, change agent, conflict management, teamwork, collaboration, nurse manager and leader competencies.

NURSE MANAGER AND NURSE EXECUTIVE BEHAVIORS: Managing oneself successfully, relating effectively to others, leading change initiatives, understanding and working with organizational politics, promoting teamwork and collaboration, and managing conflict will all be strengthened with greater concentrations of emotional competencies. Executive-level leaders select and develop nurse middle managers, and middle managers select and develop members of their staff.

Introduction

Effective leadership in organizations requires numerous talents, skills, and types of knowledge, as the existence of this textbook demonstrates. At its core, leadership is about relationships with other people. Leaders' accomplishments are largely achieved through the individual and coordinated efforts of others. Without followers, there are no leaders.[1]

Leadership theories have developed since before the time of Machiavelli, but the most recent theories originated in the industrialized world of the 20th century. In the works of scholars, researchers, exemplary leaders, and undistinguished nonleaders alike, there are few topics in management about which more has been written. Since the 1950s, research has tended to focus on western methods of leadership in traditional industries. More recently, leadership research has expanded our traditional understanding by focusing on leadership behaviors at different levels and within different functional areas of organizations, women's leadership styles, leader diversity as a competitive advantage to organizations, multicultural and global leadership,[2] the role of leaders in attaining quality outcomes, and an acknowledgement that "no one size fits all" practicing leaders. But consistently throughout time and across cultures, leadership has been recognized as a people-oriented business.

This chapter is devoted to exploring the people skills of good leaders—leaders who enable "their people" to be happy and productive workers and committed employees, who allow workers to grow and develop to their full potentials, and who themselves work successfully as committed organizational agents. As the standard bearers for high performance, effective leaders enable good performers but also counsel irretrievably poor employees to leave a setting where they perform poorly. The leadership framework discussed in this chapter is emotional intelligence,[3] a composite of 18 intra- and interpersonal competencies that predicts successful leadership at work.

What Is Emotional Intelligence?

Emotional intelligence (EI) is defined as "the capacity for recognizing our own feelings and those of others, for motivating ourselves, and for managing emotions well in ourselves and in others."[4] EI includes capabilities distinct from, but complementary to, academic intelligence or the purely cognitive capacities measured by IQ. *Emotional competencies* are defined as "learned capabilities based on emotional intelligence that contribute to effective performance at work."[4] Based on extensive research conducted by Goleman and his associates and by the Hay Group of Boston, emotional competence has been found to matter twice as much as IQ and technical skill combined in producing superior managerial job performance.

Emotional intelligence develops in human beings as a result of genetic inheritance and the socializing influences of childhood, adolescence, and adulthood; emotional competencies are a result of emotional intelligence *plus* opportunities we have to develop those competencies. They are capabilities we can learn and expand. Thus an individual born with average emotional intelligence might become exceptionally emotionally competent in adulthood if she had parents who, during her upbringing, tuned in well to her feelings; practiced leadership in college through her sorority; and worked with emotionally competent managers (positive role models) in her early work experiences. Similarly, it is possible to have life experiences that erode one's emotional intelligence. An individual born with high natural emotional intelligence could become limited in emotional competencies if she came from a home in which a parent was an alcoholic, suffered taunting or hazing in school, or had previous bosses who were abusive (negative role models).

The nursing profession requires a high degree of emotional labor—the ability of nurses to regulate their own emotions and the expression of emotions for the sake of their patients' needs. Nurses are expected to display emotions that convey caring, understanding, and compassion toward patients while regulating their own feelings. For newly graduated nurses, the added emotional burdens of coping with the transition from school to work are enormous.[5] The role of the nurse leader, then, becomes critical "in creating a supportive and positive work environment to help nurses cope with the stress of managing their own and others' emotions" concurrently.[6] Emotional intelligence provides a framework for understanding the ways in which leader behaviors are necessary for the creation of a positive emotion-intensive work environment.

The Emotional Intelligence Framework

The emotional intelligence framework consists of two dimensions: the ability to understand and manage oneself and the ability to understand and relate well to others. These dimensions are further subdivided into self-awareness and self-management, and social awareness and relationship management. In each dimension, the ability to manage oneself or others is predicated on the awareness one has of self and others. Exhibit 2-1 shows the framework of the emotional intelligence dimensions.

Self-awareness can be considered the inner barometer, or rudder, people have to understand and direct the moment-to-moment and situation-to-situation variation in internal emotions. Human beings are emotional, constantly reacting to internal and external stimuli. These stimuli may cause feelings that are positive or negative, uplifting or discouraging, threatening or pleasing, exciting or boring, and so on. An emotionally intelligent individual is aware of feelings as they emerge, understands them accurately, and has the self-confidence to continue activity in the world regardless of his or her emotions. *Self-management* extends one's emotional intelligence by

EXHIBIT 2-1
Framework of Emotional Intelligence

SELF	OTHERS
Self-Awareness	Social Awareness
Self-Management	Relationship Management

allowing for self-control of emotions, maintenance of one's integrity, and adaptability to emerging situations. Individuals low in self-awareness or emotional self-management or both may "blurt" reactions in social situations, show rigidity or brittleness when faced with differences of opinion, be defensive to criticism, act contrary to their espoused values, or project insecurity when around others (see Exhibit 2–2).

Emotionally intelligent interactions with other people depend and build on an individual's strengths in self-awareness and self-management. Without a solid base of self-understanding, self-control, emotional security, trustworthiness, and adaptability, it is virtually impossible to be open to others and constructive in work relationships. Thus good leaders must know themselves well and be able to *choose* how they will respond in social situations. These strengths then provide the foundation for working well with others.

Good relationships with others are shown through social awareness and relationship management. They are considered "social radar"—the ability to understand others and work with them productively. *Social awareness* is founded, most directly, on the skills of empathy: sensing others' feelings, needs, and concerns, and taking an active interest in them. Social awareness in work settings extends into the ability to use good political skills and an active, principled orientation to service toward customers or patients. To exhibit political astuteness at work and to serve patients with sensitivity, the nurse draws on his or her empathy for others, whether they are individuals or people who are part of groups. *Relationship management* includes areas frequently depicted in books and journal articles about leadership. Of all the emotional competencies, these are the most readily learned, either through study, reading, and practice or through leadership development programs. Relationship management encompasses capabilities in inspiring and influencing others, visioning, developing others, collaboration and teamwork, leading change initiatives, and managing conflict. The effective use of relationship management at work involves leadership that builds individual, group, and organizational engagement toward future accomplishments (see, for example, Exhibits 2-2 and 2-3).

EXHIBIT 2-2
The New Nurse Manager

Tiffany worked in a large university medical center. She completed her BSN 3 years ago, and in her first job as a staff nurse on a complex surgical unit rapidly proved herself to be a competent staff nurse. Because of her capabilities and positive attitude, she was promoted to charge nurse after one year. In her third year, she was promoted to unit manager when the previous manager left to direct an ambulatory surgery center within the medical center system. Although a "quick study" in managing the logistics of her unit, she lost trust among the nurses in the unit when she reacted defensively and impatiently to criticisms and complaints from the staff, tended to give summary orders, and projected an "I'm too busy to talk to you now" response to staff concerns. For the first time since she started on the unit, Tiffany began to dread going to work. She felt that her previous colleagues had turned against her and didn't appreciate how hard she worked for them. She often saw their concerns as petty and viewed them as not taking enough responsibility for their own roles on the unit. She talked to her nursing director regularly about the staff issues, but the director just laughed and told her that the "honeymoon was over," and that things would even out in time. After six months, her relationship with her staff had deteriorated to the point that Tiffany, feeling betrayed, scapegoated, and disillusioned, left the medical center to work in a position with an insurance agency.

The Emotional Competencies

Emotional competencies are developed from life experiences in combination with an individual's innate emotional intelligence. Human beings tend to become increasingly emotionally competent with age as we accumulate experiences that help us understand ourselves and others better. We learn from positive as well as negative experiences. Who has not made political mistakes in a job early in a career? How many haven't suffered through a performance appraisal that found us less than perfect? Who has not failed to influence a peer group to do something we thought was an obvious "no-brainer?" To our benefit or detriment, we learned from these experiences. Similarly, almost everyone can identify a teacher who helped us come to know ourselves better and, in the process, improved us or a leader whom we would follow "anywhere." Parenting, socialization experiences, role models, and the practice of new behaviors all help (or hinder) us in developing emotional competence. The positive or negative influence on any individual is dependent on the quality of the experience and how it is processed by that person. The fields of child and adult development focus on how one's natural endowment, culture, and life experiences interact to create the unique mature individual.

Eighteen work competencies, depicted in Exhibit 2-4, constitute the emotional intelligence framework. Four clusters—self-awareness, self-management, social awareness, and relationship management—contain lists of the emotional competencies relevant to self and others. Though all competencies are considered important for leadership effectiveness, five are core competencies on

EXHIBIT 2-3

The Quality Manager

Joe had worked as a staff nurse on medical floors at two different institutions for 6 and 5 years, respectively. When his first child was born, he decided to accept a job offer as the quality manager for a suburban community hospital so that he could enjoy regular hours and arrange his schedule to coordinate with the working hours of his wife. The position he accepted turned out to have more challenges than he anticipated: uneven patient quality outcomes on different nursing units, physicians angry with implied "report cards" on their medical practices, a new nurse executive who was trying to surmount the multiple demands of her position, a recently completed Joint Commission on Accreditation of Healthcare Organizations (JCAHO) survey that enumerated more than a dozen deficiencies that needed correcting within 6 months, and declining patient satisfaction scores in many areas. His first meeting with the executive team of the hospital, in which his charge to "fix things" was laid out, was a demoralizing and overwhelming experience. For a day, Joe regretted having left the comfort of staff nursing, where he knew what to do and how to do it. As a staff nurse, problems could be addressed one patient at a time.

After talking with several nurse manager colleagues from his previous place of work and with a nurse educator at a local university where he had enrolled for master's study, Joe began to get a handle on how to approach his new responsibilities. He understood hospitals. He trusted his own ability to learn what he needed to learn and to move forward one step at a time, and he recognized that the amount he needed to accomplish required a systematic and comprehensive plan. Over the next week, he talked to many different employees of the hospital and some of the physicians in leadership positions. Some of his meetings involved listening to people venting about the problems they faced in their work or the people they worked with; several included angry accusations about the perceived "quality agenda" of the CEO. Joe made no attempt to counter the comments he heard, nor did he allow himself to get defensive and angry in return. Instead, he reiterated frequently that he was just trying to learn about the issues the hospital faced so that he could put together some ideas on how to move forward.

Within several weeks, Joe had identified the areas in the hospital with the most pressing quality challenges; these, combined with the JCAHO deficiencies, were the areas of greatest priority on which he planned to work the hardest immediately. He identified types of processes and interventions that would be needed in various areas: some required setting up QI or process teams, others needed new measurement methods, and still others required a change of personnel. In some cases, he determined that he would need to coach individuals and groups on their work to improve quality. Additionally, Joe envisioned possible structural and facility changes that would be slower to implement but ultimately bring significant improvements. Joe took his plan around to key formal and informal leaders in the institution for their input and then revised the plan. He next took it to the executive team for review, their suggestions, and, once complete, approval. Within 6 weeks, Joe had an approved working plan for the first 12 months of his work at the community hospital. He subsequently found little resistance—and a good degree of cooperation—for moving forward on all of his proposed initiatives.

EXHIBIT 2-4

The Emotional Intelligence Framework & 18 Competencies[7]

PERSONAL COMPETENCE	SOCIAL COMPETENCE
Self-Awareness	*Social Awareness*
Emotional Self-Awareness*	Empathy*
Accurate Self-Assessment*	Organizational Awareness
Self-Confidence*	Service Orientation
Self-Management	*Relationship Management*
Emotional Self-Control*	Developing Others
Transparency	Inspirational Leadership
Adaptability	Change Catalyst
Achievement Orientation	Influence
Initiative	Conflict Management
Optimism	Teamwork & Collaboration

*Core competencies, on which the remaining 13 competencies depend.

which all the other competencies depend. For knowing and managing oneself, core competencies include *emotional self-awareness*, *accurate self-assessment*, *self-confidence*, and *emotional self-control*, and for working effectively with others, *empathy*. Without these core competencies, one cannot effectively exercise leadership. For example, one must be self-aware—in tune with one's own emotions—in order to practice emotional self-control. Emotional self-control is essential to collaborate with others, build teamwork, or manage conflict. Empathy is required to develop others constructively, understand organizational politics, or respond proactively to customer needs.

In Exhibit 2-2, Tiffany's behavior as a new nurse manager reflects limitations in emotional self-awareness, self-control, adaptability, and self-confidence in how she understands and manages herself; in working with others, empathy, organizational awareness, developing others, inspirational leadership, conflict management, and teamwork and collaboration all appear to be weak. Although she has been a competent and effective staff nurse, Tiffany lacks the skills and emotional competencies to move effectively into a management role. It is common in all industries, including health care, for good workers to be promoted into management positions with little or no additional training or mentoring. Sometimes these promotions work well, but often they do not. It is a management myth that the best staff workers make the best leaders. Leading people requires skills and knowledge that even the most talented employees can lack.[8] Emotional intelligence is just one of many areas in management in which plans for human resource development are critical for leader success.

Because the core emotional competencies are essential leadership traits, they are the areas in which leadership development should, in the case of deficiencies, begin. Once integrated well into leadership behavior, the core competencies can be used to support or leverage further emotional competency development.

Exhibit 2-3 gives the scenario of Joe, the new quality manager at a community hospital. Like Tiffany, Joe came from a staff nurse position to a management role. Unlike Tiffany, Joe demonstrates a number of emotional competencies as he takes on a difficult work assignment: although initially overwhelmed and discouraged by his new responsibilities, he is aware of his emotional reactions to those responsibilities. Rather than recede into self-doubt and make a choice to resign, he shows confidence in his own abilities to learn and move forward. He adapts to the magnitude of the job, seeks counsel from others (initiative and optimism), and sets out to gather information necessary for him to succeed (achievement orientation). His meetings with others in the organization are conducted with good political insight (organizational awareness) and empathy. He avoids responding emotionally to the comments he hears (emotional self-control). Joe recognizes that the job requires him to be a champion of change and that it will take collaboration and teamwork, plus development of others, to be effective. Within a reasonable period of time, Joe creates a vision for quality improvements at the hospital. In the near future, he stands a good chance of becoming an influential and inspirational leader for quality improvement.

Why was Joe so much more effective than Tiffany? We cannot say for sure, but some combination of innate emotional intelligence, socialization, positive role models, and age and experience probably provided him with the opportunities to develop his emotional competencies. In contrast, Tiffany came to her new position with serious limitations and, presumably, less positive prior growth opportunities relative to leadership. Nurse leaders who are responsible for selecting, hiring, and promoting personnel need to be aware of the great variation in emotional intelligence that exists among employees. Though Joe needed some coaching in his new position, which he obtained primarily from external sources, Tiffany required far greater in-house development to become a successful nurse manager. At a minimum, management classes and good mentoring would have provided Tiffany with some necessary initial support for her to face the challenges she encountered in her new position. In her organization, Tiffany's development needs were not identified, so she floundered and failed, carrying negative views of leadership with her to future jobs. Most likely, the harm done to her as a potential leader will need to be "unlearned" before she can develop leadership capabilities later in her career.

The 18 emotional competencies that constitute emotionally intelligent leadership are summarized in Exhibit 2-5. In the upper left cell are the competencies of *self-awareness*: emotional self-awareness, accurate self-assessment, and self-confidence. They are the foundation for effective leadership. Self-awareness gives an individual a constant internal monitoring system. It reports feelings and reactions to experiences in the present but also includes knowing and anticipating situations in which one is apt to feel stress, joy, anger, insecurity, defensiveness, impatience, etc. Self-awareness is a prerequisite for the social competency of empathy. The individual who is emotionally self-aware or has accurate self-assessment knows his or her strengths and weaknesses and is comfortable "owning" them around other people. Comfort with one's own capabilities, values, and skills—both those that are strong and those that are limited—leads to self-confidence and the potential for behavioral integrity. The self-confident leader uses these competencies to support his or her self-assurance, self-efficacy, and often the courage to voice unpopular views in the workplace. Any leader in today's health care settings needs to have some toughness to survive; self-confidence is a core component of a good survival strategy.

The capacity for good *self-management*, shown in the lower left cell, includes the emotional competencies of emotional self-control, transparency, adaptability, the drive to achieve, initiative, and optimism. Emotional self-control prevents us from being hijacked by our feelings, but it does not imply that the expression of all emotions at work is undesirable. There are many experiences in the workplace that call for the appropriate expression of feelings, such as events that stimulate anger, sadness, frustration, humor, or happiness. The key to self-control is that the individual is aware of his or her feelings and makes a choice as to whether to express them or keep them submerged. Thus a nurse might choose to let a manager know when he is frustrated with an ongoing lack of supplies to care for patients but decide not to express

EXHIBIT 2-5

Emotional Competencies Constituting Emotionally Intelligent Leadership[9]

PERSONAL COMPETENCE

Self-Awareness

One's "inner barometer," rudder

Emotional Self-Awareness*

A fundamental & essential emotional competence

Recognizing your own emotions and their effects

Knowing where your "buttons" are

Accurate Self-Assessment*

Knowing your strengths & weaknesses

Seeking out & "taking in" feedback from others

Self-Confidence*

Sense of self-worth & capabilities that can sustain you during failures & defeats; having "presence"

Self-Management

Enables one to resist the tyranny of emerging moods

Emotional Self-Control*

Being unfazed in stressful situations; influenced by biochemistry & neurologic system

Transparency

Trustworthiness, credibility, accountability for self; others can count on you. High integrity: acting consistently with your own values

Adaptability

Ability to let go of previous ways of doing things, willingness to try new ways

Achievement Orientation

A drive to accomplish goals, stretch for high performance; sets apart high achievers

Core for entrepreneurs

Initiative

Motivation; seeking out new ideas & methods; taking responsibility; readiness to act

Optimism

Persisting despite obstacles & setbacks; not fearing failure

SOCIAL COMPETENCE

Social Awareness

One's "social radar"

Empathy*

Sensing others' feelings, needs, concerns & perspectives, and taking an active interest

Organizational Awareness

Reading a group's emotional/political currents & power relationships, and acting on this awareness

Service Orientation

Anticipating, recognizing, & meeting customers' needs, and the motivation to do so

Relationship Management

Enables one to act in the interests of others without tripping over his or her own ego

Developing Others

Sensing others' development needs & bolstering the development of others' abilities

Giving timely feedback

Inspirational Leadership

Having vision; inspiring & guiding; communicating often & effectively

Change Catalyst

Recognizing the need for change; removing barriers; communicating widely; modeling

Influence

Winning people over; indirectly building consensus & support; orchestrating effective tactics of persuasion; good communication

Fine-tuning presentations/appeals to fit the audience

Conflict Management

Understanding all perspectives & negotiating with these in mind; does not mean suppressing conflict

Teamwork & Collaboration

Working toward shared goals using individual strengths & group synergy; nurturing relationships, building esprit de corps, sharing credit lavishly

Includes managing meetings well

*Core competencies

indignation when a coworker makes a mistake with a patient, as the latter case may be more constructively dealt with through rational discussion.

The rules for emotional expression or emotional control vary greatly across ethnic groups, cultures, national origins, social class, organizations, and other contexts. Some organizations enable both staff and leaders to be frank and open in the expression of feelings, while others maintain codes of formality that tend to limit the sharing of feelings. Leaders need to understand the norms of their own workplaces and use these to guide how they manage their own feelings and those of others.

Transparency—being honest, open, trustworthy, and authentic—is the competency that most expresses an individual's integrity. Transparent leaders can be depended upon and trusted. They model ethical behavior. When pressured to do something they believe to be wrong, transparent leaders will demonstrate courage by standing up against it, even when taking a stand may be personally risky. Almost everyone would like to have a transparent leader because he or she will engender trust. Such leaders live and model the behaviors they expect of others,[10] in the process enabling others to act with integrity. Trust in a leader gives rise to positive emotions in employees, and positive emotions are what attach people to their work.

The emotional competency of adaptability enables leaders to be flexible in changing situations or in overcoming obstacles to getting work done. It provides for emotional resiliency in the face of multiple demands, complex or ambiguous situations, shifting priorities, and painful realities. Though people who lack adaptability may be ruled by anxieties and fears about change, it is also true that an adaptive response to every challenge is not always desirable. There are values and principles to which leaders should adhere, and too much flexibility on these may be the wrong choice. Examples include nurse executives who hold to a floor of safe staffing, rather than agree to cut budgets that could result in dangerously low nurse-to-patient ratios; an agency director who rejects requests for special treatment for family members of local politicians; or the medical department head who refuses gifts to his department offered by pharmaceutical representatives in exchange for promotion of specific brand-name drugs. Because health care organizations are complex, fast-moving, and concerned with the health of human beings, adaptability is important for any nurse leader, but equally important is knowing those areas in which existing practices should be maintained.

The ability to harness internal motivation, the readiness to take responsibility and to persist, and the drive to stretch for high performance, take risks, and accomplish goals typify leaders high in achievement orientation and initiative. High achievers are inwardly directed, holding challenging standards for themselves. They are proactive, love to learn, seek challenges, and are willing to bend rules. In the business world, entrepreneurs tend to have these characteristics to an extreme degree, although they often lack some of the other important leadership competencies associated with social awareness and relationship management. In health care, high achievers/initiators operate in a constant state of readiness. They are frequently results-oriented and focus on performance improvements by mobilizing themselves and others.

People at work take their emotional cues from their leader(s). Because positive or negative emotions from a leader powerfully penetrate the work climate, the presence of the former is clearly preferable to the latter. An optimistic leader is one who carries a "can do" attitude and who persists despite obstacles and setbacks. Optimism enables a leader and his or her employees to learn from mistakes and move forward. He or she is a carrier of hope.

Displayed in the upper right cell of Exhibit 2-5 are the competencies of *social awareness*: empathy, organizational awareness, and service orientation. As a core competency, empathy provides the foundation for the remaining two competencies in this cell as well as the ability to manage relationships (as shown in the lower right cell). Empathy is the "sine qua non of all social effectiveness in working life,"[11] a critical competency for working with a diverse group of people and those from different cultures. Every organization has an invisible nervous system of connection and influence.[12] Political astuteness, a part of the competency of organizational awareness, derives from being attuned to individuals, groups, and organizational power dynamics; detecting social networks and unspoken rules; and knowing how to use other people and processes to advance one's own interests. For middle managers, awareness of politics needs to include those above and below them. The politically aware leader tends to have an organizational, as opposed to subunit or departmental, perspective. Even for empathetic leaders, this perspective may be the most difficult of emotional competencies to learn. As an educator, I have found that the competency of organizational awareness is best learned by my graduate students through mentoring experiences with politically gifted leaders.

Service orientation, whether customers are patients or members of other departments, draws on the ability of the leader to grasp the customer's perspective and to create systems responsive to that perspective. He or she seeks ways to increase satisfaction and loyalty.[13]

The lower right cluster of Exhibit 2-5 lists the emotional competencies of *relationship management*: development of others, inspirational leadership, change catalyst, influence, conflict management, and teamwork

EXHIBIT 2-6
The Remote Nursing Agency Director

Victoria was the director of nursing for a large, multidisciplinary home health agency serving 12 acute care hospitals in a multicounty region. Her boss, the chief operating officer (COO), was a physician who worked offsite because of numerous other responsibilities with one of the medical centers. Victoria saw the COO about 1–2 times per month; otherwise, they communicated by telephone, e-mail, and fax. The COO was erratic in his oversight of the agency. Most of the time he let it "run itself," but at other times he would arrive unannounced and demand data and financial reports all at once, often grilling the directors about what he found. Victoria and the other directors of the agency didn't like the COO's style, but they were content because, most days, he didn't meddle with them. While not yielding much profit, the agency nonetheless covered its costs, had reasonable patient and family satisfaction scores, and continued to have a steady flow of referrals.

As time went on, Victoria focused on her staff nurses and team leaders, patient care needs, interdisciplinary coordination, and referring hospitals. She attended to accreditation preparedness and compiled required reports in collaboration with her codirectors. Staff at the agency were reasonably content, although scheduling and salary complaints never seemed to go away. E-mails and faxes from the COO came frequently but were primarily concerned with issues of regulation, quality developments in health care, and cost-saving ideas. Victoria responded to these when she had something to share back with the COO, but mostly she filed or saved his communications for future reference. He knew little about home nursing care, and was not much of a team player when he interacted with others, so she tended to avoid discussions with him when possible.

After 18 months in her position, Victoria came in on a Friday morning to find the COO and the director of human resources waiting for her. They took her into the conference room, where the COO informed her that she was being relieved of her duties. He had completed a performance review about her which stated that he had found her resistant to direction, aloof, unwilling to innovate, and stuck in a "narrow nursing frame of mind." He indicated he had lost confidence in her. Shocked, Victoria responded as calmly as she could manage, noting that the agency's referrals, nursing statistics, cost per visit, patient satisfaction, profitability, turnover rates, and staff satisfaction ratings were all as good as, if not better than, those of similarly-sized home health agencies. Since her departmental outcome measures were better than acceptable, how could he justify firing her? He told her the nursing department needed a change of leadership, so that's what he was doing. He then gestured to the director of human resources, who had said nothing to this point, and indicated that she and the director could work out her termination arrangements. Following their meeting, the director walked Victoria to her office for her personal items and then to her car, collecting the agency's keys before she indicated that Victoria should leave and not return to the premises.

and collaboration. These too are built on a foundation of the core competencies of emotional self-awareness, accurate self-assessment, self-control, self-confidence, and empathy.

Healthy organizations cultivate formal and informal leadership throughout the system by developing leaders. Nurse executives, for example, play a pivotal role in the development of nurse managers.[14] In performance-oriented cultures, all staff are considered worthy of development. This can be informally addressed through coaching and feedback—giving accurate, specific, timely, descriptive feedback that the receiver can use effectively and from which he or she can grow.[15] Such cultures disparage the singular use of "overly nice" feedback that excludes critical, but important, appraisal information.

To guide others, leaders must first have a clear sense of their own direction, values, and priorities. Inspiring leaders rely on core values to orient decisions; they are intentional and authentic,[16] leading by example, whether supporting people through day-to-day work challenges or episodes of difficult change. They value and nurture the relationship between leader and followers,[17] typically creating an empowered staff. Honest, authentic, frequent two-way communication[18] enables trust development and is the hallmark of the inspirational leader. It is an "emotional craft".[19] Some research has found that the intent of staff nurses to leave is negatively correlated with their leader's transformational leadership style[20]—that is, transformational leadership contributes to nurse retention.

Any leader in health care is a change agent: it comes with the job. Most health care leaders essentially lead change all the time. No longer is most change "planned"; it usually originates outside of health care organizations in the form of government regulations, alterations in reimbursement, technological innovation, shifts in the economy and demographics, and so on. More often than not, we respond to changes beyond our control. All changes in organizations evoke some resistance. The best change agents do not give ultimatums; they use the competencies of self-awareness and self-management, as well as empathy, politicking, influence, visionary leadership, conflict management, and teamwork and collaboration, to engage employees and lead successful change efforts. Because changes are always occurring, the skills and abilities of change management need to be fully integrated into the daily practices of managers.

The desire to exert influence can be directed at individuals or groups. Skills in influencing others in the workplace are not routinely taught in nursing school, nor do staff nurses typically learn to be influential through their work except in the area of patient care. Influence skills are built on self-awareness and empathy—being in touch with your own agenda and sensing how others are likely to respond, then fine-tuning your appeal to engage others. Nurses use these skills frequently to influence the medical and administrative staffs. The persuasive leader intentionally uses his emotions and body language to affect the emotions of others. This requires good communication skills,[21] a collaborative stance, trust, and both direct and indirect methods of influencing others. Indirect methods may be especially useful, as when one builds support for an idea before presenting it to the intended audience.

Managing conflict in organizations can include such actions as intervening in interpersonal or group frictions, confronting one's boss, addressing interdepartmental conflicts, facilitating a restructuring, and bargaining with labor unions.[22] Facility in handling difficult people and tense situations constructively is not a widely distributed skill in American society. It is one of the most demanding of emotional intelligence competencies, requiring all of the competencies of self-awareness and self-management, as well as empathy, organizational awareness, the ability to develop others and exert influence, and collaboration. Although organizations rife with conflict are unhealthy work environments, it is often the organization in which differences are suppressed and conflicting views are disallowed that is the most dysfunctional. Differences of opinion and the emotions that accompany them can become toxic if not addressed. In most cases, conflicting views can be expressed, acknowledged, and addressed in positive ways. Part of Victoria's difficulty in Exhibit 2-6 was that she never surfaced and addressed differences in perspectives between the COO and herself. A politically savvy leader often anticipates where and when conflicts are likely to surface and prepares to address them. The insightful use of varying viewpoints can enable the leader to channel strong feelings into problem solving and creative solutions.

Across all types of industries, teamwork is one of the most consistently valued attributes of managers. Teamwork and collaboration are related to the emotional intelligence of groups[23] and are the means by which virtually all work is accomplished in health care organizations. Collaborative styles typically reflect an equal focus on task accomplishment and concern for relationships. Individuals able to function effectively as team players do so as a result of emotional intelligence, especially the competencies associated with self-awareness and self-management, plus empathy and service orientation. Cognitive intelligence, technical expertise, or ambition alone do not make people collaborative. Well-functioning teams consistently outperform the collective contributions of skilled individuals as a result of the synergy of "social intelligence." Combined talents and knowledge on a team interactively and unpredictably catalyze the best in everyone, leveraging the full capabilities of the team members.[24] Thus leaders who are good team builders and facilitators (i.e., running meetings well, building *esprit de corps* greatly enhance work performance while generating an atmosphere of friendly collegiality. Group cohesion has been found to be partially predictive of nurse job satisfaction,[25] as has nurse/physician collaboration.[26]

It is important to note that all forms of interactions at work need to be considered relevant to emotionally intelligent behaviors. This means that e-mails, faxes, voice mails, and written memos or reports are subject to the same sensitivities that the emotional competencies address. An example of this is using empathy when sending an e-mail or writing a memo; the emotionally intelligent sender is aware of what the recipient knows and thinks before framing the message. Often providing a sentence or two of background before stating a message or stating at the outset what the sender wants from the receiver helps the message reach the receiver. For example, as a nurse educator, it is not unusual for me to get e-mails from my undergraduate students that contain no signature at the end of the message. If I don't recognize the e-mail address, I often have no idea who sent me the message. In these cases, clearly the student is focused entirely on his or her needs and not thinking about my ability to receive the message.

No leaders, good or bad, have equal strengths (or equal weaknesses) in all of the 18 emotional competencies. Leaders and managers have their own unique constellations of the components of emotional intelligence.

Best and Worst Bosses

In training individuals in emotional intelligence, I have worked with health care professionals from many different organizations. I have often asked people to list the characteristics of their "best" and "worst" bosses, and I have found that the results of this exercise are very consistent across settings. People tend to list variations of the behaviors shown in Exhibit 2-7.

Note that the characteristics of best and worst bosses tend to be opposites of each other: creative vs rigid, gives credit vs takes credit, shares information vs withholds information, advocates vs sells out, etc. What people report seeing and valuing in a best boss includes the competencies associated with emotionally intelligent leadership.

Although we know that knowledge, skills, and capabilities in addition to those characteristics listed in

EXHIBIT 2-7
Characteristics of My "Best" and "Worst" Boss

"BEST" BOSSES	"WORST" BOSSES
Understands my strengths and weaknesses	Poor listener
Always has an open-door policy	Micro-manager
Is available and accessible	Is too busy to help me
Is genuinely interested in others	Gives orders and expects them to be carried out without question
Works with me on difficult projects	Gives negative feedback but rarely says anything positive
Has a good sense of humor	Gets angry easily; tends to "shoot the messenger"
Admits to her own mistakes; open to feedback	Has no insight into himself
Expects effort and conscientiousness but not perfection	Gives unclear instructions and then blames others when it's done wrong
Willing to change plans based on input from me and others in my workgroup	Doesn't want to know my opinion
Gives an assignment and then lets us do it; doesn't meddle	Prefers to fire off e-mails rather than sit down & talk
Is positive and upbeat	Incompetent; can't acknowledge own weaknesses; is insecure
Often brings in bagels or fruit for us	Wants to look good to her boss at all costs
Is quick to give credit to others for good work	Is unavailable, inaccessible, never "around"
Takes a lot of stress from upper management but never brings it back to us	Is often in a bad mood
Always has our department's best interests at heart	Lazy; I have absolutely no idea what he does all day
Really cares about how our patients are treated	Is unethical
Will "handle" anyone who is abusive to one of us on the unit; won't back down or let us down	Will lie or misrepresent things rather than admit she made a mistake
Works harder than anyone else	Takes credit for the work that others do
Has high standards, sticks to her values	Is clueless about our feelings about things
"Walks the talk"	Can't deal with conflict, so he avoids it
Understands the "big picture;" is visionary	Seems unhappy with her home life, and brings a lot of that into work
Always looks for new and better ways to do things; is open	Changes direction all the time
Knows a lot about what's going on in other organizations like ours and brings new ideas back to us	Is rigid & defensive
Treats everyone fairly and equally	Is cold & distant
Gives feedback—all kinds—frequently; is collaborative	Holds grudges
Encourages us to have different points of view and to express them; helps us find resolutions	Doesn't advocate for us at higher levels or with other departments; "sells out"
Will sit down with two people who are not working well together and get them to work it out	Doesn't tell me how she thinks I'm doing until I get slammed in my annual performance evaluation (which is usually months late)
Shares information; is upfront with us when something can't be changed	Listens to gossip (and selectively believes it)
Encourages us to come up with our own solutions to problems; will intervene if we're stuck	Has "favorites" (who get special treatment)
Is creative; willing to take risks	Is not a team player
Is very well liked and respected by people in other departments	Doesn't deal well with office politics
Makes us want to follow him	Doesn't address important issues, even when they go on for months or years
	Talks all the way through meetings without letting anyone else say anything
	Doesn't want to change anything—or the opposite: makes changes willy-nilly without thought
	Poor/no communication
	Has no vision, no charisma

Exhibit 2-7 are necessary for good leadership and management (for example, the ability to secure and distribute resources for work tasks, or the use of sound staffing and scheduling principles), it is noteworthy that *how others evaluate their leaders rests disproportionately on the followers' perceived relationships with those leaders*. This strikingly illustrates the basis for the importance of emotionally competent leaders.[27] Since nursing in all its forms is a people-oriented business, top-performing nursing work groups are powered by their leaders' abilities to manage themselves and work well with others.

Research and Professional Support for Emotionally Intelligent Nursing Leadership

The American Organization of Nurse Executives (AONE) sets research and education priorities that address critical issues facing the profession.[28] AONE, which represents the perspective of nursing leaders across the United States, consistently calls for professional leadership and leadership development at all levels of nursing activity. Strong, effective executive leaders in nursing can be scarce commodities, but even where they exist, their organizations frequently have inconsistent leadership strength throughout the ranks.

The American Nurses Association (ANA) publishes a booklet outlining the scope and standards for nurse administrators[29] that includes nurse executive and nurse manager levels. Both levels of nursing leadership call for knowledge and qualifications that, in part, fall within the domain of the emotional competencies framework: customer service; ethical conduct; effectiveness in communication; developing and fostering relationships; negotiation and conflict resolution abilities; organizational behavior and development; performance appraisal and improvement; strategic visioning; advocacy for patients and staff; collaboration with other disciplines and leaders; leadership in human resources management and development; facilitation of continuous quality improvement; change agentry; innovation; accountability; empowerment of staff and nurse participation in decision making; maintenance of a healthy climate and culture; competence with diversity; supervision; recruitment, selection, and retention of staff; self-assessment and openness to constructive feedback; and transmission of values. The standards reflect the values and priorities of the profession, direct the leadership of professional nursing practice, and identify areas in which nurse leaders are accountable to the public.

A growing research base documents the relationship between nursing, environments of care, staffing ratios, and nurse education levels and patient outcomes.[30] Most of this research focuses on hospital nursing and appears in journals such as *Health Affairs*; the *Journal of Nursing Administration*; *Nursing Economics*; and *Policy, Politics, & Nursing Practice* as well as in specialty nursing journals. Additionally, national foundations, such as the Robert Wood Johnson Foundation, and government agencies, such as the Agency for Healthcare Research and Quality (AHRQ) (part of the US Department of Health and Human Services), periodically issue reports on patient safety and outcomes research they have funded.[31] The documented importance of nursing to quality care is evident throughout these studies and with it, the necessity for effective nursing leadership at all levels of health care organizations.

Several areas of need for emotionally intelligent nursing leadership are especially prominent in the research literature: recruiting and retaining qualified staff, and limiting stress, transfer, grievance, turnover attrition, and nurses leaving the profession;[32] promoting positive work climates;[33] promoting nurse participation in decision making and enhancing power and control;[34] improving nurse recognition, advancement opportunities and life long learning;[35] enhancing management responsiveness to and communication with nurses; and providing better administrative support for nursing activities.[36] These areas of need are especially critical because of the shortage of nurses nationwide, the costs of turnover (replacement costs for a RN are estimated to average $42,000–64,000[37]), and the disruptions in organizational effectiveness and patient care quality associated with unstable staffing.

In spite of the common practice of promoting non-management-prepared staff nurses into charge and leadership positions, the need for well-prepared managers is well established in the nursing literature.[38] Nurse leaders make a significant difference in how nurses perceive and perform in their jobs. Repeatedly, effective behaviors and practices of nurse leaders have been found to influence work environments in innumerable ways, resulting in greater levels of staff nurse job satisfaction and organizational commitment. Exceptional nurse executive leadership will, with the proper infrastructural support,[39] positively influence the entire climate of nursing work in an organization. And because nurse middle managers can "make or break" the care delivery process, there is growing evidence that well-run nursing units provide higher levels of care quality.

Nurse executives in any health care setting establish standards, provide resources, buffer staff nurses from the effects of ongoing uncertainties in the health care industry, lead with high expectations, and negotiate with other professional groups for control over nursing practice. Additionally, top-level emotionally intelligent nursing leadership is necessary to support the effective selection and development of nurse middle managers. In

EXHIBIT 2-8
Emotional Intelligence at Work

For nearly 30 years, until the managed care decade of the 1990s,

> the Beth Israel (BI) Hospital in Boston served as an icon for the empowerment of nursing. With its chief nurse executive Joyce Clifford working in a unique partnership with CEO physician Mitchell Rabkin, the BI helped to pioneer an innovative model of nursing care. . . . The hospital . . . employed an almost all registered nurse staff, hired only RNs with bachelor's degrees, and was committed to enhancing the collaboration between nurses and physicians and giving nurses a greater voice in their institution. . . . [T]hose nurses received institutional support from the highest levels. . . . [N]ursing care does not depend on the personal kindness or the moral virtuousness of the nurse. Instead it depends on education and experience and on the institutional support that nurses receive from the hospital in which they are employed. . . . Nurses there [at BI] were among the most satisfied in the nation.[40]

Historically, Beth Israel had been one of the best hospitals in the world in which to practice as a nurse. Organizational features that both enhanced nurses' work satisfaction and improved patient outcomes included support for nurses' stature and representation in the hospital, control over the resources required to perform their work, autonomy in decisions about how to care for their patients, and teamwork and collegiality with physicians.[41] This did not happen by chance—all of its great accomplishments were voluntary creations constructed over years[42] by the collaborative relationship between the CEO and CNO.

I interviewed Dr. Rabkin in 1992 as part of Beth Israel's participation in the program *Strengthening Hospital Nursing*, a national initiative funded by the Robert Wood Johnson Foundation and the Pew Charitable Trusts. His support for nursing and nurses was both seriously and humorously relayed through the following comments:

> There are very few places, I think, where other than by some dictatorial policy, nursing is deemed to be co-equal with medicine, surgery, etc. My argument is that nursing is a clinical service just like medicine and surgery, OB/GYN, and so on. . . . Hospitals—not this place alone—are *nursing institutions* primarily, not doctoring institutions. Now if you don't have a truly professional nursing service, [empowering nurses] is not going to work. You need two things: one, you need nurses who are *smart*, because doctors don't tolerate people as colleagues who are not as smart as they are. You need to have smart nurses. The other thing is that they have to be true colleagues, and that comes about not only in nurses' education but also with their image of themselves, the capacity to understand what nursing really is, and I see that here [at Beth Israel].
>
> In fact, there was a marvelous incident a number of years ago, with a head nurse who couldn't have weighed more than 90 pounds, and this was with a new resident on the orthopaedic service; these kids [residents] rotate through all of the Harvard hospitals. This one had spent some 6 months at [another hospital], and literally within 30 minutes of his arrival at BI, he had some floor nurse in tears. The head nurse manager asked him to come into her office, and she said to him, 'You're new here, you've been [at the other hospital] for 6 months, and I've got to tell you that the way we do things around here is rather different, and what you've done is completely unacceptable. *This* is the way we work here [and she went on to explain the co-equal role of nurses at BI]. This is your first day and I realize it and we're certainly going to give you time to learn.' Then this pipsqueak put her finger on this guy's chest—he's about 6′2″—and she said, 'If you do *not* learn, we will send you back to the minor leagues where you came from.' The guy got beet red, stormed out, and then went to see the senior orthopaedic surgeon, who said, 'Well, maybe you've got something to learn.' About 3 or 4 days later he came back and asked to speak to the head nurse in private. 'I have to apologize,' he said, 'I had no idea that nurses were so good and so confident, and so capable, I really had no idea at all.' So they [new residents] learn. They also learn from role modeling by the other physicians. It's not only the nurses standing up for themselves; the nurses know that the administration backs them up.[43]

Rabkin's story suggests many aspects of the BI culture that support nursing practice, but it also illustrates an EI characteristic of "best bosses"—"handling" anyone who is abusive to nurses.

turn, nurse executives need support from their executive colleagues in order to create work environments that enable professional practice by nurses. Nationally, the strongest nursing organizations have tended to be those in which the chief executive officer (CEO) understands and values nursing and "gets it" in regard to what is needed to maintain a strong base of nursing practice. He or she trusts and grants full authority to the nurse executive to run the nursing operation (see Exhibit 2-8).

How to Develop Your Emotional Competencies

All emotional competencies can be learned and developed. The core competencies—emotional self-awareness, accurate self-assessment, self-confidence, emotional self-control, and empathy—are the most important because they are fundamental. A leader deficient in the core competencies will encounter difficulty mastering any of the remaining 13 competencies. In Exhibit 2-6, Victoria appears to have the competencies associated with self-awareness and self-management. She knows that she doesn't like the COO and his leadership style, is able to maintain self-control in his presence, and is confident of her abilities to run the nursing component of the home health agency. Her crucial mistake, however, is her lack of empathy for the COO. She didn't really know what motivated him or what was important to him, nor did she have any idea how he might be viewing her performance. It is likely that the COO, though not often present, had expectations that his direct reports would demonstrate attention and responsiveness to his communications, regardless of how important (or irrelevant) his direct reports felt those communications were. When Victoria ignored or deflected a good number of his e-mails and faxes, the COO probably found her behavior disrespectful, perhaps even offensive. As a result, he interpreted her behavior as resistant, aloof, and not innovative. Had Victoria been more aware of the COO's expectations and what his unique leadership behaviors meant to *him*, she could have been more astute in managing the politics between her and her boss. The competency of organizational awareness, which concerns one's political savvy at work, cannot be developed without first having the ability to empathize with the needs and feelings of other individuals and groups. Victoria used her own frame of reference to determine what was important in her job, giving little thought to what her COO viewed as important. She also let his relatively infrequent appearances onsite lull her into a false sense of security.

Developing emotional competencies first requires an awareness of areas of strength and weakness, and then an identification of what ideal behavior would be in a targeted area of weakness (see Exhibit 2-9). The individual needs to assess honestly his or her motivation to change and willingness to practice new behaviors. From a feasibility standpoint, it is important to focus changes on just one or two competencies.

Behavior change is most effective when it connects to activities in the individual's work life that are most in need of and likely to show improvements. Many young

EXHIBIT 2-9

Steps to Developing Emotional Competencies[44]

1. Determine your behavioral goals.
   - Ground them in your assessment of your emotional strengths and weakness, and use feedback from others who know you well. Make sure you understand the gaps between your actual and your preferred "ideal" behavior.
   - Build on and engage your strengths.
   - Develop clear, manageable goals; have them reflect your personal vision for self-development.
   - Pick no more than one or two areas (competencies) at a time. Determine whether your plans for self-directed change will fit smoothly into your life: are there day-to-day events that can be used as a learning laboratory?
   - Honestly assess your commitment to working on self-development.
2. Create a plan to reach your behavioral goals.
   - Select a coach and establish a verbal contract.
   - Identify and agree on the developmental priorities and behavioral indicators.
   - Identify how behavioral development will facilitate your career goals.
   - Identify opportunities for trials and action, using ways that fit your learning style.
   - Identify times and places for the coach (and any others you choose to involve) to observe you and provide feedback.
   - Identify role models you would like to emulate.
   - Understand that self-development will take time and sustained focus. It doesn't happen overnight!
3. Monitor your progress regularly.
   - Practice, practice, practice; use work and outside settings.
   - Tune in to behaviors you need to *unlearn* in order to learn new ones.
   - Meet and talk with your coach. Ask questions to help clarify issues.
   - Seek feedback from others as possible.
   - Identify in which situations it is easier or harder for you to improve.
   - Don't "slip" in other strength areas of emotional competency while you are focused on development in new areas; avoid relapses.
   - Do reading and thinking on your own behavior and developmental goals.
   - Keep a written record of thoughts, feedback, insights, difficulties, and successes.
   - Assess your continued commitment.
4. Celebrate successes.
   - Give yourself credit for evidence of developmental improvements; reinforce your growth.
   - Seek ways to further sharpen your developmental progress.
   - Assess your continued commitment to behavior change.

and inexperienced nurses, for example, are uncomfortable approaching physicians with recommendations for changes in patient management. Reticence with physicians can be a good starting point for behavior change: more self-assertion leads to high payoffs for both the nurse and his or her patients. Self-development in such a situation might focus on self-awareness (exactly what is the staff nurse afraid of?) and self-confidence (with a peer, practice strategies for managing the conversation). Nurse managers who are uncomfortable standing up and addressing groups might choose to work on empathy (anticipate what the members of the group might be thinking and feeling) and self-confidence (plan the presentation thoroughly, rehearse with a peer, and actively seek responses from the group members during the presentation). Even minor successes in self-directed behavior change can be highly motivating for continuing development efforts.

Change in behaviors driven by emotional habits requires that, as we practice new behaviors, we actively seek to *unlearn* the old behaviors. The old behaviors become a source of resistance and backsliding unless they are identified, acknowledged, and actively transformed. This kind of change depends on the ability to engage one's own emotions in order to change them. For example, use self-awareness to monitor how you are reacting emotionally to giving up an old habit (avoiding conflict, for example) while trying a new one (asking conflicting parties to express their differences).

The engagement of an emotionally competent coach, mentor, or friend to aid self-development efforts is essential. We cannot change what we do not see or know, so external observation and feedback provides indispensable data. A coach will also enable the individual to learn by talking over the situation, exploring alternatives, and reflecting on behavioral options. Importantly, the coach can also function as a motivator, encouraging and holding the person accountable for his or her self-development plan.

Behavior change requires practice, typically sustained over weeks and months—often up to six months—to develop a new competency. With extended practice, reflection, reinforcement, and success, mastery is possible. Supplementary activities can facilitate behavior change: reading and studying about leadership or emotional intelligence, self-reflection (journals, discussion, reflective learning groups),[45] experiential learning exercises,[46] and measurement feedback.[47] Like athletic performance, proficiency development requires ongoing cycles of practice-trial-feedback and correction.

Finally, even without intentional behavior change, there is evidence that human beings intuitively develop emotional competencies with age and experience.[48]

Summary

Throughout life, we observe leaders and learn about what makes them good. A complex phenomenon, leadership occurs in all work settings and is enacted through countless individual behaviors. In this chapter, I have focused on those aspects of leadership that involve relationships between leaders and other people—the "people" skills of leaders. Using a framework of emotional intelligence, I address the relevance of 18 emotional competencies to the successful intra- and interpersonal work lives of nurse leaders. Evidence is presented that emotionally competent organizational leadership raises the level of performance for everyone and enhances the patient experience.

NOTES

1. Safire & Safire, 1982.
2. See, for example: Shipper, Rotondo, and Hoffman, IV, 2003; Rahim and Psenicka, 2002.
3. D. Goleman, 1995; D. Goleman, 1998a; and Goleman, Boyatzis, and McKee, 2002.
4. The Hay Group, 2004.
5. Duchscher, 2001.
6. Vitellow-Cicciu, 2002.
7. Goleman, 1995, 1998a; Goleman et al., 2002; The Hay Group, 2004.
8. Wellins & Weaver Jr., 2003.
9. Goleman, 1995, 1998a; D. Goleman et al., 2002; The Hay Group, 2004.
10. Dickenson-Hazard, 2004.
11. D. Goleman et al., 2002, p. 50.
12. D. Goleman, 1998a, p. 160.
13. D. Goleman, 1998a.
14. Corning, 2002.
15. See, for example, Michaelsen & Schultheiss, 1988–1989.
16. Dickenson-Hazard, 2004.
17. Institute of Medicine & Page, 2003.
18. Woolf, 2001.
19. D. Goleman, 1998a, p. 197.
20. Larrabee, et al., 2003; Laschinger, Almost, and Tuer-Hodes, 2003.
21. R. Woolf, 2001; O'Connor, 2001.
22. Forman & Grimes, 2002.
23. Druskat & Wolff, 2001; Rapisarda, 2002.
24. Goleman, 1998a; p. 205; Druskat & Wolff, 2001.
25. Larrabee et al., 2003.
26. Boyle & Kochinda, 2004.
27. Goleman, 1998b.
28. American Organization of Nurse Executives (AONE), 2002; Ritter-Teitel, 2003.
29. American Nurses Association (ANA), 2004.
30. See, for example: Aiken, Clarke, Sloane, Sochalski, and Silber, 2002; Aiken, et al., 2001; Aiken, Smith, and Lake, 1994; Benner, Sheets, Uris, Mallock, Schwed, and Jamison, 2002; Blegen, Vaughn, and Goode, 2001; Blegen, Goode, and Reed, 1998; Institute of Medicine & Page, 2003; Mullan, 2001.
31. See, for example, the AHRQ-funded study by Kaissi, Johnson, and Kirschbaum, 2003.

32. Nurse job satisfaction and retention: Beecroft, Kunzman, Taylor, Devenis, and Guzak, 2004; Brodeur & Laraway, 2002; Cowin, 2002; Duffield, Aitken, O'Brien-Pallas, and Wise, 2004; Foley, Kee, Minick, Harvey, and Jennings, 2002; Goode & Williams, 2004; Holtom & O'Neill, 2004; HSM Group, Ltd., 2002; Ingersoll, Olsan, Drew-Cates, DeVinney, and Davies, 2002; Irvine & Evans, 1995; Jeffries, 2002; Kalisch, 2003; Kalliath & Morris, 2002; Kleinman, 2004; Kupperschmidt, 1998; Letvak, 2002; Ma, Samuels, and Alexander, 2003; McKinnon, 2002; Manion, 2003; Mark, 2002; McNeese-Smith, 1995; Navaie-Waliser, Lincoln, Karuturi, and Reisch, 2004; Neuhauser, 2002; Nikolaou & Tsaousis, 2002; O'Brien-Pallas, Thomson, Alksnis, and Bruce, 2001; Ohio Nurses Association, 2004; Roberts, Jones, and Lynn, 2004; Robinson, Eck, Keck, and Wells, 2003; Sochalski, 2002; Sullivan, Kerr, and Ibrahim, 1999; Tzeng & Ketefian, 2002; Upenieks, 2002; Wagner & Huber, 2003.
33. Positive work climates: ANA, 2004; Garrett & McDaniel, 2001; Stevens, 2002; Watson, 2002.
34. Empowerment: Larrabee et al., 2003; Laschinger et al., 2003; Manojlovich & Laschinger, 2002.
35. Improving recognition, advancement, and lifelong learning: Carroll & Austin, 2004; Manion, 2003; O'Hara, Duvanich, Foss, and Wells, 2003; The Robert Wood Johnson Foundation, Kimball, and O'Neil, 2002; Robinson et al., 2003.
36. Management responsiveness to and communication with nurses, and improving administrative support for nursing activities: Aiken et al., 2001; Bingham, 2002; Buerhaus, Needleman, Mattke, and Stewart, 2002; Corning, 2002; Cathcart, et al., 2004; Dickenson-Hazard, 2004; Fletcher, 2001; Garrett & McDaniel, 2001; Institute of Medicine & Page, 2003; Kahn, 1993; Laschinger, 2004; MacPhee & Scott, 2002; McNeese-Smith & Crook, 2003; Snow, 2001.
37. Aiken, Clarke, Sloane, Sochalski, and Silber, 2002.
38. Selection and development of nurse managers/leaders: Corning, 2002; de Ruiter & Saphiere, 2001; Hill, 2003; Horton-Deutsch & Wellman, 2002; Kahn,1993; Kleinman, 2003; Krugman & Smith, 2003; McNeese-Smith, 1995; Neuhauser, 2002; Nierenberg, 2003; Noyes, 2002; Ritter-Teitel, 2003; The Robert Wood Johnson Foundation, Kimball, and O'Neil, 2002; Russell & Scoble, 2003; Smeltzer, 2002a; Smeltzer, 2002b; Snow, 2001; Sullivan, Bretschneider, and McCausland, 2003; Tourangeau, 2003; Upenieks, 2003; Upenieks, 2002a; Vitello-Cicciu, 2002; Watson, 2004; Wellins & Weaver Jr., 2003.
39. See, for example, Cooper, Frank, Gouty, and Hansen, 2002.
40. Weinberg, 2003, pp. ix–x.
41. Ibid, p. 13.
42. Ibid, pp. 2 & xii.
43. S. Taft, Interview with Mitchell Rabkin, personal communication, Boston, MA, July, 1992.
44. Based on research conducted by Goleman, 1995, 1998a; Goleman et al., 2002; The Hay Group, 2004.
45. Brewer & Cadman, 2000.
46. de Janasz, Dowd, and Schneider, 2002.
47. See, for example, the Emotional Competency Inventory, available at http://ei.haygroup.com/about_ei/ (Boston, 9/30/04).
48. Goleman, 1995, 1998a; Goleman et al., 2002; The Hay Group, 2004.

REFERENCES

Aiken, L.H., Clarke, S.P., Sloane, D.M., Sochalski, J., & Silber, J.H. (2002). Hospital nurse staffing and patient mortality, nurse burnout, and job dissatisfaction. *Journal of the American Medical Association, 288*, 1987–1993.

Aiken, L.H., Clarke, S.P., Sloane, D.M., Sochalski, J., Busse, R., Clarke, H., et al. (2001). Nurses' reports on hospital care in five countries. *Health Affairs, 20*(3), 43–53.

Aiken, L.H., Smith, H.L., & Lake, E.T. (1994). Lower medicare mortality among a set of hospitals known for good nursing care. *Medical Care, 32*(8), 771–787.

American Nurses Association. (2004). *Scope and Standards for Nurse Administrators* (2nd ed). Washington, DC: Author.

American Organization of Nurse Executives (AONE). (2002). AONE 2002 research and education priorities. *The Journal of Nursing Administration, 32*(5), 228.

Beecroft, P.C., Kunzman, L.A., Taylor, S., Devenis, E., & Guzak, F. (2004). Bridging the gap between school and workplace: Developing a new graduate nurse curriculum. *Journal of Nursing Administration, 34*(7/8), 338–345.

Benner, P., Sheets, V., Uris, P., Mallock, K., Schwed, K., & Jamison, D. (2002). Individual, practice, and system causes of errors in nursing. *Journal of Nursing Administration, 32*(10), 509–523.

Bingham, R. (2002). Leaving nursing. *Health Affairs, 21*(1), 211–217.

Blegen, M.A., Vaughn, T., & Goode, C. (2001). Nurse experience and education: Effect on quality of care. *Journal of Nursing Administration, 31*(1), 33–39.

Blegen, M.A., Goode, C.J., & Reed, L. (1998). Nurse staffing and patient outcomes. *Nursing Research, 47*, 43–50.

Boyle, D.K. & Kochinda, C. (2004). Enhancing collaborative communication of nurse and physician leadership in two intensive care units. *Journal of Nursing Administration, 34*(2), 60–70.

Brewer, J. & Cadman, C. (2000). Emotional intelligence: Enhancing student effectiveness and patient outcomes. *Nurse Educator, 25*(6), 264–266.

Brodeur, M.A. & Laraway, A.S. (2002). States respond to nursing shortage. *Policy, Politics, & Nursing Practice, 3*(2), 228–234.

Buerhaus, P.I., Needleman, J., Mattke, S., & Stewart, M. (2002). Strengthening hospital nursing. *Health Affairs, 21*(5), 123–132.

Carroll, T.L. & Austin, T. (2004). Career coaching: A hospital and a university link hands to retain nursing talent. *Reflections on Nursing Leadership, 30*(3), 30–31.

Cathcart, D., Jeska, S., Karnas, J., Miller, S.E., Pechacek, J., and Rheault, L. (2004). Span of control matters. *Journal of Nursing Administration, 34*(9), 395–399.

Cooper, R.W., Frank, G.L., Gouty, C.A., & Hansen, M.C. (2002). Key ethical issues encountered in healthcare organizations: Perceptions of nurse executives. *Journal of Nursing Administration, 32*(6), 331–337.

Corning, S.P. (2002). Profiling and developing nursing leaders. *Journal of Nursing Administration, 32*(7/8), 373–375.

Cowin, L. (2002). The effects of nurses' job satisfaction on retention: An Australian perspective. *Journal of Nursing Administration, 32*(5), 283–291.

de Janasz, S.C., Dowd, K.O., & Schneider, B.Z. (2002). *Interpersonal skills in organizations*. Boston: McGraw Hill.

de Ruiter, H-P & Saphiere, D.H. (2001). Nurse leaders as cultural bridges. *Journal of Nursing Administration, 31*(9), 418–423.

Dickenson-Hazard, N. (2004). Cultivating effective leadership skills for nurses: A commentary. *Policy, Politics, & Nursing Practice, 5*(3), 145–146.

Druskat, V.U. & Wolff, S.B. (2001). Building the emotional intelligence of groups. *Harvard Business Review, 79*(3), 81–90.

Duchscher, J. E. B. (2001). Out in the real world: Newly graduated nurses in acute-care speak out. *Journal of Nursing Administration, 31*(9), 426–439.

Duffield, C., Aitken, L., O'Brien-Pallas, L., & Wise, W.J. (2004). Nursing: A stepping stone to future careers. *Journal of Nursing Administration, 34*(5), 238–245.

Fletcher, C.E. (2001). Hospital RN's job satisfactions and dissatisfactions. *Journal of Nursing Administration, 31*(6), 324–331.

Foley, B.J., Kee, C.C., Minick, P., Harvey, S.S., & Jennings, B.M. (2002). Characteristics of nurses and hospital work environments that foster satisfaction and clinical expertise. *Journal of Nursing Administration, 32*(5), 273–282.

Forman, H. & Grimes, T.C. (2002). Living with a union contract. *Journal of Nursing Administration, 32*(12), 611–614.

Garrett, D.K. & McDaniel, A.M. (2001). A new look at nurse burnout: The effects of environmental uncertainty and social climate. *Journal of Nursing Administration, 31*(2), 91–96.

Goleman, D. (1998a). *Working with emotional intelligence*. New York: Bantam Books.

Goleman, D. (1998b). What makes a leader? *Harvard Business Review, 76*(6), 93–102.

Goleman, D. (1995). *Emotional Intelligence*. New York: Bantam Books.

Goleman, D., Boyatzis, R., & McKee, A. (2002). *Primal leadership: Realizing the power of emotional intelligence*. Boston: Harvard Business School Press.

Goode, C.J. & Williams, C.A. (2004). Post-Baccalaureate nurse residency program. *Journal of Nursing Administration, 34*(2), 71–77.

The Hay Group, (2004). *Emotional Intelligence Services*. Retrieved November 30, 2004, from http://ei.haygroup.com/about_ei/.

Hill, K.S. (2003). Development of leadership competencies as a team. *Journal of Nursing Administration, 33*(12), 639–642.

Holtom, B.C. & O'Neill, B.S. (2004). Job embeddedness: A theoretical foundation for developing a comprehensive nurse retention plan. *Journal of Nursing Administration, 34*(5), 216–227.

Horton-Deutsch, S.L. & Wellman, D.S. (2002). Christman's principles for effective management: Reflection and challenges for action. *Journal of Nursing Administration, 32*(11), 596–601.

HSM Group, Ltd. (2002). Acute care hospital survey of RN vacancy and turnover rates in 2000. *Journal of Nursing Administration, 32*(9), 437–439.

Ingersoll, G.L., Olsan, T., Drew-Cates, J., DeVinney, B.C., & Davies, J. (2002). Nurses' job satisfaction, organizational commitment, and career intent. *Journal of Nursing Administration, 32*(5), 250–263.

Institute of Medicine and Page, A. (2003). *Keeping patients safe: Transforming the work environment of nurses*. Washington, D.C.: The National Academies Press.

Irvine, D.M. & Evans, M.G. (1995). Job satisfaction and turnover among nurses: Integrating research findings across studies. *Nursing Research, 44*(4), 246–253.

Jeffries, E. (2002). Creating a great place to work: Strategies for retaining top talent. *Journal of Nursing Administration, 32*(6), 303–305.

Kahn, W.A. (1993). Caring for the caregivers: Patterns of organizational caregiving. *Administrative Science Quarterly, 38*, 539–563.

Kaissi, A., Johnson, T., & Kirschbaum, M.S. (2003). Measuring teamwork and patient safety attitudes of high-risk areas. *Nursing Economics, 21*(5), 211–218.

Kalisch, B.J. (2003). Recruiting nurses: The problem is the process. *Journal of Nursing Administration, 33*(9), 468–477.

Kalliath, T. & Morris, R. (2002). Job satisfaction among nurses: A predictor of burnout levels. *Journal of Nursing Administration, 32*(12), 648–654.

Kleinman, C.S. (2004). Workforce issues: Leadership strategies in reducing staff nurse role conflict. *Journal of Nursing Administration, 34*(7/8), 322–324.

Kleinman, C.S. (2003). Leadership roles, competencies, and education: How prepared are our nurse managers? *Journal of Nursing Administration, 33*(9), 451–455.

Krugman, M. & Smith, V. (2003). Charge nurse leadership development and education. *Journal of Nursing Administration, 33*(5), 284–292.

Kupperschmidt, B.R. (1998). Understanding Generation X employees. *Journal of Nursing Administration, 28*(12), 36–43.

Larrabee, J.H., Janney, M.A., Ostrow, C.L., Withrow, M.L., Hobbs, G.R., & Burant, C. (2003). Predicting registered nurse job satisfaction and intent to leave. *Journal of Nursing Administration, 33*(5), 271–283.

Laschinger, H.K.S. (2004). Hospital nurses' perceptions of respect and organizational justice. *Journal of Nursing Administration, 34*(7/8), 354–364.

Laschinger, H.K.S., Almost, J., & Tuer-Hodes, D. (2003). Workplace empowerment and magnet hospital characteristics. *Journal of Nursing Administration, 33*(7/8), 410–422.

Letvak, S. (2002). Retaining the older nurse. *Journal of Nursing Administration, 32*(7/8), 387–392.

Ma, C-C., Samuels, M.E., & Alexander, J.W. (2003). Factors that influence nurses' job satisfaction. *Journal of Nursing Administration, 33*(5), 300–306.

MacPhee, M. & Scott, J. (2002). The role of social support networks for rural hospital nurses. *Journal of Nursing Administration, 32*(5), 264–272.

Manion, J. (2003). Joy at work! Creating a positive workplace. *Journal of Nursing Administration, 33*(12), 652–659.

Manojlovich, M. & Laschinger, H.K.S. (2002). The relationship of empowerment and selected personality characteristics to nursing job satisfaction. *Journal of Nursing Administration, 32*(11), 586–595.

Mark, B.A. (2002). What explains nurses' perceptions of staffing adequacy? *Journal of Nursing Administration, 32*(5), 234–242.

McKinnon, C. (2002). You can do it too in 2002: Registry reduction. *Journal of Nursing Administration, 32*(10), 498–500.

McNeese-Smith, D. (1995). Job satisfaction, productivity, and organizational commitment: The result of leadership. *Journal of Nursing Administration, 25*(9), 17–26.

McNeese-Smith, D.K. & Crook, M. (2003). Nursing values and a changing nursing workforce. *Journal of Nursing Administration, 33*(5), 260–270.

Michaelsen, L.K. & Schultheiss, E.E. (1998–1989). Making feedback helpful. *The Organizational Behavior Teaching Review, 13*(1), 109–113.

Mullan, F. (2001). A founder of quality assessment encounters a troubled system firsthand. *Health Affairs, 29*(1), 137–141.

Navaie-Waliser, M., Lincoln, P., Karuturi, M., & Reisch, K. (2004). Increasing job satisfaction, quality care, and coordination in home health. *Journal of Nursing Administration, 34*(2), 88–92.

Neuhauser, P.C. (2002). Building a high-retention culture in healthcare. *Journal of Nursing Administration, 32*(9), 470–478.

Nikolaou, I. & Tsaousis, I. (2002). Emotional intelligence in the workplace: Exploring its effects on occupational stress and organizational commitment. *The International Journal of Organizational Analysis, 10*(4), 327–342.

Nierenberg, R.J. (2003). The use of a strategic interviewing technique to select the nurse manager. *Journal of Nursing Administration, 33*(10), 500–505.

Noyes, B.J. (2002). Midlevel management education. *Journal of Nursing Administration, 32*(1), 25–26.

O'Brien-Pallas, L., Thomson, D., Alksnis, C., & Bruce, S. (2001). The economic impact of nurse staffing decisions: Time to turn down another road? *Hospital Quarterly, 4*(3), 42–50.

O'Connor, M. (2001). Reframing communication: Conversation in the workplace. *Journal of Nursing Administration, 31*(9), 403-405.

O'Hara, N.F., Duvanich, M., Foss, J., & Wells, N. (2003). The Vanderbilt Professional Nursing Practice Program, part 2: Integrating a professional advancement and performance evaluation system. *Journal of Nursing Administration, 33*(10), 512–521.

Ohio Nurses Association. (2004). Creating a compelling workplace. *Ohio Nurses Review, 79*(7), 6.

Rahim, M.A. & Psenicka, C. (2002). A model of emotional intelligence and conflict management strategies: A study in seven countries. *The International Journal of Organizational Analysis, 10*(4), 302–326.

Rapisarda, B.A. (2002). The impact of emotional intelligence on work team cohesiveness and performance. *The International Journal of Organizational Analysis, 10*(4), 363–379.

Ritter-Teitel, J. (2003). Nursing administrative research: The underpinning of decisive leadership. *The Journal of Nursing Administration, 33*(5), 257–259.

The Robert Wood Johnson Foundation, Kimball, B., & O'Neil, E. (2002). Health care's human crisis: The American nursing shortage (2002). Retrieved September 30, 2004, from http://www.rwjf.org/publications/publicationspdfs/nursing_report.pdf

Roberts, B.J., Jones, C., & Lynn, M. (2004). Job satisfaction of new baccalaureate nurses. *Journal of Nursing Administration, 34*(9), 428–435.

Robinson, K., Eck, C., Keck, B., & Wells, N. (2003). The Vanderbilt Professional Nursing Practice Program, part 1: Growing and supporting professional nursing practice. *Journal of Nursing Administration, 33*(9), 441–450.

Russell, G. & Scoble, K. (2003). Vision 2020, part 2: Educational preparation for the future nurse manager. *Journal of Nursing Administration, 33*(7/8), 404–409.

Safire, W. & Safire, L. (1982). *Good advice*. New York: Wing Books.

Shipper, F., Rotondo, D.M., & Hoffman, R.C. IV. (2003, August). *A cross-cultural study of linkage between emotional intelligence and managerial effectiveness*. Paper presented at the Academy of Management, Seattle, WA.

Smeltzer, C.H. (2002a). The benefits of executive coaching. *Journal of Nursing Administration, 32*(10), 501–502.

Smeltzer, C.H. (2002b). Succession planning. *Journal of Nursing Administration, 32*(12), 615.

Snow, J.L. (2001). Looking beyond nursing for clues to effective leadership. *Journal of Nursing Administration, 31*(9), 440–443.

Sochalski, J. (2002). Trends: Nursing shortage redux: Turning the corner on an enduring problem. *Health Affairs, 21*(5), 157–164.

Stevens, S. (2002). Nursing workforce retention: Challenging a bullying culture. *Health Affairs, 21*(5), 189–193.

Sullivan, J., Bretschneider, J. & McCausland, M.P. (2003). Designing a leadership development program for nurse managers: An evidence-driven approach. *Journal of Nursing Administration, 33*(10), 544–549.

Sullivan, T., Kerr, M., & Ibrahim, S. (1999). Job stress in health care workers: Highlights from the National Population Health Survey. *Hospital Quarterly, 2*(4), 34–40.

Tourangeau, A.E. (2003). Building nurse leader capacity. *Journal of Nursing Administration, 33*(12), 624–626.

Tzeng H-M. & Ketefian, S. (2002). The relationships between nurses' job satisfaction and inpatient satisfaction: An exploratory study in a Taiwan teaching hospital. *Journal of Nursing Care Quality, 16*(2), 39–49.

Upenieks, V.V. (2003). What constitutes effective leadership? Perceptions of magnet and nonmagnet nurse leaders. *Journal of Nursing Administration, 33*(9), 456–467.

Upenieks, V.V. (2002a). What constitutes successful nurse leadership? A qualitative approach utilizing Kanter's theory of organizational behavior. *Journal of Nursing Administration, 32*(12), 622–632.

Upenieks, V.V. (2002b). Assessing differences in job satisfaction of nurses in magnet and non-magnet hospitals. *Journal of Nursing Administration, 32*(11), 564–576.

Vitellow-Cicciu, J. M. (2002). Exploring emotional intelligence: Implications for nursing leaders. *Journal of Nursing Administration, 32*(4), 208.

Wagner, C.M. & Huber, D.L. (2003). Catastrophe and nursing turnover: Nonlinear models. *Journal of Nursing Administration, 33*(9), 486–492.

Watson, C.A. (2004). Evidence-based management practices: The challenge for nursing. *Journal of Nursing Administration, 34*(5), 207–209.

Watson, C.A. (2002). Understanding the factors that influence nurses' job satisfaction. *Journal of Nursing Administration, 32*(5), 229–231.

Weinberg, D.B. (2003). *Code green: Money-driven hospitals and the dismantling of nursing*. Ithaca, NY: Cornell University Press.

Wellins, R. & Weaver, P.S. Jr. (2003). See-level leadership. *Training and Development* (September 2003), 58–65.

Woolf, R. (2001). How to talk so people will listen. *Journal of Nursing Administration, 31*(9), 401–402.

CHAPTER 3

Ethical Principles for the Nurse Administrator

Linda Roussel, RN, DSN

I firmly believe that the most important factor is our attitude and human motivation . . . genuine human love, human kindness and human affection . . . True love or compassion is actually . . . a strong sense of care and concern for the happiness of the other; that is, genuine love. Such true love automatically becomes a sense of responsibility; we will never love our hope or our determination.

Tenzin Gyatso, His Holiness
The Fourteenth Dalai Lama

LEARNING OBJECTIVES AND ACTIVITIES

- Identify core bioethic terms and basic ethical principles for the nurse administration in health care agencies.
- Describe professional ethics and a code of ethics for nursing.
- Define critical aspects of an ethics committee and the role of the nurse administrator.
- Identify major ethical dilemmas as they relate to managing health care services.

CONCEPTS: Bioethic terms, professional ethics, code of ethics, ethical dilemmas, ethical principles, ethics committee, managerial ethics.

NURSE MANAGER BEHAVIORS: Maintains privacy and confidentiality of patients/consumers/staff, and organizational data. Advocates for nonjudgmental and nondiscriminatory behaviors in serving patients/consumers/staff in culturally diverse environments.

NURSE EXECUTIVE BEHAVIORS: Advocates for patients/consumers/personnel who are recipients of services. Adheres to Code of Ethics with Interpretive Statements (ANA, 2001). Complies with regulatory and professional standards, as well as integrity of health care business practices. Maintains processes to identify and address ethical issues and dilemmas.

Introduction

Ethics is the discipline involved in the judgment of rightness or wrongness, unfairness or fairness, virtue or vice, ends, objects, or states of affairs. "Professions are defined in part by the ethics that govern their practice."[1] Morals and principles are incorporated into any discussion about ethics, ethical decision making, and ethical dilemmas.

Professional Ethics and Integrity

True professional status implies a code of ethics. Ethics has always been significant in professional nursing practice. This commitment has been further intensified with the establishment in 1990 of the Center for Ethics and Human Rights under the umbrella of the American Nurses Association (ANA). The Center's guiding mission is to address the complex ethical and human rights confronting nurses and to designate activities and programs that serve to increase ethical competence and human rights sensitivity of nurses.[2] Professional integrity reinforces the Code of Ethics for Nurses with Interpretive Statements and can be defined as strict adherence to a code of conduct.

Standard 11 in the *Scope and Standards for Nurse Administrators* describes the decisions and actions made by nurse administrators that are based on ethical principles. Measurement criteria are identified as follows:[3]

1. Advocates on behalf of recipients of services and personnel.
2. Maintains privacy, confidentiality, and security of patient/client/resident, staff, and organization data.
3. Adheres to the Code of Ethics for Nurses with Interpretive Statements.[4]
4. Assures confidentiality with regulatory and professional standards, as well as integrity in business practices.

5. Fosters a nondisciplinary climate in which care is delivered in a manner sensitive to sociocultural diversity.
6. Assures a process to identify and address ethical issues within nurses and the organization.

This standard and the code of ethics provide a framework for decision making and managing health care systems.

Ethical Principles

Biomedical ethicists have described three primary principles—respect for persons, beneficence, and justice—that are sometimes stated as rules or obligations. Ethics addresses three types of moral problems: moral uncertainty (unsureness about moral principles or rules that may apply, or the nature of the ethical problem itself); moral dilemma (conflict of moral principles that support different courses of action); and moral distress (inability to take the action known to be right because of external constraints).[5]

The principle of respect for persons describes individuals' ability to take rational action and make moral choices. Autonomy, veracity (truth telling), confidentiality, and informed consent evolve from the principle of respect for persons.[6]

The principle of beneficence has a twofold purpose: first, do no harm; and second, promote good. This principle is basic to those providing health care services and is often contradictory. For example, aggressive treatment causes pain and complications as it possibly promotes a positive outcome.[7]

The principle of justice involves fairness, rights, and obligation. The possible rationing of scarce resources may create ethical dilemmas and be perceived as promoting or neglecting the principle of justice. For example, Mickey Mantle's liver transplant (given his history of alcoholism and later diagnosis of cancer) may have been perceived as preferential treatment and an unfair allocation of this limited resource.[8]

Ethical Theories

There are a number of ethical theories that are foundational to health care and biomedical ethics. These theories provide principles and guidelines for ethical discussion and debates centered on ethical dilemmas. Using a theoretical framework when forming an ethics committee can further guide discussion and decision making. Useful theories include the utilitarianism theory of Jeremy Bentham (1748–1832) and John Stuart Mill (1806–1873), the natural rights theory of John Locke (1632–1704), and the contractarian theory of Thomas Hobbes (1588–1679). The consequentialist, or utilitarian, view purports that the consequences of our acts are of primary concern, that the means justify the ends, that one should consider the greatest good for the greatest number, and that the concepts of good and bad are personalized for each of us. John Locke's theory provided guidelines for the US Declaration of Independence, which discusses our inalienable rights and the government's obligation to respect these rights. The contractarian theory states that morality involves a social contract, which provides the principles of what an individual can and cannot do.[9]

Other theoretical approaches, which are more traditional from a health care perspective, include the deontologic style (from the Greek root meaning "knowledge of that which is binding and proper") and teleologic style (from the Greek root meaning "knowledge of the end"). The deontologic approach assigns duty or obligation based on the intrinsic features of the act; the teleologic approach assigns duty or obligation based on the consequences of the act (its extrinsic nature).[10]

Holistic ethics has also been proposed as an ethical framework. "Holistic ethics is a philosophy that couples both reemerging and rapidly evolving concepts of holism and ethics".[11] Unity and integral wholeness of all people and of all nature is identified and sought out for unity and wholeness of self and within humanity. Dossey, Keegan, and Guzzetta further note that within this framework, "acts are not performed for the sake of law, precedent, or social norms; they are performed from a desire to do freely in order to witness, identify, and contribute to unity of the self and of the universe, of which the individual is a part."[12] Raising consciousness and being concerned about the effect of the act on an individual's larger self is the focus of holistic ethics. Decision making, problem solving, and the management of health care services can be guided by a holistic perspective, which considers all aspects within systems.

Ethical Terms

Ethical terms that are used in ethical discussions with health care providers provide a common language. Such terms may include the following:[13]

- Autonomy: One's actions are independent from the will of others. *Moral autonomy* denotes freedom to reach one's own values about what is right and wrong.
- Beneficence: Engaging in an act that is good or that brings about good effects.
- Competence: Capacity to make decisions about the provision of medical care for oneself (decision-making capacity). Competence is also considered the legal capacity to make decisions.
- Confidentiality: Not divulging information that an individual considers secret.
- Consent: One person voluntarily agrees to allow another to do something.

- Decision-Making Capacity: One's ability to make decisions about the provision of medical care for oneself. This is a clinical determination that is specific to the decision at hand and, as such, may vary from time to time or from decision to decision (see Competence).
- Euthanasia: "Happy death" (Greek); has come to mean the deliberate ending of a human life. *Active euthanasia* refers to the direct killing of a patient. *Passive euthanasia* involves the withdrawal of medical technologies in order to allow the underlying disease to take its natural course. *Voluntary euthanasia* means that the act is undertaken at the behest of the patient, and should be distinguished from *nonvoluntary euthanasia*, in which the patient has made no such request, and *involuntary euthanasia*, in which the action is performed against the patient's wishes.
- Informed Consent: Generally, a formal written consent patients give to health care professionals expressing their complete understanding and agreement and allowing tests, procedures, or experimentation.
- Nonmaleficence: Not performing actions that cause harm to patients.
- Obligations: Responsibilities assumed by human beings toward one another by law, morality, custom, or tradition.
- Rights: Justified claims upon others for actions or nonactions.
- Slippery Slope Argument: If X is allowed, Y will follow, and Y is ethically unacceptable.
- Utilitarianism: A normative ethical theory that advocates bringing about the greatest good for the greatest number of people. Originally advocated by John Stuart Mill.
- Value: Any object or quality that is found to be desirable or worthwhile.

Other terms that may be useful to understand include the following:

- Natural Law: Human good cannot be reduced to a mere function of what people desire; this theory considers the fulfillment of natural purpose, design, or essence.[14]
- Feminist Ethics: An ethical framework that considers concepts that link relational autonomy, contextual reasoning, and indeterminate boundaries and that underscores caring.[15]
- Rights-Based Ethics: An ethical theory that emphasizes the role of rights. One of the three kinds of ethics developed by R. Dworkin; the others are goal-based ethics (utilitarianism) and duty-based ethics (Kantian ethics).[16]
- Virtue-Based Ethics: Recognizes the reality of the moral agent.[17]

It is important to have a working knowledge of the above terms in discussing ethical concerns and issues. This serves as a foundation to working with ethics committees and provides some foundational information for this critical work.

Developing a Health Care Ethics Program

A health care ethics program can be instrumental in developing ethical competence and creating a climate conducive to ethical practice. Clinical practice, research, and administration can reinforce ethical competence. "Competence in ethics requires moral sensibility, moral responsiveness, moral reasoning, and moral leadership."[18] A sound health care ethics program should support the mission, philosophy, strategic plans, and policies related to human resource management and patient care. The Joint Commission on Accreditation of Health Care Organizations' standards address ethical issues, specifically focusing on respect for patients, responding to patient values and preferences, and patient responsibilities.[19]

Elements of an ethics program include education, consultation, and policy development and review.[20]

1. *Education* includes classes and information on such topics as natural law, deontology, utilitarianism, emotionalism, feminist ethics, and others. Developing a glossary of terms useful to understanding the vocabulary of an ethics committee is also important and may include principles such as autonomy, justice, beneficence, nonmaleficence, veracity, and confidentiality. Discussing clinical topics related to services offered in the facility helps to make the information disseminated applicable to the management of ethical dilemmas within the organization.
2. *Consultation* requires individuals skilled in assessment, process, and interpersonal competencies. "Ethics consultation is often assigned to an individual or group with demonstrated competency and skill in ethics consultation."[21] The American Society for Bioethics and Humanities provides core competencies for successful ethics consultation.[22]
3. *Policy development* provides guidance to organizations in addressing ethical dilemmas. "Tasks that must be assigned are (a) reviewing existing policies from an ethical perspective; and (b) developing and writing policies on such topics as informed consent, withholding/withdrawing treatment, advance directives, surrogacy, DNR, medical futility, privacy, confidentiality, organ transplant, donation, and procurement, research, conflict of interest, impaired providers, conscientious objectors, and the use of reproductive and other technologies."[23]

Jones found that offering ethics consultation reduces nonbeneficial life-sustaining treatments and that those patients receiving ethics consultation had fewer hospital, ICU, and ventilation days than those who received usual care.[24]

Developing a health care ethics program gives support and a foundation to an organization's ethics committee, which responds to the many challenging dilemmas facing health care providers. Hospital ethics committees began to appear in the 1970s and gained a high profile in 1982, when two Kaiser Permanente physicians were charged with first-degree murder. The physicians were adhering to a family's wishes to remove intravenous feeding tubes from a comatose, severely brain-damaged patient. At the time of the investigation, the judge found no guidelines within the organization to handle these issues.[25] Ethics committees' responsibilities include the following:[26]

- Defuse existing fears within an institution;
- Educate caregivers on how ethics committees can be used for personal and professional benefit;
- Be knowledgeable and nonthreatening;
- Serve in an advisory role to aid and assist decision-makers;
- Make available diverse values, knowledge, and experience; and
- Not usurp authority from a primary physician.

Along with ethics committees, ethics networks and ethics centers are also important. Ethics quality indicators are particularly important to end-of-life care and caring for individuals who are seriously ill. Trinity Lutheran's medical staff put forth four performance improvement indicators related to end-of-life care:[27]

1. The patient's record contains physician documentation of the rationale for the patient's code status.
2. If the patient resuscitation category was changed during the patient's hospital stay, there is physician documentation by the physician about the reason for the charge and patient/surrogate agreement.
3. If the patient has an advance directive, the wishes of the patient were followed.
4. For patients placed on life support, the record reflects
   a. That a meaningful discussion took place with the patient/surrogate;
   b. That the treatment decision supports the patient's known values and goals of life.

These guidelines and other types of protocols provide useful information in managing a clinical practice.

Ethical Implications for Managing a Clinical Practice Discipline

Many ethical issues are directly related to the providing of patient care services. These have become more important since the 1990s because of several factors: the increased sophistication of medical science and technology; interprofessional relationships; organ donations and transplants; special concerns relating to patients with AIDS, the uninsured, the aged, and high-risk neonates; concern about practical limits on financial resources for health care; changes in society; and growing emphasis on the autonomy of the individual.[28]

Professional nurses implement the employer's policy concerning the moral responsibility of health care. Nurses have responsibility for supervising and reviewing patient care, meeting quality standards, making certain that decisions about patients are based on sound ethical principles, developing policies and mechanisms that address questions of human values, and responding to social problems and dilemmas that affect the need for health care services.[29]

To fulfill this responsibility, professional nurses support nurses confronted with ethical dilemmas and help them think through situations by open dialogue. Nurse managers establish the climate for this discussion. Davis recommends ethics rounds as a means of discussing ethical dilemmas. Such discussions can stem from hypothetical cases, case histories, or a case based on a current patient. Ethical reasoning requires participation by a knowledgeable person. Ongoing awareness and reinforcement of ethical principles and reasoning increases the organization's awareness of the nature of professional practice. Davis describes four ethical principles:[30]

1. *Autonomy.* Personal freedom of action is an ethical principle to be applied by nurse managers toward professional nurses, who in turn apply the principle in the care of their patients. The professional nurse is given autonomy to deliberate about nursing actions and has the capacity to take nursing actions based on this deliberation. Hospitalized or ambulatory patients may have diminished autonomy, and the professional nurse becomes an advocate or autonomous agent for these patients' rights. The patient is responsible for making decisions about his or her care, and the family may be involved with the patient's consent.
2. *Nonmaleficence.* Avoidance of intentional harm or the risk of inflicting harm on someone is termed nonmaleficence. The use of restraints is an area that pits the principle of autonomy and self-determination against that of nonmaleficence. When risks outweigh costs, one must protect the patient. Side rails, safety

vests, tranquilizers, and wrist restraints all have the potential for abuse. Discharge planning can prevent negative outcomes and potential errors. When errors occur, the nurse should acknowledge them to the patient or a surrogate, with full and immediate disclosure to the physician and the institution's administration. Nurses can protect patients from incompetent practitioners and protect their own rights at the same time.
3. *Beneficence.* Beneficence is the principle of viewing persons as autonomous, not harming them, and contributing to their health and welfare.
4. *Justice.* Justice involves giving people what is owed, deserved, or legitimately claimed.

The four ethical principles of autonomy, nonmaleficence, beneficence, and justice are being studied and debated in relation to nursing research and practice, to drug trials (including the use of placebo controls), and to cost-cutting in provider organizations.[31]

Many ethical issues relate to nursing and health care, including the issue of the right to health care. However, the United States does not provide health care as a matter of law. The following are some other ethical issues:

1. The rights of individuals and their surrogates versus the rights of the state or society. This issue creates confrontations between consumers and practitioners and may lead to management efforts to cut costs by cutting services (staff) or closing treatment centers. A survey of the Association of Community Cancer Centers indicated that 84% of these institutions staffed oncology units higher than other medical/surgical units.[32]
2. The rights of patients unable to make their own decisions weighed against the rights of patients' families and the rights of institutions.
3. The rights of patients to forgo treatment versus the rights of society.
4. Issues related to the following:
   a. Reproductive technology and preselection of desired physical characteristics of children; genetic screening.
   b. Organ harvesting and transplants.
   c. Research subjects.
   d. Confidentiality.
   e. Restraints.
   f. Disclosure.
   g. Informed consent.
   h. Patient incapacity.
   i. Court intervention.
5. Reporting of ethical abuse of patients and staff.

The ANA Committee on Ethics has published several position statements and guidelines that seek to assist nurses in making ethical decisions in their practice. These guidelines are based on ethical theory and the ANA Code for Nurses, an expression of "nursing's moral concerns, goals, and values." They are designed to provide nurses with guidance on a range of ethical issues, including the withdrawing or withholding of food or fluid; risk versus responsibility in providing care; safeguarding client health and safety from illegal, incompetent, or unethical practices; nurses' participation in capital punishment; and nurses' participation and leadership in ethical review practices.[33]

Nurse managers need to know the legal framework for their actions. They should help clinical nurses to balance teaching, research, clinical investigation, and patient care. All should work for social justice to ensure a desirable quality of life and health care services. Nurses may promote compassion and sensitivity through protest of public policies that reduce quality of or access to health care for the poor. Nurses should pursue human values, wholeness, and health values.[34] This does not mean that nurses must subsidize health care by working for lower salaries; rather they should work to have the cost shared by all of society.

A study of ethical issues and problems encountered by 52 nurses in their work in one hospital used a 32-item ethical-issues-in-nursing instrument. Results indicated that nurses encountered few ethical issues. The five most common issues were inadequate staffing patterns, the prolonging of life through heroic measures, inappropriate resource allocations, situations in which patients were being discussed inappropriately, and irresponsible activity of colleagues. Ethical issues were more frequent in critical care units than in medical or surgical units. The study group recommended institutional ethics committees and nursing ethics rounds to sensitize nurses to ethical issues.[35]

A 1988 survey of institutions in the metropolitan New York area studied how nurses addressed ethical concerns in their practice. In this survey, 71 of 116 hospitals responded. Topics addressed by hospital ethics committees included allocation of resources, patients' rights, death and dying, abortion, prison health, and institutional issues. Formats used to address ethical issues included nursing meetings, in-service hospital committees, hospital ethics committees, and interdisciplinary rounds. All ethics committees had nursing representatives, mostly from administrative and management positions. It was concluded that a majority of institutions do not adequately address nursing issues and concerns.[36]

Among the ethical dilemmas seldom addressed by nurse managers are ethical boundaries, particularly those involving sex. Nurse managers and administrators should provide continuing education to increase nurses' awareness of improper nurse/patient relationships, including accepting gifts and favors, doing business with patients and their families, being coerced or manipulated by patients, visiting patients at home while off duty, and making nontherapeutic disclosures. Risk environments include inpatient psychiatric services and chemical dependency treatment programs.[37]

Patients are sometimes denied pain relief by lazy or policy-focused providers, despite mandates for a patient right to freedom from pain and pain management. Although letters to Ann Landers are not scientific, their anecdotes can be revealing. One writer wrote that a physician would not give her father pain medication the night before he died of terminal cancer because that physician would have had to walk to another unit for a small needle. In another letter, the wife of a terminal cancer patient requesting relief of intense pain was told by a nurse, "He has to wait another 30 minutes." The ethical and professional answer to such incidents is for assertive nurses to obtain adequate pain medication orders and implement them.[38]

One of the leading experts in nursing ethics, Leah Curtin, advocates creation of moral space for nurses to preserve their integrity. A nurse who believes an action to be wrong should not be forced to take that action. Curtin states that since ethics deals with values as well as with facts and interests, answers to ethical questions do not fall strictly within the bounds of any one discipline. Because ethical questions are complex, they are puzzling, even bewildering. Since any answer we frame touches many areas of concern, we cannot foresee all the consequences of the answers we choose. To solve an ethical problem, Curtin recommends that we do the following:[39]

1. Gather as much information as possible to understand precisely what the problem is.
2. Determine as many possible ways to resolve the problem as they present themselves.
3. Consider the arguments for and against each alternative we can discover or imagine.

The nurse has an obligation to protect the welfare of patients and clients by virtue of his or her legal duties, the code for nurses, and nurses' social role. From a moral perspective, one must not knowingly harm another person. Any freely chosen human act is right insofar as it protects and promotes the human rights of individual nurses. Professionals have duties to guide their young colleagues, and nurses on all levels have mutual duties to support and guide one another.[40]

Values-based management stems from the actions of CEOs who set the stage for using a values credo of shared beliefs that govern the decisions and actions of top management. Two companies that do this are Levi Strauss & Company and Holt Companies. Their values include openness, teamwork, diversity, ethical behavior, and honest communication. Their priorities are ethics, human dignity, and self-fulfillment. The employees believe that they make important contributions to the company, customers, and the community. Such companies find that productivity and products increase as a result of this attention to ethics.[41]

Ethics committees should be established to prevent burnout. Their goals should include being a forum for expressing concerns, promoting awareness and education, participating in clinical decision making and policy and procedure development, developing professional identity, and communicating with other committees. Issues that are often reviewed by ethics committees are described in the following sections.[42]

Advance Directives

An advance directive is "a written instruction, such as a living will or a durable power of attorney for health care, recognized under state law (whether statutory or as recognized by the courts of the state) and relating to the provision of such care when the individual is incapacitated." Advance directives are mandated by the Patient Self-Determination Act (a provision of the Omnibus Budget Reconciliation Act of 1990).[43] Advance directives are considered necessary because people face choices about procedures to prolong life. Studies related to advance directives indicate the following:[44]

1. Use of proxies for persons with serious mental illness is neither meaningful nor beneficial.
2. Increased use of advance directives reduces use of health care services without affecting satisfaction or mortality of persons in nursing homes.
3. Elderly persons can use an interactive multimedia CD-ROM program to learn about advance directives.

The advance directive is a directive to physicians and other health care providers given in advance of incapacity with regard to a person's wishes about medical treatment. As an example, the Texas Natural Death Act gives a person the right to provide instructions about care when faced with a terminal condition. It covers such procedures as cardiopulmonary resuscitation (CPR), tube feeding, respirators, intravenous therapy, and kidney dialysis. A durable power of attorney for health care allows a person to name another person to make medical decisions for the incapacitated person.

A directive to physicians may be called a living will. The attending physician and another physician certify that a person has a terminal condition that will result in death in a relatively short time and that the person is comatose, incompetent, or otherwise unable to communicate.

An advance directive is a legal document. In Texas, for example, it does not have to be drawn up by a lawyer or notarized but does have to be witnessed. An oral statement suffices when made in the presence of two witnesses and the attending physician. Witnesses cannot be physicians, nurses, hospital personnel, fellow patients, or persons who will have claim against a person's estate.[45]

Under Texas law (Consent to Medical Treatment Act), the following people have the option to make medical decisions for an incompetent person: spouse, sole child who has written permission from all other children to act alone, majority of children, parents, a person whom the patient clearly identified before becoming ill, any living relative, or a member of the clergy (surrogate).[46]

Ethics in Business

Lee writes that all organizations should develop a policy on ethics. Business ethics helps people find the best way to satisfy the demands of competing interests. Ethics is part of corporate culture. Ethical organizations try to satisfy all of their stockholders, are dedicated to high purpose, are committed to learning, and try to be the best at whatever they do. Leaders of ethical organizations have the moral courage to change direction, hire brilliant subordinates, encourage innovation, stick to values, and persist over time. Polaroid established internal conferences on ethics in 1983 and 1984. These included philosophers, ethicists, and business professors who looked at the language and concepts of ethics. The conferences were broadened to include leadership and dilemma workshops to apply the knowledge to company cases.[47]

Nurse managers can explore similar modes of studying ethics. They can do so with clinical nursing staff. This will include looking at how business *is* done versus how it *should* be done. Such a study will set the organizational climate for ethical decision making. Ethics can be built into orientation, management development, participative management, and policies and procedures.

According to Beckstrand, "The aims of practice can be achieved using the knowledge of science and ethics alone."[48] To apply Beckstrand's theory to nursing management, nurse managers would apply their knowledge to change the nursing work environment to realize a greater good where and when needed.

Donley states that a health care system should be based on values that promote both the individual and the common good.[49] Limitations in nursing management knowledge can cause dilemmas for nurses. There could be a hierarchy of values in managing practice. Nurse managers need to determine how much decision making power clinical nurses want and how much managers can delegate. A theory of ethics should be meshed with a theory of nursing management that is congruent with a theory of ethical conduct for clinical nurses.

Both clinical nurses and managers use scientific knowledge to determine whether conditions support change. The intrinsic value of the management actions should be given careful thought and should be debated by nurse managers who consciously attempt to practice management that realizes the highest good. The manager is more apt to be successful if scientific management knowledge is applied.

Ethics in management translated into nursing theory can be summed up as follows:

1. Nurse managers can influence the ethical behavior of nursing personnel by treating them ethically.
2. Nurse managers have a code of ethics on which peers have agreed. They enter into ethical dilemmas when they go against that code.
3. Nurse managers fall into moral dilemmas when they go against their internal values.
4. Although ethical and moral dilemmas differ, an ethical nurse manager is a moral nurse manager.
5. Ethical decisions can be clarified by three questions:
   a. *Is it legal?* This question resolves some dilemmas but not when questionable laws and policies are involved.
   b. *Is it balanced?* The nurse manager should aim for a win–win solution.
   c. *How will it make me feel about myself?* The nurse manager should consider the impact of each action on his or her self-respect.
6. Nurse managers with positive self-images usually have the internal strength to make the ethical decision.
7. An ethical leader is an effective leader.
8. Nurse managers should apply six principles of ethical power:
   a. The chief nurse executive promotes and ensures pursuit of the stated mission or purpose of the nursing division, since this statement reflects the vision of practicing nurses. Although the mission statement should be reviewed periodically, goals or objectives are set for yearly achievement.
   b. Nurse managers should build an organization to succeed, thereby building up employees through pride in their organization.
   c. Nurse managers should work to sustain patience and continuity through a long-term effect on the organization.
   d. Nurse managers should plan for persistence by spending more time following up on education and activities that build commitment of personnel.
   e. Nurse managers should promote perspective by giving their staff time to think. They should practice good management for the long term.
   f. Nursing service managers should consider developing an organization-specific code of ethics expressed in observable and measurable behaviors.[50]

A code of ethics should be ingrained in employees to create a strong sense of professionalism. Such a code should be the basis of a planned approach to all management functions of planning, organizing, leading, and evaluating. Nursing employees can help develop the code of ethics, help implement it, and determine its associated rewards and punishments. A code of ethics should be read and signed by employees and regularly reviewed and revised.

Contents of a code of ethics include definition of ethical and unethical practices, expected ethical behavior, enforcement of ethical practices, and rewards and punishments. To be objective, a code of ethics specifies rules of conduct. To be effective, it should be applied to all persons.[51]

Summary

The American Nurses Association's *Scope and Standards for Nurse Administrators* identifies ethics and ethical principles as critical to the nurse administrator's decisions and actions. This includes adherence to the Code of Ethics for Nurses with Interpretive Statements as well as compliance with regulatory and professional standards. Integrity in business practices requires that there be checks and balances to decisions and actions taken within health care systems. Ethics committees, ethics networks, and ethics centers heighten awareness of patients' rights and consumer protection. Understanding ethical theories and principles guides thinking and decision making. Developing a health care ethics program requires education, consultation, and policy review. Identifying ethics quality indicators further advances a health care ethics program and increases the competency of those involved in analyzing ethical dilemmas. As technologies of patient treatment develop and the health care delivery system evolves around managed care, nurses need avenues to pursue the ensuring ethical dilemmas.

APPLICATION EXERCISES

EXERCISE 3-1

Form a group of six to eight peers. Each group member identifies and describes, orally or in writing, an ethical dilemma. Discuss each dilemma from the viewpoints of care for the patient and support for the caregiver. What are the implications for interpersonal relationships among caregivers and care recipients?

EXERCISE 3-2

Set up two teams to debate the following issue:

Professional nurses should intervene in instances in which they observe unethical conduct or illegal or unprofessional activities.

versus

Professional nurses should not *intervene in instances in which they observe unethical conduct or illegal or unprofessional activities.*

Select a moderator. Decide on rules for selection and then decide on rules of procedure. For example, each speaker from each side may be allowed to speak to a question for three minutes.

Consider the following questions:

1. What is the individual responsibility of the professional nurse employee in instances where he or she observes unethical conduct or illegal or unprofessional activities by the employer?
2. What is the responsibility of professional nursing organizations once they are made aware of such instances?
3. What is the responsibility of community organizations if they are made aware of such instances?

Consider the following issues:

- Accreditation action
- Government action (Medicare)
- Publicity (media)
- Prevention

EXERCISE 3-3 Examine organizational policies related to patients' rights as well as statements made by nursing associations and hospital associations and articles in professional journals. What authority or source would lead one to believe that the patient has a right to know his or her nursing diagnosis, the goals of care related to that diagnosis, and the nursing actions prescribed to meet those goals? What authority or source would lead one to believe that the patient has a right to assist in the planning of his or her nursing care? What authority or source would lead one to believe that the patient has a right to know what to expect as a result of his or her nursing care?

NOTES

1. Baker, L. & Marquis, B. (Eds). (2003). *Nursing administration review and resources manual*. Washington, DC: Institute for Research, Education, and Consultation at the American Nurses Credentialing Center, 67.
2. Ibid.
3. American Nurses Association. (2004). *Scope and standards for nurse administrators* (2nd ed.). Washington, DC: Author.
4. Ibid, p. 27.
5. Dossey, B. M., Keegan, L., & and Guzzetta, C. E. (2005). *Holistic nursing: A handbook for practice* (4th ed.). Sudbury, MA: Jones and Bartlett Publishers, 94.
6. Veatch, R. M. (Ed.). (2002). *Medical ethics*. Upper Saddle River, NJ: Prentice Hall.
7. Orentlicher, D. (2001). *Matters of life and death: Making moral theory work in medicine and the law*. Princeton, NJ: Princeton University Press.
8. Fowler, M. (1989). Ethical decision making in clinical practice. *Nursing Clinics of North America*, *24*(4), 955–965.
9. Milner, S. (1993). An ethical practice model. *Journal of Nursing Administration*, *23*(3), 22–25.
10. Ibid.
11. Dossey, Keegan, & Guzzetta, 2005, 96.
12. Ibid., p. 96.
13. Ibid.
14. Kantor, J. E. (1989). *Medical ethics for physicians-in-training*. New York: Plenum Medical Book Company.
15. Wolf, S. (1996). Introduction: Gender and feminism in bioethics. In S. Wolf (Ed.), *Feminism and bioethics: Beyond reproduction* (pp. 3–45). New York: Oxford University Press.
16. Bandman, E. & Bandman, B. (2002). *Nursing ethics through the life span* (4th ed.). Upper Saddle River, NJ: Prentice Hall, 294.
17. Veatch, 2002.
18. Turner, M. (2003). A toolbox for healthcare ethics program development. *Journal for Nurses in Staff Development*, *19*(1), 9–15.
19. Joint Commission on Accreditation of Healthcare Organizations. (1996). *Comprehensive accreditation manual for hospitals*. Oakbrook Terrace, IL: Author.
20. Turner, 2003.
21. Ibid.
22. Worthley, J. A. (1999). *Organizational ethics in the compliance context*. Chicago, IL: Health Administration Press.
23. Pellegrino, E. D. (2000). Interview with Edmund D. Pellegrino, M. D. In M. Boylan (Ed.), *Medical ethics* (pp. 25–36). Upper Saddle River, NJ: Prentice Hall.
24. Jones, T. (2004). Ethics consultations reduced hospital, ICU, and ventilation days in patients who died before hospital discharge in the ICU. *Evidence-Based Nursing*, *7*(2), 53.
25. Eckberg, E. (1993). The continuing ethical dilemma of the do-not-resuscitate order. *The Association of Perioperative Registered Nurses*, *67*(4), 784.
26. Ibid.
27. Christopher, M. (2001). Role of ethics committees, ethics networks, and ethics centers in improving end-of-life care. *Pain Medicine*, *2*(2), 162.
28. Special Committee on Biomedical Ethics. (1985). *Values in conflict: Resolving ethical issues in hospital care*. Chicago, IL: American Hospital Association.
29. Ibid.
30. Davis, A. J. (1982). Helping your staff address ethical dilemmas. *Journal of Nursing Administration*, 9–13.
31. Flaherty, M. (1999, August 30). Search for answers: Drug trials create ethical balancing act. *HealthWeek*, 1, 10; Noble-Adams, R. (1999). Ethics and nursing research, 1: Development, theories and principles. *British Journal of Nursing*, 888–892; Dwyer, M. L. (1998). Genetic research and ethical challenges: Implication for nursing practice. *AACN Clinical Issues*, 600–605; Kawas, C. H., Clark, C. M., Farlow, M. R., Knopman, D. S., Marson, D., Morris, J. C., et al. (1999). Clinical trials in Alzheimer disease: Debate on the use of placebo controls. *Alzheimer Disease & Associated Disorders*, 124–129; Brommels, M. (1999). Sliced down to the moral backbone? Ethical issues of structural reforms in healthcare organizations. *Acta Oncology*, *38*(1), 63–69.
32. Mortenson, L. E. (1984). Are oncology nurses too expensive? *Oncology Nursing Forum*, 14–15; Committee on Ethics, American Nurses Association. (1988). *Ethics in nursing: Position statements and guidelines*. Kansas City, MO: Author.
33. American Nurses' Association. (1988). Ethics in nursing: Position statements and guidelines. Kansas City, MO: Author.
34. Sauer, J. E. (1985). Ethical problems facing the healthcare industry. *Hospital & Health Services Administration*, 44–53.
35. Berger, M. C., Seversen, A., & Chvatal, R. (1991). Ethical issues in nursing. *Western Journal of Nursing Research*, 514–521.
36. Scanlon & Fleming, C. (1990). Confronting ethical issues: A nursing survey. *Nursing Management*, 63–65.
37. Pennington, S., Gafner, G., Schilit, R., & Bechtel, B. (1993). Addressing ethical boundaries among nurses. *Nursing Management*, 36–39.
38. Landers, A. (1994, June 17). Pain-free death is a right worth defending. *San Antonio Express-News*, p. 5J.
39. Curtin, L. L. (1993). Creating moral space for nurses. *Nursing Management*, 18–19.
40. Curtin, L. L. (1992). When the system fails. *Nursing Management*, 21–25.
41. Konstam, P. (1992, December 12). Values-based system focuses on ethics. *San Antonio Light*, p. D1.
42. Buchanan, S. & Cook, L. (1992). Nursing ethics committees: The time is now. *Nursing Management*, 40–41.
43. United States. Cong. House. 101st Congress, 2nd Session. S. 4206, Medicare Provider Agreements Assuring the Implementation of the Patients Right to Participate in and Direct Health Care Delivery Affecting the Patient [introduced in the US House; 26 October 1990]. 101st Congress. Congressional Record-House, H12456–H12457.

44. Murphy, C. P., Sweeney, M. A., & Chiriboga, D. (2000). An educational intervention for advance directives. *Journal of Professional Nursing*, 21–30; Molloy, D. W. et al. (2000). Systematic implementation of an advance directive program in nursing homes: A randomized controlled trial. *JAMA*, 1437–1444; Geller, J. L. (2000). The use of advance directives by persons with serious mental illness for psychiatric treatment. *Psychiatric Quarterly*, 1–13; Burt, J. G. (1999). Compliance with advance directives: A legal view. *Critical Care Nursing Quarterly*, 72–74.
45. Bexar County Hospital District (1991). Understanding advance directives: Your rights as a patient. San Antonio, Texas: Author.
46. Premack, P. (1993, July 23). Medical OK law has a key change. *San Antonio Express-News*, p. 11D.
47. Lee, C. (1986). Ethics training: Facing the tough questions. *Training*, 30–33, 38–41.
48. Beckstrand, J. (1978). The need for a practice theory as indicated by the knowledge used in the conduct of practice. *Research in Nursing and Health*, 175–179.
49. Donley, R. (1993). Ethics in the age of health care reform. *Nursing Economic$*, 19–23.
50. Fernicola, K. C. (1988). Take the high road . . . to ethical management: An interview with Kenneth Blanchard. *Association Management*, 60–66.
51. Mizock, M. (1986). Ethics: The guiding light of professionalism. *Data Management*, 16–18, 29.

REFERENCES

American Society for Bioethics and Humanities. (1998). *Core competencies for health care ethics consultation*. Glenview, IL: Author.

Arras, J. D. & Steinbock, B. (1999). *Ethical issues in modern medicine* (5th ed.). Mountain View, CA: Mayfield.

Ashley, B. M. & O'Rourke, K. D. (1994). *Ethics of health care: An introductory textbook* (2nd ed.). Washington, DC: Georgetown University Press.

Bell, S. E. (2003). Ethical climate in managed care organizations. *Nursing Administration Quarterly*, *27*(2), 133–139.

Beauchamp, T. L. & Childress, J. F. (2001). *Principles of biomedical ethics* (5th ed.). New York: Oxford University Press.

Malpas, P. & M. Schaffner. (2000). Managerial ethics: Arriving at decisions we can live with. *Gastroenterology Nursing*, *23*(5), 239–240.

Marshall, M. F. (1997). Treatment refusals by patients and clinicians. In J. C. Fletcher, P. A. Lombardo, M. F. Marshall, & F. G. Miller (Eds.), *Introduction to clinical ethics* (2nd ed.). Frederick, MD: University Publishing Group.

CHAPTER 4

The Components of Change: Creativity and Innovation, Critical Thinking, and Planned Change

Elizabeth Simms, RN, MSN

Something unforeseen and magnificent is happening. Health care, having in our time entered its dark night of the soul, shows signs of emerging, transformed.

Barbara Dossey and Larry Dossey

LEARNING OBJECTIVES AND ACTIVITIES

- Define and differentiate between *creativity* and *innovation*.
- Develop plans for recognizing and increasing the creativity, critical thinking skills, and innovation of clinical nurses.
- Identify methods of critical thinking.
- Perform a concept analysis of critical thinking.
- Identify reasons or need for change in nursing practice and management.
- Identify and differentiate between theories of planned change: Redding, Lewin, Rogers, Havelock, Lippitt, and Spradley.
- Identify reasons for resistance to change; develop strategies to overcome that resistance.
- Describe the need for nursing research in a service setting; develop a plan for a research project within that setting.

CONCEPTS: Creativity, innovation, critical thinking, change theory, nursing research.

NURSE MANAGER BEHAVIORS: The manager promotes an environment in which creativity, innovation, and critical thinking are recognized and rewarded. He or she considers change the domain of executive nursing and initiates all efforts for planned change accordingly.

NURSE EXECUTIVE BEHAVIORS: A leader encourages all nursing employees to think freely, considers creative ideas critically, and recommends innovations in the practice of nursing and in the environment in which nursing is practiced. He or she involves nurses in implementing planned change and encourages nurses to be involved in the change process and in nursing research activities.

Introduction

In a climate of chaos and change within the health care industry, the trends at the forefront of the competitive market are based upon the creativity and innovations of organizations. "Today's most sought-after talent is the ability to originate."[1] The creative process is not limited; it encompasses a range from organizations reaching out to develop new market strategies to bedside clinicians searching for new and better ways to provide care. Critical thinking skills must be applied to creative ideas, with successful innovations as the outcome, accomplished through planned change within an organization's stated policies and procedures. Changing organizations for excellence must afford opportunities and must change the ways people think and interact to create workplaces and systems that are purposeful and aligned with evidence-based results.

Creativity and Innovation

Creativity and Innovation Defined

Creativity is defined in *Webster's New Twentieth Century Dictionary, Unabridged* (2nd edition) as "artistic or intellectual inventiveness." Innovation is defined as "the introduction of something new." These definitions suggest that the terms are interchangeable. Creativity is the mental work or action involved in bringing something new into existence, whereas innovation is the result of that effort.[2] To differentiate between the two, one might say that a nurse can create or invent a new nursing product, process, or procedure (creativity) and then can effect change by putting a new product, process, or procedure into use (innovation). Creativity is a way of using the mind.[3] Creativity is a special talent and an important tool for survival in the 21st century. Research indicates that creativity is separate from intelligence.[4]

Creativity is the fuel of innovation.[5]

Why Creativity?

A constant flow of new ideas is needed to feed the mandate for change in every aspect of our lives. Business leaders argue that creativity yields profits. With creativity, new products can be developed and a company can compete. New methods (innovations) are the fruits of that creativity. For many years nurses have tended to think of selling their services like a product as mercenary or unethical; this thinking has changed as nurses have acquired a higher level of education and have become more autonomous, with professional nurses becoming entrepreneurs in establishing businesses of their own. Sister Reinkemeyer predicted this development as early as 1968 when she wrote, "university programs try to produce independent personalities and thinkers capable of facing some of the modern scientific and psychosocial changes in nursing."[6]

Innovation is key to the survival and growth of both health care and nursing. Entrepreneurs create the new and different; entrepreneurial nurses create new businesses with new products and services, from which both the nurse and the organization benefit. The nurse gains personal satisfaction, rewards, and recognition while the organization survives, thrives and prospers.[7]

Establishing a Climate for Creativity

For creativity to prosper, the organization should provide an intellectual environment that gives employees recognition, prestige, and an opportunity to participate. Employees will gain a sense of ownership and commitment by being involved in planning their work and making decisions. Nurse managers promote creativity through sensitivity, giving people the attention they want and treating them as distinct individuals. Competent managers inspire creativity by taking risks, as well as by showing confidence, giving praise and support, being nourishing, using tact, and having patience.[8]

Creative thinking can be developed with the intent of increasing the creative capacity and/or behavior of individuals or groups. Techniques of creativity training can include brainstorming, synectics, morphological analysis, forced fit, forced relationships, brainwriting, visualization, cueing, lateral thinking, and divergent thinking.[9] These techniques can be utilized when nurse leaders encourage free thinking and allow nurses to express their ideas openly.

Other motivators of creativity in nursing include the following:[10]

- providing assistance to develop new ideas,
- encouraging risk taking while buffering resistant forces,
- providing time for individual effort,
- providing opportunities for professional growth and development,
- encouraging interaction with others outside the group,
- promoting constructive intragroup and intergroup competition,
- recognizing the value of worthy ideas, and
- exhibiting confidence in workers.

With motivators in place, leadership is able to allow the creative process to evolve. The following are actions that facilitate the production of goal-oriented ideas:[11]

1. Assemble the separate elements that will be creatively combined to produce a product or a new procedure. The problem must be identified in terms of usefulness of this product or process. If a known element is missing, what is available to replace it?
2. Use the available and assembled elements in combinations that produce original ideas.
3. Remove inhibitions to creativity such as excess motivation, anxiety, fear of taking risks, dependence on authority, and habitual modes of thinking and speaking. Creativity is not confined to a small, exclusive set of gifted people. Language contains the potential for creative thought, and everyone has this potential.
4. Study techniques of creativity so that the elements can be used.

Metamanagement

Metamanagement describes a cooperative effort of entrepreneurial or creative managers, strategic planners, and top management. It is a planning framework that cuts across organizational boundaries and facilitates strategic decision making about current practices and future directions. It is a flexible and creative planning process that stimulates in-house entrepreneurial thinking and behavior, and it is a consistent and accepted value system that reinforces management's commitment to the organization's strategy. Metamanagement stresses teamwork, organizational flexibility, open communication, innovation, risk taking, high morale, and trust.[12]

Nurse managers practicing metamanagement will plan the organizational structure: its dynamics, nature, and position. They will perform as an innovative, committed, enlightened, and disciplined group willing and able to restructure thinking and organizations and to generate and execute successful plans for a profitable nursing business. They will stimulate the input of the clinical staff, thereby generating direction for the nursing organization and occupation.

The following task-related actions by nurse managers will help to develop and maintain a creative climate:[13]

1. Providing freedom to experiment without fear of reprimand.
2. Maintaining a moderate amount of work pressure.
3. Providing challenging yet realistic work goals.
4. Emphasizing a low level of supervision in performance tasks.
5. Delegating responsibilities.
6. Encouraging participation in decision making and goal setting.
7. Encouraging use of a creative problem-solving process to solve unstructured problems.
8. Providing immediate and timely feedback on task performance.
9. Providing the resources and support needed to get the job done.

Creative Problem Solving

Creative problem solving starts by using vague or ill-defined problems as challenges. Problems can be attacked intuitively to generate as many ideas as possible. Solutions may create new challenges and new cycles of creative problem solving. The creative and innovative approaches to situations involve literacy and an exchange of ideas, perhaps more familiar to "right-brained" thinkers; in analytical thinking, an almost mathematical twist guides the process, stemming from "left-brain" thinking. Research indicates that both the right and left cerebral hemispheres contribute to the maintenance of multiple word meanings in highly creative persons.[14]

There are several theories of creative problem solving. Lattimer and Winitsky suggest the following:[15]

1. Thinking: Identifying factors to be used in solving an issue or developing a strategic plan; the choice is between a risk-free alternative and an alternative that involves risk.
2. Decomposing: Breaking the situation into components—alternatives, uncertainties, outcomes, and consequences—working with each component, and combining the results for a decision.
3. Simplifying: Determining the important components and concentrating the most crucial factors and the most essential relationships, then making intuitive judgments.
4. Specifying: Establishing the value of key factors, the probabilities for the uncertainties, and the preferences for the outcomes.
5. Rethinking: Examining the original analysis regarding omissions, inclusions, order, and emphasis.

Godfrey recommends an alternative theory of creativity with the following five steps:[16]

1. Perception: Realizing there is a problem.
2. Preparation: Research, data collection, and arrangement of information to define the problem.
3. Ideation: Analysis and structure of a variety of formats that stimulate analogies and images; brainstorming.
4. Incubation: Withdraw and relax when the flow of ideas ends. The unconscious takes off and forms images of possible solutions.
5. Validation: Test a solution.

Drucker indicates that every corporation needs a strategy for innovation. He suggests four strategies for innovation, as follows:[17]

1. The first with the most. Be first in the market and first to improve a product or cut its price. This discourages prospective competitors.
2. The second with the most. Let someone else establish the market. Satisfy markets with narrow needs and specific capabilities. Provide excellent products for big purchasers with narrow needs. Offer new features. This strategy can be seen in the competitive health care market, in which certain corporations have specialized in psychiatric services, rehabilitation services, or drug-dependency services.
3. The niche strategy. Corner a finite market, making it unprofitable for others. When the niche becomes a mass market, change the strategy to remain profitable.
4. Making the product your carrier; one product carries another. This strategy is used by medical supply companies whose electronic thermometers are the basis for sales of disposable covers and intravenous pumps, which are in turn the basis for sales of fluid administration sets.

Creativity in the Workplace

Creative people, including nurses, have a broad background of knowledge. They have the mental skills of curiosity, openness, sensitivity to problems, flexibility, ability to think in images, and capability of analysis and synthesis.[18] Creative nurses use their knowledge to stimulate their sensory perceptions. In addition to solving problems, they identify new problems to solve by formulating questions about the hows and whys of established practices. Creative people are sometimes considered different from other people. This difference has been described by Levinson (1965): "The public would have him nearsighted but farseeing, brilliantly innovative but absentminded, widely acclaimed but impervious to applause, capable of highly involved abstract thinking but naive and eccentric in his everyday reasoning. The truth of the matter is that the creative person is different but is not a monster strangely mysterious and incomprehensible."[19] An individual may appear to have been gifted with a brilliant intellect. During childhood this individual may have been the curious type who searched for books to read and tasks to do that satisfied his or her curiosity. Searching for the approval and encouragement of parents, friends, or teachers but not receiving it, he or she may have become something of a loner.

Creative individuals value the work and association of other creative individuals; they stimulate each other to think and perhaps even to be competitively creative. They can tolerate ambiguity; they have self-confidence, the ability to toy with ideas, and persistence.[20]

Nursing leaders possess the attributes of teamwork, global thinking, multitasking, creativity, and flexibility that are so important to the health care marketplace. They have integrated clinical and business principles and are a source of knowledge and skills to make their organizations prosper.[21] To foster independence and creative talents, nurse managers should assume that creative nurses are not odd or eccentric. As a consequence, barriers will not be erected among peer groups. Nurse managers should communicate and cooperate with clinical nurses to set new goals or new practices for achieving goals.[22] Performance appraisals of creative employees should reward unconventional, intelligent efforts toward innovation, even if those efforts have failed. Evaluation must keep pace with human judgments resulting from complexity, uncertainty, theory, change, and control.[23]

Managing creativity can be challenging. Nurse managers must build an environment in which interpersonal relationships and trust are established to allow for the maximal creative effort among staff. With a willingness to listen and a spirit of cooperation, staff will accept differing behaviors and ideas without defensiveness or fear of losing control. Nurse managers can plan to nourish creativity in nursing personnel by doing the following:

1. Noting the creative abilities of those who develop new methods and techniques and enhancing employees' self-esteem.
2. Providing time and opportunity for creative work; this can be planned for during performance appraisals and included in scheduling. Permitting time for educational offerings.
3. Recognizing expertise in clinical practice, teaching, research efforts, and management skills.
4. Encouraging nursing personnel to become involved in progress in the workplace, in community endeavors, and in professional organizations.
5. Encouraging calculated risk taking and acceptance of personal responsibility; allowing for the freedom to fail.

To encourage creativity, hire creative people! Frequently, they are the ones who have taken time off to learn and explore; sometimes considered "off-the-wall," they bring fresh viewpoints to their chosen profession. Weed out the complacent. Support generous sabbaticals. Model, measure, and teach curiosity; seek out curious work. Change the pace, and make it fun![24]

Critical Thinking

> **The ideal critical thinker is habitually inquisitive, well informed, trustful of reason, open minded, flexible, fair minded in evaluation, honest in facing personal biases, prudent in making judgments, willing to reconsider, clear about issues, orderly in complex matters, diligent in seeking relevant information, reasonable in the selection of criteria, focused in inquiry, and persistent in seeking results which are as precise as the subject and circumstances of inquiry permit.**
>
> **P. A. Facione[25]**

The term *critical thinking* has been prominent in the field of education since the early 1980s. While some believe that the term is applicable across all genres, others believe that the term is best defined as discipline-specific.[26] This idea is particularly pertinent to nursing because the discipline is continuously concerned with purposeful, goal-directed thinking toward making judgments on evidence-based practice rather than on conjecture.[27] On a daily basis, nurses are required to assimilate an abundance of data and information to make decisions within their practice for which there are frequently no absolute or singly correct responses.[28]

Nurses use critical thinking for several purposes, including applying professional and technical knowledge and skills in caring for clients. In these applications, critical thinking is the best guarantee that nurses will have successful outcomes. In the tenth edition of their book entitled *Argumentation and Debate*, Freeley and Steinberg claim that competence in critical thinking is necessary for developing one's ability to participate effectively in human affairs, pursue higher education, and succeed in the highly competitive world of business and the professions. These authors also indicate that the ability to reach successful decisions is based on accurate evidence and valid reasoning.[29] Behaviors based on critical thinking are essential to a nurse's role as clinician, manager, researcher, or teacher.

Freeley identifies seven methods of critical thinking:

1. Debate: Debate involves inquiry, advocacy, and reasoned judgment on a proposition. A person or

group may debate or argue the pros and cons of a proposition in coming to a reasoned judgment. A debate usually entails opposing positions and specific rules.
2. Individual decisions: An individual may debate a proposition in his or her mind using problem-solving or decision-making processes. When consent or cooperation of others is needed, the individual may use group discussion, persuasion, propaganda, coercion, or a combination of these methods.
3. Group discussion: Five conditions for reaching decisions through group discussion are that "the group members (1) agree that a problem exists, (2) have comparable standards of value, (3) have compatible purposes, (4) are willing to accept the consensus of the group, and (5) are relatively few in number."[30]
4. Persuasion: Persuasion is communication to influence the acts, beliefs, attitudes, and values of others by reasoning, urging, or inducement. Debate and advertising are two forms of communication whose intent is to persuade.
5. Propaganda: Propaganda can be good or bad; it is multiple media communication designed to persuade or influence a mass audience. Propagandists may debate and argue. Their tactics need to be subjected to critical analysis.
6. Coercion: Threat or use of force is coercion. An extreme example is brainwashing, in which subjects are completely controlled physically for an indefinite period of time.
7. Combination of methods: Some situations require a combination of the foregoing communication techniques to reach a decision.[31]

A consensus is emerging that critical thinking should underlie the nursing process within nursing education programs. Critical thinking generally is regarded by academics as essential to the educated mind and superordinate to problem solving in the nursing process.[32]

The rudiments of critical thinking are recalling facts, principles, theories, and abstractions to make deductions, interpretations, and evaluations in solving problems, making decisions, and implementing changes.

Research

In 2000, an international panel of 55 expert nurses was utilized for a study to define critical thinking. A Delphi technique with 5 rounds of input identified and defined 10 "habits of the mind" (affective components) and 7 skills (cognitive components) associated with critical thinking in nursing.[33] They are as follows:

Habits of the Mind (affective components)

1. Confidence, or the assurance of one's own reasoning abilities.
2. Contextual perspective, or the ability to synthesize components relative to the whole.
3. Creativity, or intellectual inventiveness.
4. Flexibility, or the ability to adapt or accommodate.
5. Inquisitiveness, or seeking to explore possibilities and alternatives.
6. Intellectual Integrity, or truth seeking, with acceptance of findings contrary to the expected.
7. Intuition, or an insightful sense of knowing.
8. Open-mindedness, or receptivity to divergent views and recognition of personal bias.
9. Perseverance, or the determination to pursue a course of action.
10. Reflection, or the ability to contemplate toward a deeper understanding.

Skills (cognitive components)

1. Analyzing, or the ability to grasp the relationships of the parts to the whole.
2. Applying Standards, or appropriate application of personal or professional criteria.
3. Discriminating, or recognizing similarities and differences.
4. Information Seeking, or gathering data from relevant sources.
5. Logical Reasoning, or drawing conclusions from evidence presented.
6. Predicting, or envisioning a course of action and its outcome.
7. Transforming Knowledge, or the ability to convert the form or function of concepts among contexts.[34]

A number of research studies have examined critical thinking and nursing education. Using the Health Care Professional Attitude Inventory to measure professionalism and the Watson-Glaser Critical Thinking Appraisal (CTA) to measure general critical thinking abilities, Brooks and Shepherd sampled 200 associate's degree, diploma, generic, and upper-division baccalaureate nursing students and found the following:

- Seniors in upper-division and generic programs exhibited significantly more advanced critical thinking abilities than did seniors in associate's degree and diploma programs.
- A positive correlation between critical thinking abilities and professionalism was almost as strong in seniors with generic and associate's degrees as it was in seniors in upper-division programs.
- Seniors in diploma programs exhibited the lowest levels of professionalism and critical thinking.

- Seniors in upper-division programs achieved higher professionalism scores than did seniors in the four-year generic programs; these two groups showed almost identical levels of critical thinking abilities.[35]

Other research studies reached the following conclusions:

1. A study was conducted to determine the relationship between critical thinking skills and clinical judgment in baccalaureate nursing (senior) students; using the California Critical Thinking Skills Test (CCTST), researchers found a positive relationship between critical thinking skills and clinical judgment abilities. Predictors of clinical judgment were the CCTST subscales *inductive reasoning* and *inference*.[36]
2. Critical thinking skills increased among sophomore and senior collegiate nursing students as measured by the CCTST. Significant increases also were seen in the overall scores of these same students, and in subtest scores in truth seeking, analyticity, self-confidence, and inquisitiveness, as measured by the California Critical Thinking Disposition Inventory.[37]
3. In a study to examine the relationship between critical thinking and clinical competence, May and colleagues used an exploratory nonexperimental design with a heterogeneous sample consisting of two graduating nursing classes (N = 143).

   While the group of participants was able to think critically and practice competently according to set standards, there were no statistically significant correlations between critical thinking and clinical competence total scores. One conclusion for these findings is that critical thinking may not emerge as an associated factor with clinical competence until some time after nursing students become practicing nurses.[38]
4. In another study involving 15 qualified nurses, Bell and Procter came to the following conclusion: "Engaging in research activities does not always result in the development of practice; however, there appears to be a link between practice development and critical thinking."[39]

More descriptive research studies are needed in nursing management. Fulfilling this need will require that more nurse managers be trained in nursing research and suggests that the members of the nursing community should unify to implement a theory of nursing management that encompasses critical theory. Nurse managers employing a critical thinking approach would determine how their subordinates interpret organizational phenomenon. They would discuss possible falsities of interpretations with their associates, bringing out illusions and delusions.[40]

Applications of Critical Thinking

Concept analysis is frequently advocated as a strategy for promoting critical thinking.[41] Concept analysis uses critical thinking to advance the knowledge base of nursing management and nursing practice.

A class of master's-level nursing students at Louisiana State University developed a method of concept analysis in their nursing management course using critical thinking. The students did literature searches before each class in preparation for concept analysis. In their first session, they developed the following format for concept analysis:

1. Identify and clarify the concept, including the philosophy and content analysis.
2. List the characteristics and attributes of the concept—for example, concrete/abstract, quality, and quantity.
3. Obtain perceptions, that is, what people think or their interpretations about selling, marketing, and customers (determine whom the concept affects and what is perceived as needed).
4. Identify the use or application and the policies, procedures, practices (skills), and knowledge required.
5. Perform a researchable and synergistic evaluation to promote change, create energy, and validate theory.[42]

This format was used to study and analyze concepts such as organizational climate, legal and ethical nursing practices, nursing care delivery systems, theory of nursing management, standards of nursing practice, evaluation of patient care, and research in nursing administration.

Application of critical thinking theory to nursing management requires that the nurse manager have knowledge of the theory. Nursing staff development faculty also must have knowledge of the theory and the teaching skills that will stimulate critical thinking and test it at the highest cognitive, affective, and psychomotor domains, not only in process but also in outcomes. Lectures are the least effective method for teaching critical thinking. Teaching methods to develop and test the higher level of the cognitive domain and competencies of the affective and psychomotor domains should be a part of the staff development process.[43] Critical thinking skills can be developed through the study of logic, problem-solving observation, analytic reading of books and articles about nursing and management, and group discussion.[44] (See Exhibit 4-1.)

Critical thinking is consistent with the nursing process and should be evident in higher level learning objectives in the cognitive, affective, and psychomotor domains.

Futurist John Naisbitt describes high tech as technology that embodies both good and bad consequences. "High touch is embracing the primeval forces of life and death. High touch is embracing that which acknowledges all that is greater than we."[45] Professional nurses are

EXHIBIT 4-1
Activities and Strategies for Promoting Critical Thinking

Activities and strategies for promoting critical thinking include problem solving, decision making, clinical judgment, reflective thinking, questioning, dialogue, dialectical thinking, concept mapping, concept analysis, inquiry-based learning, script theory, two-way talks, case studies, clinical pathways, research findings, clinical rounds, peer review, shift reports, information processing, skills acquisition theory, conferences, context-dependent test items, and cognitive apprenticeship.

Models for studying critical thinking include the following:

- Loving's competence validation model.[46]
- The cognitive apprenticeship model.[47]

high-tech-high-touch people whose work requires the cognitive abilities of synthesis and analysis; professional nurses *are* critical thinkers.

Planned Change

Machiavelli said, "There is nothing more difficult to take in hand, more perilous to conduct, or more uncertain in its success, than to take the lead in the introduction of a new order of things."[48] With a few notable exceptions, such as the weather, most of the change that takes place in our society is planned. This means that nurse managers can plan with clinical nurses to implement change, first deciding that a new skill or technique using a new apparatus or technology is needed to improve patient care. Then nurse managers and clinical nurses can plan and carry out the changes they want to make.

Let us consider the philosophy embodied in theories of human resource management, theories based on assumptions about human nature and human motivation. Has the nurse organized money, materials, equipment, and personnel in the interests of providing quality services to patients and thereby giving them their money's worth? Have nursing employees had experiences of supervision that have made them passive and resistant to organizational needs? Or do nursing employees work under conditions that inspire them to develop their potential, assume increased responsibility, and work to achieve their personal goals as well as those of the organization? Are clinical nurses able to direct their own efforts?

Spradley defines planned change as "a purposeful, designed effort to bring about improvements in a system, with the assistance of a change agent."[49] Peters writes that planned change is the exception rather than the rule.[50] Change occurs whether one wants it to or not. New technology is developed and new treatments result, causing personnel and organizational adjustments. These changes need to be controlled or managed; we refer to this process as *planned change*.

The Need for Change

Four general reasons for designing orderly change have been defined by Williams:[51]

1. To improve the means of satisfying economic wants.
2. To increase profitability.
3. To promote human work for human beings.
4. To contribute to individual satisfaction and social well-being.

To these reasons one must add the concerns of the new millennium: the structures of health care organizations will continue to change as will the structures of other industries. These changes encompass higher standards and superior performance, constant innovation in technology and corporate structure, the accomplishment of doing more for less, teamwork, customer preference, employee versus employer loyalties, industry regulations, corporate ownership, increased opportunities, shrinking resources, increased competition, and increasing complexity.[52] The need for organizational change may involve not only the whole system but also each of its units. This change will require management of the political dynamics and transition as well as motivation of constructive behavior.[53]

Change can help achieve organizational objectives as well as individual ones. The status quo of nursing will change with new models of patient care. Nurses are certainly aware of changes in relationships with those who hold authority and power, changes in responsibility and status, and changes in organizational, departmental and unit objectives. Increased mobility within society at large has given rise to the creation of highly profitable travel nurses' agencies, creating increased staffing turnover as nurses leave to travel, and as travel nurses are temporarily employed. Some employees resist change, but others welcome it as an opportunity to make adjustments in existing work situations, alter their relationships with their associates, and achieve personal growth and goals.

Structural change will greatly affect central staffers; these changes will include those in human resource development as well as those in nursing staff development. Central staffers will need to become project creators and network builders for the primary business units—the direct patient care units and the product sales units. As consultants to these units, central staffers can help develop the expertise necessary for success. If not involved in consulting for the existing structure, they can develop independent service centers, selling their services to the business units within the organization and to outside markets.[54] All of this change is needed because of increasing competition, technological advancements, and human resource concerns.[55]

The end of the 20th century saw significant changes in the nature of health care organizations, the demands placed on nurse managers, and the needs and motivations of nursing personnel. Successful nurse managers have learned to manage change and have publicly related the role of nursing to being an involved and concerned member of society. They recognize the growing complexity of the health care organization, particularly in the division of nursing, and they recognize the changing values of nurses within the profession.

Nurses want opportunities for advancement or promotion, recognition for their work, and more help from their peers and supervisors to improve their job skills. One dramatic change for nurses has been the impetus to develop their professional standards to higher levels by raising their credentials, particularly with regard to education. Nurses have also recognized the need for continuing education to deliver up-to-date services. Evidence suggests that technological innovation can cause scientists' and engineers' knowledge to become obsolete in 10 years or fewer if they do not pursue further education; parallel evidence could be developed to support the same conclusion about nursing. A glance at the plethora of nursing journals shows nurses' awareness of society's current problems and their increasing involvement with them. These include problems of health, environmental pollution, poverty, ethnic equality, education, civil rights, religion, and advances in genetics.

Today's nurses are more committed to task, job, and profession than they are loyal to an organization; they are no longer bound by threat or ritual. Younger nurses, like other younger professionals, are mobile and have salable skills. They want to use all of their skills and to be collaborative and democratic.[56] They look at the kind of services provided (short-term, critical, or chronic), management's philosophy (participative versus authoritarian), experimental outlook, and physical and geographical location. Nurses are willing to work hard; they desire an environment in which there is humor and the opportunity to use imagination, and in which they can exert some control.

Nurse managers must change their behavior to suit the profile of this new breed of worker; they must be constantly aware of cues for the need for change. They must become more flexible and individualized in dealing with employees, and they must be candid, confronting conflict by allowing nurses to express their feelings, thoughts, and reactions. Management styles change, as do policies, procedures, relationships with subordinates, and employment and compensation practices. Individual needs and group motivations should be considered. The changes in nursing management aim to promote the ideas of all people, to encourage attentive listening, and to reward people for becoming personally involved and committed to their work. Nurse managers see themselves as agents of change functioning within a profession that draws its basic support from society. ". . . [T]he nurse manager will have to act as change agent in moving the organization forward, utilizing human-intensive skills to mobilize the resources available to her and her professional nursing peers. All of this effort will serve to define, implement, and evaluate the strategies and processes that will meet the health care needs of the future."[57]

Adaptation to change has always been a job requirement for nursing. Change is the key to progress and to the future; often that change begins with a focus on technology, without consideration for human relationships and political sensitivities. It will be the task of nursing management to develop complimentary nursing systems that will encompass new technology, improve patient care, and ultimately give greater satisfaction to nursing workers.

Change Theory

Some widely used change theories are those of Reddin, Lewin, Rogers, Havelock, Lippitt, and Spradley.

Reddin's Theory

Reddin has developed a planned change model that can be used by nurses. He has suggested seven techniques by which change can be accomplished:

1. Diagnosis
2. Mutual setting of objectives
3. Group emphasis
4. Maximum information
5. Discussion of implementation
6. Use of ceremony and ritual
7. Resistance interpretation

The first three techniques are designed to give those who will be affected by the change an opportunity to influence its direction, nature, rate, and method of introduction. These individuals are then able to have some control over the change, to become involved in it, to express their ideas more directly, and to propose useful modifications.

Diagnosis (the first technique) is scientific problem solving. Those affected by the change meet and identify problems and the probable outcomes. *Mutual objective setting* (technique number 2) ensures that the goals of both groups, those instituting the change and those affected by it, are brought into line. It may be necessary for groups to bargain and compromise. *Group emphasis* (number 3) is sometimes referred to as team emphasis. Change is more successful when supported by a team rather than by a single person. "Groups develop powerful standards for conformity and the means of enforcing them."[58]

Maximum information (number 4) is important to the success of change. Discussion of implementation (number 5) by the use of ceremony and ritual (number 6) considers the culture of the organization, particularly the use of rewards to reinforce the change. Interpretation of any resistance to change (number 7) takes into account the processes and systems in place which may require a revisiting of the group's work and objectives set for implementation (numbers 3, 4, and 5). Management should make at least four announcements with regard to a proposed change:[59]

1. That a change will be made.
2. What the decision is and why it was made.
3. How the decision will be implemented.
4. How implementation is progressing.

Lewin's Theory

One of the most widely used change theories is that of Kurt Lewin. Lewin's theory involves three stages:

1. The unfreezing stage: The nurse manager or other change agent is motivated by the need to create change. Affected nurses are made aware of this need. The problem is identified or diagnosed, and the best solution is selected. One of three possible mechanisms provides input to the initial change: (a) individual expectations are not being met (lack of confirmation), (b) the individual feels uncomfortable about some action or lack of action (guilt anxiety), or (c) a former obstacle to change no longer exists (psychologic safety). The unfreezing stage occurs when disequilibrium is introduced into the system, creating a need for change.[60]
2. The moving stage: The nurse manager gathers information. A knowledgeable, respected, or powerful person influences the change agent in solving the problems (identification). A variety of sources give a variety of solutions (scanning), and a detailed plan is made. People examine, accept, and try out the innovation.[61]
3. The refreezing stage: Changes are integrated and stabilized as part of the value system. Forces are at work to facilitate the change (driving forces). Other forces are at work to impede change (restraining forces). The change agent identifies and deals with these forces, and change is established with homeostasis and equilibrium.[62]

Rogers's Theory

Everett Rogers modified Lewin's change theory. Antecedents included the background of the change agent and the change environment. Rogers's theory has five phases: Phase 1, awareness, corresponds to Lewin's unfreezing phase; phase 2, interest, phase 3, evaluation, and phase 4, trial, correspond to Lewin's moving phase. Phase 5, adoption, corresponds to the refreezing phase. In the adoption phase the change is accepted or rejected. If accepted, it requires interest and commitment.[63]

Rogers's theory depends on five factors for success. These factors are as follows:[64]

1. The change must have the relative advantage of being better than existing methods.
2. It must be compatible with existing values.
3. It must have complexity—more complex ideas persist even though simple ones get implemented more easily.
4. It must have divisibility—change is introduced on a small scale.
5. It must have communicability—the easier the change is to describe, the more likely it is to spread.

Havelock's Theory

Havelock's theory is another modification of Lewin's theory, expanded to six elements. The first three correspond to unfreezing, the next two to moving, and the sixth to refreezing. Havelock's phases are as follows:[65]

1. Building a relationship.
2. Diagnosing the problem.
3. Acquiring the relevant resources.
4. Choosing the solution.
5. Gaining acceptance.
6. Stabilization and self-renewal.

Lippitt's Theory

Lippitt added a seventh phase to Lewin's original theory. The seven phases of his theory of the change process are as follows:[66]

- Phase 1: Diagnosing the problem. The nurse as change agent looks at all possible ramifications and involves those who will be affected. Group meetings are held to win the commitment of others. To ensure success, key people in top management and policy-making roles are involved.
- Phase 2: Assessing the motivation and capacity for change. Possible solutions are determined, and the pros and cons of each are forecast. Consideration is given to implementation methods, roadblocks, factors motivating people, driving forces, and facility forces. Assessment considers financial aspects, organizational aspects, structure, rules and regulations, organizational culture, personalities, power, authority, and the nature of the organization. During this phase the change agent coordinates activities among a number of small groups.

- Phase 3: Assessing the change agent's motivation and resources. The change agent can be external or internal to the organization or division. An external change agent may have fewer bases but must have expert credentials. An internal change agent, however, knows the people. The process could involve both. The change agent must have a genuine desire to improve the situation, knowledge of interpersonal and organizational approaches, experience, dedication, and a personality to suit the situation. The change agent should be objective, flexible, and accepted by all.
- Phase 4: Selecting progressive change objectives. The change process is defined, a detailed plan is made, timetables and deadlines are set, and responsibility is assigned. The change is implemented for a trial period and evaluated.
- Phase 5: Choosing the appropriate role of the change agent. The change agent will be active in the change process, particularly in handling personnel and facilitating the change. The change agent will deal with conflict and confrontation.
- Phase 6: Maintaining the change. During this phase emphasis is on communication, with feedback on progress. The change is extended in time. A large change may require a new power structure.
- Phase 7: Terminating the helping relationship. The change agent withdraws at a specified date after setting a written procedure or policy to perpetuate the change. The agent remains available for advice and reinforcement.

Exhibit 4-2 compares these theories.

It should be noted that all five theories are similar to the problem-solving process itself, indicating that the latter could be used to implement planned change. The nurse manager should select the theory he or she feels most comfortable with after identifying the change to be made. A management plan is then made to cover the phases of making the change. The planning phase requires gathering data to support a decision for change. To set objectives, the nurse manager would work with the nursing staff who will be affected by the change. Thus, the entire group becomes aware of and interested in the need for change. A relationship is built between the nurse manager and nursing employees. The plan can then become an opportunity made cooperatively, implemented by an enthusiastic group, and evaluated and maintained by the group. Decision making is implemented by planned change.

Spradley's Model

Spradley has developed an eight-step model based on Lewin's theory. She indicates that planned change must be constantly monitored to develop a fruitful relationship between the change agent and the change system. Following are the eight basic steps of the Spradley model:[67]

1. Recognize the symptoms. There is evidence that something needs changing.
2. Diagnose the problem. Gather and analyze data to discuss the cause. Consult with the staff. Read appropriate materials.
3. Analyze alternative solutions. Brainstorm. Assess the risks and the benefits. Set a time, plan resources, and look for obstacles.
4. Select the change. Choose the option most likely to succeed that is affordable. Identify the driving and opposing forces, using challenges that include assimilation of the opposition.
5. Plan the change. This will include specific, measurable objectives, actions, a timetable, resources, budget,

EXHIBIT 4-2
Comparison of Change Theories

REDDIN	LEWIN	ROGERS	HAVELOCK	LIPPITT
1. Diagnosis	1. Unfreezing	1. Awareness	1. Building a relationship	1. Diagnosing the problem
2. Mutual objective setting	2. Moving	2. Interest	2. Diagnosing the problem	2. Assessing motivation and capacity for change
3. Group emphasis	3. Refreezing	3. Evaluation	3. Acquiring the relevant resources	3. Assessing change agent's motivation and resources
4. Maximum information		4. Trial	4. Choosing the solution	4. Selecting progressive change objective
5. Discussion of implementation		5. Adoption	5. Gaining acceptance	5. Choosing the appropriate role of the change agent
6. Use of ceremony and ritual			6. Stabilization and self-renewal	6. Maintaining change
7. Resistance interpretation				7. Terminating the helping relationship

an evaluation method such as the Program Evaluation Review Technique (PERT), and a plan for resistance management and stabilization.

6. Implement the change. Plot the strategy. Prepare, involve, train, assist, and support those who will be affected by the change.
7. Evaluate the change. Analyze achievement of objectives and audit.
8. Stabilize the change. Refreeze; monitor until stable.

In a study of a nursing center for the community elderly, results showed that the use of change theory could determine a client's readiness to change health behaviors.[68]

The New Management Theory

Dunphy and Stace describe a differentiated contingency model for organizational change. It includes two contrasting theories of change (incremental and transformational) and two contrasting methods of change (participation and coercion).

Incremental change assumes that the effective manager moves the organization forward in small, logical steps. The long time frame plus the sharing of information increases confidence among employees and reduces the organization's dependence on outsiders to provide the impetus and momentum for change. The incremental model is similar to the systems approach to change and organizational development. It is used when the organization is ready for predicted future environmental conditions, but adjustments are needed in mission, strategy, structure, and/or internal processes.[69]

An organization may require transformational change on a large scale when there is environmental "creep," organizational "creep," diversification, acquisition, merger, shutdowns, industry reorganization, or major technological breakthroughs. Transformational strategies embody large-scale adjustments in strategy, structure, and process requirements.

Participative methods of change are used to overcome work force resistance. Coercive methods are authoritarian and use force. The contingency model uses a mixture of methods as dictated by conditions.[70]

The new theory of management is one of transformation or change. Today the fundamental sources of wealth are knowledge and communication, not natural resources and physical labor. Change means opportunity and danger. Information technology and the computer are the enablers of productivity. Customers have much more power; computers have replaced middle managers. Success requires quick responses to changing circumstances. Organizational design should be reconfigurable on an annual, monthly, weekly, daily, or hourly basis. Organizations should be able to develop new products rapidly, have flexible production systems, and use team-based incentives. Big companies are outsourcing many functions and paying for intellectual labor. Intellectual assets—networks and databases—have replaced physical assets. The most valuable devices will help people cope with change.[71]

Management theory is going through a massive transformation, referred to in management literature as a revolution. The new theory of change process has three steps:

1. The awakening. This is when the need for change is realized. During step 1 the leadership articulates why the change is necessary.
2. Envisioning. This is a group effort that addresses technical, political, and cultural resistance. During step 2, resistance is dealt with. There will be technical resistance, political resistance related to resource allocation and powerful coalitions, and cultural resistance related to the chain of command, media, and training.
3. Re-architecting. This eliminates boundaries and compartments. To get rid of boundaries or ceilings, the hierarchy is de-layered, perks for executives are reduced, and gain-sharing incentive systems are broadened. To get rid of horizontal boundaries or internal walls, cross-functional teams, project teams, and partnership are used. To get rid of external boundaries, alliances are created, customer satisfaction is measured, and teams are built with customers and suppliers.

Leadership skills for the change include the following:[72]

1. Identify changes in the environment that will affect the business.
2. Lead others to overcome fear and uncertainty in making change.
3. Visualize the business through the eyes of the customer.
4. Have a clear vision of the future of the business.
5. Assume responsibility for own mistakes.
6. Build coalition and network across organizational lines to achieve important goals.
7. Lead the change.

Transformation is the process of reinventing an organization. Leaders create an atmosphere of continual change. Evaluation is done by peers, superiors, and subordinates. Transformed organizations have no boundaries; employees work up and down the hierarchy, across functions and geography, and with suppliers and customers. Goals center on numbers, total quality, and unity. Celebration is crucial, with emphasis on teamwork and using people's brains, imagination, and dedication. Let the team map the work to do it better and faster. The transformational manager views any process as susceptible to improvement. Reorganization focuses on customer segments and needs.[73]

In this transformation, leadership requires courage, judgment, and visibility. It requires a burning desire to change as health care organizations move to meet a world standard of quality. Managers need to motivate, empower, and educate employees. Managers may practice seven steps to being the best:[74]

1. Determine the world standard in every part of the process of providing care.
2. Use process mapping for the system's parts. Redesign to get rid of inefficiencies. Survey customers.
3. Communicate with your employees as though your life depended on it.
4. Distinguish what needs to be done from how hard it is to do it.
5. Set stretch targets. Let people decide how to reach them. Do not punish.
6. Never stop.
7. Pay attention to your inner self: recreation.

The Change Agent

As one studies change theory, one notes that its application tends to mimic the problem-solving process. The nurse, operating as a change agent, uses change theory to identify and solve problems. This nurse learns to anticipate impending change, including that arising from interdependent systems, responds to change, and takes action to direct its course.

Nurses can compete successfully in the world of health care by doing things a new way. Professional nurses are expected to have the vision to change things and to be change agents.[75]

Examples of the Application of Change Theory

Retrenchments involving layoffs do not always use appropriate change theory. As a consequence, considerable unnecessary pressures, including unfavorable publicity, are placed on nurses. The organizational climate becomes tense and disruptive and gives personnel a sense of loss of security. Nurse executives feel tired and drained.

Causes of such problems include policies and plans that are developed after the fact, with few policies developed to deal with employees remaining with the organization. The media can be used to inform the public of changes in the health care system that necessitated the layoff.

The following are among the positive responses that will minimize resistance to the change of retrenchment:[76]

1. Have a strong orientation toward reality, preparedness, knowledge of human behavior, stress management, and openness and honesty in dealing with employees.
2. Develop organization-wide retrenchment plans and policies with the advice of the personnel or human resource management department and legal counsel.
3. Consider the use of consultants.
4. Evaluate the criteria for layoffs: seniority, performance appraisal, and job categories. The principle of last hired, first fired should be weighed against the principle of keeping the most qualified employees.
5. Have the public relations department (or a consultant) handle publicity.
6. Deal positively with rumors through newsletters, informal discussions, and open meetings.
7. Reassure remaining employees by being visible and available. Make frequent rounds.
8. Do team building with chaplains, psychiatric specialists, and human resource specialists.
9. Form a nurse manager support group that includes families, friends, colleagues, and nonnursing professional peers.
10. Be fair and honest and handle people with dignity and care.

Transformational change brings radical change to the mission, structure, and culture of an organization. This change may be managed with consultation and employee participation. The nurse manager should keep training personnel abreast of organizational changes. Empowerment is a key factor in managing change, because empowered employees become change agents. Some coping strategies are problem-focused; some are emotion-focused.

Employees need time to adjust to change, sometimes as long as several years. They can use this time to learn new skills and should become well trained. If they are to leave the organization, they need time to prepare résumés and do a job search. All employees should be treated with respect and concern. Whenever possible, change should give employees choices.[77]

Resistance to Change

Resistance to change, or attempting to maintain the status quo when efforts are being made to alter it, is a common response. Change evokes stress that in turn evokes resistance.

Resistance is often based on a threat to the security of the individual, as change upsets an established pattern of behavior. If the problem-solving approach is used, answers should be provided to questions about the impact of the change, including the following:

- Will the change affect the work standard and subsequent employment, promotion, and raises?
- Will it mean an increased work load at an accelerated pace?
- Do employees visualize how they will fit into the picture if this change occurs?

In-service education and continuing education may help provide the answers.

Factors that stimulate resistance to change include habits, complacency, fear of disorganization, set patterns of response to change, conservatism, perceived loss of power, ego involvement, insecurity, perceived loss of current or meaningful personal relationships, and perceived lack of rewards.[78]

People are afraid of change because of lack of knowledge, prejudices resulting from a lifetime of personal experience and exposure to others, and fear of the need for greater effort or a higher degree of difficulty.

People have developed fears, biases, and social inhibitions from the cultural environment in which they live. Since they cannot be separated from these cultural factors, it is necessary to find ways of managing them within a system.

Barriers to change include a perception of implied criticism. "You are changing the system because you don't like the way I do it." Employees perceive that machines and systems are replacing them or making their jobs less interesting. For example, a programmed system could be used by patients to take their own nursing histories.

Change may demand the investment of a great deal of time and effort in relearning. If nurses are to be independent practitioners, what happens to those who are not prepared? "Probably the greatest single personal barrier is that individuals do not understand or refuse to accept the reasons for the change or the need for it. Unfortunately, it is not always easy to equate the reasons and the needs and to communicate them in meaningful and compelling language."[79]

People are members of a social system in a community and will resist change if it affects that social system. Social changes that threaten social customs, values, self-esteem, and security are resisted more than technical changes. One member of the social system may influence others even if that person is unaffected by the change.

Other causes of resistance to change include time and pace; different generations of nurses have different rates of change.

Values and Beliefs

Cognitive frameworks are based on values and beliefs about the effective means of achieving these values. Nurse managers who value the chain of command, policies, and procedures, and who believe their management experience does not need input from clinical nurses, may not look for problems needing change. So long as they are successful, these nurse managers are strengthened by success that builds their self-respect. This success fosters resistance to any change that threatens the integrity of the framework. People resist discarding their own ideas. Accepting another's idea reduces their self-esteem. They may consider a good idea a unique event to be preserved. Ideas should have life cycles. They shine and then dim and need to be replaced. Ideas need to be considered a depreciable.[80]

Change is affected by the crucial differences among geographic regions. Some regions are more open to fast change, whereas others accept slow changes. Cultural changes are affected by religious or political beliefs. People hold fast to meaningful beliefs.[81]

Gillen claims that change stimulates increased levels of energy, which is called *hyper-energy* and is not stress. Hyper-energy is the heightened drive a person feels in response to a perceived challenge or threat. If not managed, hyper-energy is used by employees to think of surreptitious ways of preventing change. Hyper-energy can be pooled for collective resistance to change. It distracts employees, causing errors and accidents.[82] Skilled nurse leaders bring employees into the change process so the employees do not view the change as a threat. Employees' hyper-energy is then channeled into involvement in the change process.

One reason for resistance to change is that hierarchical, bureaucratic frameworks with rules achieve stability. It should be kept in mind that both individuals and organizations need such stability through continuity in policies and procedures so that recurring needs can be dealt with routinely and problems do not have to be resolved anew each time they appear.

The major symptoms of resistance to change are refusal, confrontation, covert resistance such as nonpreparation for meetings or misunderstandings of the place or time, incomplete reports, refusal to accept responsibility, uncooperative employees, passive aggressiveness, absenteeism, and tardiness.[83]

Strategies for Overcoming Obstacles to Change

According to Drucker, "One cannot manage change. One can only be ahead of it."[84] Drucker suggests that the manager lead change and view it as an opportunity. Change can be led with nurse managers acting as change agents. One of the strategies a nurse manager can use is to hire a consultant to make the diagnosis and recommend programs that will improve the productivity of nurse personnel while giving them job satisfaction. Such measures can include educational programs to improve the areas in which problems exist.

Effectively led change leads to improvement of patient care services, raised morale, increased productivity, and meeting of patient and staff needs. Change is an art, the mastery of which can be exhilarating, refreshing, challenging, and exciting, because it represents opportunity. Change is facilitated when nurse employees are assigned to adapt to changing job requirements.

Collection and Development of Data

Nurse managers need to gather data about work so that it can be discussed, analyzed, and used to effect change when indicated. Personnel, particularly managers, can be educated to make and manage change. They will learn about labor power planning and utilization rather than leave this entirely to the human resources department. They will learn about financial management rather than depend on the accounting office personnel to take care of it. These are areas in which effective strategies can be developed to foster external cooperative efforts among chief nurse executives of similar institutions and organizations within a community. Such concepts can be expanded to clinical services. If a division of nursing cannot afford to use such specialists as a full-time mental health nurse practitioner, several organizations can collectively contract for the services of one. Thus change becomes a cooperative venture.

Integration of computers and automated equipment is essential to the change process, particularly when managers are competing for professional nurses as well as for health care dollars. Within this domain, nurse educators can elicit the advice and skills of nursing management system personnel as impartial third-party critics of the change being effected. These personnel will give nurse educators effective feedback while providing management information support systems.

Preparation for Planning

Planning will help overcome many obstacles to change. Planning will keep interpersonal relationships from being disrupted if persons with common frames of reference are brought together. The planner can assist people to meet their goals while minimizing their fear and anxiety. Fear is stimulated by the external threat of change. Anxiety, which is self-induced dread, is internally stimulated. Planning will help people accept change without fear or anxiety.

In making changes, nurse managers should plan to help people unlearn the old (unfreeze) and use the new (refreeze). Implementation and updating of nursing management information systems can refine much of the unfreezing and refreezing. Often nurse managers help their staff learn the new without having them unlearn the old. This is a major problem in nursing because of the changing role of nurses.

To prepare a plan carefully, the nurse manager should share information and decision making, work for common perception and understanding, and support and reinforce the nursing staff's effort to effect change. Clear statements of philosophy, goals, and objectives are needed in preparing for change.

Beyers recommends that nurse executives be involved in the following elements of strategy planning:[85]

1. Product/market planning
2. Business unit planning
3. Shared resource planning
4. Shared concern planning
5. Corporate-level planning

Nursing in all areas, both clinical and managerial, must consider competition. The patient will go where there is higher-quality nursing care, which results from effectively planned and managed change. Nurse educators should perform market surveys to determine the nursing products and services that consumers want.[86] This activity itself will constitute change and will result in changes.

Looking at the theory of the business of the health care organization and of nursing, what needs to be abandoned? This may include products, services, markets, distribution channels, and every end user who does not fit the theory of the business. End users do not need many organizations to get information; they use the Internet to obtain information on providers and services. Nursing's goal is to improve this information and these services in the interest of survival and progress. The opportunity is with maintaining physical and mental functioning of individuals and populations. Drucker suggests that managers look at windows of opportunity:[87]

- The organization's own unexpected successes and failures, as well as the unexpected successes and failures of the organization's competitors.
- Incongruities, especially incongruities in the process, whether of production or distribution, and incongruities in customer behavior.
- Process needs.
- Changes in industry and market structures.
- Changes in demographics.
- Changes in meaning and perception.
- New knowledge.

Plans will list every person on whom the change depends and the level of involvement of each. Who will oppose and who will support the change? The dominant coalition in the organization and the forces that will stimulate change should be identified and their support enlisted. Appropriate current events should be noted through reading and meetings; those that will enhance the mission of the organization and for which the clinical nurses will claim or share ownership should be highlighted.[88] This activity brings new ideas and new knowledge to stimulate and justify the need for change.

Planning will also require thinking in multiple time frames: changes to be effected in six months, one year, and so on. The nurse manager should identify the trade offs between nursing and other departments, between clinical and management staffs, and within the change process itself, and he or she should list ways to enlist support.[89]

Nurse managers need to be careful not to overplan. They should leave some room for the people who will implement the change to exercise intelligent initiative. They need to be sure that the rewards or benefits to individuals and to the group are carefully communicated. If people want a change to work, they will make it happen. Change leads to real innovation and, although it creates uncertainty and discomfort, requires nurse leaders to have the knowledge and skills to manage it.[90]

Training and Education

The frequency of training and education should match the frequency of change. Nursing personnel will require constant staff development programs to keep from depreciating in knowledge and competence. From initial hiring and orientation, change should be portrayed as an integral part of the nurse's job.[91] Nurse managers should inform employees of the pressures that make change necessary.

Rewards

Rewards for old behavior patterns should be removed after the individuals have been helped to see the reasons for the proposed change. Employees need to see the necessity for the new behaviors and should be given real incentives, financial or nonfinancial. Here is where job standards come in. The job standards should incorporate the new methods or skills and phase out the old ones. To provide an incentive, performance appraisal can be based on the new standards. Time must be allowed and opportunity provided for retraining. Nonfinancial rewards include enriching jobs and encouraging self-development. Such activities can satisfy individual needs.

Using Groups as Change Agents

Groups in themselves are often effective change agents. When the group appears to work in harmony and to have well-understood goals, it may be used to institute the change. If the idea can be planned in the group, it will be implemented more successfully. A group is more willing to assume risks than most individuals are. Planning should make clear the need for change and provide an environment in which group members identify with such need. Objectives should be stated in clear, concise, and qualitative terms. Administrative policy should contain broad guidelines with understandable procedures for achieving the objectives, and these guidelines and procedures should be communicated to the group.

As agents of change, nurse managers need to utilize staff talents by using temporary work teams to solve specific problems and effect change. They need to participate on interdisciplinary task forces and prepare people for job mobility through experiences planned to facilitate it. Third-party critics may help diagnose and solve problems.

The informal group can promote and support change. It can be formed by enlisting the help of a strong leader and by forming a strong group that will communicate its perception of needed change to nurse managers and educators.[92]

Communications

Too often change is announced by rumor when it should be clearly introduced. Since changes split teams and kill friendships, causing productivity to drop, employees should be told about upcoming changes before they become rumors.[93] Announcements should be factual and comprehensive and should state objectives, nature, methods, benefits, and drawbacks of the change. An announcement made face-to-face will be better received.

Discussion of implementation should give people maximum information. The discussion should cover the rate and method of implementation, including the first steps that will be taken and the sequence and people involved in each element.

Ceremonies may be effective in various aspects of the change. They are useful for retirement; promotion; introduction of a new coworker, superior, or subordinate; a move to a new job; start of a new system; and reorganization. When used well, ceremonies focus on the importance of the ongoing institution and underline the importance of individual loyalty to that institution and its positions. They convey that the organization and the employees are both needed.

As change agent, the nurse manager discusses with people reasons for resisting change. When people understand the real reasons for the change, they are not as resistant to it. They should be encouraged to sound off.

Planned change needs to be successfully communicated to all employees, even those who are not directly or immediately involved. Verbal announcements can be followed up with written ones and progress reports. Change occurs smoothly in direct proportion to the positive and democratic behavior that demonstrates management's philosophy and practice at all levels from the top down. Communication includes body language and tone of voice as well as words.[94]

The Organizational Environment

Nurse managers could be more successful if they paid attention to the organizational environment into which change is introduced and the manner in which it is done. Managers need to be committed to a change and to support it by actions that express their attitudes.

When the nurse leader attempts to impose change in an authoritarian manner, people often resist it. Concern for employees is as important as concern for patients. Managers can establish an environment for change by doing the following:

1. Emphasizing relationships with and between groups.
2. Bringing out mutual trust and confidence.
3. Emphasizing interdependence and shared responsibility.
4. Containing group membership and responsibility by preventing individuals from belonging to too many groups and ensuring that the same responsibilities are not given to several groups.
5. Having a wide sharing of control and responsibility.
6. Resolving conflict through bargaining or problem-solving discussions.[95]
7. Permitting job movement to facilitate careers.
8. Anticipating and rewarding change, thus institutionalizing it.[96]
9. Modifying the nursing organizational structure to accommodate changes that provide growth and development.
10. Promoting a can-do attitude.
11. Providing predictability and stability by maintaining job security, sharing bad news early, and shifting concern to teamwork and process improvement.[97]

When the organizational climate changes, employees change behaviors. A desired organizational climate fosters high-quality patient care.[98]

Anticipating Potential Failures

Although preparation is the key to successful change, it should include anticipation of potential failure. Three questions need to be answered before actions for change begin. First, nurse leaders should determine what the risks are and how much they are willing to expend in terms of resources. Second, they should decide who would do the work. Third, they should have a flexible agenda and plan what will be done when it goes wrong.

Mistakes will happen. The importance of the change will determine how much risk the nurse leader is prepared to take. For example, one might risk a great deal and reorganize an entire unit to achieve the goal of having professional nurses perform as case managers. Changes can be introduced in one unit, evaluated, and modified before being extended to other units.

The positive aspect of resistance to change is that it pushes the change agent to plan more carefully, listen with sympathetic understanding, and reexamine goals, functions, priorities, and values. When properly addressed, resistance uses less of people's energy. Other effective responses to resistance are showing respect for honest questions and differences of opinion, altering strategy and tactics, altering composition of groups, and proceeding in an objective, firm, assertive, and nonjudgmental manner.[99]

Managing Creativity

The nurse manager can encourage creativity through interpersonal relationships that establish trust. This requires acceptance of differing behaviors and ideas and a willingness to listen. It requires friendliness and a spirit of cooperation. It will also require respect for the feelings of others and a lack of defensiveness.[100]

Creative nurses produce a lot. They are unconventional and individualistic. Their critical skills are problem awareness and specification, skills that lead to problem resolution.[101]

Nurse managers can plan to nourish creativity in nursing personnel by doing the following:

1. Noting the creative abilities of those who develop new methods and techniques.
2. Providing time and opportunity for people to do creative work. This can be planned during the performance appraisal process.
3. Recognizing those who are masters or experts in nursing work in clinical practice, teaching, research, and management.
4. Encouraging nursing personnel to become involved in new nursing endeavors at work, in the community, and in professional organizations, as well as undertaking other activities that increase knowledge and skills.
5. Encouraging risk taking and acceptance of personal responsibility.

Successful companies hire and keep creative employees who will create and market new products. They keep people by knowing how to manage, motivate, and reward them. Venture teams composed of persons with diverse expertise and experiences usually accomplish more than individuals alone. Human resources planning includes recruitment of employees with this expertise and experience. Venture teams are used by such firms as Motorola and the 3M Company.

Creative venture team members include those with technical skills and people skills. They have members who are practical problem solvers and team players. They include artists, scientists, and businesspersons. They must be decisive.

Successful companies do extensive interviewing before hiring. They then do extensive training. They seek people who are genuine in their desire to create new products and serve the customer.

Performance appraisal rewards risk taking and intelligent effort that may result in failure.

Innovation results in profitability. Successful companies reward generation of new ideas from within and adoption from without. Performance evaluation should help marginal performers do better. Six-month evaluations are recommended. Peer evaluation and feedback are effective.

Innovative companies do technical audits of individual units to rate them on technical factors, business factors, and overall viability. Reward systems include freedom for creative individual research; freedom to fail; fellowships; in-house grants; autonomy; choice of own venture team; pay raises based on performance, not on seniority; three-track career systems—scientific, managerial, and research; in-house promotions; peer recognition awards; banquets; plaques; and letters of appreciation. Reward teams to foster cooperation. Research confirms results. Reward individuals when someone has gone "the extra mile," to encourage the newcomer, to thank someone who is leaving, when someone's contribution has been ignored by the team, to stir up the team from groupthink, and when members differ greatly in their choice of rewards.

Encourage careers through empowerment to raise self-esteem, leading by example, continuing education, and sabbaticals. Motorola spent $60 million on training and $60 million on lost work time to reeducate its employees in 1989.[102]

The Relationship of Nursing Research to Change

The Need for Nursing Research

Although there are many predictions of the coming directions of health care, the future will probably differ from all of them. Nursing research is essential to preparing for the future and for competition within the health care system. Nurse managers should have good information to keep nursing competitive with other caregivers in providing patient care. They should also have the knowledge to be competitive among employers and in a global economy. This requires the development and employment of nursing scientists who are researchers. Employment of these nursing researchers will commit nurses to developing research in managing human beings to their full potential. It is an investment that keeps people, the future human capital, from depreciating.[103]

Nursing research improves nursing practice. A profession grounds practice in scholarly inquiry. Nurse educators will improve the quality of nursing practice when they promote nursing research and the application of the findings of nursing research. Nursing research will validate the discipline of nursing.[104]

Nurse managers, clinical nurses, instructors, and others are often eager to effect change. They like to try something new, to apply the latest technologies; they can do so through the nursing research process. There are two kinds of research activities: those in which nurses are the subjects and those in which they develop their own nursing research program. Real research requires preparation and time.

Nursing Research in the Service Setting

It follows, then, that if there is to be research in nursing, and if it is to be part of the organizational goals, there must be planning. Plans incorporate a budget, a staff, and defined problems for research. Staff nurses working in clinical jobs and management personnel usually do not have time for this kind of research. They can use the results of such research and apply them to their situation to build better health care delivery systems.[105]

A nursing position filled by a scholar will enhance the chances that a nursing research program will be successful. A scholar will have the knowledge to increase nursing research of a high intellectual and professional caliber. A nurse researcher can promote the reunification model of nursing education and nursing service through joint appointments and joint nursing research endeavors, supporting cooperation between service and education.

Nursing faculty tend to disengage from practice because of the numerous demands of their teaching roles. One reason that faculty focus on wellness may be their disengagement from practice. Since nursing faculty are often well-prepared scientists, nursing managers should find ways to budget money for released time from faculty duties. Faculty may then do clinical practice, and the service agency reimburses the school for the faculty member's work. A coalition will benefit all nurses because faculty will be recognized for research activities that keep them up-to-date, and managers will benefit from improved patient care.[106]

Nursing administration scholars will allow clinicians adequate time to develop their projects. They will provide a resource link to help clinicians find research partners with whom they can pursue relevant nursing research.[107]

A survey of nursing deans indicated increased demand for well-prepared nurse researchers. Researchers were most highly needed in the psychosocial and biophysical domains. Also needed were those in health care delivery systems and administration, education, and methodology and instrumentation. All areas of research are important to the profession and the development of its theoretical-base.[108] The National Center for Nursing Research has focused on funding for training in biological theory and measurements in nursing research.[109]

Nurse managers and administrators can improve the use of nursing research findings by encouraging replication of nursing studies, having research findings translated into understandable language, and rewarding nurses for implementing research findings. Otherwise, too much new nursing knowledge will continue to be unused.[110]

Nurse managers can facilitate the implementation of nursing research findings through specific continuing education programs and by providing sources of help in developing research activities, identifying available library services, and using computer networks. They should keep clinical nurses informed on institutional review policies. Seed money can often be found by institutional administrators. Research forums may be held once or twice a year. Research awards are excellent forms of recognition. They are even better when supported by funds for presentation that come from professional organizations.[111]

Establishing a research program in a clinical institution requires administrative support, including funds for staffing, supplies, and equipment. The program coordinator may be established in the nursing division or the research and development department. Goals and priorities need to be established for the types of research to be done: education, administration, program evaluation, methodology, case study, and clinical nursing. A nursing research program requires a budget, funding, and strategies. One strategy may be to focus on research and not be distracted by other activities. Nursing research should focus on outcomes that will have values for clients and for nurses and nursing.[112]

Efforts are being made to use research findings to change nursing practice. Laschinger and others designed a project to use the findings of research in nursing administration. Students chose the area of job satisfaction. They presented themselves as an external consultant team and chose the Conduct and Utilization of Research in Nursing (CURN) model as an approach. One project was to develop a program using research findings for nurse managers in an agency.[113]

To build a nursing research culture, nurse managers should create an environment that fosters it. This can be achieved by using the learning process. Resource individuals are academic nursing faculty and nurses prepared in research methodology at the graduate level. The nurse leaders provide continuing education to promote interest in nursing research. They support this interest with internal and external funding as pay for performance in productive research activities.[114]

The Nursing Research Process

The nursing research process includes both scientific and technical steps. The format for writing up research is a problem-solving one and includes the following sections:[115]

1. Introduction. Includes an overview of the problem and tells why the research is being done.
2. Statement of the problem. An explicit and precise expression of the research question.
3. Purpose of the study. Answers the question, "What is the long-term goal of the research, the ultimate purpose that will be achieved by the findings?" The statement also relates to current nursing concerns and the motivation for the study. If readers of a study cannot determine its purpose, they should read no further.
4. Review of the literature. A summary of the studies previously published and their results and a statement indicating what this study will add. The review should present a conceptual framework for the study, concepts and theories documented in previous studies, and evidence to support the approach. It should also indicate how the proposed study goes beyond what has already been achieved. The dependent variables to be measured and the independent variables to be manipulated should be identified.
5. Hypothesis. A formal statement of the research question, of what relationships are being tested and how they are to be measured. The variables are specifically defined.
6. Methodology or design. Describes the setting, the subjects, method of choosing the subjects, procedures, analysis, and data collection. Measurement techniques used will be those appropriate to the hypothesis.
7. Analysis. A statistical test that measures the effect of the independent variable.
8. Results. Answers the research question objectively. The presentation of results stays within the parameters of the designed study.
9. Discussion. Includes any unexpected results as well as the conclusions reached.

This format can be used to evaluate research reports. Steps 1 through 5 indicate how to develop a research proposal; plans for steps 6 through 9 should be included in the proposal.

The Research Question

The research question comes from many intensive hours of thought, literature review, and reflection. It avoids value judgments and opinions. The research question needs more than one variable. It may be a question or a statement. The researcher begins by getting thoughts down on paper and by writing an annotated statement of the question without concern for grammar, which will be refined later. A literature search is undertaken to find out what facts are known about the subject, including relationships and their level of confidence.

Written abstracts are made by the researcher, including types of studies and categories of variables. The researcher also defines the independent and dependent variables and has peers critique them. Questions answered include the following: Are these variables related so that change in one is apt to produce change in the other? What variables other than the one to be tested could influence the variable(s) to be measured?[116]

According to Lindeman and Schantz, a good research question will meet the following criteria:[117]

1. It can be answered by collecting observable evidence or empirical data.
2. It contains reference to the relationship between two or more variables.
3. It follows logically and consistently from what is already known about the topic.

Lindeman and Schantz state that experimental studies should not be done if no descriptive ones exist.[118]

The Research Design

The research design is the blueprint created to answer the research question. It follows development of the research question, the literature search, and statement of the hypothesis. The following are six elements of a good research design for quantitative studies:

1. Setting. This is the place where research will be done. There must be enough cases or variables specific to the intent of the research, thereby strengthening internal and external validity and the ability to generalize.
2. Subjects. Subjects should be profiled and limited to those most useful in answering the research question. Their human rights will be protected. When there is a lack of consensus among the research community on the relative efficacy of the treatments, the equipoise standard can be used. Equipoise is a standard to be used when treatment interventions confer benefit regardless of the subject's perception.[119]
3. Sampling. This is the method for choosing the sample size or number of subjects. Increasing the size of a sample adds strength, power, and meaningfulness.
4. Treatment. Subjects of the sample are assigned to groups—experimental or control—randomly. Variables are manipulated to increase the difference between the groups.
5. Measurement. Statistical tests are selected to measure the differences between the groups. A reliable instrument produces consistent results. A valid instrument measures what it claims to measure.
6. Communication of the results. Data are analyzed and results reported to others. Findings related to the research question are given first, followed by surprise data.[120]

Research Strategies

Nursing Research in a Health Care Agency

Utilization of nursing research findings is poor in all spheres of nursing. This is improving as nurse administrators establish nursing research programs within their organizations. Once the nurse administrator, with input from practicing nurses, defines the objectives of a nursing research program, a decision can be made regarding the organizational design for it. If resources are so scarce that additional budgeted personnel cannot be hired, a standing research committee can be established. A standing committee will promote stability by maintaining effective protocols and standards. The committee chair should have research expertise.

Since program resources are a determinant of the scope of the research program, the nurse administrator will need to establish a budget related to the objectives. This may include reallocation of money, generation of external funding, or revenue-generating activities by the professional nursing staff.

Budget permitting, the nurse administrator may hire a research specialist, full- or part-time. Sometimes a budgeted position is shared by another nurse specialist. It could be a joint appointment with the college of nursing faculty.[121]

A research consortium can be established as a cooperative venture with other organizations within the community. This can include such organizations as hospitals, home health care agencies, and nursing homes.

Given a larger budget, the nurse executive can establish a research department as a separate cost center. Such a department will have direct accountability and clearly structured authority. It can even be self-supporting. Success will reflect strong commitment and will give increased visibility.

The ultimate purpose of service-based nursing research is to improve patient care through evidence-based practice. Nursing management research will answer questions related to the management of resources used in providing patient care. As practicing nurses become aware of the availability of competent nurse researchers, they will refer research questions to them.

Four phases occur in the application of research findings to practice:[122]

1. Evaluation of the strength of the research design.
2. Evaluation of the feasibility and desirability of making the change in practice.

3. Planning the introduction and implementation of the change.
4. Using a pretest and posttest to evaluate the effect of the proposed change on practice.

Milieu

A University of Michigan study of the Conduct and Utilization of Research in Nursing (CURN) model included participating hospitals with milieus that supported research. These milieus were found to include an active clinical faculty for such resources as undergraduate and graduate students, existing research programs, influential nurse administrators, and librarians. Each facility had experienced, degree-prepared nurses with flexible, autonomous roles that facilitated research. These nurses perceived nursing research to have increased the status and visibility of nursing on both the education and practice sides.[123]

Organizational Considerations

Once nurse administrators decide that nursing research will be a component of the nursing organization, they must plan the program design within the organizational structure. The mission, philosophy, and objectives will give direction to a nursing research program design. Input can be obtained from interested professional nurses at the planning stage. This can be done through an ad hoc committee that defines clear objectives for both clinical and administrative research activities. These objectives can include those for research conducted to satisfy departmental, personal, and interdisciplinary needs of the institution, graduate students, staff, faculty, and others. Other ad hoc committees can be formed to conduct research studies or to evaluate and implement research findings. Their composition will be determined by their objectives and by interest and expertise of participating nurses.

Research Strategies

Protocols can be developed to benefit the entire institution. A hospital-wide research department or committee can include nurses. Such a committee can standardize procedures for approval, evaluation, and implementation of all research.

Staff development programs can support interest in the nursing research program. Instructors can communicate to the nursing staff the relevance of nursing research studies and teach nursing staff their roles. The nursing staff can be provided with rewards of nursing research in the form of money, improved care, and prestige. This will be supplemented with consistent communication in memoranda, study abstracts, literature, references, presentations, seminars, and conferences.[124]

Pressure is increasing to produce research that is congruent with societal need. This pressure reflects the public's view of costs versus benefits and of societal need versus scientific interest. Heads of US corporations indicate that most innovation today is coming from industry rather than from the research community. Americans tend to waste research money. Five major international research priorities are "human resources, cultural concerns (effect of socioeconomic status and culture on health practices, patterns of illness, and styles of intervention), health of women and children, models for delivery of nursing care, and models for education." Nursing research should result in a significant payoff to the public.[125]

Summary

Ability to manage planned change is a necessary competency of all nurses, as it represents viability of the nursing organization. Because planned change is a necessity, nurse managers create the climate for its receptivity by nursing personnel. Change, the key to innovation and the future, has its basis in change theory.

Lewin's change theory is widely used by nurses and involves three stages: unfreezing, moving, and refreezing. In the unfreezing stage, employees are made aware of needed changes. A plan for change is made and tested in the moving stage. During the refreezing stage, the change becomes a part of the system, establishing homeostasis and equilibrium.

Rogers, Havelock, and Lippitt each modified Lewin's original change theory. Reddin's theory has many similarities, and all have common elements of problem solving and decision making.

Resistance to change is evoked by stress from threatened security of affected employees. It can be overcome by planning that involves those who will be affected, particularly if they can see a benefit. Established values and beliefs, imprinting, time perspectives, and hyper-energy all stiffen resistance to change.

The nurse as change agent is the manager of change and thus requires knowledge of the theory of change. Education and training are necessary for nursing personnel who will be affected. Intrinsic and extrinsic rewards are another management tool. Using groups to effect change will help absorb the risks of change; risks are part of the process.

Creativity and innovation are important aspects of nursing that lead to better practice as new knowledge and skills are applied. The result is change that leads to maintenance of a competitive share of the health care market, thus ensuring the position of nursing.

Nursing educators can promote change through nursing research, thus committing nursing to a clinical practice based on scholarly inquiry. Promotion of nursing research effects change through application of research findings. Nursing research can be financially beneficial when it produces more effective and efficient nursing prescriptions.

Change involves nursing managers in many functions of nursing. It requires planning. The organization is adapted to accommodate the changes. The nurse manager uses communication, leadership, and motivation theory to overcome resistance and gain support in making the change work. The implemented change is continually evaluated to keep it working and effective.

APPLICATION EXERCISES

EXERCISE 4-1 In your own words, write a definition of critical thinking. Relate it to your use of the nursing process in caring for clients.

EXERCISE 4-2 We all make personal decisions daily that relate to work, home, family, community, or other aspects of our lives. State a personal problem facing you. Identify the outcome that you want. Determine the means available to achieve this outcome. List the pros and cons of each means, and decide which you will use. Do it!

EXERCISE 4-3 Refer to your daily newspaper. Identify an issue being discussed related to local (city or county) government.

- What are the arguments involved?
- Which do you support?
- What can you do about them?

Debate the issue. Form a group of your peers and do the following:

1. Determine the pros and cons of the issue.
2. Elect a team captain for each side of the issue.
3. Identify the members of each team.
4. Set rules for the debate: decide on a monitor, determine the speaking sequence and length of time each team member may speak, decide whether the team captains will give summaries, determine who will judge the debate, and decide when and where the debate will take place.
5. Evaluate the debate.

Note: If you wish to do a more formal debate, refer to the Freeley and Steinberg book of note 29, particularly pages 310–311.

EXERCISE 4-4 Select a change that needs to be made in managing nursing personnel or in nursing care of patients. The needed change may originate from the results of research or from a notable problem. Decide which change theory or theories to use and make a plan for the change.

EXERCISE 4-5 Ascertain whether your unit of employment has a business plan. If not, develop one with your peers. If there is a business plan, note whether it needs updating, and if so, update it. Will this process result in any changes within the unit?

EXERCISE 4-6 Organize a group of professional nurses to do the following:

- Explore the theory of the nursing business within an organization (hospital, nursing home, home health care, professional organization).
- Identify products and activities to be abandoned.
- Identify products or activities to be developed. Select one for a pilot test.

EXERCISE 4-7 You may complete the following exercise as an individual or as a group.

Scenario: It was obvious to the entire nursing staff of a community hospital that the work load was decreasing. There were empty beds on every unit. Deliveries on the obstetrical unit were down to an average of one per day, and the daily census of the postpartum unit and newborn nursery was four to six patients. Work load and patient census on the pediatric unit were low as well. Rumors were rampant. One was that the pediatric and obstetrical units would be combined. Another was that they would both be closed and their patients would be combined with medical-surgical patients on other units. A third rumor was that the other community hospital was having similar problems and that negotiations were under way to combine several specialty services between the two institutions. It was even rumored that one would become an extended-care facility and that the management of both hospitals would be combined. Worries of nursing staff gave way to gossip among various groups in corridors, at coffee breaks, in the dining room, and everywhere employees chanced to meet, including areas to which patients were transported, such as the x-ray lab, the physical therapy room, and the medical laboratory. Employees were concerned most about job security and institutional stability—whether there would be jobs for all of them and whether the job benefits would be the same if they worked at either hospital. At a clinical nurse managers' meeting, the director of nursing was asked if any of the rumors were true. She stated that the administrator would make an announcement at the appropriate time and that until then the staff should continue with its work. That afternoon the local newspaper announced a merger of the two hospitals, describing in detail the missions and services each would provide to the community. No reference was made to the plans for employees.

Prepare a business plan (management plan) that embodies application of change theory that would be best under the preceding scenario.

EXERCISE 4-8 Scan the previous year's issues of ten different nursing journals and answer the following.
How many articles report research in:
Management or administration? ______________
Teaching? ______________
Practice? ______________

EXERCISE 4-9 Identify a published research study from one of the journals you used for Exercise 4-8. What was the research question? How does it meet the criteria of Lindeman and Schantz? Evaluate the study, using the steps of the research process outlined in this chapter.

EXERCISE 4-10 Identify a published research study from one of the journals used for Exercise 4-8 and apply the results. Use change theory to make a business or management plan for doing this.

EXERCISE 4-11 Form a group of your peers and have each member identify something that can be improved in nursing. This may be a policy or a procedure; a change in a form to make its use more effective; an interdepartmental protocol, such as how tests are scheduled or patients transported or handled; or a change in clinical practice. Using change theory, each person makes a plan for improvement and discusses it with the peer group. When the group decides the plan merits implementation, present it to nursing administration where you work or are assigned as a student.

EXERCISE 4-12 Scan several nursing journals for the past year. Select research findings you would like to use in clinical nursing. Select a model for implementation such as the Conduct and Utilization of Research in Nursing (CURN) model. (See Horsley, J.A., Crane, J., & Bingle, J. (1978). Research utilization as an organizational process. *Journal of Nursing Administration, 8* (7, 4–6). Prepare a plan and implement the findings.

EXERCISE 4-13 Explore the idea of creating a nursing research council. Consider its mission, philosophy, and objectives. If there is enough interest among the nurses in the organization in which you work, make a management plan to launch the council as an organizational entity.

EXERCISE 4-14 Use the Internet to look at some of the practices of highly profitable companies. What business practices do they use that could be used in the health care industry? Pay particular attention to practices related to creativity, innovation, and research. Is there evidence of the application of change theory?

NOTES

1. Wynett, C., Fogarty, T., & Kadish, R. (2002). Inspiring innovation. *Harvard Business Review*, 39–49.
2. Newcomb, D. P. & Swansburg, R. C. (1971). *The team plan: A manual for nursing service administrators* (2nd ed.). New York: Putnam, 136–172.
3. Lattimer, R. L. & Winitsky, M. L. (1984). Unleashing creativity. *Management World*, 22–24.
4. Gordon, J. & Zemke, R. (1986). Making them more creative. *Training*, 30.
5. Gilmartin, J. (1999). Creativity: The fuel of innovation. *Nursing Administration Quarterly*, 1–8.
6. Reinkemeyer, M. H. (1968). A nursing paradox. *Nursing Research*, 8.
7. Manion, J. (1991). Nurse intrapreneurs: The heroes of health care's future. *Nursing Outlook*, 18–21.
8. Godfrey, R. R. (1986). Tapping employees' creativity. *Supervisory Management*, 16–20.
9. Gordon & Zemke, 1986.
10. Van Gundy, A. G. (1984). How to establish a creative climate in the work group. *Management Review*, 24–25, 28, 37–38.
11. Glucksberg, S. (1968). Some ways to turn on new ideas. *Think*, 24–28.
12. Lattimer & Winitsky, 1984.
13. Van Gundy, 1984.
14. Atchley, R. A., Keeney, M. & Burgess, C. (1999). Cerebral hemispheric mechanisms linking ambiguous word meaning retrieval and creativity. *Brain Cognition*, 479–499.
15. Lattimer & Winitsky, 1984.
16. Godfrey, 1986.
17. Drucker, P. F. (1985). Creating strategies of innovation. *Planning Review*, 8–11, 45.
18. Godfrey, 1986.
19. Levinson, H. (1965). What an executive should know about scientists. *Notes & Quotes*. Hartford, CT: Connecticut General Life Insurance Company, 1.
20. Godfrey, 1986.
21. Kleinman, C. S. (1999). Nurse executives: New roles, new opportunities. *Journal of Health Administration Education*, 15–26.
22. Newcomb & Swansburg, 1971.
23. Southon, G. (1999). IT, change and evaluation: An overview of the role of evaluation in health services. *International Journal of Medical Information*, 125–133.
24. Peters, T. (1990, August 11). Lack of curiosity may kill business. *San Antonio Light*, p. B2.
25. Facione, P. A. (1990). *The Delphi Report. Critical Thinking: A Statement of Expert Consensus for Purposes of Educational Assessment and Instruction* (Executive Summary). Milbrae, CA: The California Academic Press, 2.
26. Scheffer, B. K. & Rubenfeld, M. G. (2000). A consensus statement on critical thinking. *Journal of Nursing Education*, 352–359.
27. Simpson, E. & Courtney, M. (2000). Critical thinking in nursing education: Literature review. *International Journal of Nursing Practice*, *8*, 89–98.
28. Ibid.
29. Freeley, A. J. & Steinberg, D. L. (1999). *Argumentation and Debate* (10th ed.). Belmont, CA: Wadsworth, 1–3.

30. Ibid., p. 8.
31. Ibid., p. 9–12.
32. Jones, S. A. & Brown, L. N. (1993). Alternative views on defining critical thinking through the nursing process. *Holistic Nurse Practitioner*, 71–76.
33. Scheffer & Rubenfeld, 2000.
34. Scheffer & Rubenfeld, 2000.
35. Brooks, K. L. & Shepherd, J. M. (1992). Professionalism versus critical thinking abilities of senior nursing students in four types of nursing curricula. *Journal of Professional Nursing*, 87–95.
36. Bowles, K. (2000). The relationship of critical-thinking skills and the clinical-judgement skills of baccalaureate nursing students. *Journal of Nursing Education*, 373–376.
37. McCarthy, P., Schuster, P., Zehr, P., & McDougal, D. (1999). Evaluation of critical thinking in a baccalaureate nursing program. *Journal of Nursing Education*, 142–144.
38. May, B. A., Edell, V., Butell, S., Doughty, J., & Langford, C. (1999). Critical thinking and clinical competence: A study of their relationship in BSN seniors. *Journal of Nursing Education*, 100–110.
39. Bell, M. & Procter, S. (1998). Developing nurse practitioners to develop practice: The experience of nurses working on a nursing development unit. *Journal of Nursing Management*, 61–69.
40. Steffy, B. D. & Grimes, A. J. (1986). A critical theory of organizational science. *Academy of Management Review*, 332–336.
41. Kemp, V. H. (1985). Concept analysis as a strategy for promoting critical thinking. *Journal of Nursing Education*, 382–384.
42. Graduate students in the master's program in nursing management at Louisiana State University School of Nursing, New Orleans, LA, Fall 1993.
43. Woods, J. H. (1993). Affective learning: One door to critical thinking. *Holistic Nurse Practitioner*, 64–70.
44. McKenzie, L. (1992). Critical thinking in health care supervision. *Health Care Supervisor*, 2.
45. Naisbitt, J. (1999). *High Tech High Touch*. New York: Broadway Books, 24–26.
46. Bos, S. (1998). Perceived benefits of peer leadership as described by junior baccalaureate nursing students. *Journal of Nursing Education*, 189–191.
47. Taylor, K. L. & Care, W. D. (1999). Nursing education as cognitive apprenticeship: A framework for clinical education. *Nurse Educator*, 31–36.
48. Reddin, W. J. (1969). How to change things. *Executive*, 22–26.
49. Spradley, B. W. (1980). Managing change creatively. *The Journal of Nursing Administration*, 32–37.
50. Peters, T. (1991, May 7). Vote for change but follow through. *San Antonio Light*, p. B2.
51. Williams, E. G. (1969). Changing systems and behavior. *Business Horizons*, 53–58.
52. Kanter, R. M. (1989). *When Giants Learn to Dance*. New York: Simon & Schuster, 9–26.
53. Nadler, D. A. & Tushman, M. L. (1989). Organizational frame bending: Principles for managing reorganization. *Executive*, 194–204.
54. Peters, T. (1991, November 19). Winds of change hit central staffs. *San Antonio Light*, p. E3.
55. Covin, T. J. & Kilmann, R. H. (1990). Participant perceptions of positive and negative influences on large-scale change. *Group & Organizational Studies*, 233–248.
56. Brynildsen, R. D. & Wickes, T. A. (1970). Agents of changes. *Automation*.
57. Porter-O'Grady, T. (1986). *Creative nursing administration: Participative management in the 21st century*. Norcross, GA: AffiliatedDynamics, Inc, 109.
58. Reddin, 1969.
59. Ibid.
60. Spradley, 1980; Welch, L. B. (1979). Planned change in nursing: The theory. *Nursing Clinics of North America*, 307–321.
61. Ibid.
62. Ibid.
63. Welch, 1979.
64. Ibid.
65. Ibid.; Oates, K. (1997). Models of planned change and research utilization applied to product evaluation. *Clinical Nurse Specialist*, 270–273.
66. Welch, 1979.
67. Spradley, 1980.
68. Kreidler, C. M., Campbell, J., Lanik, G., Gray, V. R., & Conrad, M. A. (1994). Community elderly: A nursing center's use of change theory as a model. *Journal of Gerontological Nursing*, 25–30.
69. Dunphy, D. C. & Stace, D. A. (1988). Transformational and coercive strategies for planned organizational change: Beyond the O. D. model. *Organizational Studies*, *9*(3), 317–334.
70. Ibid.
71. Stewart, T. A. (1993). Welcome to the revolution. *Fortune*, 66–80.
72. Tichy, N. M. (1993). Revolutionize Your company. *Fortune*, 114–118.
73. A master class in radical change. (1993). *Fortune*, 82–96.
74. Ibid.
75. Roach, J. V. (1988, April 4). U.S. business: Time to seize the day. *Newsweek*, 10; Beyers, M. (1984). Getting on top of organizational change: Part 1, process and development. *Journal of Nursing Administration*, 32–39; Freed, D. H. (1998). Please don't shoot me: I'm only the change agent. *Health Care Supervision*, 56–61.
76. Feldman, J. & Daly-Gawenda, D. (1985). Retrenchment: How nurse executives cope. *Journal of Nursing Administration*, 31–37.
77. Rosenberg, D. (1993). Eliminating resistance to change. *Security Management*, 20–21.
78. Williams, 1969.
79. Ward, M. J. & Moran, S. G. (1984). Resistance to change: Recognize, respond, overcome. *Nursing Management*, 30–33.
80. Hunt, R. E. & Rigby, M. K. (1984). Easing the pain of change. *Management Review*, 41–45.
81. Ibid.
82. Gillen, D. J. (1986). Harvesting the energy from change anxiety. *Supervisory Management* , 40–43.
83. Ward & Moran, 1984.
84. Drucker, P. F. (1999). *Management challenges for the 21st century*. New York: HarperCollins, 73.
85. Beyers, M. (1984). Getting on top of organizational change. Part 2. Trends in nursing service. *Journal of Nursing Administration*, *14*(11), 31–37.
86. Ibid.
87. Drucker, 1999.
88. Beyers, 1984; Gillen, 1986.
89. Gillen, 1986.
90. McPhail, G. (1997). Management of change: An essential skill for nursing in the 1990s. *Journal of Nursing Management*, 199–205.
91. Hunt & Rigby, 1984.
92. Ward & Moran, 1984.
93. Report on Victor E. Dowling's change theory, "How to wage the war on change." (1990). *Electrical World*, 38–39.
94. Levick, D. (1996). How do you communicate? Managing the change process. *Physician Executive*, 26–29.

95. Endres, R. E. (1972). Successful management of change. *Notes & Quotes*, 3.
96. Hunt & Rigby, 1984.
97. Report on Victor E. Dowling's change theory, 1990.
98. Beyers, 1984.
99. Ward & Moran, 1984.
100. Van Gundy, A. G. (1984). How to establish a creative climate in the work group. *Management Review*, *73*, 24–25, 28, 37–38.
101. Gordon, J. & Zemke, R. (1986). Making them more creative. *Training*, *23*(5), 30–34.
102. Gupta, A. K. & Singhal, A. (1993). Managing human resources for innovation and creativity. *Resource Technology Management*, *36*, 41–48.
103. Horton, T. R. (1987, October 5). Poised for tomorrow. *Newsweek*, S-4.
104. McClure, M. L. (1981). Promoting practice-based research: A critical need. *Journal of Nursing Administration*, 66–70; American Hospital Association (AHA). (1985). *Strategies: Integration of nursing research into the practice setting*. Chicago: AHA Nurse Executive Management Strategies.
105. Swansburg, R. C. (1968). *Management of patient care services*. St. Louis, MO: C. V. Mosby, 334.
106. McClure, 1981.
107. Krone, K. P. & Loomis, M. E. (1982). Developing practice-relevant research: A model that worked. *Journal of Nursing Administration*, 38–41.
108. Sherwen, L. N., Bevil, C. A., Adler, D., & Watson, P. G. (1993). Educating for the future: A national survey of nursing deans about need and demand for nurse researchers. *Journal of Professional Nursing*, 195–203.
109. Cowan, M. J., Heinrich, J., Lucas, H., Sigmon, H., & Hinshaw, A. S. (1993). Integration of biological and nursing sciences: A 10-year plan to enhance research and training. *Research in Nursing & Health*, *16*(1), 3–9.
110. Bock, L. R. (1990). From research to utilization: Bridging the gap. *Nursing Management*, 50–51.
111. Krouse, H. J. & Holloran, S. D. (1992). Nurse managers and clinical nursing research. *Nursing Management*, 62–64; Retsas, A. (2000). Barriers to using research evidence in nursing practice. *Journal of Advanced Nursing*, 599–606.
112. Marchette, L. (1985). Developing a productive nursing research program in a clinical institution. *Journal of Nursing Administration*, 25–30.
113. Laschinger, C. A., Foran, S., Jones, B., Perkin, K., & Boran, P. (1993). Research utilization in nursing administration: A graduate learning experience. *Journal of Nursing Administration*, *23*(2), 32–35.
114. Polk, G. C. (1989). Building a nursing research culture. *Journal of Psychosocial Nursing*, *27*(4), 24–27.
115. Lindeman, C. A. & Schantz, D. (1982). The research question. *Journal of Nursing Administration*, 6–10; Schantz, D. & Lindeman, C. A. (1982). Reading a research article. *Journal of Nursing Administration*, 30–33.
116. Lindeman & Schantz, 1982.
117. Ibid.
118. Ibid.
119. Olsen, D. P. (2000). Equipoise: An appropriate standard for ethical review of nursing research? *Journal of Advanced Nursing*, 267–273.
120. Schantz, D. & Lindeman, C. A. (1982). The research design. *Journal of Nursing Administration*, 35–38.
121. AHA, 1985.
122. Hefferin, E. A., Horsley, J. A., & Ventura, M. R. (1982). Promoting research-based nursing: The nurse administrator's role. *Journal of Nursing Administration*, 34–41.
123. Krone & Loomis, 1982.
124. AHA, 1985.
125. Larson, E. (1993). Nursing research and societal needs: Political, corporate, and international perspectives. *Journal of Professional Nursing*, 73–78.

REFERENCES

Adams, M. H., Stover, L. M., & Whitlow, J. F. (1999). A longitudinal evaluation of baccalaureate nursing students' critical thinking abilities. *Journal of Nursing Education*, 139–141.

Ayers, A. F. (1988–1989). Defined objectives helping management to reach for stars. *Presidential Issue*, 70–72, 74.

Barker, S. B., & Barker, R. T. (1994). Managing change in an interdisciplinary inpatient unit: An action research approach. *Journal of Mental Health Administration*, 80–91.

Barry-Walker, J. (2000). The impact of systems redesign on staff, patient, and financial outcomes. *Journal of Nursing Administration*, 77–89.

Beasley, P. (2000, May 7). Ways to boost creativity in the workplace. *The Knoxville News Sentinel*, p. J1.

Beitz, J. M. (1998). Concept mapping. Navigating the learning process. *Nurse Educator*, 35–41.

Bittner, M. P., & Tobin, E. (1998). Critical thinking: Strategies for clinical practice. *Journal of Nursing Staff Development*, 267–272.

Blake, L. (1992). Reduce employees' resistance to change. *Personnel Journal*, 72–76.

Bolster, C. (1991). Work redesign: More than rearranging furniture on the Titanic. *Aspen Advisor* 6, 4–7.

Bolton, L. B., Aydin, C., Popolow, G., & Ramseyer, J. (1992). Ten steps for managing organizational change. *Journal of Nursing Administration*, 14–20.

Bradshaw, M. J. (1999). Clinical pathways: A tool to evaluate clinical learning. *Journal of the Society of Pediatric Nurses*, 37–40.

Brink, P. J. & Wood, M. J. (1994). *Basic steps in planning nursing research* (4th ed.). Sudbury, MA: Jones and Bartlett Publishers.

Brock, A., & Butts, J. B. (1998). On target: A model to teach baccalaureate nursing students to apply critical thinking. *Nursing Forum*, 5–10.

Brockopp, D. Y. & Hastings-Tolsma, M. T. *Fundamentals of nursing research* (2nd ed.). Sudbury, MA: Jones and Bartlett Publishers.

Brothers, J. (1994, April 10). Some techniques that can help you . . . turn a drawback into a strength. *Parade*, 4–6.

Brown, H. N. & Sorrell, J. M. (1998). Connecting across the miles: Interdisciplinary collaboration in the evaluation of critical thinking. *Nursing Connections*, 43–48.

Buckley, D. S. (1999). A practitioner's view on managing change. *Frontier Health Service Management*, 38–43, 49–50.

Coeling, H. V. E. & Wilcox, J. R. (1990). Using organizational culture to facilitate the change process. *ANNA Journal*, 231–236.

Collucciello, M. L. (1999). Relationships between critical thinking dispositions and learning styles. *Journal of Professional Nursing*, 294–301.

Drenkard, K. (1997). Executive journey: From 1,300 FTEs to none. *Nursing Administration Quarterly*, 57–63.

Dumaine, B. (1993). Payoff from the new management. *Fortune*, 103–104, 108, 110.

Fowler, L. P. (1998). Improving critical thinking in nursing practice. *Journal of Nursing Staff Development*, 183–187.

Golembienski, R. T. & Ben-Chu Sun. (1991). Public-sector innovation and predisposing situational features: Testing covariants of successful QWC applications. *PAQ*, 106–131.

Greenwood, J. (2000). Critical thinking and nursing scripts: The case for the development of both. *Journal of Advanced Nursing*, 428–436.

Hanson, E. J., Tetley, J. & Clarke, A. (1999). Respite care for frail older people and their family caregivers: Concept analysis and user group findings of a pan-European nursing research project. *Journal of Advanced Nursing*, 1396–1407.

Helle, P. F. (1999). Creativity: The key to breakthrough changes, how teaming can harness collective knowledge. *Hospital Materials Management Quarterly*, 7–12.

Ingersoll, G. L., Kirsch, J. C., Merk, S. E., & Lightfoot, J. (2000). Relationship of organizational culture and readiness for change to employee commitment to the organization.

Journal of Nursing Administration, 11–20.

Jones, D. C. & Sheridan, M. E. (1999). A case study approach: Developing critical thinking skills in novice pediatric nurses. *Journal of Continuing Education in Nursing*, 75–78.

Keenan, J. (1999). A concept analysis of autonomy. *Journal of Advanced Nursing*, 556–562.

Lane, A. J. (1992). Using Havelock's model to plan unit-based change. *Nursing Management*, 58–60.

Leppa, C. J. (1997). Standardized measures of critical thinking. Experiences with the California Critical Thinking Tests. *Nurse Educator*, 29–33.

Lesic, S. A. (1999). Using instrumental leadership to manage change. *Radiology Management*, 44–52, 53–56.

Lynn, M. R. (1989). Poster sessions: A good way to communicate research. *Journal of Pediatric Nursing*, 211–213.

Lyth, G. M. (2000). Clinical supervision: A concept analysis. *Journal of Advanced Nursing*, 722–729.

Manz, C. (1990). Preparing for an organizational change: The managerial transition. *Organizational Dynamics*, *19*, 15–26.

Marshall, Z. & Luffingham, N. (1998). Does the specialist nurse enhance or deskill the general nurse? *British Journal of Nursing*, 658–662.

Marszaleck-Goucher, E. & Eelsenhans, V. D. (1988). Intrapreneurship: Tapping employee creativity. *Journal of Nursing Administration*, 20–22.

Massarweh, L. J. (1999). Promoting a positive clinical experience. *Nurse Educator*, 44–47.

McGregor, D. (1966). *Leadership and motivation*. Cambridge, MA: M.I.T. Press.

McGuire, D. B. & Ropka, M. E. (2000). Research and oncology nursing practice. *Seminar in Oncology Nursing*, 35–46.

Merchant, J. (1991). Task allocation: A case of resistance to change? *Nursing Practice*, *4*(2), 16–18.

Munhall, P. L. & Boyd, C. O. (2000). Nursing research: A qualitative perspective (2nd ed.). Sudbury, MA: Jones and Bartlett Publishers.

Muir, N. (2004). Clinical decision-making: Theory and practice. *Nursing Standard*, *18*(36), 47–52, 54–55.

Murphy, F. A. (2000). Collaborating with practitioners in teaching and research: A model for developing the role of the nurse lecturer in practice areas. *Journal of Advanced Nursing*, 704–714.

Noble-Adams, R. (1999). Ethics and nursing research. 2: Examination of the research process. *British Journal of Nursing*, 956–960.

Peters, T. (1991, February 12). Ingersoll-Rand tetools the way it makes tools. *San Antonio Light*, p. D1.

Oermann, M. H. (1998). How to assess critical thinking in clinical practice. *Dimensions of Critical Care Nursing*, 322–327.

Oermann, M. H. (1999). Two-Way talks. *Nursing Management*, 56–58.

Petro-Nustas, W. (1996). Evaluation of the process of introducing a quality development program in a nursing department at a teaching hospital: The role of a change agent. *International Journal of Nursing Studies*, 605–618.

Platzer, H., Blake, D., & Ashford, D. (2000). An evaluation of process and outcomes from learning through reflective practice groups on a post-registration nursing course. *Journal of Advanced Nursing*, 689–695.

Redfern, S., Christian, S. & Norman, I. (2003). Evaluating change in healthcare practice: Lessons from three studies. *Journal of Evaluation in Clinical Practice*, *9*(2), 239–249.

Rempusheski, V. F. (1991). Incorporating research role and practice role. *Applied Nursing Research*, 46–48.

Rodger, M. A. & King, L. (2000). Drawing up and administering intramuscular injections: A review of the literature. *Journal of Advanced Nursing*, 574–582.

Ryan, M., Carlton, K. H., & Ali, N. S. (1999). Evaluation of traditional classroom teaching methods versus course delivery via the World Wide Web. *Journal of Nursing Education*, 272–277.

Schell, K. (1998). Promoting student questioning. *Nurse Educator*, 8–12.

Sedlak, C. A. & Doheny, M. O. (1998). Peer review through clinical rounds. A collaborative critical thinking strategy. *Nurse Educator*, 42–45.

Smith, L. S. (1998). Concept analysis: Cultural competence. *Journal of Cultural Diversity*, 4–10.

Thurston, N. E., Tenove, S. C., & Church, J. M. Hospital nursing research is alive and flourishing. *Nursing Management*, 50–53.

Wade, G. H. (1999). Professional nurse autonomy: Concept analysis and application to nursing education. *Journal of Advanced Nursing*, 310.

Whitley, G. G. (1999). Processes and methodologies for research validation of nursing diagnosis. *Nursing Diagnosis*, 5–14.

Wilson, H. S. & Hutchison, S. A. (1986) *Applying research in nursing: A resource book*. Menlo Park, CA: Addison Wesley.

Zeira, Y. & Aredisian, J. (1989). Organizational planned change: Assessing the chances for success. *Organizational Dynamics*, 31–45.

CHAPTER 5

Decision Making and Problem Solving: Communication Practices and Skills

Linda Roussel, RN, DSN
Russell C. Swansburg, Phd, RN

> Between two beings there is always the barrier of words. Man has so many ears and speaks so many languages. Should it nevertheless be possible to understand one another? Is real communication possible if word and language betray us every time? Shall, in the end, only the language of guns and tanks prevail and not human reason and understanding?
>
> Joost A.M. Meerloo

LEARNING OBJECTIVES AND ACTIVITIES

- Define decision making.
- Distinguish among different models of decision making.
- Describe the steps in the decision-making process.
- Apply the decision-making process.
- Identify ways to make decision making more effective.
- Describe the place of intuition in the decision-making process.
- Describe the steps in the problem-solving process.
- Describe group problem-solving techniques.
- Illustrate the components of communication as it relates to decision making and problem solving.
- Interpret the elements of communication, evaluating the climate for effective communication.
- Distinguish between communication as perception and communication as information.
- Compare communication with feedback to communication without feedback.
- Distinguish among causes of listening habits and techniques to improve listening.
- Distinguish among media of communication.
- Contrast future impacts on communication on decision making and problem solving.

CONCEPTS: Decision making, normative model, decision-tree model, descriptive model, strategic model, cost-benefit analysis, intuition, organizational decision, personal decision, problem solving, communication, elements of communication, communication climate, perception, feedback, information, listening, media of communication, questions, oral communication, written communication, interviews, human capital.

NURSE MANAGER BEHAVIORS: A manager applies decision-making theory and the problem-solving process in achieving the mission of the nursing agency, supports the notion that all communication takes place within the principle of channel of communication, facilitates staff participation in decision making, considers the development and implementation of organizational systems, and specifies resources necessary to implement the plan.

NURSE EXECUTIVE BEHAVIORS: A leader coaches and involves team members and associates when applying decision-making theory and the problem-solving process to achieve the mission of the nursing agency and collaborates in the design and improvement of systems and processes that assure interventions and implemented by appropriate staff member.

Introduction

Collaborative decision making and problem solving are often praised as the best management practices in successful organization. These strategies incorporate staff members' feedback and involvement in the organization and its work. "Frequent, ongoing communication through multiple media is a key ingredient of successful organization change initiatives."[1] Research in magnet hospitals on attracting and retaining nurses as well as maintaining positive patient and organizational outcomes further advances this notion, identifying excellent communication, collaborative relationships, and participation in decision making as assets.[2–4] Keeping patients safe by transforming the work environment for nurses, a major initiative, underscores the critical nature of communication, collaborative decision making, and problem solving.[5] *Nursing's Agenda for the Future: A Call to the Nation*, further strengthens these directives.[6] The nurse administrator's ability to meet these challenges requires an understanding of decision making, problem solving, and communication.

This chapter explores the answers to these questions. Complex decision making is a part of any level of nursing. To function successfully, the nurse must consistently demonstrate the ability to solve problems in rapidly changing and uncertain situations in which indecisiveness or poor decisions are costly. The ability to foster organizational decision making and problem solving is an essential personal skill for nurses. This chapter deals with models and strategies that nurses can use to successfully strengthen personal skills and further develop the decision-making and problem-solving abilities of staff members. The theory of decision making, a required competency for all professionals, is an essential component of the nursing process and the management process. Good decisions require outside information on how other people view the world of nursing and make decisions about their care.

The Decision-Making Process

Definition

Since everyone is involved at some time in making decisions, it may be assumed that innate abilities, past experience, and intuition form the basis for making successful decisions. Decisions are often made by choosing among known alternatives. But what about unknown alternatives? Making a choice is not the only element of decision making. The process, which usually involves a systematic approach of sequenced steps, should be adaptable to the environment in which it is used. Lancaster and Lancaster define decision making as a systematic, sequential process of choosing among alternatives and putting the choice into action. This definition acknowledges natural and learned abilities while providing order and continuity to the process of decision making.[7]

Empirical evidence shows that speedy decision makers are needed in today's environment. Such decision makers consider more alternatives, more batches of options, at one time. They are experienced mentors, or they rely on older, experienced mentors. Speedy decision makers thoroughly integrate strategies and tactics. They juggle budgets, schedules, and organizational options simultaneously. They constitute the winning culture in decision making.[8]

Clinical Decision Making

In the clinical decision-making arena, clinical nurses manage patients' histories and physical data, nursing diagnoses, nursing interventions, and nursing outcomes data to effect therapeutic results.[9] Many decision support systems are available in the medical treatment of patients. Research has shown that a majority of patients prefer to leave decision making to their physicians. This is, however, changing with the widespread use of the Internet, which can inform patients of their illness and their health care and treatment options. Evidence-based practices have also influenced patients' decision-making ability, giving sound information on which to base decisions.

Patients' decision-making activity decreases with age and severe illnesses and increases with education.[10] Information on decision making related to individual protocols abounds. This literature includes decision making about cancer treatments, cardiovascular disease, growth hormone (GH) therapy, triage practices, and computer systems related to clinical decision-making models in general.[11] Nurse practitioners use these decision support systems while developing additional ones. Such nurse practitioner support systems are being studied in relation to general practice.[12]

A review of the literature yields a number of decision-making models. Four models are covered in this chapter.

The Normative Model

This model is at least 200 years old. It is assumed to maximize satisfaction and fulfills the "perfect knowledge assumption" that in any given situation calling for a decision, all possible choices and the consequences and potential outcome of each are known.[13] Seven steps are identified in this analytically precise model:

1. Define and analyze the problem.
2. Identify all available alternatives.
3. Evaluate the pros and cons of each alternative.
4. Rank the alternatives.
5. Select the alternative that maximizes satisfaction.
6. Implement.
7. Follow up.

The normative model for decision making is unrealistic because it assumes that there are clear-cut choices between identified alternatives.

The Decision-Tree Model

Various adaptations of decision-tree analysis are found in the literature; the essential elements described in the 1960s are standard. All factors considered important to a decision can be represented on a decision tree. Vroom arranged answers to seven diagnostic questions in the form of a decision tree to identify types of leadership style used in management decision-making models. The questions focus on protecting the quality and acceptance of the decision and deal with adequacy of information, goal congruence, structure of the problem, acceptance by subordinates, conflict, fairness, and priority for implementation.[14] Magee and Brown depict decision trees as starting with a basic problem and using branches to represent *event forks* and *action forks*. The number of branches at each fork corresponds to the number of identified alternatives. Every path through the tree corresponds to a possible sequence of actions and events, each with its own distinct consequences. Probabilities of both positive and negative consequences of each action and event are estimated and recorded on the appropriate branch. Additional options (for example, delaying the decision) and consequences of each action–event sequence can be depicted on the decision tree. Computer simulations of decision trees are now available and can be adapted to a limited number or a highly complex network of branches involved in the decision making process. Normal analysis of the tree is conducted by computing predicted consequences of all event forks (the right-hand edge of the tree), substituting that value for the actual event fork and its consequences, and selecting the action fork with the best expected consequences. Both the optimal strategy and its expected consequences will be determined. Quantitative analysis in the form of decision trees can be used for any type of problem but may be unnecessary in simple problems involving limited consequences.[15]

The Descriptive Model

Simon developed the descriptive model based on the assumption that the decision maker is a rational person looking for acceptable solutions based on known information. This model allows for the fact that many decisions are made with incomplete information because of time, money, or personnel limitations; it also allows for the fact that people do not always make the best choices. Simon wrote that few decisions would ever be made if people always sought optimal solutions. Instead, he contended, people identify acceptable alternatives. The following are the steps in the descriptive model:[16]

1. Establish an acceptable goal.
2. Define subjective perceptions of the problem.
3. Identify acceptable alternatives.
4. Evaluate each alternative.
5. Select an alternative.
6. Implement a decision.
7. Follow up.

The descriptive model may lend itself well to nurses faced with daily decisions that must be made rapidly and that will have significant consequences. Steps in the model are not unlike those in the familiar nursing process, although the sequencing is different. Readers may readily identify conditions in their own environments similar to those described by Simon and see immediate application of this model.[17] Lancaster and Lancaster illustrated the use of this model for nursing administrators.[18]

Exhibit 5-1 has been developed by Swansburg (one of this chapter's authors) after many years of experience using the descriptive model.

The Strategic Model

Strategic decision making usually relates to long-term planning. As an example, hospitals merge, and nursing departments are affected. Among the decisions that are made are whether to hire one top manager or department head versus two or more, whether to decentralize and eliminate middle managers, and what operational strategies will prevent duplication and maximize the use of scarce resources and provide for their efficient use. Nagelkerk and Henry used a model by Mintzberg, Raisinghani, and Theoret (the MRT model) to design and test the nature of strategic decision making that entails substantial risk. They worked with chief nurse executives employed in 6 acute care hospitals with 400 or more beds each.[19] In applying this model, participants used mixed scanning of general and specific information from subordinates to identify complex problems. To develop potential solutions they gathered facts from hospital documents. They made their selection of the best single solution by "(1) screening solutions using predetermined criteria, (2) identifying the costs and benefits as nearly as possible, and (3) selecting the single best solution."[20]

It was concluded that top managers make these final choices using intuition, formal analysis, and knowledge of organizational politics. In making good choices, top managers do extensive planning, communicating, and politicking.

In this research project, successful strategies for decision making were reported as follows:[21]

1. Building extensive networks of individuals and groups who would provide resources at local, state, and national levels.
2. Searching the nursing, hospital, and business literature.
3. Being knowledgeable and involved in the politics of one's organization and professional organizations.

EXHIBIT 5-1

The Decision-making Process Including Cost-Benefit Analysis

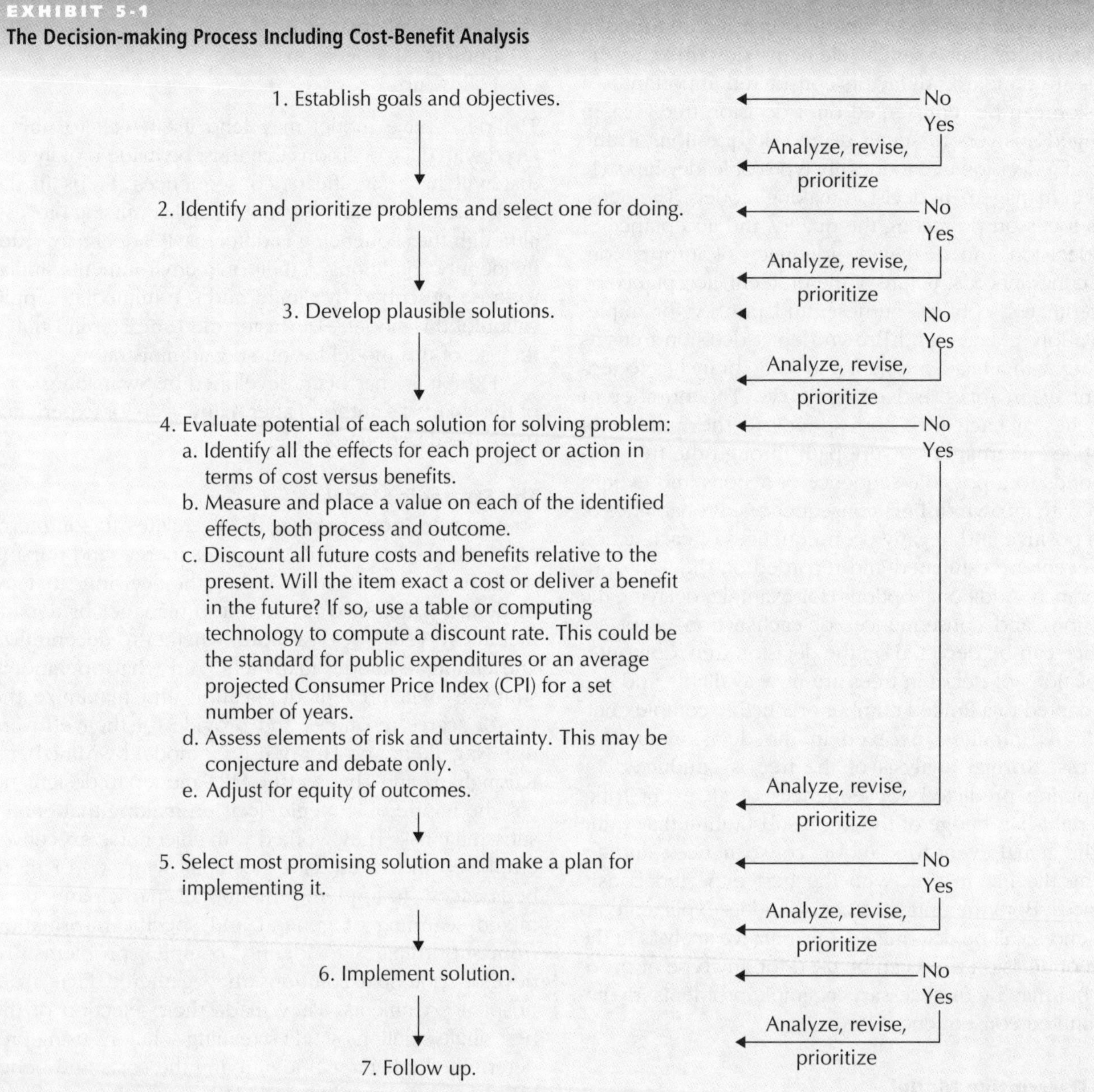

Establishing goals and objectives requires that decisions be made as to how they will be achieved. A first decision may be setting the priority in which the goals will be carried out. Decisions do not relate only to problems. They relate to development of plans and programs to accomplish nursing goals and objectives. When the best alternative does not work, another decision on whether to start over from step 1 is required, especially if other alternatives have less chance of success. The cost versus the benefit of the solution is introduced at step 4.

4. Communicating regularly and repeatedly about decision-making activities to organization members, especially those in the hospital's dominant coalition—usually the chief executive officer, finance manager, and chief of the medical staff.
5. Directing most of their time and energy toward the accomplishment of their plans.

Because the model proved promising in strategic decision making, it needs further testing, particularly in the area of human resource development and investment in human capital. As described in this work, strategic decision making was the domain of top management. With health care organizations becoming flatter and leaner, input from self-managed work teams may be profitable.

Steps in the Process

From these and other models of decision making, seven general steps of the process have been identified. Goals and objectives may be set prior to beginning the general process. They will answer the question, "What do we want the outcome or results of this decision to be?" When new products or services are the outcome, the goals and objectives are established first and problems or decisions are then forecast (step 1 of Exhibit 5-1). (Managers who wish to reverse steps 1 and 2 may do so.)

The problem must be identified (step 2 of Exhibit 5-1). Although this step may seem simple, recognizing and defining the problem is complex because of the diversity of individual perceptions. Because all individuals affected by the problem should be involved in discussing it, authority for decision making should be delegated to individuals at the level of impact. When this is impossible, representatives of various affected groups may provide input. Each representative may have a different perspective as to what the outcome should be. Nurses should make certain that the identified problem is one that requires their attention and cannot be handled alone by those involved. Collecting factual information in addition to subjective perceptions is essential. Logical and systematic fact finding includes questioning all sources for divergent opinions and objective data. When the difference between desired and present situations or outcomes is significant, it may signal recognition of the problem.

Once the problem has been identified, the nurse must then evaluate the potential for a solution and determine the priority of the problem. Reitz suggests three approaches to setting priorities for problems:[22]

1. Deal with problems in the order in which they appear.
2. Solve the easiest problems first.
3. Solve crises before all other problems: A decision will depend on the time and energy that can be devoted at that time. When a high-priority problem with limited potential for resolution is identified, the decision maker may be forced to give it lower priority until more information is collected and acceptable alternatives can be found. The fact that needed information is missing may help define the real problem underlying the perceived one.

The third step in decision making is gathering and analyzing information related to the solution (step 3 of Exhibit 5-1). This step involves defining, through a series of activities, the specifications to be met by the solution. A thorough information search may be needed to validate that the problem has been correctly identified. This search should include knowledge of organizational policy, prior personal experience or training, or the experience of others. Externally, the nurse begins to identify alternatives, comparing the potential solutions to the desired outcome and the desired outcome to available resources. In organizational settings, database information systems may provide this information quickly. Establishing goals with measurable objectives helps focus the search for alternatives. When comparing potential alternatives, one should certainly consider the cost, the time required and available, and the capabilities of those who will be involved in implementing a decision.

Once again, it is essential to involve in these discussions the individuals who will be affected by the choice. Irrelevant, insignificant, and extraneous factors must be eliminated from consideration. Gaining a commitment to implement a decision before the choice is made supports the process. It is possible to reach a point of overload when the searcher has received information too quickly or in too great a quantity to process. Research indicates that the quantity of information sought has a direct, positive correlation with the degree of anticipated risk in the decision to be made. The personal confidence of the decision maker also affects the amount of information required to support decision-making choices. Less searching is required by the nurse who recognizes patterns or similarities to previously encountered problems and confidently makes a choice of alternatives.

The fourth and fifth steps in decision making are evaluating all alternatives and selecting one for implementation. In the evaluation of alternatives, possible positive and negative consequences and the estimated probability of each choice are identified. A common approach involves identifying the best and worst possible outcomes to an alternative and then the outcomes that fall between the two extremes. As each alternative is evaluated, additional options may become apparent. Disagreement may stimulate the imagination and produce better solutions.

The effects of making no decision must be weighed against the effects of each proposed solution. Each alternative must be systematically evaluated for its efficiency and effectiveness in accomplishing the desired outcome and for the likelihood of achieving it with available or obtainable resources. The advantages and disadvantages of each alternative are identified during these steps to determine risk factors in possible outcomes. One should identify the solution that best satisfies specifications before any compromises, concessions, or revisions are made by involved parties. The alternative that provides the greatest probability of an acceptable desired outcome using available resources is most likely to be selected.

A sixth step in the decision-making process is to act on or implement the selected alternative (step 6 of

Exhibit 5-1). The knowledge and skills of the decision maker transform the alternative into action by completing any necessary plans involving sequencing steps and preparing individuals to implement the solution while effectively communicating the process with all involved.

Orton suggests asking seven questions to increase the success of one's decision:[23]

1. Does the quality of the decision really make a difference?
2. Do I have all the information I need to make the decision alone?
3. Do I know what I'm missing? Do I know where to find the information? Will I know what to do with the information I'm given?
4. Do I need anybody's commitment to make sure this succeeds?
5. Can I gain commitments without offering participation in the decision?
6. Do those involved in the decision share the organization's goals?
7. Is there likely to be conflict about the available alternatives?

A final step in the process of decision making is to monitor the implementation and evaluate the outcomes (step 7 of Exhibit 5-1). The nurse compares actual results with anticipated outcomes and makes modifications as needed to accomplish the desired outcome. Evaluation criteria obtained from measurable objectives provide feedback for testing the validity and effectiveness of the decision against the actual sequence of events in the process. Determination of flaws or gaps in the process may assist the decision maker to monitor the process more closely in the future and prevent the recurrence of problems. The effective decision maker consciously follows these seven steps in a logical sequence.

Cost-Benefit Analysis

Cost-benefit analysis has a major role to play as a decision-making tool. Is the expenditure justified in terms of the return or benefit on the investment? Exhibit 5-1 illustrates the addition of cost-benefit analysis to the decision making process. Additional reference to cost-benefit analysis is found in Chapter 11. Cost-benefit analysis should be as objective as possible. Many actions can be quantified and a value placed on them. Others are qualitative and should be evaluated on a rational basis.[24]

Prescriptive Decision Theory

Prescriptive decision theory uses decision-making rules that are more clearly related to the rational modes of thinking (left-brain thinking). Descriptive decision theory, on the other hand, looks for patterns, regularities, or principles related to the process by which people actually make decisions.

The defining attributes of a decision are the following:[25]

1. Making a deliberate mental choice.
2. Taking action based on indication or evidence.
3. Choosing between two or more options.
4. Bringing doubt or debate to an end by committing to certain actions or inactions.
5. Expecting to accomplish certain goals.

The antecedents of a decision are the following:

1. Consideration of a matter that causes doubt, wavering, debate, or controversy.
2. Awareness of choices or options.
3. Gathering information about alternatives.
4. Examination and evaluation of the feasibility of the various alternatives.
5. Weighing the risks and possible consequences of each option.

The consequences of a decision are the following:

1. A stabilizing effect, with an end to the doubt, wavering, debate, or controversy.
2. An action with one of the following goals: to reaffirm the decision with full implementation, to reverse the decision, to stand by the decision but to curtail full implementation, and to consider subsequent decisions in response to ever-changing circumstances and desires.

Pitfalls of Decision Making

Although information technology increasingly affects decision making, pitfalls in the process originate more frequently in individuals than in computers. Individuals are still resistant to change involving risk and new ideas. Such attitudes stifle not only individuals but also groups. When nurses find themselves resisting, they should analyze their behavior with the goal of becoming more imaginative and creative. It is important to move away from becoming authoritarian and controlling. If the nurse chooses to control decision making and omit from the process those affected by the decision, a weaker commitment to implementing the decision is a natural result. When feasible, the nurse may use a team approach to decision making, as in a matrix organization. Group decision making usually produces greater commitment to putting the selected alternative into action and working for success. Team decision making is especially effective in patient care.

Other pitfalls of decision making include inadequate fact finding, time constraints, and poor communication. Failing to systematically follow the steps of the decision making process will likely result in unanticipated results.

Improving Decision Making by Improving Communication

Basic precepts other than those already mentioned include educating people so they know how to make decisions, securing top management support for decision making at the lowest possible level, establishing decision-making checkpoints with appropriate time limits, keeping informed of progress by ensuring access to first-hand information, using statistical analysis when possible to pinpoint problems for solution,[26] and staying open to the use of new ideas and technologies to analyze problems and identify alternatives. Computers can be used to support decision making through databased management systems. Numerous strategies and tools are available to improve decision-making abilities.

A successful nurse is one who stays informed about decisions being made at different levels of the organization after appropriately delegating these responsibilities, who deals only with those decisions requiring his or her level of expertise, who supports implementation of decisions, and who credits the decision maker. McKenzie states that managers who make all decisions themselves convey a lack of trust in the ability or loyalty of their subordinates. Selective delegation of decision making gains the support of staff members and raises their self-esteem. They gain a sense of belonging and develop loyalty. Delegation leads to leadership. Leaders share authority and power rather than impose it. This is not to say that leaders never make decisions without input from associates. This may be necessary on occasion and is acceptable to associates who know they participate in decisions that rely on their level of knowledge and experience.[27]

Wrapp wrote that good managers don't make policy decisions. Instead, they concentrate on a limited number of significant issues, identify areas in which they can make a difference, judge how hard to force an issue, give a sense of direction to the organization through open-ended objectives, and spot opportunities that permit others to "own" their own ideas and plans for implementation. Wrapp's description of the successful manager portrays a motivator, knowledgeable and skilled in both decision making and problem solving, who serves as a role model for others.[28]

Consensus Building

One of the strong points of decision making by Japanese leaders is consensus building. When a major change is to occur, Japanese leaders may spend months and even years gaining consensus of internal customers and even of some external customers such as suppliers. When the change is initiated, all concerned parties have had input into the decision-making process and so get behind it to make it successful. They are stakeholders with a perception of a shared future. Kanter would probably label this a synergy, since it encourages cooperation of all groups. Partnerships among groups require consultation and cooperation. Such partnerships are egalitarian, with members talking about work and its tasks. These members search for consensus on goals that lead to successful outcomes for the corporation, the employees, and the shareholders.[29]

Groupthink and consensus building are somewhat in conflict. To build consensus, one listens to all parties, uses their ideas, and brings them onto the team by involving them in critical thinking and realistically considering their ideas. Groupthink aims for fast solutions with minimal critical thinking and participant input.

The Role of Intuition

Intuitive reasoning abilities have a place in the decision-making process. Intuition is a powerful tool for guiding decision making. So-called left-brain activities, such as analytical and logical thinking, mathematics, and sequential information processing, are essential in decision making and problem solving. But right-brain functions allow people to simultaneously process information, conceive and use contradictory ideas, fantasize, and perceive intuitively. Intuition is defined as the power to apprehend the possibilities inherent in a situation. It is a subspecies of logical thinking and integrates information from both sides of the brain—facts and feeling cues.[30] Nurses who can think intuitively have a sense of vision; they generate new ideas and ingenious solutions to old problems. Agor reported research involving 2000 managers using a Myers-Briggs Type Indicator (MBTI). The MBTI is widely used to measure intuition. Initial findings showed intuitive ability varying by managerial level, with higher ability in top-level managers than in middle- or lower-level managers.

Factors cited by middle- and lower-level managers that impeded the use of intuition included lack of confidence, time constraints, stress factors, and projection mechanisms such as dishonesty and attachment. Followup of the 200 top executives who scored in the top 10% of the first study revealed that all but one used intuitive ability as a tool in guiding decisions. These managers stated that their intuitive ability stemmed from years of knowledge and experience. From this research, Agor identified eight conditions in which intuitive ability seems to function best:[31]

1. A high level of uncertainty exists.
2. Little previous precedent exists.
3. Variables are less scientifically predictable.
4. Facts are limited.
5. Facts don't clearly point the way to go.

6. Analytical data are of little use.
7. Several plausible alternative solutions exist to choose from, with good arguments for each.
8. Time is limited, and there is pressure to come up with the right decision.

Nurses can certainly identify with each of these decision-making situations. It should be gratifying to know that research has supported the use of intuition in decision making. Research findings suggest that decision making in clinical practice is both a rational and intuitive process.[32] Research also indicates "that intuition occurs in response to knowledge, is a trigger for action and/or reflection and thus has a direct bearing on analytical processes in patient/client care."[33] Intuition is based on rational factors of knowledge and experience.[34] However, it is stressed that there are appropriate times for using intuition as an adjunct to the logical steps of decision making—not situations in which objective data are complete. Because basic nursing education stresses the need for assessing facts and avoiding personal opinions, it may be difficult for some nurses to activate intuition for decision making. Agor has identified techniques and exercises used by executives to activate and expand their intuitive decision-making abilities, including relaxation and mental/analytical techniques. A full account of Agor's research is beyond the scope of this chapter; the reader is referred to Agor's extensive writings on the subject of intuitive decision making.[35]

Intuition is observed in individuals and in groups and is a creative and powerful attribute. Groups use intuition to reach consensus, particularly when information is incomplete. Consensus in a group leads to selection of a solution to a problem or to the making of a decision. Intuition can be developed through group brainstorming sessions, group visualization, and quiet thinking time.[36]

The human brain has a specialized region for making personal and social decisions, which is located in the frontal lobes at the top of the brain and is connected to deeper brain regions that store emotional memories. Injury or stroke damage to this area causes personality changes, and the injured person can no longer make moral decisions. This knowledge has implications for behavior related to intuitive versus rational decision making.[37]

Decision making involves critical thinking. As the nurse becomes more expert, the process becomes more intuitive, and the expert nurse automatically processes the decision-making action as a consequence of a high level of knowledge and experience. The decision-making process is fostered by training, feedback, and the expansion of nursing knowledge. Case studies are good vehicles for teaching critical thinking.[38]

Nurses make critical decisions about resources affecting patient care. Resources include staff, equipment, supplies, bed space, time, and patient assignments to staff. Expert nurses make different decisions than do novice nurses. Nurses make decisions requiring intelligence and judgment, personal and professional values, ethics, law, political reality, organizational culture, norms of classes, and economics.[39] Intuitive nurses have clinical skills, incorporate a spiritual component in their practice, are interested in the abstract nature of things, are risk takers, are extroverted, and express confidence in their intuitions.[40]

Organizational Versus Personal Decisions

Organizational decisions relate to organizational purpose; constant refinement of organizational purpose is required because the organizational environment changes. This process provides opportunities for participative management styles, thereby giving subordinates the prerogative and responsibility of professional decision making.[41]

When are organizational decisions necessary? It would be easy to say we deal with professionals who are capable of making decisions related to their practice. An effective manager would not make decisions for competent professionals. However, incapacity of associates, uncertain instructions, novel conditions, conflicts, or failure of authority to make effective decisions or to make decisions at all may cause decisions to be appealed to a higher authority. Effective organizational decisions require collaboration and consultation with those having specialized knowledge.

From an organizational standpoint, decisions may be analyzed on the basis of futurity, impact, or qualitative (or value) factors, and on whether the decision is recurrent, rare, or unique. *Futurity* is defined as the length of time over which the decision will affect the organization in the future and the time required to reverse its impact. *Impact* refers to the number of individuals or departments affected and is a determinant of the level at which the decision is made. When *qualitative* or *value* factors of philosophy or ethics are involved, decisions must be made at a higher level. The last characteristic refers to the uniqueness of the decision; recurrent decisions are made following a rule or principle already established.[42]

But what about institutional policy? Historically, decision making in nursing has been authoritarian, with minimal input from nursing staff, particularly when it involves institutional policy. Nurses have also been limited in their professional autonomy. Literature on the sociology of professions has indicated that a professional person has an ultimate or independent decision-making authority granted by society on the basis of unique knowledge and skill. This viewpoint gives physicians control over nurses. The traditional definition of autonomy no longer applies: patients now demand more input in decision making, and, increasingly, patient care technology requires nurses to make independent life-and-death decisions. McKay redefined professional autonomy as "both independent and interdependent practice-related decision making based on a complex body of knowledge and skill."[43] Primary nursing promotes nurse accountability, intraprofessional and interprofessional consultation, and an assertive synthesis of nursing and medical care plans. Interdependent decision making promotes professional autonomy.

Since nurse caregivers are functioning with increasing professional autonomy, nurse managers are moving into more executive positions in health care administration. Nurse managers recognize the advantages of nurses being involved in strategic institutional decisions such as those concerning major programs, policies, promotions, personnel, and budgets. In addition to enhancing professional autonomy, the involvement of nurses in decision making has resulted in higher job satisfaction, better morale, lower turnover, improved communication, improved professional relationships with peers and colleagues from other disciplines, and higher productivity.[44]

Blegen and others at the University of Iowa studied nurses' preferences for decision-making autonomy in Iowa hospitals. They found that nurses wanted a more independent level of authority and accountability in 12 of 21 patient care decisions, including those that concern patient teaching, pain management, preventing complications, clarifying and advancing orders, scheduling and discussing the plan of care with the patient, consulting with other providers, and arranging daily assignments and schedules. They also found that nurses wanted to make group decisions about such matters as setting policies, procedures, unit goals, job descriptions and standards, quality improvement, and job performance. Nurse managers wanted to increase decision making by staff nurses. It would appear that nurse managers should provide the impetus for more involvement in decision making by staff nurses by asking them what they want and actively involving them. The latter would include training and education. Staff nurses may want decision making autonomy in areas in which they are expert and competent.[45]

Many nurses equated decision-making autonomy with nurse professionalism. Most nurses are nonautonomous since they are not self-employed. Research studies do not always support the premise that decision-making autonomy increases job satisfaction or performance or decreases nurse turnover.[46]

The nurse manager can maximize the opportunity for staff nurses to be involved in interdependent decision making by involving them at all levels of patient-care decision making, especially on interdisciplinary institution-wide committees. Strategies that have proven successful in involving nurses in accomplishing this include decentralization to the unit level, committee systems, and governance systems.[47]

Nurses who pursue holistic nursing practice encourage clients to make decisions about health and health care issues. Decisions about health care policy are not controlled by health care professionals. They are made by the business sector and according to sociopolitical and economic variables. Nurses need to become policy analysts, since analysts use communication networks or structures as strategy to action. Communication with decision makers is crucial to effecting decision making. Nurses use networking and professional relationships to influence decision makers. They arrive at positions on health care policy through interest groups. Membership in professional associations, committees, and interest groups, plus communication with or as analysts, leads to participation in policy decision making and changes in the primary health care system.[48]

Shared governance is an organizational administrative model that has been used as a vehicle for increasing staff-nurse participation in decision making and problem solving. It often involves multidisciplinary groups. Shared governance has as its object the provision of a trusting and nonjudgmental environment in which nurses, along with others, use the decision-making and problem-solving processes to make productive changes in organizations. Improved communication is a product of the shared governance process.[49]

Research indicates that promotion of decision making by nurse managers is a factor in retention of critical care nurses.[50] Research also indicates that increased academic education is associated with better decision making in practice.[51]

The Problem-Solving Process

At this point, you may be wondering about the relationship between decision making and problem solving. The first step in decision making is to identify the problem. But problem solving can involve making several decisions. The best way to define the relationship between the two is to define the steps of problem solving.

Steps in the Process

The steps of the problem-solving process are the same as the steps of the nursing process and the decision-making process: assess and analyze, plan, implement, and evaluate. Assessment includes systematic collection, organization, and analysis of data related to a specific problem or need. It involves logical fact finding, questioning all sources, and differentiating between objective facts and subjective feelings, opinions, and assumptions. Knowledge and experience guide the data collection and analysis of data. Before the process goes any further, assessment should also determine whether a commitment exists to implement a decision or an action.[52] Making certain that there is no readily apparent solution also saves the time of all the people who may become involved in problem solving. Once the problem is identified, it must be determined whether it requires other than routine handling—that is, whether it is a rare or unique situation rather than a recurrent one.

This leads to the second step of problem solving: planning. Planning involves several phases. In nursing terms, we determine priorities, set goals and measurable objectives, and plan interventions. Management literature essentially describes the same process: break the problem down into components and establish priorities; develop alternative courses of action; determine probable outcomes for each alternative; decide which course is best in relation to resources, goals, risks, and the like; and decide on and make a plan of action with a time table for implementation.[53]

When determining priorities, nurses should relate the problem to the corporate mission. Decisions involve choosing among alternative courses of action. They must have an acceptable effect on those directly involved, other areas affected, and the entire organization. Plans should include when and how to alter a course of action when undesired results occur.

The third step is implementation of the plan. The nurse should keep informed of the status of the process because it is unlikely that he or she will be directly involved. This is the one step in the process most likely to be delegated to associates. Implementation requires knowledge and skills appropriate to the specific alternatives selected.

Evaluation, the final step in problem solving, includes determining how closely goals and objectives were met, the success or failure of actions taken in resolving the problem, and whether the plan should be terminated because the problem has been resolved or whether it should be continued with or without modification.

Effective problem solving requires that the practitioner frequently work at a high cognitive level: the level of abstract thinking. The essential difference between problem solving and decision making is that in the former, the thinking process works to solve a problem, whereas in the latter, it serves to reach a goal or condition. Students learn to do problem solving by actually solving client's problems. In doing so, student and client collaborate. Computer simulations are available for problem solving. Students progress through several levels of cognitive problem solving and practice: novice, advanced beginner, competent, and proficient. Interactive videos are available for practice in solving clinical problems.[54] Many strategies are available through the Internet.

Group Problem Solving

While each step of the problem-solving process can be approached by an individual, input from all affected individuals or areas promotes more complete data collection, creative planning, successful implementation, and evaluation indicating problem resolution. Managerial problem solving groups are often formed in organizations, with the expectation that the group's effectiveness will prove to be greater than that of its individual members. Brightman and Verhoeven state that "[a] team of problem solvers has greater potential resources than an individual, can have a higher motivation to complete the job, can force members to examine their own beliefs more carefully, and can develop creative solutions."[55]

Grounded in decision-making and problem-solving skills, the nurse administrator uses expert communication skills to advance the organization's mission and goals.

Communication to Enhance Decision Making and Problem Solving

To answer the question of who is involved in communication, one could simply say, "everyone." However, several aspects must be considered. The first of these is that the person who wants to be heard is involved in communication. For example, the Bantam fried chicken facility wants to sell chicken and wants people to know that it has chicken to sell. Its manager will therefore advertise in an effort to communicate this desire to sell an appetizing product. The manager will advertise through media such as newspapers, billboards, radio, television, and the Internet. All kinds of tempting pictures will be portrayed in these advertisements. If the manager is successful and people buy lots of Bantam fried chicken as a result of the advertisements, then the people have received the message and the manager has communicated to them.

A second aspect of communication occurs when a person seeks out desired information. Suppose a working person is just plain tired of cooking and wants Bantam fried chicken to serve the family for Sunday dinner. That person knows where the nearest store is, having heard or seen it advertised. He or she may have driven past the facility and seen the sign that identify the product. That person may have been reminded of the product in the Sunday paper that morning. Even if the person cannot remember the address, he or she can always refer to the Yellow Pages for an address and phone number or call directory assistance. When a person wants information, there are many sources from which to obtain it. All these sources are media of communication.

Elements of Communication

At least two people are involved in communication: a sender, or provider, and a receiver. A sender usually has something he or she wants to communicate, even if the information is distasteful. A receiver usually has need of some information, whether good or bad. Regardless of the medium, information is transmitted from sender to receiver, and a communication occurs.

Whether or not money is exchanged, communication always involves a "buyer" or a "seller." The buying or selling is based on a need. Sometimes the receiver's need to hear is not as acute as the sender wants it to be. An example of this is the communication between a parent and a child. A parent can tell the child to be in by midnight on Saturday. The parent has said the same thing before, however, and when the child did not return by midnight, there were no consequences. As a result, now the child does not even hear the parent, because he or she has no reason to listen. When the child returns after midnight and is then told that curfew the next four weeks will be 8:00 P.M., however, the child does have a reason to listen. Communication now takes place, because the child finds sufficient reason for listening.

Communication is a human process involving interpersonal relationships, and therein lies its difficulty. In the workplace, some managers view their knowledge of events as power; sharing knowledge through communication is sharing power, and the manager does not want to share. Other managers do not realize the importance of communication in an information age because they are not up-to-date on the advantages of decentralization and participatory management. These managers frequently fall into crisis management, treating the symptoms of poor communication and never identifying the root causes. A third group of managers recognizes that communication is like the central nervous system in that it directs and controls the management process.

More than 80% of a higher-level manager's time is spent on communication: 16% of that time is spent reading, 9% on writing, 30% on speaking, and 45% on listening. Is there any question that communication skills are absolutely essential to career advancement in nursing?[56] Effective communication has three basic principles:

1. Successful communication involves a sender, a receiver, and a medium.
2. Successful communication occurs when the message sent is received.
3. Successful nurse managers achieve successful communication.

Climate for Communication

Organizational climate and culture are discussed in Chapter 6, *Organizational Structure and Analysis*. The communication climate should be in harmony with the corporate culture and should be used to encourage positive values, such as quality, independence, objectivity, and client service, among nursing employees. Communication is used to support the mission (purpose or business) and vision of the nursing organization and to tell the consumers or clients that nursing is of high quality. The media used will include performance, nursing records, and marketing. Communication will be objective when it is accurately portrayed with descriptions of factual outcomes judged on the basis of objective outcome criteria.

Nursing literature abounds with evidence of nurses' desire for autonomy and knowledge that they may use to communicate their support of autonomy. Nurses also may provide a climate in which the nursing business remains as free as possible of political constraints. When political considerations are imperative, the imperative will be communicated to employees, who make decisions based on the institution's values and beliefs.

Organizational culture is more difficult to change than organizational climate, but both can be modified with managerial effort and skill. The first step for nurse managers is to sample employees' attitudes or ideas of how they receive information and effect communication. Managers and employees know the formal structure, including roles and modes of operation used to inform and communicate. What is the informal structure? It involves people who are heroes or role models who can be involved in communication if they are positive and enthusiastic. Otherwise, they may have to be replaced, particularly if these role models are destructive.

Cultural Agendas

Cultural agendas publicize the mission or business of the organization. They tell what the organization stands for and on what the nursing division, department, or individual unit places value.

Cultural agendas are used to communicate promotions, new hires, marriages, deaths, and other news about personnel. Heroes are highlighted with features that illustrate support of desired values and beliefs: the nurse who presents a paper, authors a book, or achieves prominence in the profession or the community; the nurse who is a champion bowler, an elected officer in an organization, or an appointed official in the health care system; and the nurse who is a volunteer in community activities. The cultural agendas also are used to publicize nursing units and special achievements such as ongoing research in burn care or rehabilitation.

Cultural agendas are publicized using various media, including newsletters, memorandums, awards ceremonies, and external communications, such as publications, radio, television, and organizational meetings. Such communications are most effective when they depict the people who are directly involved in the publicized events.

Cultural agendas can be effectively used to change the organizational climate and culture.[57] The nurse leader must establish the climate for effective communication. Wlody recommends the following:[58]

- Step I: Review your own communication technique.
- Step II: Concentrate the staff's attention on communication as a needed skill that everyone can develop.
- Step III: Lead the staff into more positive interaction within the unit.
- Step IV: Make daily rounds with the whole team.
- Step V: Form a group to reduce stress.

To be an effective communicator, a manager should develop close professional relationships with customers on their own turf. Nurse managers can do this by identifying their customers and visiting them. Their customers include their employees, other professionals, patients, families, suppliers, and others. Being a role model shows that the manager cares. Success is ensured through partnerships between managers and front-line employees.[59]

The Nature of an Effective Climate for Communication

Important communication occurs between supervisor and employees at the work level, where climate is set. A supportive climate encourages employees to ask questions and offer solutions to problems. Additionally, a supportive climate facilitates equality, spontaneity, empathy, and respect. Conversely, a defensive climate emphasizes control, traditional hierarchical structures, superiority, and one-way communication. Nurse leaders should strive for a supportive climate.

Although research in the area of organizational attributes has been limited and the results inconclusive, some evidence shows that organizational size (number of employees) influences communication among associates but not between supervisors and associates. The climate is more open at the top, where higher-level supervisors are more likely to involve associates in decision making.

Openness decreases as organizations increase in size, particularly in those with more than 1,000 employees. With increased organizational size, communication increases but is perceived by employees to be increasingly closed. That is, more communication occurs but with less openness. Although a narrow span of control increases communication between supervisor and associates, an increased span of control is not perceived to decrease openness, thus indicating that the quality of interaction may be more important than is quantity.[60]

A supportive climate will produce clear communication to support productive nursing workers and effective teamwork. It will provide for identification of communication problems by designing instruments to collect data during specified periods of time. Real communication patterns and problems will be diagnosed from analysis of the data and can be related to the communication climate and solved by using problem-solving techniques.

A strong relationship exists between good communication skills and good leadership.

Communication problems have been described as a major source of job dissatisfaction. Organizational communication systems are powerful determinants of an organization's effectiveness. Communication rules are organization-specific and are either explicit or implicit. Explicit rules are codified. They govern formal activities such as access to managers or supervisors. Violation of explicit rules may result in sanctions. Implicit rules mimic norms of behavioral expectations and are not codified but mutually shared. Conformation to rules reduces dissonance and maintains stability. A questionnaire may be used to assess communication in six areas:

- accessibility of information
- communication channels
- clarity of messages
- span of control
- flow control/communication load
- the individual communicators.[61]

Negotiation

When disagreements about the intent of a communication occur, negotiation is needed to prevent conflict, resignation, or avoidance between supervisor and employee. Negotiation requires knowledge of human behavior and is based on human needs. When there is lack of confidence between supervisor and employee or among employees, nurse managers can solve the communication problem through a climate of openness that restores confidence through agreement and promotes individual autonomy as well as *esprit de corps*.[62]

Communication and change require negotiation; two basic types are cooperative and competitive. Agreement is the objective in both types. For nurse managers, cooperative or win–win negotiation is best. Nurse managers and employees negotiate cooperatively for win–win outcomes for employees and the institution.

The principles of negotiation are as follows:

- Maintaining self-identity and insight into your own motives, values, perceptions, and skills.
- Understanding others' values without judging them to be better or worse but only different from your own.
- Viewing issues potentially solvable.
- Using personal flexibility in analyzing and reacting to issues and behaviors.
- Using skills to repair damaged relationships, including the ability to retreat and regroup in a manner that allows for perceptual openness.

In the win–win negotiation process, the nurse manager will state these principles so that both manager and employee are on equal footing.

The following are the steps of the negotiation process:[63]

1. Preparing for negotiation (e.g., introducing a topic at a meeting)
2. Communicating a general overview of what is to be accomplished during the process
3. Relating the history of why negotiation is required
4. Redefining the issue to be addressed
5. Selecting when issues will be worked on
6. Encouraging discussion during the conflict stage of the issue
7. Addressing the fallback or compromise for both parties on the issue
8. Agreeing in principle during the settlement stage
9. Recapping and summarizing the agreement
10. Monitoring subsequent compliance of the agreement (after settlement)

During the negotiation process, the nurse manager is always positive in explaining ideas, suggestions, and benefits. The nurse manager actively listens to employee responses, gaining perceptions, identifying concerns, and explaining obstacles to these ideas. The manager encourages explanations and suggests ways of overcoming obstacles. Questions are phrased to obtain doubtful discussion and answers.

Successful negotiators achieve win–win outcomes that indicate progress, maintain self-respect, leave positive feelings, are sensitive to each other's needs, achieve a majority of each other's objectives, and facilitate future negotiation.

Change theory is involved in negotiation.[64]

Open-Door Policy

Communication climate influences the success of an open-door policy. An open-door policy of a nurse manager implies that an employee can walk into the manager's office at any time. Because nurse managers follow schedules, however, it usually is more convenient for both parties when the employee makes an appointment.

The communication climate associated with some organizations has made employees wary of the open-door policy. Line managers sometimes feel threatened when they see their employees in the boss's office. They find out the reason for the visit by any means possible. Some managers punish the employee by telling them to use the chain of command, adjusting performance evaluations, ostracizing the employee, adjusting pay increases, or working to fire the employee. This climate quickly teaches the employee not to use the open-door policy.

During negotiation, a supportive environment includes a favorable location.

A nurse manager who believes in the open-door policy will clearly state the rules, including whether the employee needs someone else's permission to make an appointment with the manager. A democratic manager who believes in setting a climate for open communication will encourage visits. Such a manager knows how to deal with confidential communication to protect employees and their supervisors.

Communication as Perception

In nursing, as in other disciplines, communication is perception. A person perceives only that which he or she is capable of hearing. A communication must be uttered in the receiver's language, and the sender must have knowledge of the receiver's experience or capacity to perceive.

Conceptualization conditions perception; a person must be able to conceive to perceive. In writing a communication, the writer must work out his or her own concepts first and ask whether the recipient can receive them. The range of perception is physiological, because perception is a product of the senses. However, the limitations to perception are cultural and emotional. Fanatics, for instance, cannot receive a communication beyond their range of emotions.

Different people seldom see the same thing in a communication, because they have different perceptual dimensions. Drucker has said that to communicate, the sender must know what the recipient, the true communicator, is able to see and hear, and why. Perhaps if we focus on the recipient as the "true" communicator, we will improve communications. The unexpected is not usually received at all or is ignored or misunderstood. The human mind perceives what it expects to perceive; to communicate, the sender must also know what the recipient expects to see and hear. Otherwise, the recipient has to be shocked to receive the intended message.[65]

People selectively retain messages because of emotional associations and receive or reject messages based on good or bad experiences or associations. Communication makes demands on people. It is often propaganda and so creates cynics. It demands that the recipient become somebody, do something, or believe something. This is powerful when the demand fits aspirations, values, and goals. Communication is most powerful when it converts, because conversion demands surrender.

Communication as perception indicates the value of a stated mission, philosophy, and goals. If statistical quality control (SQC) is practiced, it should be applied to organizational communication as part of the total system and to prevent misconceptions.

Communication is the process by which time management, skills, prioritization, planning, and personal involvement are transmitted by managers to establish an SQC program that implements change effectively. As managers effectively implement SQC, they inspire conviction, commitment, and conversion of their workers. The workers are first motivated with conviction of the desirability of change; they are inspired by the leader's attitudes. This leads to commitment to the change and internal conversion to a personal attitude that results in high productivity.

Statistical quality control succeeds in a climate that fosters open communication among all managers and workers, commitment to employee involvement, and recognition of individuals and the unit or organization. The climate should be nonthreatening and positive.[66]

There is a major difference in perceptions between patients and clinic managers of patients' accessibility to health care clinics.[67] Patients with less education, a history of chronic heart disease, and a diagnosis of stable angina need special followup.[68]

Leveling with Employees

Leveling is being honest with employees. Managers make all information, both good and bad, known to the employees. Being honest gives employees a chance to improve. Managers can control the content of negative information, not by concealing it but by sharing ideas, feelings, and information with employees. Nurse managers address issues as they arise. They focus on employee needs, offering help as indicated. Communication is a major factor in a performance evaluation.[69]

Conflict Management

Conflict is often a result of poor communication. Supervisors sometimes react to employee outbursts in any of the following ways:

- Overriding their better judgments.
- Becoming defensive.
- Reprimanding the individual.
- Cutting off further expression of feelings.
- Monopolizing the conversation.

The result is increased frustration for both the employee and the manager.

Baker and Morgan suggest the following techniques for dealing with employee outbursts:[70]

1. Tune into the real message the employee is trying to communicate. Interpret it correctly, and direct a response at the feeling level of the employee.
2. Determine the nature of the feelings being expressed. Be sensitive to them because they are subjective and express the employee's values, needs, and emotions. Feelings are neither right nor wrong, but they represent absolute truth to the individual and usually are disguised as factual statements. Determine if they disguise anger, frustration, hurt, or disappointment.
3. Let the feelings subside by encouraging venting. Listen and give emotional support, and then summarize what you have heard and interpreted from the outburst.
4. Clarify issues with questions that can be answered yes or no.
5. When impasses occur try linking the ideas or feelings the employee has expressed.
6. Allow the employee to save face.
7. Be sure perceptions are accurate by summarizing them and checking them with the employee.
8. Verbalize your feelings as a supervisor by using positive "I" statements.

Communication Direction

For effective communication, start with the perceptions of the recipients. Listeners do not receive the communication if they do not understand the message. Nurse managers need to know what listeners are able to perceive before formulating a message. Many nurse managers focus on what they want to say and then cannot understand why the recipient does not understand the message.

The information load should be kept to a minimum to help increase communication. Management by objectives focuses on perceptions of both recipients and senders. Recipients have access to the experience of the manager. The communicative process focuses on aspirations, values, and motivations: the needs of the subordinates. Performance evaluation or appraisal should focus on the recipient's concerns, perceptions, and expectations. Communication then becomes a tool of the recipient and a mode of organization for the employee to use.

Feedback

Feedback completes or continues communication, making it two-way. Today's workers are better managed in a climate that promotes theory, participation, or involvement. Most workers are more affluent and better educated than workers of the past, have increased leisure time, and retire earlier—all indications of their changed values.

Feedback is one of the most important factors influencing behavior. People want to know what they have accomplished and where they stand. Feedback works best when specific goals are set to note the improvements sought, measurable targets, deadlines, and specific methods of attaining goals.

Communication requires mutual respect and confidence.

Effective communication includes giving and receiving suggestions, opinions, and information. If this two-way interaction does not occur, little or no communication takes place.

One-way communication prevents input or feedback and interaction. It causes nurses to depersonalize their relationships with patients and families and serves as a barrier between nurses and physicians. It causes distorted communications that result in distorted and inaccurate feedback; scapegoating of peers, patients, and families; emotional blowups, skepticism of all messages; frustration and stress; delay of therapeutic interventions; and negative socioeconomic consequences.[71]

Research on Feedback

Research shows that feedback increases productivity. One study showed an 83% increase in productivity as measured by staff treatment programs and client hours, using the technique of private group feedback. Using the technique of public group feedback, productivity increased 163% in 38 weeks.[72]

When suggestions were answered promptly in a mental health organization of 80 employees, the number of suggestions increased by 222.7% over a 32-week period. In other studies, feedback plus training have been found to be even more effective. A review of 27 empirical studies indicated that objective feedback worked in virtually every case.

A study was done to test the effect of feedback on process versus outcomes of reality orientation in a psychiatric hospital serving elderly patients. Subjects were psychiatric nurses and were divided into three groups: two groups were given appropriate feedback, whereas the third group did not receive any feedback. The nurses in the process feedback group showed "substantial increases" in process behavior over the control group that did not receive feedback. The nurses in the feedback group had increased patient contacts, but it was not determined whether their patients had increased reality orientation.[73]

Innovation and experimentation may be reduced by feedback that causes people to concentrate on process, methods, and procedures. Nurse managers should focus on outcomes or accomplishments that show that clinical nurses have been creative. New ideas as well as application of results of nursing research should be encouraged, and clinical nurses should be supported to develop proposals and conduct new nursing research. Levenstein recommends the following:[74]

1. Be clear in your own mind about the criteria you are using to assess staff performance.
2. Clarify the ends, and the means are more likely to fall into place.
3. Emphasize flexibility in getting results rather than ritualistic observance of rules and procedures.

Successful synergies require leadership, cooperative management plans, joint incentives, information sharing, computer networks, face-to-face relationships, shared experiences, mutual need, and a shared future.[75] Communication is involved in almost every one of these activities. Kanter goes on to say that the communication imperative is that "[m]ore challenging, more innovation, more partnership-oriented positions carry with them the requirement for more communication and interaction."[76]

Information

Although they are interdependent, communication and information are different. Communication is perception; information is logic. Information is formal and has no meaning. It is impersonal and not altered by emotions, values, expectations, and perceptions.

Computers allow us to handle information devoid of communication content (for example, personnel information). Information is specific and economical, based on a need of a person and for a purpose. Information in large amounts beyond that which meets a person's needs is an overload.

Communication may not be dependent on information; it may be shared experience. Information should be passed to the person who needs to know it, and that person must be able to receive it and act on it. Perception and communication are primary to information, and as information increases, the communicator or receiver must be able to perceive its meaning.[77] In the interest of time management, nurse managers need skills that sort information according to its importance. These skills require clear communication and acute perception.

Listening

Communication takes place between employer and employee. To have satisfied, productive employees, an employer must hear what employees are saying as well as what they are not saying. To really hear someone requires concentration. Consider, for example, what happens in church on Sunday: the preacher speaks, but the congregation hears only by concentrating on what the preacher is saying. Otherwise, the people supposedly listening to the preacher are planning next week's work or the rest of the day's events. Many managers do not listen effectively to what employees are saying to them and thus discourage the person who may want to point out a problem but knows that either he or she will not be heard or that the suggestion will have no effect.

One reason nursing personnel find it difficult to listen to a change-of-shift report is that a person can listen 4 times faster than the 125 to 150 words per minute that are being spoken. The listener who is tuned out may not hear a message about an appointment or a directive regarding a patient. As a result, it is usually more efficient for the person to read a change-of-shift report or listen to it on a tape recorder.

Most working persons are engaged in some form of verbal communication 70% of the waking day, or approximately 11 hours and 20 minutes out of 16 hours. Of that time, 45% is spent listening to what will be 50% forgotten within 24 hours. Another 25% is forgotten in the next 2 weeks.[78] If this is true of nursing personnel, they will forget 75% of what they hear today within the next 2 weeks. Some researchers claim that immediately after a 10 minute speech we remember only 50% of what we hear; 25% is considered a good retention level.[79]

By learning the art of listening and observing, managers better understand what employees mean by what they say. They receive cues from employees' words and actions. Managers learn that men and women communicate differently. Learning the art of listening creates a better organization with better relationships and better outcomes.[80]

Causes of Poor Listening Habits

Remember that it is a bad habit to call a subject uninteresting or boring. Listen for useful information from what is considered a dull subject. Sift and screen, separate wheat from chaff, and look for something useful. Be an interested person, and make the subject interesting. Good listeners attempt to hear what is said.

It is a bad habit to criticize the delivery. Concentrate on finding out what the speaker has to say that is interesting or useful. Keep from being overstimulated by the subject. Otherwise, you mentally prepare an argument or rebuttal and miss what the speaker says. Hear the speaker out before making judgments. Listen for the main idea rather than the facts; identify principles, concepts, and generalizations. Facts merely support the generalizations. Accept the face value of the message rather than evaluate it.

Avoiding eye contact with the speaker is a bad habit that decreases trust. Remember that 60% of a message is nonverbal.

Defensive listening occurs when the speaker's message threatens the listener with blame or punishment for something. It prevents accurate listening and perceptions. Defensive listening is stimulated when a person's speech implies that a listener's behavior is being evaluated. Defensive response is reduced when the speaker describes behavior objectively. Speech that indicates the sender is trying to control the receiver evokes defense. People don't want their values and viewpoints controlled and will shut out such messages. They want to have freedom to choose. When the sender solicits the collaboration of the receiver in solving mutual problems, the receiver responds positively.

Receivers defend themselves against perceived strategies to change their behaviors or control them, which they regard as deceitful. They respond to spontaneity and honesty, which they perceive as free of deceit.

Speech perceived as being unconcerned about the group's welfare evokes defense, whereas speech perceived as being empathetic evokes acceptance. People want to hear speech that indicates they are valued. Gestures can also communicate neutrality or empathy.

Communication, verbal or nonverbal, that indicates superiority evokes defense, whereas speech indicating equality is accepted and supported. Certainty indicates dogmatism and evokes defense. A defensive reaction is reduced by professionalism; such speech indicates the sender wants help, information, data, or input from the listener.[81]

Other reasons supervisors give for not listening include the following:[82]

- Employees do not expect them to listen.
- Employees have nothing of value to say.
- Listening is not part of their jobs.
- Employees should listen to them.

Active listening is a skill for recognizing and exploring patients' clues, thereby giving health care providers a deeper understanding of the true reasons for the visit, which should result in increased patient satisfaction and improved outcomes.[83]

The speech-comprehension difficulties of aging persons primarily reflect declines in hearing rather than in cognitive ability.[84]

Techniques to Improve Listening

Improving listening ability can be accomplished in many ways. One method is to summarize what is being said for better understanding and retention. The listener should give empathetic attention to the speaker and try to understand the substance of what is being said; seek to be objective and to apply creativity; go beyond the speaker's dialect, stance, gestures, and attire to understand the meaning of the speaker's words; and try to counter his or her own emotions or prejudice even though the speaker may have opposite convictions.

It is important to discriminate among those to whom one listens. Listen to people who keep you informed and lighten your workload or save time. Listen to those who argue constructively and use those judgments to sharpen your own judgment. Know the kind of people who want to listen to you and the situation in which they will try to make you hear. Learn to recognize when you are prone to listen and when you are not.

Some people give good information, and others should listen to them. These people are trusted troubleshooters, line managers in charge of the bread-and-butter functions of primary patient care, staff specialists who have been delegated special tasks, or reliable decision makers. Graciously avoid exaggerators, opportunists, office politicians, gossips, and chronic complainers.[85]

The speaker's appearance, facial expression, posture, accent, skin color, or mannerisms can turn off the listener. A person who wants to hear must thus put aside all preconceived ideas or prejudices and give the speaker full attention so that the speaker will be motivated to do a better job of communicating. While the person is talking, the listener analyzes what is said for ideas and facts. The receiver must also listen for feelings, which are the background to the performance—tone of voice, gestures, and facial expressions.

Mnemonics

A mnemonic is a device used to help one remember. The following are two examples of mnemonics:

1. AIDA: Capture **a**ttention, sustain **i**nterest, incite **d**esire, and get **a**ction.
2. PREP: **P**oint, **r**eason, **e**xample, and **p**oint.[86]

Such formulas are useful for preparing impromptu comments. The AIDA formula causes the speaker to focus on the listener's needs, interests, and problems. The PREP formula is ideal for spur-of-the-moment speaking. The first point reminds the speaker to clearly express a point of view on the subject. In giving the reason, the speaker explains why this is his or her point of view. These reasons should be illustrated with specific examples to clarify and substantiate the point: statistics, personal experiences, authoritative quotes, examples, analogies, anecdotes, and concrete illustrations. In the final point, the speaker brings the speech to a close with a restatement of the initial point of view. These formulas are intended to gain the attention of the listener and to elicit a positive response.

The following are some practical suggestions for encouraging people to listen:

1. Be prepared by answering the questions *Who?* and *What?*
2. Identify and evaluate the purpose of your remarks.
3. Organize and outline the report or speech to convey the facts.
4. Make efficient notes, and use them.
5. Remember that you are part of the presentation.
6. Make your voice work for you with proper breathing and pitch.
7. Communicate with your eyes.

Because critical thinking skills require interpretation of events based on present experience and factual data collection, they are also communication skills. Conceptualizing, which is a part of both communication and critical thinking processes, supports this conclusion. Also, the set of information, belief-generating, and processing skills and abilities and the habit (based on intellectual commitment) of using these skills and abilities to guide behavior support the integration of critical thinking ability and communication skills. Managers use their critical thinking ability to identify feelings and become aware of beliefs, values, and attitudes of employees to communicate and respond to their needs. Active listening through use of all the senses is required of managers who need to recognize and respond to verbal and nonverbal messages from employees.[87]

Peters says that managers should become obsessed with listening.[88]

To become a good listener requires practice. Listening to the patient can prevent errors. For example, during a patient's temporary stay in a skilled nursing facility, a medication error was made because the nurse refused to listen to the patients, a husband and wife admitted to the same room. The nurse communicated with a physician who did not know either patient. Unneeded laboratory tests were done and reported late. A further irony was the wife was an RN, the husband was a medical doctor, and both were mentally alert. Every nurse manager and practicing nurse should work at improving his or her listening skills.

Good listeners get out from behind the desk and circulate with their customers. Good listening turns people on. Good listeners provide quick feedback, and act on what they hear, and listen intensely and without preconceived notions.

Listening provides information that facilitates work, notes changes in patients' conditions more quickly and speeds up responses to changes. It brings closure to action and problems, and it involves everyone.[89]

Managers who are good listeners may want to reward acts of meritorious listening.

People tend to change the focus from listening to talking and telling. They perceive education as a solution to communication problems, whereas listening and adapting are the real solutions.

Listen informally at meals and coffee breaks, and listen formally to feedback from informative newsletters. Listen at no-holds-barred meetings. Listen rather than preach. Train people to listen. Provide employees with opportunities and places to talk and solve problems.

Listening to employees empowers them. A good listener is an engaged listener and takes notes. It is okay to ask "dumb" questions when one needs information. Knowledge is power and should never be hoarded. Because information is frequently leaked before it happens, managers should provide it to the first-line people who need it. Providing information does many things:[90]

- Motivates employees by making them potent partners.
- Facilitates continuous improvement.
- Discourages unneeded controls and delays.
- Speeds up problem solving and decision making.
- Stirs competition by stimulating ideas.
- Begets more information.
- Abets the flattened organizational pyramid.

To get information flowing requires extensive training in basic management skills.[91]

Techniques to improve communication and prevent malpractice claims include documenting telephone advice to patients, determining when and how to terminate patients, improving communication and listening styles, knowing how to effectively obtain the patient's consent, and implementing careful oversight mechanisms with the receipt of outside diagnostic test results.[92]

Some providers are being taught active listening techniques because malpractice suits are considered an expression of anger about some aspect of patient-provider relationships and communications.[93]

Results of Effective Listening

The results of effective listening are that two people hear each other, beneficial information is furnished on which to base right decisions, a better relationship between people is established, and it is easier to find solutions to problems.[94]

Communication across settings is needed to understand nurses' contribution to the care of elderly patients making the transition from hospital to home.[95] Knowledge of the communication dynamics of caring for patients may help providers to design strategies to attain the basic goals of continuity of care.[96]

Communication Media

Meetings

Meetings of all kinds are a medium for communication, often for purposes of information dissemination as well as true communication.

To make his company successful, Robert Davies, founder and president of SBT Corporation, changed his management style. To keep his employees motivated, he decided to include two employees in all management meetings to provide ideas from the production level of the organization. Davies encourages employees to risk telling what they really think through an e-mail suggestion system. This computer suggestion box is connected to all employees via more than 100 stations. It assures anonymity and in 6 months it has spawned more than 100 suggestions, which must be read and answered. For example, employees kept requesting relaxation of the dress code, which was done and is successful. Even Robert Davies dresses casually, and employees are more comfortable talking with him. Technology, combined with listening, results in consensus, support for decisions, and a company in which employees do their best.[97]

Supervisors

Supervisors or managers at all levels are also a medium for communication. To be successful in a complicated work environment, the nurse manager should be out and about. Communication includes gathering information for decision making, spreading the management vision, and letting employees know that leaders care for them. Communication is visibility. By walking around among employees and other customers, the nurse manager can prevent information distortion. This requires visiting and chatting with these knowledgeable people. The vision stamp is applied on the front line. By walking around, managers facilitate and coach; they do not give orders and conduct inspections. That is the work of the hands-on team.

Peters recommends the following actions for increasing management visibility:[98]

1. Put a note card in your pocket that says, "Remember, I'm out here to listen."
2. Take notes, promise feedback, and deliver. Fix things.
3. Cycle your actions through the chain of command and give managers the credit for fixing things.
4. Protect informants.
5. Be patient.
6. Listen, but preach a little, too, by killing unneeded red tape.
7. Give some, but not much, advance notice and travel alone. Take your own notes.
8. Work some night shifts; take a basic training course.
9. Watch out for the subtle demands you put on others that cut down on their practice of visible management.
10. Use rituals to help force yourself and your colleagues to get out and about.

We live in an information society; communication is the necessary ingredient for accomplishing missions and objectives. An effective communicator is an effective leader. Some managers use models or drawings to get their meanings across. Use synesthesia, the technique of transforming one sense to another, to communicate. Synesthesia helps one think "outside the box" by involuntarily joining real information from one of our senses to a perception in another sense. It stretches the mind to perceive reality from a more vivid sphere and range. Learn to express ideas graphically to engender employees' understanding, trust, and support. Use symbols of success, not symbols of defeat.

Some corporate executives have dismantled their offices. They maintain work areas at unit levels, with a system to correspond on the phone or computer and handle mail. They are visible.

Effective communication creates meaning. It should be an act of persuasion. The right metaphor connects with the listener. The effective manager as leader acts and personifies the message transmitted via the metaphor. This leader transmits the message over and over.[99]

Effective nurse leaders share all the information possible. Employees cannot have too much information about the company. The only information a manager does not share is that protected by law, ethics, and decency.

A nurse manager who holds information as a source of power is not an effective manager or leader.

Recognition programs promote communication. Nurse managers recognize fairly mundane actions, send written notes for work well done, and offer special recognition, such as serving a box of doughnuts or a cake to celebrate an individual or a group achievement. Nurse managers should be sure that all acts of special effort are heartfelt, that is, they should not be phony. Nurse managers should do a few big rewards and many small ones, be systematic, and celebrate events they would like repeated.[100]

Questions

Asking questions is an important method of communicating. Questions are asked to obtain information; the goal is mutual understanding. The tone of voice must encourage confidence and trust from the person questioned. Facial expression is important as the physical conduct of the questioner. The nurse manager should always go beyond the answer to a primary question and not flatly agree or disagree with the question.

The following types of questions should be used:

1. Open questions that give the other person the opportunity to freely express thoughts and feelings, rather than closed questions that force the receiver to become the sender of information. Questions that can be answered *yes* or *no* do not give information or explanation. In the courtroom, attorneys use these questions to trap people or clarify a point.
2. Leading questions that give direction to the reply, rather than loaded ones that restrict by putting the respondent on the spot.
3. Cool questions that appeal to reason, rather than heated ones reflecting the emotional state of asker and answerer.
4. Planned questions that are reflective and asked in logical sequence, rather than impulsive ones that just happen to occur to the asker.
5. Complimentary or "treat" questions that tell the respondent that he or she can make an important contribution to the asker's views, rather than trick ones that place the respondent on the spot.
6. "Window" questions that elicit the respondent's true thoughts and feelings, rather than "mirror" ones that reflect the point of view of the questioner.

Successful questioning consists of creating and maintaining a climate for communication, asking the right questions in the right way, and listening to the responses.

Questions can be used to improve listening, with their use serving to clarify unclear statements. The questioner should take care not to overawe or threaten the speaker. Questions should be worded and spoken in a nonthreatening way, for example: *I am sorry I did not hear your comment clearly. Would you mind repeating it, please?* or *I do not quite understand what you mean by "capital resource." Would you explain further, please?*

A listener should never be embarrassed to ask questions that improve his or her understanding of a person's communication. Serious questions that result in clarification of or additional information increase comprehension and clear up misperceptions, thus helping senders and receivers. If the medium is an oral presentation, questions can be written down for use at appropriate times, such as during question periods and breaks, after meetings, and even later at an interview. Thus the listener can construct thoughtful questions.

When questions are used to clarify a point made by the sender, they can be closed yes-or-no questions. An example is, *Do you support the position on nurse autonomy you have just described?*[101]

Oral Communication

Oral communication is the most common form of communication used by executives, who spend 50%–80% of their time communicating. Because oral communication takes so much time, a nurse manager should use the most effective words. Verbal messages are said to be 7% verbal (word choice), 38% vocal (oral presentation), and 55% facial expression.[102]

An advantage of face-to-face communication is that a person can respond directly to another or others. The larger the group, the less effective is face-to-face communication. An effective message requires knowledge of words and their various meanings as well as of the contexts within which the words can be used. Thus, effective communication may depend on use of the dictionary for correct vocabulary.

When giving a speech, one needs to keep in mind that the members of the audience are usually informed and sophisticated and have access to information. The members of the audience want the speaker to talk things over with them, not to talk to them. The speaker must be sincere and respect the listeners.

To present an effective speech, the speaker needs to do the following:

- Develop an outline and hold to four or five main ideas.
- Put other ideas under the main topic as subordinate ones.
- Open with an introduction.
- Close with a brief summary.
- Type the speech for easy reading.
- Practice by reading the speech.
- Maintain eye contact during the speech.
- Keep voice and manner informal and conversational.

A speaker should know the audience and its members' knowledge of the subject, intellectual level, attitudes, and beliefs. Former Vice President Hubert Humphrey said, "The necessary components to build a speech are full understanding of the facts of the subject, thorough understanding of the particular audience, and a deep and thorough belief in what you are saying."[103]

Exhibit 5-2 lists other techniques to use in preparing and giving an effective oral presentation.

Interviews

An interview is essential to practicing management by objectives. When good counseling and guidance techniques are practiced, interviews also are used to apprise current employees of their performance as well as to interview prospective employees. In disciplining an employee, it is necessary to interview the individual. When an employee leaves, an exit interview is desirable to learn why the person is leaving and to gain ideas for strengthening the personnel management program. Interview questions should be worded to obtain the most beneficial information. The following are suggestions for conducting effective interviews:

1. Use plain and direct language rather than technical, professional, or slang terms.
2. Keep questions short.
3. Use familiar illustrations.
4. Do not assume that the person being interviewed knows what you mean or are saying. Check the extent of the interviewee's knowledge beforehand.
5. Avoid improper emphasis so as not to indicate the answer you hope to elicit.
6. Be sure the interviewee attaches the same meaning to words that you do.
7. Be precise in choosing words. Use accurate synonyms and words with one pronunciation.

Written Communication

Writing is a common medium of communication. It comes in massive quantities: memos to be read and passed on, even if they go into someone else's wastebasket; letters and e-mail that need to be answered; newspapers and

EXHIBIT 5-2

Techniques for Effective Public Speaking

1. Prepare carefully. What is the goal of your presentation? Is it to inform? Persuade? Entertain? It can be a combination of these and, to be effective, should probably combine at least two, such as entertainment with information or persuasion.
2. Prepare the presentation carefully. Make an outline and develop the content to fit the outline. Start well in advance so that you can read and adjust the material for a smooth flow of ideas.
   a. What is the purpose of the presentation? Did you select the topic, or was it given to you? In either instance, clarify the purpose with the organizers of the event or whoever engaged you to do the presentation.
   b. Prepare an introduction that will gain the attention of the audience. Spark their interest. Humor often helps, but be careful of using cynicism or making derogatory remarks. References to religion, sex, and other controversial subjects should be carefully selected, if used at all. They are better avoided if you wish to persuade or inform, unless they are a part of your topic. Remember, words convey feelings, attitudes, opinions, and facts. Use them to turn the audience on, not off.
   c. Make the main points in the body of the presentation. Support them with appropriate and specific examples.
   d. Prepare or select visual aids to support the key points of the presentation. They are an extension of your presentation designed to appeal to the senses and increase reception.
   e. Know who the audience will be and tailor the message to it. Provide useful material.
   f. Plan for audience participation with questions or appropriate exercises to involve listeners.
   g. Tie the message together with interval summaries and an effective conclusion. How do you want to leave the audience?
   h. If you plan to speak extemporaneously, make notes on cards or put outlines on a visual aid such as a poster, a chalkboard, an overhead transparency, or a slide projection screen.
3. Prepare the environment beforehand. Surroundings are important and should be as attractive as possible. Bear this in mind when you have input into selection.
   a. If you want to speak from a podium, make sure it is in place. If you want to sit, have a table and chair in place.
   b. Check lighting and sound equipment.
   c. Check audiovisual equipment.
   d. Remove unneeded barriers such as screens, furniture, and other movable objects. If pillars are in the way, rearrange your position or the audience seating, if this is possible. Arrange your proximity to the group to facilitate a feeling of closeness.
   e. Prepare your person for the presentation. Wear clothes that present you best. Conventional clothes are best because the audience should focus on your words and not your appearance. Be well groomed.
   f. Good preparation will help you to be relaxed. Get a good night's sleep the night before the presentation. Plan your schedule so as not to be excited beforehand. Eat and drink moderately. Sit and do deep-breathing exercises immediately before.
4. Be on time and use time effectively.
5. Speak to be heard.
   a. Use your voice, varying pitch, volume, rate, and tone for planned effect.
   b. Practice pronouncing words with which you have trouble.
   c. Pause to enhance your delivery. Short silences emphasize points and allow the audience to think about them.
   d. Make your presentation sound natural even if you read it.
6. Use body language effectively.
   a. Slowly develop the audience's awareness of your nonverbal behavior. Be aware of it yourself.
   b. Maintain eye contact.
   c. Plan your movements: walking, standing. Your posture should convey energy, interest, approval, confidence, warmth, and openness.
   d. Keep the space between you and the audience open.
   e. Use positive gestures.
   f. Use head movements for effect.
   g. Use facial expression for effect.
   h. Know where your hands and feet are at all times.
   i. Be genuine! An audience can quickly identify a fake.
7. Adapt to audience feedback, being sensitive to listeners' interests and moods.
   a. Listen for unrest, shifting in seats, whispering, muttering.
   b. Watch for nonverbal responses. Pay attention to body language, facial expressions, gestures, and body movements. Leaning backward or away is perceived as a negative response.
   c. Be prepared to answer questions if there are breaks in the presentation. You may want to plan for them. Repeat them before answering, regardless of whether they are oral or written. You are giving additional information.
   d. Treat your audience with respect in every way, and they will view you as genuine.

magazines that collect in stacks; junk mail; posters and flyers; and notices and newsletters. How should one handle all this material? First, make a mental decision to deal with each piece of paper. Establish a system for assigning priorities to the mass of written communications; skim through everything, and then answer or delegate that which can be handled immediately. Put aside whatever can be taken care of at a future date, but do not put things where they will be forgotten. Papers can be placed in a folder according to priority.

When writing, remember that you are writing for a receiver: a reader, viewer, listener, observer, or member of an audience. The receiver is not interested in you as a writer, but only in the message being conveyed. Direct your message to the reader, use good marketing techniques, and sell your product.[104]

Exhibit 5-3 lists nine rules to follow when writing.

The writer should put the reader's interest first, begin with a provocative question or striking statement, and get right to the point: the purpose of the written

EXHIBIT 5-3

Nine Rules to Follow When Writing

1. Empathize. Be sensitive to the needs and desires of those who will read what you are writing. Arouse and maintain the reader's interest by appealing to the mind and emotions. For example, compose a message that will transmit respect for the nurse while offering a credible and unique inspiration to taking nursing histories or preparing nursing care plans. When giving orders, explain why you are asking for the task to be done. You-centered (rather than I-centered) communications are interesting to the reader or listener. Give people honest and deserved praise, the kind of flattery that makes them feel that they are worth flattering. If you are addressing a particular person, put that person's name in the salutation as well as in the body of the letter or memo. Make an effort to please the receiver by using tact, respect, good manners, and courtesy.
2. Attempt to avoid the COIK ("clear only if known" to the reader or listener already) fallacy. Think of the misunderstandings that could occur in a written message that uses abstract terms. Your aim should be to create mental pictures using language that is suitable to the experience and knowledge level of the receiver.
3. Do not repeat anecdotes frequently, or the reader will be insulted. Avoid overcommunication, overdetailing, and redundancy. Necessary repetition can be achieved by using pleasant and meaningful examples, illustrations, paraphrasing, and summaries. Repetition is essential to the mastery of a skill.
4. Express yourself in clear, simple language. Lincoln's Gettysburg Address contains 265 words, three fourths of them with just one syllable. Abstract, technical-sounding jargon, clichés, and trite platitudes may cover up insecurity in a writer afraid of committing herself or himself in writing. Avoid archaic commercial expressions, specialized in-house jargon, and fading "journalese" by writing clearly and concisely.
5. Make yourself accessible to the reader by positively and courteously requesting a response. You can ask a direct question and expect a reply by a certain date. You can also encourage response by giving a special return address, a private box or phone number, writing instructions, a postcard, or a return envelope. Make it easy, desirable, and pleasant for the reader to reply.
6. Use the format of the newspaper story: accuracy, brevity, clarity, digestibility, and empathy. Arouse the reader with a headline opener. Follow it with a summary that tells significant highlights in the opening paragraph. Then tell the details. Here is an example of a memo form that has worked for others.

   Date ____________ Time ____________

   To: ____________ Subject: ____________

   From: ____________

   Objective: ____________

   1. ____________

   ____

   2. ____________

   ____

   3. ____________

   ____

7. Break up a solid page of print with a variety of forms: underline, space, italicize, capitalize, enumerate, indent, box, summarize, and illustrate. Make your reading attractive and digestible.
8. Back up what you write by what you do; build a reputation for integrity.
9. Organize your material.
   a. Outline key points.
   b. Compile data into groups according to commonality.
   c. Arrange materials in a logical sequential order:
      (i) Chronological
      (ii) Cause-effect relationship
      (iii) Increasing complexity
   d. Tie the groups together using transitional devices:
      (i) Time-order words (first, later, finally)
      (ii) Guide words (as a result, therefore, on the other hand)
   e. Link the communication with the previous message by referring to the following:
      (i) Date
      (ii) Subject
      (iii) Sender of correspondence
   f. Furnish appropriate excerpts from past correspondence.

communication, and the request for action. A personal letter is always better than a form letter. One should use a friendly tone, with first names and personal pronouns, which express an interest in the reader.

The following are some simple suggestions for communicating effectively through writing:[105]

- Use the active voice to give strength to written communication. About 10% of total words should be verbs.
- Use strong nouns.
- Use the subject and main verb early in the sentence.
- Avoid overuse of adjectives and adverbs; be specific when using adjectives. State a specific amount such as 100 instead of *much, any,* or *a lot.*
- Be as brief as possible.
- Use short words.
- Use sentences that contain one idea and are no longer than 16 to 20 words. Vary sentence length.
- Write naturally, using friendly conversational language. Use contractions such as *didn't* and *aren't* with discretion.
- Reread and revise your written communication. Look at the nouns and verbs. Evaluate your sentences; they should be simple, not complex. Determine whether you have said what you mean. Eliminate unneeded words.
- You may want to add a personal handwritten note at the bottom.

Written Reports

Written reports should indicate how the nursing objectives are being met. If a 24-hour nursing report is made from the patient units to the director of nursing, the information provided should show progress in relation to the achievement of unit and department objectives. The information should be provided in a simple, functional or practical, and qualitative (rather than complex and quantitative) manner. In providing information, the reporter should consider its relative value and purpose, eliminate overlap and duplication, and put the report in perspective. The report should indicate the work load and state pertinent facts describing the patients' status, the reason for hospitalization, and the nursing diagnosis and prescription. The following are other factors to consider in writing useful reports:

1. Size and cost should not exceed the need or strength of the objective or operation.
2. A strong report will not be contaminated with individual bias. For that reason, a computer printout has value over a hand-prepared report.
3. A strong report will be useful to many people, providing them with vital information to run the operation.
4. A strong report will have authentic and reliable sources of information, that is, people with the knowledge and skills required to judge what information needs to be transmitted. Some information can be given by clerks, some by technicians, and some, of necessity, by the nurse manager.
5. If the report is going to a group of people with limited time, such as a board of directors, the writer should add an executive summary at the beginning of the report and highlight items on which he or she wants the readers to act. This may speed up the response.

Sometimes managers have a tendency to eliminate reports. Although the busy nurse manager may hope that all reports would be eliminated, doing so without consensus sometimes drives reports underground. Because reports and forms tend to proliferate, each should have an elimination date, at which time it will be eliminated unless it is rejustified.

Time is an element common to all reports. The perpetual report shows up-to-date events for a full year. As the latest month or quarter is added, the oldest is dropped. This time base deals with the realities of the present and provides consistency, completeness, and effectiveness in reporting.

If top management cannot extract the information it wants from reports, then either the information is unnecessary or the procedures need to be improved. Persons who design reports and reporting procedures should do the following:

1. Gain access to all documents listing the short- and long-term objectives of the unit, department, division, and institution. Objectives should be in agreement and clearly stated in writing. Progress is reported.
2. Establish priorities for reports.
3. Categorize reports, indicating which objectives are supported by each.
4. Determine what top management needs and wants to know, and then screen reports.
5. Test reports for logical patterns that avoid complexity and unwieldy clumsiness.
6. Classify reports according to frequency.
7. Determine the levels through which reports will pass.
8. Determine the point of origin.
9. Coordinate reports with the organizational structure.
10. Check for accuracy and consistency.
11. Account for the total cost of reporting.
12. Obtain the concurrence of all levels of management.

Reports form the nucleus of all management communications, and successful communications depend on an intelligently conceived report structure. The reader should be able to read from top to bottom and laterally, as well as from bottom to top.

Organizational Publications

Barnard states that the first function of an executive is to develop and maintain a system of communication.[106] The bigger the organization, the more difficult it is for the director of nursing to communicate with the employees who give direct care to patients. This problem is further complicated by the requirement that services be provided 24 hours a day, seven days a week. One medium for communication between nurse executives and employees is an organizational publication such as a newsletter or in-house magazine. This procedure does not have to be confined to nursing but can be supported and used by nursing staff. Certainly, the nurse executive will have input into the development and evaluation of such an organizational publication.

According to Tingey, a successful organizational publication will fulfill six requirements:[107]

1. It will meet clearly stated objectives related to the process of communications. These objectives will state what the executives of the institution or organization, including those in nursing, want to accomplish through the publication.
2. The publication will need a competent editor who can provide professional editing and who will ensure that the objectives are met.
3. The editor will need access to the ideas of top management. The nurse executive must provide the editor with the information needed to inform nursing personnel of changes in policy and procedures.
4. The objectives of the publication will be developed into a master management plan. This plan will indicate articles and story themes to be used to accomplish each objective.
5. Information about future events will provide personnel with articles that give an anticipatory viewpoint. In nursing this could include the organization's role in supporting continuing education, expected problems involved in collective bargaining, changes in organizational structure, and changes that will affect practice, such as new equipment, new supply products, and new support activities.
6. The editor should know the audience, including its members' educational level, interests, problems, and attitudes. The publication should be interesting to family members and contacts. An unread publication is useless.

Specific objectives of the publication will be related to the internal technologic environment, the internal social environment, the external environment, company social responsibilities, and organizational dynamics.

Electronic Media

Electronic media are key to a successful management strategy. To increase productivity in the workplace, nurse managers need to be aware of development within the telecommunications industry. For example, fax machines provide quick and accurate transmission of orders from physicians to nurses. Nurse managers should consider the following questions:

- Will fax machines improve the output of clinical nurses if they can use faxes to get drugs from the pharmacy more quickly and accurately?
- Will fax machines improve response times and the accuracy of diagnostic testing by providing an electronic link to the medical laboratory, radiology, and other departments?
- Will fax machines increase therapeutic response times among clinical nurses, physicians, physical therapists, respiratory therapists, and others?

Numerous other electronic media are available, including computer bulletin boards for fast memos and software programs that can be used to control supply inventories and provide just-in-time supplies. Electronic networks provide sources of instant up-to-date information about diagnoses and treatments. Cellular phones, electronic memo pads, and all the latest in telecommunications technology should be evaluated by nurse managers for use within and among patient care units. Evaluation should be a part of the strategic planning process. Adoption of new tools should be evaluated on the basis of value added to individual and corporate performances and cost-benefit analysis.

Even though sophisticated communications technology is in place, managers and employees often fail to communicate. Good communication is the key to achieving personal and organizational effectiveness. To be effective, information must be transferred in a timely fashion. Managers are responsible for using available information technology and therefore need to have related competencies. To communicate effectively, managers and employees need training in the skills of information technology.[108] The management information system or nursing information system should be transformed into a customer information system. Lack of electronic memos or faxes or other communications may indicate to personnel and patients that a nurse manager is not listening.

Obtaining Information

Receivers have a responsibility for obtaining information. Professional employees feel some conflict between their personal needs and the demands of the organization. Communication, the giving and receiving of information, helps an employee to control or tolerate this conflict. Assume that management controls information that will be given to employees. A conservative manager will give employees as little information as possible, because this manager believes that too much information will be distorted or misunderstood.

For example, a director of nursing stated that although the registered nurse in the recovery room was totally competent, she would not give this RN the title of nurse manager nor bring her to nurse manager meetings because she believed that the RN would misinterpret the statements made there. An enlightened manager will be direct and honest, believing that employees need all the information they can have to do their jobs. Bad news usually leaks, and trying to keep it covered up only creates distrust and anxiety.

Poor communication is caused by caution and preoccupation with running the department. Some managers treat information as private property. People tend to protect their egos and prejudices, and employees must seek out information. Geography and size of the organization or system effect communication. Communication of information is a joint responsibility of employer and employee. So if you need to know something, ask. Find out how your organization is developing and what its future prospects are. Learn whether its requirements continue to be compatible with your personal goals.

The Future

People as Capital

Specialization, division of labor, and economics of scale do not work in a service organization. People are the capital resource, and return on people is the measurable outcome, not capital in building and machines. The cost basis of service organizations will continue to be in people.

- Good employees want ownership. They want to own stock in the company. They also want psychic ownership in the company. They believe they are entrepreneurs. Within the corporation, "intrapreneurship" is already creating new products and new markets, revitalizing companies from the inside out.
- The service economy produces to meet unique human needs. Ideas come from employees, who have a rich mix of cultures. Customer demands and needs spur intuition and creativity, leading to new products and services. Medical problems, including nursing problems, are not neatly packaged. They are organic and interdependent, requiring workers who will integrate the specialties to meet the needs of the people.
- Capital must be compounded through education and software. Training and education will reduce general and administrative costs to maintain and increase competition. Information should be bought as a direct cost because a productive employee must be up-to-date and have information to be competent and productive.

Organizations

Organizations that foster personal growth will attract the best and brightest people. Work enlargement yields greater productivity from such people. They want health and fitness and education programs from their employers. They want work integrated into their lives. They want to work in environments that are democratic and that allow them to network and to work in small teams. They want work to be fun.

To grow and profit, organizations will have to eliminate their hierarchical orientation and become team-oriented. They will have to emulate the positive and productive qualities of small business. The infrastructure of the organization will give way to networking and people orientation.

Many businesses are striving for monopoly through mergers, acquisitions, and coalitions to control their environments. Though success evolves from market feedback, market forces demand change from people and are brutally destructive when people fail. The market will become the arbiter of power, obliterating layers of bureaucracy unless seized by political means.

A successful organization has effective communication at all levels, including the managerial level. Managers are skilled in managing human resources to effect communication. Communication makes employees valuable, contributing members of the corporate team (an important perception). Successful communication reduces conflict by reducing litigation and external intervention by labor unions and regulatory governmental agencies.

A good communication system does the following:

- Aids in cost savings, improves efficiency, and enhances productivity. People who know the system uncover and fix any problems.
- Keeps management better informed as it supports trust.
- Keeps employees informed of the company's plans, policies, goals, philosophies, and requirements. Informed employees act positively.
- Improves morale. Information means a satisfied employee not swayed by outside influences.
- Makes employees feel they are part of a team. Again, spirit and trust support common goals.

- Maintains a work environment free of outside adversaries and unwanted third-party influences.
- Provides some confidentiality for mutual trust and respect.
- Responds promptly and completely.
- Provides a means for employees to vent.
- Provides sufficient information.
- Recognizes employees as individuals.

Employee attitude surveys may be a means of evaluating the effectiveness of company communication. These surveys cover employees' feelings about job duties, working conditions, supervisory and managerial skills, communications, pay, benefits, training, promotional opportunities, personnel policies and procedures, morale, and job security. Analyze results, and make and implement a plan to resolve problems. Resurvey after a sufficient period.[109]

Managers

Managers should be retrained to be coaches and facilitators. Some organizations are already doing this. W. L. Gore & Associates has 38 plants, 5,000 employees, and no plant managers. Plant size is limited to 150 employees. As employees develop a following, they become the chosen leaders. Employees have sponsors when they are employed. If a job is not learned within 90 days, the employee is no longer paid. Advocate sponsors are consulted by a compensation sponsor to determine salary based on accomplishment.

Thirty-five percent of American corporations pay managers more than they deliver as value added, that is, the increased production and profit they add as a result of their performance. The manager's new role is that of coach, teacher, and mentor.[110]

Technology

Technology will be linked to the service orientation of surviving, adaptive, customer-oriented organizations. It will shift the cost curve, with labor continuing to have high income because of increased productivity. Quality will be paramount, requiring that the organizational design and the technology be brought together as enablers for human resources. Computers can supplement, not replace, human capital.

Technology will become overhead. Information technology will be used to solve problems for which there is little intelligence and very little collective knowledge. When available, information should be bought and not generated directly to decrease overhead costs and hierarchy. Otherwise, managers must establish entire teams of experts to develop and implement a system that may already be available. It will be cheaper to pay the experts by the minute, because many will be available electronically. Thus contract or consultative labor will replace hired labor, especially in the technologic sphere.

Artificial intelligence will be a key enabler that will create generalists. It replaces experts and encapsulates and capitalizes knowledge. Knowledge will be added to machines to become an extension of the user. A symbiotic relationship will exist between the manager and the expert machine.

Survival in the information age will depend on a combination of technology and strategic insights. Service organizations will have to find people who need services and deliver these services to them. During the past 6,000 years, information has belonged to the power structure, which did not trade it, market it, or give it away. The service industries of the information age will market services that are heavily information based.

People and technologic systems can quickly become obsolete. Managers should go after strategic, not technical, gains. They should not computerize what does not work or maintain obsolete technology in hiring people. Employers must be developed and updated, adjusted to the system, or they will "career hop" within and outside of the organization. Turnover is expensive because it throws away assets. Human resource assets generate more value added when they are managed, enriched, and involved in the enterprise.[111]

Summary

Decision making and problem solving occur concurrently with all major functions of nursing. Four models of the cognitive thinking skills involved in decision making are presented: the normative model, the decision-tree model, the descriptive model, and the strategic model.

Decision making involves having an objective, gathering data pertaining to the objective, analyzing the data, identifying and evaluating alternative courses of action to achieve the objective, selecting an alternative (the decision), implementing it, and evaluating the results. Nurses make the best decisions through knowledge and use of the theory of decision making combined with intuitive ability developed over years of experience.

Although problem solving is not the exact equivalent of decision making, it employs a similar thinking process. Decision making is different from problem solving in that its objective does not have to pertain to a problem. It can be an objective that relates to change, progress, research, or implementation of any operational or management plan.

Communication occurs between government and the governed, between governments, between buyers and sellers, between manufacturers and consumers, between pupils and teachers, between parents and children, and between neighbors, but most importantly, communication occurs between people only if they want it to. The products of lack of communication are too costly to accept: misinformation, misunderstanding, waste, fear, suspicion, insecurity, and low morale.

People have difficulty accepting that communication is not the answer to all problems of human relations and personnel management. A gap exists between senders and receivers that must be recognized before it can be bridged—a gap in background, experience, and motivation.

Good communication is frequently an illusion. It is not achieved only with open doors, geniality, or jokes. Communication is aided by listening to what people are really saying and perceiving what they are projecting through their words, facial expressions, tone of voice, and actions. To induce people to accept direction, one must encourage them to participate. They will listen for genuineness in the word of the boss as demonstrated by actions.

APPLICATION EXERCISES

EXERCISE 5-1

The following exercises may be done individually or as a group. You may want to work with a group of your peers.

Case Study: You are Ms. Carrie Platt. You have been director of nursing at Mason General Hospital for 1 1/2 years. Mason General is a 500-bed general hospital in a metropolitan area, serving a population of 700,000. The city has 4 other hospitals and a University Medical Center. A local ADN nursing program is affiliated with your hospital. Today is Monday, March 20. During the past week, on Thursday, March 16, and Friday, March 17, you were away from the hospital to conduct a 2-day workshop. It is 8 A.M. and you have just arrived at the hospital. You must leave the hospital at 8:50 A.M. in order to be at the airport at 9:10 A.M. There has been an unexpected death in the family and you will be gone the entire week. You notice that the in-basket contains several items. You should make decisions about these things before leaving.

INSTRUCTIONS: Three decision making exercises appear on the following pages. Each exercise is composed of a memorandum or other medium and a decision worksheet format. Use the worksheet format to list ideas for action and arrive at a decision. If the information given lacks essential details, make any assumptions necessary. Possible examples of decisions include the following:

1. Take immediate action and state what the action is.
2. Delegate the action to another person and state who the person is.
3. Postpone the action; state to what time.
4. Other course; please specify.

A. MEMORANDUM
TO: Ms. Platt
FROM: Kay Campbell, Nurse Manager–5 N
SUBJECT: Poor charting of I&O
Date: March 17

The I&O record on Mrs. East in 517 is incomplete for evening and night shifts for her postoperative period. She went into shock in the recovery room and is in renal failure. Dr. Blake is extremely upset about the lack of thorough charting of I&O. One of the evening aides heard Mr. East call his lawyer about the possibility of a lawsuit. We thought you needed to be aware of this situation.

DECISION WORKSHEET

SUBJECT DECISION ALTERNATIVES	ANALYSIS	DECISION SELECTED	DECISION

(continued)

EXERCISE 5-1 ***(continued)***

B. MEMORANDUM
TO: Ms. Platt
FROM: Mrs. Back, In-service Instructor
SUBJECT: Uniform Regulations
DATE: March 17

The meeting with the nursing assistants regarding uniform regulations has been scheduled for March 21 at 10:00 A.M. in In-service Room 406. We appreciate your offer to discuss this matter with the nursing assistants.

DECISION WORKSHEET

SUBJECT DECISION ALTERNATIVES	ANALYSIS	DECISION SELECTED	DECISION

IMPORTANT MESSAGE

FOR Ms Platt
DATE March 17 TIME 10:15 A.M. / P.M.
Ms Tonia Cole, MSN
OF Chicago
PHONE ______
AREA CODE NUMBER EXTENSION

TELEPHONED	X	PLEASE CALL	
CAME TO SEE YOU		WILL CALL AGAIN	
WANTS TO SEE YOU	X	RUSH	
RETURNED YOUR CALL		SPECIAL ATTENTION	

MESSAGE Called in reference to ad for clinical specialist. Will be in area Wed and Thurs next week and would like appt.

SIGNED ______

C. MEMORANDUM

DECISION WORKSHEET

SUBJECT ALTERNATIVES	DECISION ANALYSIS

DECISION SELECTED	DECISION

EXERCISE 5-2 Check your in box. If you are not receiving communications from your customers (clinical nursing personnel, patients, and others), start a personal listening ritual. Call three customers a day and ask how they are doing and what their problems are. Listen to their responses.

EXERCISE 5-3 From your communications (calls, memos, etc.), follow up on complaints or problems. Help resolve them.

EXERCISE 5-4 Have a group of internal and external customers meet with you to discuss communication and information problems. Listen to them. Guide them to good solutions. Facilitate action.

EXERCISE 5-5 Use a group of coworkers to evaluate your current recognition program. Discard those activities that are not working if they cannot be fixed. Infuse the others with excitement. Consider having an "attaboy" and "attagirl" award for which customers can pick up a short form and fill it out when they feel especially good about something an employee has done. Recognize the employee immediately at change-of-shift report, breakfast, lunch, dinner, or whenever. Send out 10 thank-you notes a month to employees and 10 more to customers.

EXERCISE 5-6 Make notes of calendar events and take a box of doughnuts or a cake to them.

EXERCISE 5-7 Be the first to make a contribution to the United Way or other community agency. Lead the charge when supporting a voluntary effort for a community activity. Recognize those who put forth community effort.

EXERCISE 5-8 Walk around your area of responsibility. Note at least one hassle that can be fixed each day (or week or month). Fix it!

EXERCISE 5-9 Identify and analyze your worst failure each month. How can it be fixed? Fix it!

EXERCISE 5-10 Visit customers who call you on the phone. These include employees, patients, suppliers, peers, and others.

EXERCISE 5-11 Make a list of all the information you want employees to have. Schedule meetings with all of them. Give them the information, and leave them with a printed version.

NOTES

1. Page, A. (Ed). (2004). Keeping patients safe, transforming the work environment of nurses. Washington, DC: Institute of Medicine of the National Academies, 118.
2. Ingersol, G., Fisher, M., Ross, B., Soja, M., & Kidd, N. (2001). Employee response to major organizational redesign. *Applied Nursing Research*, *14*(1), 18–28.
3. Rousseau, D. & Tijoriwala, S. (1999). What's a good reason to change? Motivational reasoning and social accounts in organizational change. *Journal of Applied Psychology*, *84*, 514–528.
4. Heifetz, R. & Laurie, D. (2001). The work of leadership. *Harvard Business Review*, *79*(11), 131–140.
5. Ibid.
6. Ibid.
7. Lancaster, W. & Lancaster, J. (1982). Rational decision making: Managing uncertainty. *Journal of Nursing Administration*, 23–28.
8. Peters, T. (1992, March 3). This is CNN: Chaos is the future of business. *San Antonio Light*, p. B9.
9. Nolan, P. (1998). Competencies drive decision making. *Nursing Management*, 27–29.
10. Arora, N. K. & McHorney, C. A. (2000). Patient preferences for medical decision making: Who really wants to participate? *Medical Care*, 335–341; Babic, S. H., Kokol, P., Zorman, M., & Podgorelec, V. (1999). The influence of class discretization to attribute hierarchy of decision trees. *Student Health Technology Information*, *68*, 676–681.
11. Shankar, R. D. & Musen, M. A. (1999). Justification of automated decision making: Medical explanations as medical arguments. Proceedings of the AMIA Symposium, 1999, 395–399; Jamieson, P. W. (1990). A new paradigm for explaining and linking knowledge in diagnostic problem solving. *Journal of Clinical Eng*, 371–380; Gerdtz, M. F. & Bucknall, T. K.

(1999). Why we do the things we do: Applying clinical decision-making frameworks to triage practice. *Accident Emergency Nursing*, 50–57; Dowie, J. (1999). What decision analysis can offer the clinical decision maker: Why outcome databases such as KIGS and KIMS are vital sources for decision analysis. *Horm Res*, *51* (Suppl. 1), 73–82; Taylor, C. A., Draney, M. T., Ku, J. P., Parker, D., Steele, B. N., Wang, K., et al. (1999). Predictive medicine: Computational techniques in therapeutic decision making. *Computer Aided Surgery*, *4*(5), 231–247; Balneaves, L. G. & Long, B. (1999). An embedded decisional model of stress and coping: Implications for exploring treatment decision making by women with breast cancer. *Journal of Advanced Nursing*, 1321–1331; Mazumdar, M. & Glassman, J. R. (2000). Categorizing a prognostic variable: Review of methods, code for easy implementation and applications to decision making about cancer treatments. *Statistical Medicine*, 113–132.

12. Offredy, M. (1998). The application of decision making concepts by nurse practitioners in general practice. *Journal of Advanced Nursing*, 988–1000; McGuinness, S. D. & Peters, S. (1999). The diagnosis of multiple sclerosis: Peplau's interpersonal relations model in practice. *Rehabilitation Nursing*, 30–33.
13. Lancaster & Lancaster, 1982, 23.
14. Vroom, V. H. (1973). A new look at managerial decision making, organizational decision making. *Organizational Dynamics*, 66–80.
15. Brown, R. V. (1970). Do managers find decision theory useful? *Harvard Business Review*, 78–89; Magee, J. (1964). Decision trees for decision making. *Harvard Business Review*, 126; Magee, J. (1964). How to use decision trees in capital investment. *Harvard Business Review*, 79.
16. Simon, H. A. (1976). *Administrative behavior* (3rd ed.). New York: The Free Press.
17. Ibid.
18. Lancaster & Lancaster, 1982.
19. Nagelkerk, J. M. & Henry, B. J. (1990). Strategic decision making. *Journal of Nursing Administration*, 18–23.
20. Ibid., 21.
21. Ibid.
22. Reitz, J. H. (1977). *Behavior in organizations*. Homewood, IL: Richard D. Irwin, 154–199.
23. Orton, A. (1984). Leadership: New thoughts on an old problem. *Training*, 28, 31–33.
24. Harrison, K. (1991). Cost benefit analysis: A decision-making tool for physiotherapy managers. *Physiotherapy*, 445–448.
25. Matteson, P. & Hawkins, J. W. (1990). Concept analysis of decision making. *Nursing Forum*, *25*(2), 4–10.
26. Graham D., & Reese, D. (1984). There's power in numbers. *Nursing Management*, 48–51.
27. McKenzie, M. E. (1985). Decisions: How you reach them makes a difference. *Nursing Management*, 48–49.
28. Wrapp, H. E. (1967). Good managers don't make policy decisions. *Harvard Business Review*, 91–99.
29. Kanter, R. M. (1989). *When giants learn to dance*. New York: Simon & Schuster, 114, 153–155.
30. Agor, W. H. (1986). The logic of intuition: How top executives make important decisions. *Organizational Dynamics*, 5–18.
31. Ibid., p. 9.
32. Watkins, M. P. (1998). Decision-making phenomena described by expert nurses working in urban community health centers. *Journal of Professional Nursing*, 22–23.
33. King, L. & Appleton, J. V. (1997). Intuition: A critical review of the research and rhetoric. *Journal of Advanced Nursing*, 194–202.
34. Easen, P. & Wilcockson, J. (1996). Intuition and rational decision making in professional thinking: A false dichotomy? *Journal of Advanced Nursing*, 667–673.
35. Agor, 1986.
36. Rew, L. (1986). Intuition: Concept analysis of a group phenomenon. *Advances in Nursing Science*, 21–28.
37. Blakeslee, S. (1994, May 30). Seat of morality inside the brain. *San Antonio Express-News*, p. 24A.
38. Casebeer, L. (1991). Fostering decision making in nursing. *Journal of Nursing Staff Development*, 271–274.
39. Botter, M. L. & Dickey, S. B. (1989). Allocation of resources: Nurses the key decision makers. *Holistic Nursing Practice*, 44–51.
40. Miller, V. G. (1995). Characteristics of intuitive nurses. *Western Journal of Nursing Research*, 305–316.
41. Barnard, C. & Beyers, M. (1982). The environment of decision. *Journal of Nursing Administration*, 25–29.
42. Swansburg, R. C. (1976). *Management of patient care services*. St. Louis: C.V. Mosby, 149–170.
43. McKay, P. S. (1983). Interdependent decision making: Redefining professional autonomy. *Nursing Administration Quarterly*, 21–30.
44. American Hospital Association (AHA). (1984). Strategies: nurse involvement in decision making and policy development. Author, 1–10.
45. Blegen, M. A., Goode, C., Johnson, M., Maas, M., Chen, L., & Moorhead, S. (1993). Preferences for decision-making autonomy. *Image*, 339–344.
46. Dwyer, D. J., Schwartz, R. H., & Fox, M. L. (1992).Decision making autonomy in nursing *Journal of Nursing Administration*, 17–23.
47. AHA, 1984.
48. Murphy, N. J. (1992). Nursing leadership in health policy decision making. *Nursing Outlook*, 158–161.
49. Anderson, B. (1992). Voyage to shared governance. *Nursing Management*, 65–67; Ide, P. & Fleming, C. (1999). A successful model for the OR. *AORN Journal*, 805–808, 811–813; Bell, H. M. (2000). Shared governance and teamwork: Myth or reality. *AORN Journal*, 631–635.
50. Boyle, D. K., Bott, M. J., Hansen, H. E., Woods, C. Q., & Taunton, R. L. (1999). Managers' leadership and critical care nurses' intent to stay. *American Journal of Critical Care* , 361–371.
51. Girot, E. A. (2000). Graduate nurses: Critical thinkers or better decision makers? *Journal of Advanced Nursing*, 288–297.
52. Scharf, A. (1985). Secrets of problem solving. *Industrial Management*, 7–11.
53. Blai, B., Jr. (1986). Eight steps to successful problem solving. *Supervisory Management*, 7–9.
54. Klaasens, E. (1992). Strategies to enhance problem solving. *Nurse Educator*, 28–30.
55. Brightman, H. J. & Verhoeven, P. (1986). Why managerial problem solving groups fail. *Business*, 24–29; Shaddinger, D. E. (1992). Digging for solutions. *Nursing Management*, 96f, 96h.
56. Morgan, P. & Baker, H. K. (1985). Building a professional image: Improving listening behavior. *Supervisory Management*, 34–36; Griver, J. A. (1979). Communication skills for getting ahead. *AORN Journal*, 242–249.
57. Corbett, W. J. (1986). The communication tools inherent in corporate culture. *Personnel Journal*, 71–72, 74.
58. Wlody, G. S. (1984). Communicating in the ICU: Do you read me loud and clear? *Nursing Management*, 24–27.
59. Bice, M. (1990). Behavior is the most effective communicator. *Hospitals*, 78.

60. Joblin, F. M. (1982). Formal structural characteristics of organizations and superior-subordinate communication. *Human Communication Research*, 338–347.
61. Farley, M. J. (1989). Assessing communication in organizations. *Journal of Nursing Administration*, 28.
62. O'Sullivan, P. S. (1985). Detecting communication problems. *Nursing Management*, 27–30.
63. Smeltzer, C. H. (1991). The art of negotiation: An everyday experience. *Journal of Nursing Administration*, 26–30; Bazerman, M. H., Curhan, J. R., Moore, D. A., & Valley, K. L. (2000). Negotiation. *Annual Review of Psychology*, *51*, 279–314.
64. Ibid.
65. Drucker, P. F. (1973). *Management: Tasks, responsibilities, practices*. New York: Harper & Row, 483.
66. Crosby, P. (1987). *Running things: The art of making things happen*. New York: NAL-Dutton.
67. Sanchez, J., Byfield, G., Brown, T. T., LaFavor, K., Murphy, D., & Laud, P. (2000). Perceived accessibility versus actual physical accessibility of healthcare facilities. *Rehabilitation Nursing*, 6–9.
68. Missik, E. (1999). Personal perceptions and women's participation in cardiac rehabilitation. *Rehabilitation Nursing*, 158–165.
69. St. John, W. D. (1984). Leveling with employees. *Personnel Journal*, 52–57.
70. Baker, H. K. & Morgan, P. (1986). Building a professional image: Using "feeling-level" communication. *Supervisory Management*, 25.
71. Wlody, 1984.
72. Levenstein, A. (1984). Feedback improves performance. *Nursing Management*, 64, 66.
73. Levenstein, A. (1984). Back to feedback. *Nursing Management*, 61.
74. Ibid.
75. Kanter, R. M. (1989). *When giants learn to dance*. New York: Simon & Schuster, 108–114.
76. Ibid., p. 275.
77. Drucker, 1973, 487–489.
78. Haakenson, R. (1964). How to be a better listener. *Notes & Quotes*, 3.
79. Morgan & Baker, 1985.
80. Sousa, L. (1993, May 1). We need to teach life 101. *San Antonio Express-News*, p. 6B; Foster, N. J. (2001). Good communication starts with listening. Available at www.mediate.com/articles/foster2.cfm. Accessed July 25, 2005.
81. Gibb, J. R. (1982). Defensive communication. *Journal of Nursing Administration*, 14–17.
82. Shields, D. E. (1984). Listening: A small investment, a big payoff. *Supervisory Management*, 18–22.
83. Lang, F., Floyd, M. R., & Beine, K. L. (2000). Clues to patients' explanations and concerns about their illnesses: A call for active listening. *Archives of Family Medicine*, 222–227.
84. Schneider, B. A., Daneman, M., Murphy, D. R., & See, S. K. (2000). Listening to discourse in distracting settings: The effects of aging. *Psychology of Aging*, 110–125.
85. Stewart, N. (1963). Listen to the right people. *Nation's Business*, 60–63.
86. Guncheon, J. (1967). To make people listen. *Nation's Business*, 96–102.
87. Woods, J. H. (1993). Affective learning: The door to critical thinking. *Holistic Nursing Practitioner*, 64–70.
88. Peters, T. (1981). *Thriving on chaos*. New York: Harper & Row.
89. Ibid.
90. Ibid., pp. 524–532.
91. Ibid.
92. Irving, A. V. (1998). Twenty strategies to reduce the risk of a malpractice claim. *Journal of Medical Practice Management*, 130–133.
93. Virshup, B. B., Oppenberg, A. A., & Coleman, M. M. (1999). Strategic risk management: Reducing malpractice claims through more effective patient-doctor communication. *American Journal of Medical Quality*, 153–159.
94. Sigband, N. B. (1969). Listen to what you can't hear? *Nation's Business*, 70–72.
95. Bowles, K. H. (2000). Patient problems and nurse interventions during acute care and discharge planning. *Journal of Cardiovascular Nursing*, 41.
96. Anderson, M. A. & Helms, L. B. (2000). Talking about patients: Communication and continuity of care. *Journal of Cardiovascular Nursing*, 15–28.
97. Davies, R. (1992). Managing by listening. *Nation's Business*, 1–6.
98. Peters, 1981, 608–613.
99. Bennis, W. & Nanus, B. (1985). Leaders: The strategies for taking charge. New York: Harper & Row, 14, 33–43, 106–108.
100. Ibid., pp. 366–367.
101. Nathan, E. D. (1966). The art of asking questions. *Personnel*, 63–71; Pulick, M. A. (1983). How well do you hear? *Supervisory Management*, 27–31; Morgan & Baker, 1985.
102. St. John, W. D. (1985). You are what you communicate. *Personnel Journal*, 40–43; Caruth, D. (1986). Words: A supervisor's guide to communication. *Management Solutions*, 34–35.
103. Zelko, H. P. (1965). How to be a better speaker. *Notes & Quotes*, 3.
104. Wilkinson, R. (1986). Communication: Listening from the market. *Nursing Management*, 42J, 42L.
105. Dulik, R. (1984). Making personal letters personal. *Supervisory Management*, 37–40.
106. Barnard, C. I. (1938). *The functions of the executive*. Cambridge, MA: Harvard University Press, 226.
107. Tingey, S. (1967). Six requirements for a successful company publication. *Personnel Journal*, 638–642.
108. Nalley, E. A. & Braithwaite, J. E., Jr. (1992). Communication: Key to a vital future. *Phi Kappa Phi Newsletter*, 1–3.
109. Gilberg, K. L. (1993). Open communication provides key to good employee relations. *Supervision*, 8–9.
110. Strassman, P. A. & Zuboff, S. (1985). Conversation with Paul A. Strassman. *Organizational Dynamics*, 19–34; Rutigliano, A. J. (1985). Naisbitt & Aburdene on "re-inventing" the workplace. *Management Review*, 33–35.
111. Ibid.

REFERENCES

Argyris, C. (1967). How tomorrow's executives will make decisions. Reprint from *THINK Magazine*, IBM.

Argyris, C. (1982). *Reasoning, learning and action*. San Francisco: Jossey-Bass.

Auger, B.Y. (1967). How to run an effective meeting. *Commerce*.

Beissner, K. L. (1992). Use of concept mapping to improve Problem solving. *Journal of Physical Therapy Education*, 22–27

Collette, C. L. (2000). Understanding patients' needs is the foundation of perioperative nursing. *AORN Journal* , 629–630.

Crawford, M. J. & Kessel, A. S. (1999). Not listening to patients: The use and misuse of patient satisfaction studies. *International Journal of Social Psychiatry*, 1–6.

Davidhizar, R. E. & Brownson, K. (1999). Literacy, cultural diversity, and client education. *Health Care Management*, 39–47.

Finsher, S. (1985). Rework, revise, rewrite. *Business*, 54–55.

Foster, N. J. (2000). *Barriers to everyday communication*. Available at www.mediate.com/articles/foster2.cfm. Accessed July 25, 2005.

Gelfand, L. I. (1970). Communicate through your supervisors. *Harvard Business Review*, 101–104.

Is anybody listening? (1950). *Fortune*, 77.

Hansten, R. I. & Jackson, M. (2004). *Clinical delegation skills: A handbook for professional practice* (3rd ed.). Sudbury, MA: Jones and Bartlett Publishers.

Institute of Medicine. (2003). *Health professions education: A bridge to quality*. Washington, DC: The National Academies Press.

Iyengar, S. & Simon, A. F. (2000). New perspectives and evidence on political communication and campaign effects. *Annual Review of Psychology*, *51*, 149–169.

Kennedy, M. M. (1999). Understanding the demographics of the evolving workforce. *Clinical Laboratory Management Review*, 310–313.

Kleinman, C. S. (2004). Leadership and retention. *Journal of Nursing Administration*, *34*(3), 111–113.

Lynch, E. M. (1966). So you're going to run a meeting. *Personnel Journal*, 22+.

Macrae, C. N. & Bodenhausen, G. V. (2000). Social cognition: Thinking categorically about others. *Annual Review of Psychology*, *51*, 93–120.

Patterson, F., Ferguson, E., Lane, P., Farrell, K., Martlew, J., & Wells, A. (2000). A competency model for general practice: Implications for selection, training, and development. *British Journal of General Practice*, 188–193.

Peters, T. (1992, October 20). Listening to what's wrong and right. *San Antonio Light*, p. D2.

Severson, M. A., Leinonen, S. J., Matt-Hensrud, N. N., & Ruegg, J. A. (1999). Transcultural patient care committee: Actualizing concepts and developing skills. *Journal of Nursing Staff Development*, 141–147.

Stevens, R. D. & Katsekas, B. S. (1999). Nursing the terminally ill: Being with people in difficult times. *Home Healthcare Nursing*, 504–510.

Suding, M. J. (1984). Decision making controlling the computer input. *Nursing Management*, 44, 46, 48–52.

Watson, C. A. (2004). Evidence-based management practices. *Journal of Nursing Administration*, *34*(5), 207–209.

Willemsen, M. C., Meijer, A., & Jannink, M. (1999). Applying a contingency model of strategic decision making to the implementation of smoking bans: A case study. *Health Education Resources*, 519–531.

CHAPTER 6

Organizational Structure and Analysis

Denise Danna, RN, DNS, CNAA, CHE

Our life is frittered away by detail . . . Simplify, simplify.

Henry David Thoreau

LEARNING OBJECTIVES AND ACTIVITIES

- Define *organizing*.
- Apply or illustrate selected principles of organizing.
- Describe a bureaucracy.
- Identify the components of a organization.
- Define *team*.
- Define *committee*.
- Discuss group dynamics and the roles played by group members.
- Analyze phases of groups.
- Describe the characteristics of various group techniques.
- Distinguish between standing and ad hoc committees.
- Describe the characteristics of self-directed work teams.
- Analyze committee effectiveness.
- Analyze an organizational structure.
- Use of set of standards to evaluate an organizational chart.
- Distinguish among various forms of organizational structure.
- Describe decentralization and participatory management.
- Illustrate advantages and disadvantages of decentralization and participatory management.
- Use a set of standards to evaluate departmentation.
- Describe an informal organization.
- Identify characteristics of organizational effectiveness of a nursing organization, including symptoms of malorganization.

CONCEPTS: Organizing, bureaucracy, role theory, organizational development, autonomy, accountability, organizational culture, organizational climate, team building, committee, group dynamics, focus group, groupthink, ad hoc committee, standing committee, organizational structure, organization chart, decentralization, participatory management, autonomy, vertical integration, horizontal integration, job enrichment, personalization, entrepreneurship, shared governance, gain sharing, nursing care delivery system, departmentation, informal organization, organizational effectiveness, differentiated practice, flat organization, tall organization, organization chart, organizational effectiveness, informal organization.

NURSE MANAGER BEHAVIORS: The nurse manager maintains the nursing organization to support an organizational structure through adherence to basic principles of organizing and by appointing nursing personnel to all organization committees; collaborates in the design and improvement of systems and the identification of resources that assure interventions are safe, effective, efficient, age-relevant, and culturally sensitive; and collaborates in the design and improvement of systems and processes that assure interventions are implemented by the appropriate personnel.

NURSE EXECUTIVE BEHAVIORS: The nurse executive works with nursing employees to develop a decentralized and participatory management organizational structure that supports autonomy, accountability, shared governance through committee structure, group dynamics, and a culture and climate conducive to satisfied patients, families, nurses, physicians, and other staff; designs and improves systems and identifies resources that support interventions that are consistent with the established plans; and participates in the development, evaluation, and maintenance of organizational systems that integrate policies and procedures with regulations, practice standards, and clinical guidelines.

Organizational Theory

Organizations exist to bring people and material resources together to accomplish the work of the organization. "Organizing is the process of grouping the necessary responsibilities and activities into workable units, determining the lines of authority and communication, and developing patterns of coordination."[1] Once plans are made, the mission, purpose, or business for which the organization exists has been established; the philosophy and vision statements have been developed and adopted; the objectives have been formulated; and resources are organized to sustain the philosophy, achieve the vision, and accomplish the mission and objectives of the organization. Organizations develop as goals become too complex for the individual and must be divided into units that individuals can manage.[2]

Fayol referred to the organizing element of management as the form of the body corporate and stated that the organization takes on form when the number of workers rises to the level requiring a supervisor. It is necessary to group people, distribute duties, and adapt the organic whole to requirements by putting essential employees where they will be most useful. An intermediate executive is the generator of power and ideas.[3] The body corporate of the nursing organization includes executive management and its staff, departmental managers (middle managers), operational managers (first-line managers), and practicing professional and technical nursing personnel. Reformed organizations eliminate middle management, with operational managers becoming the department heads. Professional nursing personnel manage the performances of technical nursing personnel. In a theory of nursing management, nurse managers have as their object the development of a nursing organization that facilitates the work of clinical nurses.

Definitions of Organizing

Urwick referred to organizing as the process of designing the machine. The process should allow for personal adjustments, but these will be minimal if a design is followed. It should show the part each person will play in the general social pattern, as well as the responsibilities, relationships, and standards of performance. Jobs should be put together along the lines of functional specializations to facilitate the training of replacements. The organizational structure must be based on sound principles, including that of continuity, to provide for the future.[4]

Organizing is the grouping of activities for the purpose of achieving objectives, the assignment of such groupings to a manager with authority for supervising each group, and the means of coordinating appropriate activities horizontally and vertically with other units that are responsible for accomplishing organizational objectives. Organizing involves the process of deciding which levels of organization are necessary to accomplish the objectives of a nursing division, department or service, or unit. For the unit, it would involve the type of work to be accomplished in terms of direct patient care, the kinds of nursing personnel needed to accomplish this work, and the span of management or supervision needed.

Organizational Principles

Principle of Chain of Command

The chain of command principle states that organizations are established with hierarchical relationships, within which authority flows from top to bottom in order to be satisfying to members, economically effective, and successful in achieving goals. This principle supports a mechanistic structure with a centralized authority that aligns authority and responsibility. Communication flows through the chain of command or channel of communication and tends to be one-way—downward. In a modern nursing organization, the chain of command is flat, with line managers and technical and clerical staffs that support the clinical nursing staff. Communication flows freely in all directions, with authority and responsibility delegated to the lowest operational level.

Principle of Unity of Command

The unity of command principle states that an employee has one supervisor and that there is one leader and one plan for a group of activities with the same objective. This principle is still followed in many nursing organizations but is increasingly being modified by emerging organizational theory. Primary nursing and case management modality support the principle of unity of command, as does joint practice. Professional nurses and others frequently engage in matrix organizations in which they answer to more than one supervisor.

Principle of Span of Control

The span of control principle states that a person should be a supervisor of a group that he or she can effectively manage in terms of numbers, functions, and geography. This original principle has become elastic—the more highly trained the employee, the less supervision is needed. Employees in training need more supervision to prevent blunders. When different levels of nursing employees are used, the nurse manager has more to coordinate. In the past, most nurse managers had a narrow span of control; they were responsible for one nursing unit and a limited number of staff. More recently, span of control has increased to the point at which a nurse manager might cover several nursing units and departments with a larger number of employees. Some management experts recommend up to 75 employees answering to one supervisor.[5]

Principle of Specialization

The principle of specialization is that each person should perform a single leading function. Thus there is a division of labor: a differentiation among kinds of duties. Specialization is thought by many to be the best way to use individuals and groups.

The hierarchy or scalar chain is a natural result of these principles of organizing. It is the order of rank from top to bottom in an organization. Another concept is centrality, which relates to the position or distance the person has on the organizational chart from other workers. For example, the middle manager possesses a larger amount of centrality because he or she gives information from the top, bottom, and middle.[6] These principles of organizing are interdependent and dynamic when used by nurse managers to create a stimulating environment in which to practice clinical nursing.

Bureaucracy

Bureaucracy evolved from the early principles of administration, including those of organizing. Max Weber coined the term. Bureaucracy is highly structured and usually includes no participation by the governed. The principles of chain of command, unity of command, span of control, and specialization all support bureaucratic structures. These structures do not work in pure form and have been greatly adapted in today's organization.

Among the historic strong points of bureaucratic organizations is their ability to produce competent and responsible employees. These employees perform by uniform rules and conventions; are accountable to one manager who is an authority; maintain social distance with supervisors and clients, thereby reducing favoritism and promoting impersonality; and receive rewards based on technical qualifications, seniority, and achievement. The characteristics of bureaucracy include formality, low autonomy, a climate of rules and conventionality, division of labor, specialization, standardized procedures, written specifications, memos and minutes, centralization, controls, and emphasis on a high level of efficiency and production. These characteristics frequently lead to complaints about red tape, procedural delays, and general frustration.[7]

Using the bureaucratic model as a reference, Hall studied ten organizations evaluating the following six dimensions: division of labor, hierarchy of authority, employee rules, work procedures, impersonality, and technical competence. He found varying degrees of each of these dimensions. An organization could be highly bureaucratized in one dimension but not in others. Highly bureaucratic structures would have a high degree of bureaucracy in each of the six dimensions. Similar organizations may have similar degrees of bureaucracy.[8]

Hall also found that age and size of an organization do not relate to its degree of bureaucratization. The "technical competence" dimension did not appear to correlate with the other five dimensions. It is the rational aspect of bureaucracy. A high degree of impersonality develops in organizations that deal with large numbers of customers or clients.[9] Hall's study has significance for nursing administration; the scale can be used for testing in health care organizations and in nursing divisions.

Hall also studied the relationship between professionalism and bureaucratization. In a study using both structural aspects and attitudinal attributes of a profession, his findings were as follows:[10]

1. Attitudes are strongly associated with behavior, particularly as they related to membership in professional organizations and obtaining specialty certifications.
2. Nurses are high in professionalism in terms of belief in service to the public, belief in self-regulation, and sense of calling to the field, but are low in feeling of autonomy and using the professional organization as a reference point.
3. Nurses are high in bureaucratization, except for technical competence.
4. Autonomous organizations have less hierarchy of authority.
5. An organization's size does not affect hierarchy.
6. Autonomous organizations have less division of labor.
7. Autonomous organizations have fewer procedures.
8. Autonomous and heteronymous organizations emphasize technical competence.
9. Professionalism increases with decreased division of labor, decreased procedures, decreased impersonality, and increased autonomy. Hierarchy is accepted if it serves coordination and communication functions.
10. Bureaucracy inhibits professionalism.

The conclusion would be that the less bureaucratic the organization, the more nurses in it perceive themselves as professionals. Nurse managers need to move from bureaucratic management to transformational leadership, thereby empowering professional nurses in a world in which technology, communication, and political, economic, demographic, and social forces are constantly reshaping the health care system.[11]

Organizational Components

Role Theory

Role theory claims that when employees receive inconsistent expectations and little information, they will experience role conflict, which leads to stress, dissatisfaction, and ineffective performance. Role theory supports the chain of command and unity of command principles. Multiple lines of authority disrupt, divide authority between profession and organization, and create stress. They force employees to make choices between formal authority and professional colleagues. The result is role conflict and dissatisfaction for employees and reduced efficiency and effectiveness for the organization. Role conflict reduces trust of and personal liking and esteem for the person in authority; it reduces communication and decreases employee effectiveness. Management that provides for the following can reduce role conflict and ambiguity:

1. Certainty about duties, authority, allocation of time, and relationship with others.
2. Guides, directives, policies, and the ability to predict sanctions as outcomes of behavior.
3. Increased need fulfillment.
4. Structure and standards.
5. Facilitation of teamwork
6. Toleration of freedom.
7. Upward influence.
8. Consistency.
9. Prompt decisions.
10. Good, prompt communication and information.
11. Use of the chain of command.
12. Personal development.
13. Formalization.
14. Planning.
15. Receptiveness to ideas by top management.
16. Coordination of work plans.
17. Adaptation to change.
18. Adequacy of authority.

The implications for nurse managers are obvious. Role conflict and role ambiguity are separate dimensions; role conflict is more dysfunctional. Some employees, however, find stress rewarding.[12] In a changing work environment; nurses are required to perform in new roles and under new circumstances. Managers provide the education and support needed by nurses who are coping with their role changes. Management support addresses the potential and real need deficits nurses will confront. The goal is to prevent role insufficiency by thoroughly preparing nurses to function in new roles. Managers may opt to do this through role modeling. Clear understanding of role changes and planned programs to support them will reduce role stress and prevent role strain.[13]

Effective use of role theory has a positive impact when making changes in a nursing care delivery system. Role ambiguity, role stress, and role strain are minimized through educational programs aimed at socializing nurses into their new roles. Effective communication improves role changes.[14]

Nurses acquire more personal power and incentives as they move up the managerial hierarchy. Nurse managers are motivated by the content of their work and the tasks and responsibilities assigned to their positions. Upper-level managers and supervisory-level nurses have firm beliefs in their competence and regard their roles as meeting professional goals.[15] With the restructuring of health care organizations, particularly hospitals, a whole new approach to organizing is required. It will include applications of organizational theory as related to culture, climate, team building, and role theory, among others.

Organizational Development

Organizational development deals with changing the work environment to make it more conducive to worker satisfaction and productivity. An underlying premise is that "people planning" is as important as technical and financial planning. Organizational development allows managers to attend to the psychologic as well as the physical aspects of organizations. Change is the terrain to which organizational development applies.

Organizational development can sustain the favorable or desirable aspects of bureaucracy. Change can be employed to modify the undesirable aspects of bureaucracy. There is room for directive as well as nondirective leadership within organizations. Nurse managers have to be strong and tough in supporting the values of clinical nurses. They have to be proactive in planning, designing, and implementing new organizational structures and work environments. The object is to develop people, not to exploit them. Organizational development emphasizes personal growth and interpersonal competence.[16]

Autonomy and Accountability

Among the psychologic and personality attributes of organizational development are autonomy and accountability, both crucial elements of nursing professionalism. A professional nurse is obliged to answer for decisions and actions. This would be achieved using a management by results (MBR) approach. This approach defines performance standards incorporating acceptable behavior and results. It includes tracking for progress, performance feedback, making adjustments, and personnel accountability.[17]

Characteristics of professional autonomy include self-definition, self-regulation, and self-governance. Professional nurses respond to demographic changes in society by defining and reshaping the content of nursing practice. They address societal needs, including the needs for increased care for the elderly and the control of resources. Autonomy will be strengthened by unbundling the hospital bill and by direct reimbursement for nursing services by third-party payers.

Self-governance for nursing includes a nursing administrator hired or elected with input from nurses, self-employment of nurses, approval of nursing staff privileges by peer review with privileges revoked by the nursing staff organization, and case management.[18]

Argyris describes people as complex organizations who work for an organization for their own needs or gains. These needs exist in varying degrees or at varying depths that must be understood by organizations. People seek out jobs to meet their needs. They develop and live on a continuum from infancy to adulthood that is reflected throughout life and work and leisure.[19]

Ridderheim describes a particular hospital administrator's action to change a management style that was paternalistic, used downward communication, encouraged dependency, and inhibited management development. In an opinion survey, the hospital's employees scored high on patient care and personal pride in work but low in decision-making ability. The following are among the changes made by the administrator after organizational assessment and consultation:[20]

1. Decisions were turned back to operating managers, giving them freedom to act within broad policy guidelines.
2. Operating management was restructured in an executive operating committee (EOC) that included the administrator and assistants for medical staff affairs, operations, facilities, patient care, personnel, and finance. Each assistant had policy-making status.
3. A core group was established at lower levels of management to focus on the technical interests and objectives of the hospital.
4. Task forces were established for special projects.
5. A team was set up to monitor terminations, retirements, recruitments, advancements, and demotions.
6. Performance standards were developed for each manager.
7. Team-building seminars were held.
8. After nine months, progress was critiqued at a retreat, first by the EOC, then by subordinate managers.
9. Achievement in relation to goals, individual growth, and teamwork was stressed over seniority.
10. Subsequent surveys showed improvement in job satisfaction, supervisory concern for employees, supervisory emphasis on goal achievement, and work group emphasis on teamwork, decision-making practices, and motivational conditions.

Culture

Organizational culture is the sum total of an organization's beliefs, norms, values, mission, philosophies, traditions, and sacred cows. It is a social system that is a subsystem of the total organization. Organizational cultures have artifacts, perspectives, values, assumptions, symbols, language, and behaviors that have been effective. Organizational cultures include communication networks, both formal and informal. They include a status/role structure that relates to characteristics of employees and customers or clients. Such structures also relate to management styles, whether authoritative or participatory. Management style impacts individual behavior. In a health care setting, these structures promote either individuality or teamwork. They relate to classes of people and can be identified through demographic surveys of both employees and patients. In addition, there is a technical or operational arm for getting the work done and an administrative arm for wages and salaries; hiring, firing, and promoting; report making and quality control; fringe benefits; and of budgeting. Exhibit 6-1 illustrates aspects of organizational culture.

The artifacts of an organizational culture may be physical, behavioral (rituals), or verbal (language, stories, myths). Verbal artifacts result from shared values and beliefs. They include traditions, heroes, and the party line, and they result in ceremonies that embody rituals. These include ceremonies to reward years of service, the annual picnic, the Christmas party, and the wearing of badges and insignia.[21] Culture is created by such rites and rituals as the following:[22]

- Casual day—workers wear jeans and sport shirts on Friday to create an atmosphere of creativity and friendship.
- Birthing rooms and sibling birth participation programs to promote family health.
- Focus on quality, service, and reliability.
- A strong communication network.
- Face-to-face contacts.

A nurse manager needs to be aware of the culture of his or her unit, department and organization. A successful manager identifies and accepts the prevailing culture before making changes. It is more difficult to change a culture at the level of basic beliefs, values, and perspectives. It is easier to change technical and administrative systems. Managers and personnel who survive in a culture learn how to support the values and norms of that culture. Their conformity impedes change and innovation. The social, technical, and managerial systems are changed through organizational development. To change the culture may require changing the leader.[23]

EXHIBIT 6-1
Organizational Culture

ARTIFACT	Dress, office space, office décor, logos, pictures
VALUES, ASSUMPTIONS	Language, stories, verbal communication, nonverbal communication, rites, rituals
BEHAVIORS	Ceremonies, hiring and terminating practices

Research and Organizational Culture

Research indicates that a strong culture that encourages participation and involvement of employees in shared decision making; emphasizes customers, stockholders, and employees; and requires leadership from managers at all levels positively affects an organization's performance. Such organizations outperform competitors 2:1 in return on investments and sales. The organizational culture can be influenced by the CEO.[24]

Organizations all have cultures, and large ones have subcultures. With time and effort nurse managers can change the culture of their organization to improve performance. Culture change is accomplished through strategic planning, the first step of which is the creation of a vision of desired values and outcomes. Suggestions for culture change include the following:[25]

1. Emphasize quality.
2. Use available knowledge of processes that have worked in other organizations.
3. Create partnerships for care and an organizational structure and philosophy of shared ownership and participation.
4. Culture change requires collaboration; shared decision making, and problem-solving work experience. It includes patient and family, physicians, nurses, other caregivers, and support and administrative staff. Use clinical pathways and clinical practice guidelines. Collaboration requires joint rounds, caregiver commitment, and total commitment of top management. Information is shared and communications are free-flowing.
5. Redesign the roles and responsibilities of managers as well as caregivers and support staff. Practices that do not work should be abandoned. Patient and family become a part of the entire process.

Ideas, values, and symbols relate to and transform attitudes, feelings, and behavior. Bureaucracy has survived and expanded within organizations. Most cultural changes within organizations occur within the bureaucratic structure. Nurse leaders should initiate and support cultural changes that not only keep the enterprise profitable and economically fit but also preserve the caring behavior of nurses.

Through qualitative research Ray developed the theory of differential caring. Differential caring has multiple meanings, including the following:

- Humanistic: empathy, love, and concern.
- Political-legal and decision making, liability, and malpractice.
- Ethical-religious and trust, respect, acts of "brotherly" love, and ideals of "doing unto others."
- Economic and budget management and economic well-being.
- Technologic/physiologic and use of machinery.
- Educational and information, teaching, education programs.
- Social and communication, social interaction and support, interrelationships, involvement, intimacy, knowing clients and families, humanistic potential for compassion and concern, love and empathy.

A formal theory of bureaucratic caring emerged from the substantive theory of differential caring. The challenge for nurse managers is to create an organizational culture that supports the theory of bureaucratic caring.[26]

Fleeger studied organizational culture to arrive at the characteristics of consonant and dissonant cultures. She recommends that managers promote a consonant culture through the following:[27]

- Strategic planning sessions promoting employee's involvement.
- Identifying conflict situations as opportunities for creative change.
- Planning job redesign and job-enrichment activities in departments in which personnel demonstrate signs of stagnation.
- Increasing both formal and informal staff interactions.
- Adapting a nursing care model that promotes autonomy and responsibility.

It takes a well-planned and well-executed unit orientation to integrate new employees into the corporate culture and subculture. The object is to achieve a fit between employee and organization. The Organizational Culture Inventory (OCI) is an instrument that can be used to measure culture as perceived by employees. It was used to profile the "ideal" nursing culture as described by a small group of nurses representing several hospitals. Such instruments can be used to measure organizational culture to define what needs preservation versus what needs changing.[28]

When nurse executives from magnet hospitals were asked to identify nursing's top three current challenges, one of their responses included culture—"identifying, reassessing, changing the culture of nursing in my organization."[29] Nurse executives reported that culture issues were related to the changing role of the RN and effects of mergers and consolidations. Other notable issues identified by the nurse executives were their concern about educating new staff to the organization's culture and values, and how financial awareness and responsibility is so ingrained into health care organizations.[30]

Climate

Organizational climate is the emotional state, perceptions, and feelings shared by members of the system. It can be formal, relaxed, defensive, cautious, accepting, trusting, and so on. It is the employees' subjective impression or perception of their organization. The employees of major concern to nurse managers are the practicing nurses. Practicing nurses create or at the very least contribute to the creation of the climate perceived by patients.

Managers create the climate in which practicing nurses work. If managers trust them, practicing nurses will provide good information to keep their managers informed. This climate promotes the concept that most hands-on employees can perform routine management, accounting, engineering, and quality tasks. Well-trained, well-equipped, and self-managed work teams, the members of which are also good salespersons, can perform 90% of expert staff work. The object of expert staff is to spread knowledge quickly.[31]

Organizational climate relates to the personality of an organization and can be changed. Following are six sociological dimensions of organizational climate:

1. Clarity in specifying certification of the organization's goals and policies. This is facilitated by smooth flow of information and management support of employees.
2. Commitment to goal achievement through employee involvement.
3. Standards of performance that challenge, promote pride, and improve individual performance.
4. Responsibility for one's own work fostered and supported by managers.
5. Recognition for doing good work.
6. Teamwork and a sense of belonging, mutual trust, and respect.[32]

Practicing nurses want a climate that will give them job satisfaction through good working conditions, high salaries, and opportunities for professional growth through counseling and career development experiences and opportunities. Nurses achieve job satisfaction when they are challenged and their achievements are recognized and appreciated by managers and patients. They achieve satisfaction from a climate of collegiality with managers and other health care providers and in which they have input into decision making. Just as importantly, nurses want a climate of administrative support that includes adequate staffing and shift options. Personnel shortage, frustration, failure, and conflict in nursing have required sweeping changes in intrinsic and extrinsic rewards, including career development programs that increase the ability of professional nurses to develop their self-esteem through self-actualization. This is particularly relevant in today's environment of constrained resources and nursing shortages.

Management climate surveys measure clarity and understanding of an organization's goals, effectiveness of decision-making processes, integration, cooperation, vitality, leader effectiveness, openness and trust, job satisfaction, opportunities for growth and development, level of performance, orientation and accountability, effectiveness of teamwork and problem solving, and overall confidence in management. Surveys may be used to make a diagnosis and to achieve the following:[33]

- Establish new strategic directions.
- Clarify an organization's mission, objectives, and goals.
- Identify managers and supervisors' training and development needs.
- Reallocate resources.
- Prepare a foundation for cultural change.
- Revise hiring priorities using a patterned interview as well as peer interviewing to select the best fit for the unit and organization.

Many studies have been done to determine work climate within business, industry, and health care organizations. Climate and philosophy result from the corporate culture, and changing the culture leads to climate change. One head nurse designed and implemented a project to motivate the nursing staff of a medical unit to better service and greater self-satisfaction. She designed an "employee of the month" motivational strategy that included measurable performance criteria. Though the staff was initially disinterested, they eventually increased their interest and participation. Productivity increased, as did emergence of talents. The strategy culminated in a recognition ceremony. The employee of the month received a free lunch or dinner, and his or her picture was put on the bulletin board. By the end of 6 months, 25 of 144 employees had earned the title of employee of the month, their voluntary participation indicating that it met some of their needs.[34]

Activities to promote a positive organizational climate include:

1. Developing the organization's mission, philosophy, vision, goals, and objectives statements with input from practicing nurses, including their personal goals.
2. Establishing trust and openness through communication that includes prompt and frequent feedback and stimulates motivation.
3. Providing opportunities for growth and development, including career development and continuing education programs.
4. Promoting teamwork.
5. Asking practicing nurses to state their satisfactions and dissatisfactions during meetings and conferences and through surveys.
6. Marketing the nursing organization to the practicing nurses, other employees, and the public.
7. Following through on all activities involving practicing nurses.

8. Analyzing the compensation system for the entire nursing organization and structuring it to reward competence, productivity, and longevity.
9. Promoting self-esteem, autonomy, and self-fulfillment for practicing nurses, including feelings that their work experiences are of high quality.
10. Emphasizing programs to recognize practicing nurses' contributions to the organization.
11. Assessing unneeded threats and punishments and eliminating them.
12. Providing job security with an environment that enables free expression of ideas and exchange of opinions without threat of recrimination, which may manifest as downscaled performance reports, negative counseling, confrontation, conflict, or job loss.
13. Being inclusive in all relationships with practicing nurses.
14. Helping practicing nurses to overcome their shortcomings and to develop their strengths.
15. Encouraging and supporting loyalty, friendliness, and civic consciousness.
16. Developing strategic plans that include decentralization of decision making and participation by practicing nurses.
17. Being a role model of performance desired of practicing nurses.

Team Building

Team building is an essential process in today's health care environment. As health care organizations are faced with intense pressure to control cost and increase productivity and efficiency with continued regulatory and legislative constraints, effective team building can produce the ultimate outcome of improved health care. For example, one study concluded that the amount of involvement and interaction between the nurses in an intensive care unit and the physicians directly influenced the differences in patient mortality.[35] In the *Scope and Standards for Nurse Administrators*, interdisciplinary collaboration (team building) is threaded throughout the standards of practice: assessment, diagnosis and identification of outcomes, planning, and implementation.[36] In the *Standards of Professional Performance, Standard 12. Collaboration*, the nurse administrator is identified as the one who should collaborate with nursing staff, interdisciplinary teams, all departments, and the community.[37] Collaboration should be focused on developing, implementing, and evaluating programs and services; enhancing care delivery; and increasing employee satisfaction.[38] As the nursing work force continues to intensify and the shortages increase, nursing is called upon to develop interdisciplinary collaborative solutions.[39] One way to achieve this expectation is through team building and the effective use of interdisciplinary teams, work groups, and committees.

Team building is a method of participative management that encourages commitment, creativity, support, and growth of the individual, the unit, and the organization. The objective of team building is to establish an environment of cohesiveness among health care workers, whether among different shifts on one unit or among other units and departments throughout the facility. This cohesiveness will enable organizations to develop patient care teams, committees, or work groups that use problem solving techniques and demonstrate a commitment to the organization and each other to reach the goals and objectives of the organization.

One continually hears such remarks as "This organization does not care about the employees!" or "This organization really cares about its employees!" Nurse managers want to hear the positive statement. A person who works courageously and confidently, with the discipline and willingness to endure hardship, manifests high morale. Morale is a motivation factor related to productivity and product or service quality indicators. A person with low morale is not satisfied with his or her work. Low morale is evident in the person who is timid, cowardly, devious, fearful, disorderly, unruly, rebellious, turbulent, or indifferent as a result of job dissatisfaction and organizational milieu. Dissatisfied workers will not contribute positively to *esprit de corps*. Companies want high morale and cohesiveness among employees and they use different strategies, such as team building, to address the issue.

The principle of synergy underlies team building. Synergy puts the thinking power of a selected group together for the most effective outcome. To sustain synergy, six basic rules should be followed:[40]

1. Define a clear purpose. Each team member must clearly be knowledgeable about the reason they are together. The team members must be able to articulate the goals, objectives, and purpose of the team.
2. Actively listen. Each team member must be focused on each individual and listen to what is being said. Active listening is not judgmental and means being completely absorbed and attentive to the speaker.
3. Maintain honesty. Each team member must be objective in providing feedback to the speaker. No one should make the speaker feel belittled or that his or her views are not correct or important.
4. Demonstrate compassion. Each team member should listen in a caring manner to the other's viewpoint.
5. Commit to resolution of conflicts. Each team member must agree to disagree even though his or her view or opinion is not the same. Team members must work toward a common understanding and acceptance of the issue at hand.

6. Be flexible. Each team member must be open and flexible to another individual's perspective. Everyone works together to accomplish the goal or objective.

The value of team building is to improve such processes as goal setting, relationships among people performing the work, group collaboration, and the allocation of the work that needs to be done.[41] Nurse managers should create a humanistic environment for nursing employees, one that fosters trust and cooperation—the synergy. Such an environment treats employees, rather than technology and buildings, as the most important asset. Nurses who have high self-esteem or self-worth are energetic and confident, take pride in their work, and have genuine respect and concern for their patients, visitors, peers, and others. Their behavior reflects this self-worth expressed in high morale, job satisfaction, and a commitment to each other and to the organization.

Today's nurse managers will be effective if they are informed about nursing staff's personal values and concerns. Work conflicts, type of shifts, child care services, and family responsibilities are examples of what is important to staff nurses. By knowing such information, the nurse manager can be knowledgeable about the issues and provide whatever guidance and assistance is needed to promote a positive work climate for staff.

Before team performance can be improved, the nurse manager must assess how the current team is functioning.[42] To facilitate team building and successful teams, the nurse manager can take the following steps:[43]

1. Assess the functioning of the team through such methods as direct observation, employee interviews or meetings, and questionnaires.
2. Identify the problem(s) resulting in team dysfunction, such as negativism, poor goal setting, poor interpersonal relationships among the members, and lack of commitment and disengagement.
3. Analyze the team's strengths and weaknesses.
4. Develop an action plan to develop strategies for the team.
5. Implement the strategies that should be communicated to the entire staff.
6. Evaluate the results of the team-building effort on a continuous basis.

A nurse manager may begin team building by asking for volunteers from every shift to work together on an issue. One example could be to work on improving the response time of answering patients' call lights. The team would be asked to present its recommendations to the staff on that unit.[44] Once the team functions well, team building then can focus on work production. Some meeting time should always be dedicated to morale, motivation, and team skills and discussion of team direction.[45]

Recognition of the individual worth of each nurse is an important morale builder. It gives the individual self-esteem. Managers can stimulate self-esteem with praise that promotes a sense of competence, success, and worth. Nurse managers have to feel worthy before they can nurture that feeling in subordinates. Each nurtures each other. Managers who have self-esteem are not afraid to explore their personal feelings with their peers or subordinates.

Most professional nurses spend many hours in the workplace, and they depend on their jobs as a major source of self-esteem. For this reason, nurse managers should aspire to build a work environment that enhances the self-esteem of all nurses. Such an environment promotes outstanding performance. This is even more important in times of stress and with particular challenges: downsizing, declining patient days, and work force shortages. Recognition can be made through many avenues and even a simple "thank you" will increase the self-esteem of an individual. Nave and Thomas suggest 50 specific techniques to boost employee morale, including such strategies as snacks during breaks, potluck suppers, annual parties, birthday cards, and other strategies that acknowledge the individual and teams.[46]

Team development is a complex and tough job. The team leader identifies training needs of the team and the individual members. The team leader also runs interference for the team, acts as liaison in negotiation for scarce resources, arranges publicity for accomplishments, and keeps abreast of information on outside events affecting the team. When conflicts arise from perceptions that some team members are doing more than their share of work or that the wrong members are getting promoted, the team leader manages them. The dream team collaborates with enthusiasm to get a job done well.

Teams

The team organization has been tried in nursing since the 1950s. It has been used mainly at the operating or primary care level rather than at top or middle management levels. "A team is a number of people—usually fairly small and with different backgrounds, skills, and knowledge, and drawn from various areas of the organization (their home) who work together on a specific and defined task. There is usually a team leader or team captain.[47]

In health care institutions, patients see the physician as team leader. However, the team leader uses the resources of the entire organization; in many cases it is the nurse who identifies, recommends, and coordinates these resources.

A team must have a continuing mission, which nursing has. The team should be highly flexible without a rigid chain of command. Like all organizational structures in business, industry, or health care institutions, the team organization needs clear and sharply defined objectives. Leadership decides on decision and command authority, and the team is responsible for accomplishing the tasks or mission. Team members know each other's functions, but leadership must first establish clarity of objectives in everybody's role. Everyone on the team should know the whole work and be adaptable and receptive to innovation. The team leader gives continuing attention to clear communications and clear decision making. A team should be kept small for top management work and for innovative work. Otherwise, the team design complements the functional design. A combination may consist of employees who work in teams but produce work organized on the functional principle. This approach seems to work best in nursing and is probably better than either organizational structure in its pure form. Team organization is a difficult structure requiring great self-discipline.

EXHIBIT 6-2
Standards for Evaluating Nursing Committees

1. The committee has been established by appropriate authority: by laws, executive appointment, or other.
2. Each committee has a stated purpose, objectives, and operational procedures.
3. There is a mechanism for consultation between chairs and persons to whom they report.
4. Each committee meeting has a published agenda.
5. Committee members are surveyed beforehand to obtain agenda items, including problems, plans, and sharing of news.
6. Each committee has an effective chair.
7. Recorded minutes of each committee's meetings are used to evaluate the committee's effectiveness in meeting stated objectives.
8. Committee membership is manageable and representative of the expertise needed and the people affected.
9. Nurses are adequately represented on all appropriate institutional committees.

Committees

A committee is a group that evolves out of a formal organization structure. Committees are formed to make collective use of knowledge, skills, and ideas. They blend the good characteristics of several individuals' reason to make careful appointments or selections. Committees can serve useful functions in the organizational process of nursing and administration. In addition to being organizational entities, committees are a part of managerial planning, and, in turn, they make plans. They are directed by leaders who are appointed by management or elected by constituents determined by management. Because professional nurses want autonomy but are mostly employed by organizations, formal groups, including committees, are a medium for promoting autonomy by giving these nurses a voice in managing the organization. Research conducted on magnet hospitals in the early 1980s revealed that nursing staff was significantly involved in committees throughout the hospital. Committees included medical staff, hospital, and nursing committees in which nurses were viewed as active participants and contributors to the committees.[48] Exhibit 6-2 outlines standards for evaluating nursing committees.

Group Dynamics

Because the work of organizations is accomplished by groups, teams, or committees, many researchers have studied the dynamics of group function. Nurse managers need to be well grounded and knowledgeable about group dynamics, as group work is such a time commitment. Although not all groups are committees, the management of a group of employees whose goal is to accomplish the objectives of the enterprise is similar to the leadership and management of a committee whose goal is to accomplish selective objectives. In the 1920s, researchers at Harvard Business School found that worker morale and productivity were positively influenced by small, informal work groups.[49]

In the world of the nurse manager, work is performed by individuals and by groups. Primary nursing is a frequently-used modality of practicing nursing because it gives professional nurses more autonomy than do other modalities. It adds accountability, as nurses are continuously responsible for patients from admission through discharge. Case management adds group dynamics to the autonomy, as the case manager is responsible for functioning in a collaborative practice with other professional nurses and with physicians. Case management also uses managed care as a medium to keep the patient on the critical path from admission through discharge. Case management can extend through the illness episode to include home care, even at the critical care level.

Stevens advocates the use of groups for management and states that they can greatly increase productivity when used effectively. Nurse managers need to be able to function in groups to promote problem solving and acceptance of responsibility. The group can function within an administrative council and demonstrate its ability to manage itself by preparing agendas, reviewing status of agenda topics, obtaining and using learning aids, and handling meetings. In short, it is possible to structure the business of groups and to direct and control the behavior of group members.[50]

Each member of a group plays a role in achieving the work of the group. Since each member has a unique personality and individual abilities, the group leader needs to know how groups function to facilitate effectiveness. Original studies of group dynamics were done through observations of informal groups. The Hawthorne studies of 1924–1932 were conducted in four phases designed to discover what would make workers increase their output. The results of the studies indicate that employees respond to identification with their groups and to the interpersonal relationships with members of their small groups by increasing their output.

Through interpersonal relationships, group members perform task roles, group-building and maintenance roles, and individual roles. In the performance of these roles, the group members share the power of the organization and its management.

Group Task Roles

Each member of a group performs a role related to the task of the group or committee to arrive cooperatively with the other group members at a definition of and solution to a common problem. Benne and Sheats identify 12 group task roles, each of which may be performed by a group member or by the leader; one person may perform several roles. These roles are as follows:[51]

1. Initiator-contributor, a group member who proposes or suggests new group goals or redefines the problem. (This may take the form of new procedures or group restructuring. There may be more than one initiator-contributor functioning at different times within the group's lifetime.)
2. Information seeker, a group member who seeks a factual basis for the group's work.
3. Opinion seeker, a group member who seeks opinions that reflect or clarify the values of other members' suggestions.
4. Information giver, a group member who gives an opinion indicating what the group's view of pertinent values should be.
5. Elaborator, a group member who suggests by example or extended meanings the reason for suggestions and how they could work.
6. Opinion giver, a group member who states personal beliefs pertinent to the group discussion.
7. Coordinator, a group member who clarifies and coordinates ideas, suggestions, and activities of the group members or subgroups.
8. Orienter, a group member who summarizes decisions or actions and identifies and questions differences from established goals.
9. Evaluator critic, a group member who compares and questions group accomplishments and compares them to a standard.
10. Energizer, a group member who stimulates and prods the group to act and to raise the level of its actions.
11. Procedural technician, a group member who facilitates the group's action by arranging the environment.
12. Recorder, a group member who records the group's activities and accomplishments.

Group-Building and Maintenance Roles

Individual members of the group work to build and maintain group functioning. Again, each role may be performed by a group member or by the leader, and one person may perform several roles. The following are the seven group-building roles:[52]

1. Encourager, a group member who accepts and praises the contributions, viewpoints, ideas, and suggestions of all group members with warmth and solidarity.
2. Harmonizer, a group member who mediates, harmonizes, and resolves conflicts.
3. Compromiser, a group member who yields his or her position within a conflict.
4. Gatekeeper and expediter, a group member who promotes open communication and facilitates participation to involve all group members.
5. Standard setter or ego ideal, a group member who expresses or applies standards to evaluate group processes.
6. Group observer and commentator, a group member who records the group process and uses it to provide feedback to the group.
7. Follower, a group member who accepts the group members' ideas and listens to their discussion and decisions.

Individual Roles

Group members also play roles to serve their individual needs. To keep individual roles from disrupting the group's activities in meeting its objectives, selected group members are frequently trained in group dynamics. This training is particularly important for the group leader. These individual roles are not suppressed but are managed by the leader and the other trained leaders. The following are the eight individual roles:[53]

1. Aggressor, a group member who expresses disapproval or vetoes the values or feelings of other members through attacks, jokes, or envy.
2. Blocker, a group member who persists in expressing negative points of view and resurrects dead issues.
3. Recognition seeker, a group member who works to focus positive attention on himself or herself.
4. Self-confessor, a group member who uses the group setting as a forum for personal expression.
5. Playboy, a group member who remains uninvolved and demonstrates cynicism, nonchalance, or horseplay.

6. Dominator, a group member who attempts to dominate and manipulate the group.
7. Help seeker, a group member who manipulates members to sympathize with expressions of personal insecurity, confusion, or self-deprecation.
8. Special interest leader, a group member who cloaks personal prejudices or biases by ostensibly speaking for others.

Nurse managers with a working knowledge of group dynamics can use their knowledge to assemble groups. Such knowledge is important in the selection of chairs of committees, task forces, and other groups of clinical nurses. It is equally important in selecting nurses for organization committees if nursing is to gain power and recognition for its contributions to the mission and objectives of the corporate entity.

Group training will give members awareness of the roles they play and the opportunity to manage themselves so that they become more productive. Group training has evolved into a science that contributes to a theory of nursing practice and nursing management. Self-analysis or self-evaluation and development of sensitivity to others to make oneself productive within group settings are a part of these theories. Nurse managers benefit from training in group dynamics and may include it in a continuing staff development program for professional nurses. This can be done through actual role playing of group missions.

Group Leaders

Group leaders may be formal, informal, or specialized. Formal leaders are appointed by management or elected by management directive; they carry line authority and the power to discipline and control group members. Informal leaders emerge from the group process. Their influence inspires cooperation and mediation, and group members reach consensus about their contributions to the effective functioning of the group in their quest of goals. Specialized leaders are often temporary leaders who have a special skill or ability that is needed by the group at a particular point in time.

Participative management requires commitment of individuals to work toward shared goals as well as profitability. A dynamic leader inspires people to put spirit into working for a shared goal. The leader can use symbols, posters, slogans, T-shirts, and memorable events. The leader must believe in people and support a theory of leadership that espouses self-direction, self-control, commitment, responsibility, imagination, ingenuity, creativity, and effort. How the leader behaves toward peer group members will demonstrate these beliefs.[54] Leaders can make committees and meetings effective by having an extensive knowledge of group dynamics. They will keep the group on course by convincing each member of the genuine need for input and by personal sensitivity to group processes. They will draw in the shy and the quiet. They will politely cut off the garrulous and protect the weak. While controlling the squashing reflex in themselves, they will encourage a clash of ideas by mitigating domination by cliques. They will refrain from being judgmental. Being a group leader requires a thinking, skilled performance based on knowledge and ability acquired through management education and training.[55]

Phases of Groups

Groups have a natural history of development. The following are five generally accepted phases of a group.

1. *Forming or orientation phase.* This is the phase during which group members discover themselves. They want uniqueness; they want to belong while maintaining personal identity. They test each other for appropriate and acceptable behavior. This is the time to exchange information, discover ground rules, size each other up, and determine fit. When forming these groups, the nurse manager will include experts, affected constituencies, people who will implement the solution, persons with different problem-solving styles, and equal numbers of sensing/thinking and intuitive/feeling individuals. The group leader will develop the explicit norm of constructive conflict: disagreement, multiple definitions, minority opinions, devil's advocate, professional management, and a "group wins" psychology. Implicit norms are avoided because they bring bias to the group process by imposing individual values and beliefs. The leader helps members fit into the group, providing structure, guidelines, and norms, and making members comfortable.
2. *Conflict or storming phase.* During this phase, group members jockey for position, control, and influence. Leadership struggle and increased competition take place. The leader helps members through this phase, assisting with roles and assignments.
3. *Cohesion or norming phase.* Roles and norms are established, with a move toward consensus and objectives. Members reach a common understanding of the true nature of the opportunity to reach the group's goals. They will diagnose the root cause of the problem, the deviation from expected performance. They will be open to alternative definitions with multiple views. Morale and trust improve, and the negative is suppressed. The leader guides and directs as needed.
4. *Working or performing phase.* Members work with deeper involvement, greater disclosure, and unity. They complete the work. The leader may intervene as needed.

5. *Termination phase.* Once goals are fulfilled, the group terminates. The leader guides the members to summarize discussions, express feelings, and make closing statements. The group is reluctant to break up. A celebration can help.[56]

Group Cohesiveness

Group cohesiveness includes the forces (bundle of properties) acting on the members of a group to preserve group integrity. These forces deal with and overcome disruption and conflict. Among the forces are such beliefs as the power of influence of the group, the personality of individual members of the group, and the mission or goals of the group. Cohesiveness is demonstrated by mutual understanding and support, improvements in self-esteem, and successful completion of the mission and goals of the group. Cohesive groups have a positive valence, with the combination of members' inputs leading to a strengthening of group processes and outcomes.[57]

Knowledge of group dynamics is needed by nurse managers to improve leadership competencies and to facilitate group discussion and communication. Groups are a common feature of a majority of experiences of all nurses in such roles as outcome management, team coordination, and teaching of students, patients, and families.[58]

Selected Group Techniques

A number of group techniques have been developed to make groups effective and productive. Among these are the Delphi technique, brainstorming, the nominal group technique, and focus groups.

Delphi Technique

Originally developed by the Rand Corporation as a technological forecasting technique, the Delphi technique pools the opinion of experts. This technique can be used in nursing management to pool the opinions of a group of leaders in the field. Each round of questioning has three phases. For example, the group is polled for input, which is analyzed, clarified, and codified by the investigator and given as feedback to the experts; the experts are then polled for further commentary on the composite of the first round. This process can continue for three to five rounds.[59]

Members of the group using the Delphi technique may never have the opportunity to meet personally, since most of the activities are done through correspondence or electronically.

Brainstorming

As a group technique, brainstorming seeks to develop creativity by free initiation of ideas. The object is to elicit as many ideas as possible. The following are the steps in the brainstorming technique:

1. The leader instructs the group, giving the member the topic or problem and telling him or her to respond positively with any ideas or suggestions relative to it. No critical responses are allowed.
2. The leader lists on a poster or chalkboard all ideas and suggestions as they are given and encourages their generation.
3. Ideas and suggestions are evaluated only after each group member has contributed all possible ideas and suggestions.

One variation on brainstorming, the Gordon technique, keeps the subject area general to elicit more ideas. Success depends on the skills of the group leader. A second variation of brainstorming is the Phillips 66 buzz session, used for large groups. The large group is broken down into smaller groups of 6 members each. Each conducts a brainstorming session for 6 minutes and then reports to the large group.[60]

The Nominal Group Technique

In this technique, the problem or task is defined. Members independently write down ideas about it, trying to make the ideas more problem-centered and of higher quality. Each member presents ideas to the group without discussion. The ideas are summarized and listed. Next, the members discuss each recorded idea to clarify, evaluate, and assign a priority to each decision. The results are averaged and the final group decision is taken from the pool. The process takes about 1.5 to 2 hours and results in a sense of accomplishment and closure.[61] Nominal group technique is a reliable evaluation tool as well as an efficient group teaching technique.[62]

Focus Groups

Focus group methods stem from consumer market research. They do not provide quantitative research but a phenomenologic approach to qualitative research. Focus groups offer descriptions of the vicarious experiences of the participants. Groups of 8 to 12 participants meet as a group with a moderator who facilitates focused discussion on a topic.

Focus groups have been used to develop nurse retention programs. Some of the objectives of focus groups are as follows:[63]

1. To provide an intellectual forum for innovative solutions to chronic problems.
2. To encourage a specific communication process whereby a different breadth and depth of interaction, spontaneity, and cross-fertilization can occur, allowing participants to pick up ideas from one another. Ultimately, group ownership of ideas occurs.

3. To allow for necessary venting of workplace irritants.
4. To provide an excellent opportunity for management to hear and translate constructive criticism in a neutral, nonemotional environment.
5. To provide an environmental process whereby groups can visualize, define, and appreciate the size and complexity of the problem as well as that of the solution.[64]

Focus groups are used within qualitative research studies as a methodology. Perceptions of members of groups are frequently analyzed using focus group techniques. These perceptions include those about client-centered care, expanded roles of professional nurses, experiential learning, cultural diversity, workplace stress, community population characteristics, substance-abuse prevention, resident abuse in long-term care, and relationships between lifestyles and disease prevention.

The three phases of the focus process are as follows:

- Phase 1: Gathering data of internal and external conditions related to the group's objectives.
- Phase 2: Designing the study type and size of sample, group discussion method, and focus group format. Identify 3 to 4 groups of 8 to 12 participants. During this phase, the role of moderator is defined and the script is developed.
- Phase 3: Implementing the plan and providing participant confidentiality.[65]

Groupthink

One of the potential disadvantages of team building and working in committees or other work groups is the possibility of *groupthink* among members of the team or committee. Groupthink is inappropriate conformity to group norms. It occurs when group members avoid risk and fear to disagree or to carefully assess the points under discussion. The following are the symptoms of groupthink:[66]

1. Illusions of invulnerability, leading to overconfidence and reckless risk taking.
2. Negative feedback ignored and rationalized to prevent reconsideration.
3. A belief of inherent morality.
4. Stereotyping of the views of people who disagree as wrong or weak and badly informed.
5. Pressure on members to suppress doubts.
6. Self-censorship by silence about misgivings.
7. Unanimous decisions.
8. Protection of members from negative reactions.

Groupthink will not occur when members are aware of the potential for it. Groups are considered effective when their resources are well used; their time is well used; their decisions are appropriate, reasonable, and error-free; their decisions are implemented and supported by group members; problem-solving ability is enhanced; and group cohesion is built by promoting group norms and structuring cooperative relationships. The group's leader should teach group members cures for groupthink that include the following:[67]

1. Acting as devil's advocate.
2. Considering unlimited alternatives.
3. Thinking critically.
4. Providing increased time for discussion.
5. Changing directions.
6. Surveying people affected by the problem under discussion.
7. Seeking other opinions.
8. Constructing challenging group measures.
9. Including input from people in the group who do not agree with you.

Types of Committees

Two of the most common types of committees in which nurses participate are ad hoc/task force and standing committees. Committees are used by organizations to provide a mechanism to bridge communication gaps between departments or units. Standing committees are advisory in authority, although some may have collective authority to make and implement decisions. An example of a standing committee is the Nurse Practice Committee, or the Infection Control Committee. Ad hoc committees, or task forces, are groups of several individuals who work together on a specific project that is time-limited—for example, a group of nurses selected by their peers to develop a preceptor program for graduate nurses. Ad hoc committees are very important in health care organizations, because they bring together in a short time frame individuals who have the expertise to work on the projects.

Self-Managed (Self-Directed) Work Teams

One specific type of team that has been used effectively is the self-managed (self-directed) work team. A self-directed work team is a functional group of typically 8 to 15 employees. The team shares responsibility for a particular unit of production, including units of service or information. Members are cross-trained in all the technical skills necessary to complete the tasks assigned. Members have the authority to plan, implement, and control all work processes. Members are responsible for scheduling, quality, and costs, and responsibilities have been clearly defined in advance. The nine characteristics of a self-directed work team include bottom-up communication, consensus, big picture, ongoing diverse training, moving around, empowerment, challenge/innovation, external competition, and work and celebration. Employers indicate that self-directed work teams improve quality, increase productivity, decrease operating costs, and foster greater commitment from workers. Employees state that they feel "in on things," involved in decisions, challenged, and empowered, and they also have increased job satisfaction.

Self-directed work teams have leaders. During early phases, upper management appoints the leader. As the team grows and changes, it selects its leader. Eventually, the role rotates. The team leader is an internal facilitator. Middle managers are trained to become external facilitators.[68]

Self-managed work teams are empowered to make all decisions about the work they do. For example, Federal Express and IDS claim productivity up 40% with self-managed work teams. A survey of Fortune 1,000 companies indicates that 68% use self-managed work teams, although only 10% of workers are in them.[69]

To make self-managed teams successful, employers should do the following:

1. Empower the teams with decision making.
2. Provide teams with e-mail communication systems so teams can talk with each other.
3. Create teams only for work that can be done by teams.
4. Make teamwork the centerpiece of a pay-for-performance system.
5. Inspire teams to increase morale, productivity, and innovation.
6. Use the right team for the right job. Form a problem-solving team to solve a problem, then disband it. Use work teams to do the day-to-day work. Work teams should be self-managed, have power to change the order of things, and have budgets.
7. Create a hierarchy of teams that make decisions on the spot. To build the 777, Boeing used three layers of teams: a top management team to see that the plane was built correctly and on time, leader teams from engineering and operations to oversee the work teams, and cross-functional work teams. A fourth layer of airplane integration teams with access to everyone in the organization was added later. Problems were identified and solved early.
8. Maintain trust and morale. When restructuring, bring employees into the process. Plan for job loss by retraining, reassigning, retiring, and attrition.
9. Tackle people problems head on by spending time to get people to work together.

The change to self-managed work teams requires training of management personnel who are uncomfortable with the process and find their status and power threatened. Managers have to unlearn traditional autocratic approaches with punitive emphasis and tight controls on the work force. Managers are trained to overcome feelings of threat and resentment to change; to perceive workers as mature and responsible; to believe that workers can train each other; to believe that peer pressure can overcome absenteeism and that a self-managed team gives them time to develop key people; and to believe they can be a resource to team members and a support group among themselves. They will be facilitators who work with the group. The leaders are key to the success of self-directed work teams and their use of power is crucial in breaking down the organizational barriers preventing effective teams. Managers can make the transition to new roles with modified behavior and attitudes, but is not a simple task for them.[70]

One of the activities that self-managed work teams can do effectively is problem solving, a powerful service strategy that gets everyone working toward top performance. Employees feel that their ideas and efforts are valued. Once the self-managed work teams are formed, problem solving may be introduced in five steps as follows:[71]

1. Brainstorming to identify problems. Team members are asked to describe problems they have observed or experienced.
2. Once all problems are listed, team members are asked to vote on paper for the three problems they believe are most significant. The votes are tallied and the most important problem is presented.
3. Brainstorming for possible solutions to the problem. The most promising solution is selected. Team members are assigned to investigate the solution and gather further information to report on later. The meeting is then closed.
4. At the next meeting, the team reports their findings, which are discussed, including positive and negative aspects.
5. The team chooses the solution through discussion and general agreement. Team members share the responsibility for putting the solution to work.

Self-directed work teams and work groups are successfully used to reduce cost per unit-of-service, improve service and customer satisfaction, determine optimal staffing levels, and reduce the number of layers of organization. These teams perform tasks that require technical and management skills, thereby increasing productivity.[72]

Making Committees Effective

Purposes of Committees

Organizations promote communication through meetings. In one year the cost of meetings in US companies is several billion dollars, and executives spend as much as 60% of their time in meetings. For this reason, nurse managers should evaluate the purposes and functions of committees, particularly of standing committees.

Evaluation should be both normative and summative and should determine whether committees are accomplishing their purpose or are wasting the time and talents of many people who are required to attend the meetings. Are unnecessary meetings being held?

Meetings fulfill deep personal and individual needs. Their effective use by groups improves productivity. Types of committees are determined by organizational objectives and functions. Committees can be effectively used to implement major policy changes, to accomplish a job, and to plan strategically. Problems requiring research and planning are better assigned to individuals. Day-to-day decisions should be handled by line managers.[73]

A major purpose of using groups or committees is to involve personnel in participatory management that gives representation of employees at all levels a share in the decision-making process. According to Dixon, this goal can be accomplished by having the following:[74]

1. Enough groups to ensure representation at all levels.
2. Standing committees, ad hoc committees, town hall meetings, and small meetings so that all levels feel represented.
3. Representation by visible managers to ensure support.
4. Control of employees.
5. Planned absence of managers at selective meetings to encourage discussion.
6. Stimuli to employee participation with tangible results.
7. Members solicited as volunteers, appointed by managers, or selected by employees.
8. Technical assistance to identify problems, promote communication, and solve problems.
9. A focus on the power of the group to act on its own recommendations, have its own budget, or access company resources.

American health care organizations are confronted with a hostile and turbulent environment of expanded demands, inflation, competition, shortages of professional nurses, and intrusion by other groups. Professional nurses are more highly educated and have higher expectations for extrinsic reward and intrinsic satisfiers such as autonomy and challenge. They want to participate and to affect organizational performance and employee satisfaction positively.

Mohrman and Ledford's recommendation for successful employee participation can be used by nurse managers. Success depends on design and implementation of the participation group process. Participation groups are designed to do the following:[75]

1. Be effective in group problem solving.
2. Be effective within the larger organization as well as within the division or unit of nursing. This can be expanded to include appropriate professional and service organizations.
3. Achieve legitimacy.
4. Acquire resources and approval for their ideas.
5. Motivate others in the organization to accept, implement, and support their group solution.

Organization of Committees

Committees and work groups are effective when they are formally organized, have a purpose, designate a leader, keep written minutes of their work, and achieve results. When organizing committees, the following factors should be considered:

1. Every committee should have a purpose and short-term objectives.
2. Committee members should be chosen according to their expertise and their capacity to represent the larger group.
3. The committee members must contribute in terms of commitment, time, and energy.
4. Committees should be of manageable size for discussion and disagreement. Six to eight members are usually recommended.
5. Committee chairs should be accountable to a specific administrator who provides guidance to the chair through consultation.
6. Committees should have prepared agendas and effective chairs. Exhibit 6-2 contains standards for evaluating nursing committees.

Nursing should be represented on most health care institution committees and always on those whose activities will affect nursing. It should have representation that will be effective in determining the outcomes of a health team approach to patient care services. In effect, nurses should determine how they would practice nursing. The organizational standards presented in Appendix 6-1 meet the goals of shared governance.

Improving Committee Effectiveness

There is no one way to measure group effectiveness, but multiple indicators can provide a framework to measure effectiveness of groups and committees.[76]

1. Productivity of the work group or committee.
2. Satisfaction of group members.
3. Quality of work produced.
4. Opportunity for the work group or committee to work together toward one common goal.

Nurse managers can improve the effectiveness of standing and ad hoc committees by establishing minimal ground rules, including the following:[77]

1. Establish clearly stated objectives. For ad hoc or specialized meetings, discuss the goals before planning the meetings. Base the goals on advancing the clinical and business goals of nursing. See Appendix 6-1.

2. Establish a committee structure to support the clearly stated objectives (see Exhibit 6-2).
3. Plan all meetings and events to meet the goals and objectives.
   a. Keep the committee or event to a manageable size. Define membership. Assemblies begin at 100 and increase in size. They observe and listen but may have little participation. Councils comprise 40 to 50 persons who listen or comment. Committees should include approximately 10 to 12 persons who all participate on an equal footing.
   b. Draw up a point-by-point agenda and send it to the attendees. Include the purpose of the meeting. Because the sequence of the agenda is important, the following points are helpful:
      (i) Put dull items early and "star" items last.
      (ii) Decide whether to place divisive items early or late.
      (iii) Plan a time for starting important items.
      (iv) Limit committee meetings to 2 hours or fewer.
      (v) Schedule meetings to begin 1 hour before lunch or 1 hour before the end of the workday.
      (vi) Avoid putting extraneous business on the agenda.
      (vii) Read the agenda and write in comments before the meeting.
   c. Tailor the meeting room to the group and prepare it beforehand.
   d. Prepare for the meeting by learning the subject matter and by preparing audiovisual materials to support it. Bring input via videotaped interviews from people who do not attend. Make events memorable.
   e. Time the agenda items. New or controversial subjects usually take more time. Attention spans diminish after the first hour. Use time efficiently, including mealtimes.
   f. Referee and set the pace of the meeting. Summarize and clarify as needed.
   g. Promote lively participation by involving attendees in the program with a warm-up "getting acquainted" phase, a conflict phase, and a total collaboration phase. Bring out the personal goals of the individuals.
   h. Listen to what others say so there will be a sharing of knowledge, experience, judgments, and folklore.
   i. Bring the meeting to a definite conclusion by obtaining decisions and commitments.
   j. Follow up as necessary to eliminate loose ends. Evaluate whether the meeting's purpose was achieved.
   k. Circulate useful information with the minutes. Keep the minutes brief, listing time, date, place, chair, attendance, agenda items and action, time ended, and the time, date, and place of the next meeting. Exhibit 6-3 provides checklist for evaluating meeting effectiveness.

Developing an Organizational Structure

An organizational structure for a division of nursing must meet the needs of that division as written in the statements of mission, philosophy, vision, values, and objectives. Most existing institutions already have an organizational structure. Before the structure is changed, the nurse managers should engage in a systematic analysis as well as do some sound thinking about altering the organization's design and structure, starting with objectives and strategy.

A newer concept in the theory of organizations is that the organizational structure affects the strategic decision-making process. Historically, changes in organizational structure have followed changes in strategy such as unit volume, geographic dispersion, and vertical and horizontal integration. The organizational form determines the decision-making environment: it delimits responsibilities and communication channels, controls the decision-making environment, and facilitates information processing.[78] Strategic decision making requires wide expertise from numerous levels. In nursing, managers should seek broad input from clinical nurses. This can be done through task forces, committees, project teams, or ad hoc groups.

In developing or changing an organizational structure, results from research should be considered. In the report *To Err is Human: Building a Safer Health System*, the Institute of Medicine (IOM) found that approximately 98,000 patients who are hospitalized each year die as a result of medical errors.[79] In a response to this report, the US Department of Health and Human Services' (DHHS) Agency for Healthcare Research and Quality (AHRQ) requested that the IOM conduct a study to identify the opportunities to improve the work environment of health care staff, especially nurses, that would improve patient safety.[80] Several of the recommendations that were given by the IOM included changes in the organizational structure and culture. By analyzing the current practices and structure in organizations, recommendations such as the following can be implemented to ultimately change the structure of an organization.[81]

1. Ensure that direct-care nursing staff participates in the decisions relating to design of work processes and workflow.
2. Organizations should support and develop interdisciplinary collaboration throughout the organization.
3. Organizations should provide the resources necessary to create a work environment for nurses to reduce errors.
4. Organizations should create a culture of safety.

EXHIBIT 6-3

Checklist for Evaluating Meeting Effectiveness

STANDARDS	YES	NO
1. The meeting started on time.	____	____
2. A quorum existed.	____	____
3. The meeting agenda is on a schedule.	____	____
4. The agenda for the meeting reflects the purpose of the committee.	____	____
5. The chair acts as an equal member of the group, taking no special considerations.	____	____
6. The chair follows the agenda.	____	____
a. Dull items are scheduled early, star items last.	____	____
b. Divisive items are strategically placed.	____	____
c. Important items have a starting time.	____	____
d. The agenda avoids "any other business."	____	____
e. Meetings are scheduled for one hour before lunch or one hour before end of work day.	____	____
f. The chair is well prepared for the meeting.	____	____
g. The chair referees, paces, summarizes, and clarifies discussion.	____	____
h. The meeting concludes with definite decisions and a commitment to them.	____	____
i. The chair follows up on necessary items.	____	____
j. Useful information is circulated with the minutes.	____	____
7. The chair allows adequate time for discussion.	____	____
8. The chair facilitates participation by all members.	____	____
9. Items requiring further study are referred to smaller groups as projects. Timetables for results are established.	____	____
10. Managers attend meetings when needed to ensure support.	____	____
11. Managers plan absences from selected meetings to encourage discussion.	____	____
12. Technical assistance is provided to facilitate meeting success.	____	____

EXHIBIT 6-4

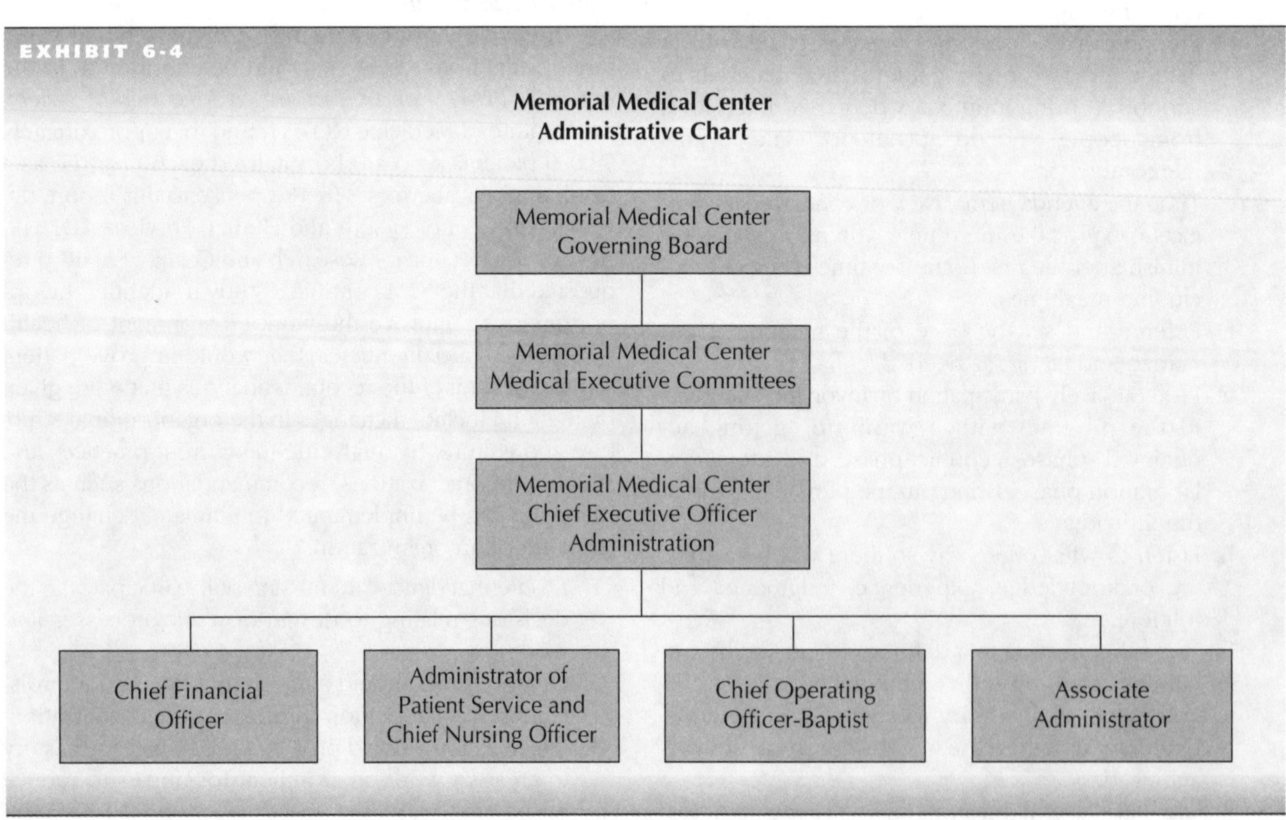

Organization Charts

Most nursing organizations have made graphic representations of the organizing process in the form of organization charts. These charts usually show reporting relationships and communication channels. Line charts show supervisor and employee relationships from top to bottom of the nursing organization. Hierarchical relationships exist on which communication channels follow the line of authority to and through the chief nurse executive. (See Exhibits 6-4, 6-5, 6-6, and 6-7.)

Staff charts show the advisory relationship of specialists or experts who are extensions of the nurse administrators. These types of charts usually depict the title or rank of each line and staff officer position in the authority relationship structure. They denote the delegation of authority and responsibility as well as the direction of accountability for the goals of the nursing division.

Organization charts distribute the nursing responsibilities, and lines connect the positions. These responsibilities may be divided according to one function or a combination of functions: contiguous geography, similar techniques, similar objectives, or similar clientele. The solid lines on an organizational chart represent line positions. Lines of authority can be either horizontal or vertical. An example would be that all the nurses in the emergency department report up to one manager who has authority over all the nurses, and these nurses are accountable to the manager.[82] The horizontal lines represent the communication patterns between individuals with similar responsibilities in the organization. For example, a solid horizontal line would exist between the nurse manager of an oncology unit and the nurse manager on the intensive care unit. Both of the nurse managers have the same responsibility in their job duties, report to the same supervisor, and have to work together to achieve the overall objectives of nursing and the organization.[83] The dotted lines on an organizational chart represent staff positions. Staff positions provide support and assistance to others. For example, the cardiovascular clinical nurse specialist and the intravenous nurse hold staff positions.[84]

Organization charts are sometimes referred to as *schemas*. Decentralized schemas are flatter because there are fewer levels of control or management. Managers have more freedom to act, and the emphasis is on results.

There are advantages to having a current organization chart. Such charts should show clear relationships. They show employees who their supervisor is and supervisors whom they supervise. They could facilitate coordination and communication. They can prevent intrigue, frustration, and duplication of effort, and promote decision making, efficiency, and adherence to policy. They can tie the structure together and show inconsistencies and complexities. Organization charts also have limitations. They will show formal authority structure only; if they are outdated and obsolete, they will show what *was* rather than what *is*. Organization charts may confuse authority with status.

The success of nursing and of health care organizations depends on service to the customer. The focus then is on job function, and the organization chart should reflect this rather than show titles or names. Look at the traditional organization chart. It tells the employee who the boss is, and it often becomes a plan for empire building and for abdication of responsibility.

A circular organizational chart may be reflective of a hospital's increased reliance on team processes throughout the organization and a significantly reduced number of reporting assignments.[85] Intertwining and interconnecting circles may be indicative of relationships of the board, councils, and committees of such an organization.[86]

A new way of drawing organizational charts is the *organigraph*, which is a map offering an overview of a company's functions and the way people organize themselves at work. The organigraph is said to help managers see untapped opportunities by showing where ideas flow, what parts are connected to one another, and how processes and people should come together.[87]

Exhibit 6-8 shows how to evaluate an organization chart of a nursing division, department, or unit.

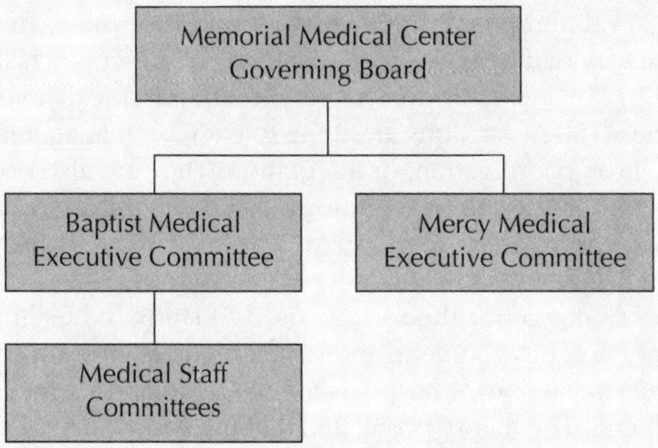

Context

There are certain contextual variables that relate to an organization's structure, such as organizational charter or social function, size, technology, environment, interdependence with other organizations, structuring of activities, concentration of authority, and line of control of workflow.[88]

EXHIBIT 6-5

Memorial Medical Center
Medical Staff Organization Chart

Memorial Medical Center Governing Board

Baptist Medical Executive Committee

Mercy Medical Executive Committee

Medical Staff Committees

EXHIBIT 6-6

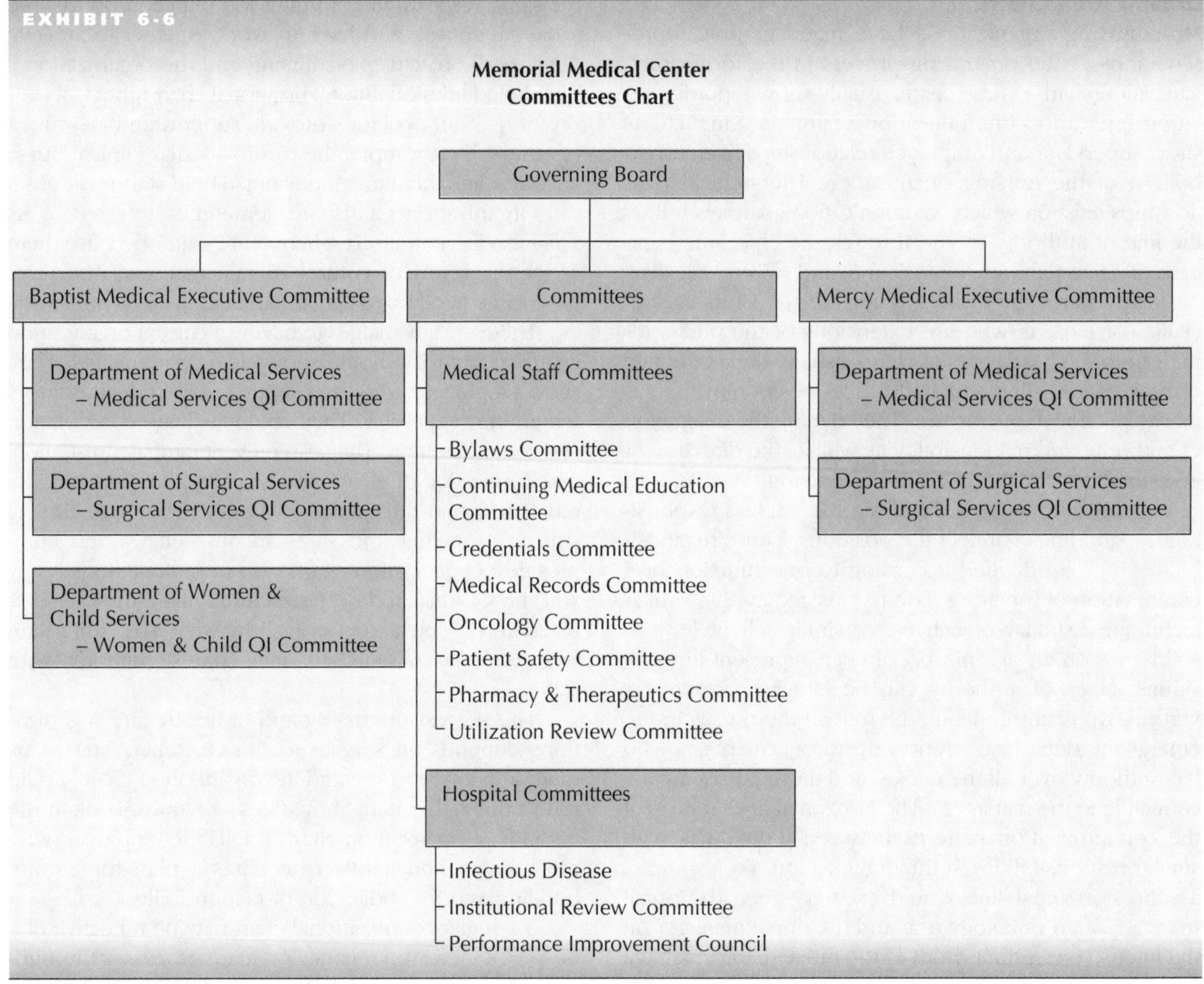

Organizational Charter or Social Function

Nursing organizations exist within institutions that are either government-owned, private not-for-profit, or private for-profit. Government-owned organizations are impersonally founded and highly centralized, with concentrated authority. Impersonality of origin increases the level of control of workflow. Since many health care organizations are impersonal in origin, they are highly centralized with increased line control of workflow of professional nurses.

Since professional nurses want autonomy of decision making in their practice, they will initiate strategies to increase and allow the desired autonomy and accountability of clinical nurses in order to increase their independence, their status, and their representation on policy-making entities.

Size

Larger organizations tend to have more specialization and more formalization than small ones. The larger the size, the more decentralized the organization and the more standardized the procedures for selection and advancement of personnel. Bureaucracy increases with size and decreased personal integration.[89]

Increased size of an organization requires that managers differentiate employees into work groups, functions, departments, or work centers with described tasks. They are also differentiated into hierarchical levels. These differentiations are done to exercise management control, coordination, or integration. They are also done to buffer the core technology of an organization and to prepare it to respond to variety in the external environment.[90]

Contingency theory was used to study the technology, size, environment, and structure in 157 nursing subunits located in 24 hospitals in the Canadian province of Alberta. The theory postulated that the wide range of differences in organizational structure varies systematically with such factors as technology, size, and environment. It was found that increased subunit beds decreased the

EXHIBIT 6-7

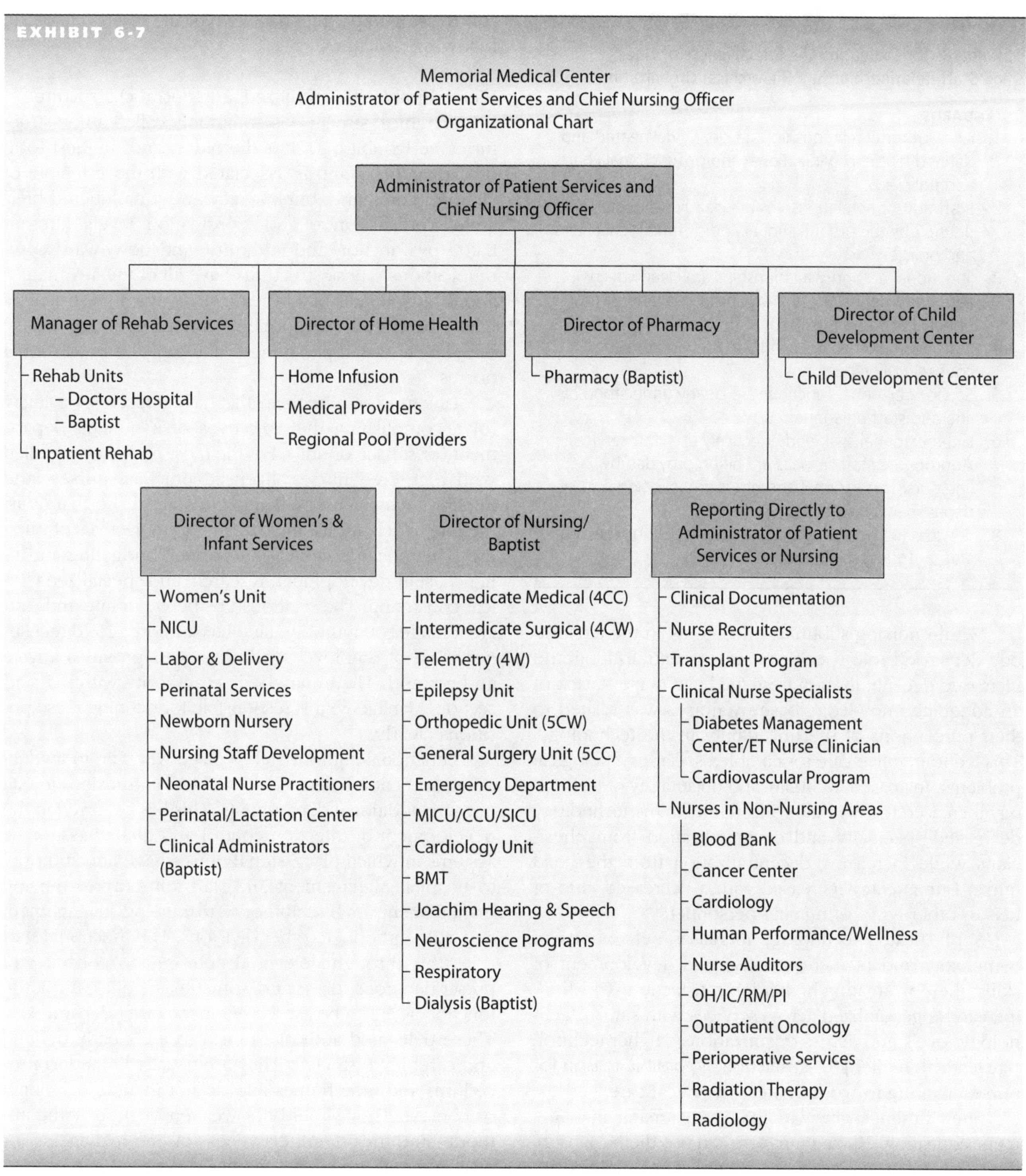

RN-ratio and increased the measure of bureaucratization of professionals. There was no relationship between decentralization of the subunit and size and little relationship between size and role specificity.[91] These findings would support those of Pugh and others who found no relationship between size and concentration of authority, between size and line control of workflow, or between size and autonomy.[92]

Technology

Technology can be defined as the steps or ordering of physical techniques used for organizational workflow, even if the physical techniques involve only the formulation of the plan. The more rigid and highly integrated the technology, the greater the structuring of activities and procedures and the more impersonal the control. Complex technology emphasizes administration.[93]

EXHIBIT 6-8

Standards for Evaluating the Effectiveness of Line and Staff Relationships in a Hierarchical Organization

STANDARDS

1. Line authority relationships are clearly delineated and defined by the organizational and/or functional charts and policies.
2. Staff authority relationships are clearly delineated and defined by the organizational and/or functional charts and policies.
3. Functional authority relationships are clearly delineated and defined by the organizational and/or functional charts and policies.
4. Staff personnel consult with, advise, and provide counsel to line personnel.
5. Service personnel functions are clearly understood by line and staff personnel.
6. Line personnel seek and effectively use staff services.
7. Appropriate staff services are being provided by line nursing personnel and other organizational departments or services.
8. Services are not being duplicated because of line and staff authority relationships.

Within nursing subunits, uncertainty in the technology decreased role specificity and decentralization and increased decentralization from the head nurse. A lack of an adequate knowledge base by nurses was related to their perceptions of the uncertainty in the technology. This led to intuitive care for complex social-psychological problems. Increased instability and uncertainty of technology increased the RN ratio. Uncertainty in the technology decreased specificity and decentralization from physicians while increasing decentralization from the head nurse. Bureaucracy increased with a decreased ratio of RNs to other types of nursing personnel.[94]

Sophisticated technology increases perceptions of complexity and of increased use and development of skills, thereby creating higher job satisfaction. This finding can be generalized across services with similar technology levels and across organizations. Higher technology leads to higher job satisfaction, a possible reason for nurses aspiring to work in areas of critical care.[95]

Such findings give credibility to nursing management education. Nurse managers can use them to justify differentiated practice, since complex technology requires more advanced education and staff development that sustains more advanced knowledge and skills. Education can thus be related to performance and pay.

Forms of Organizational Structures

A structure enables an organization to get the work done. It helps ensure that the purpose, goals, and objectives of the organization are achieved.

Nursing departments have typically used one of the following structures.

Hierarchical (Tall, Centralized, Bureaucratic) Structure

A hierarchical structure is commonly called a line structure (see Exhibit 6-4). It is the oldest and simplest form of management and is associated with the principle of chain of command, bureaucracy and a multitiered hierarchy, vertical control and coordination, levels differentiated by function and authority, and downward communications. These structures have all of the advantages and disadvantages of a bureaucracy. Most line structures have added a staff component. In nursing organizations, both line and staff personnel will usually be professional nurses.

Line functions are those that have direct responsibility for accomplishing the objectives of a nursing department (or service or unit). For the most part, they are filled with registered nurses, licensed practical nurses, and nursing technicians. Staff functions are those that assist the line in accomplishing the primary objectives of nursing. They include clerical, personnel, budgeting and finance, staff development, research, and specialized clinical consulting. The relationships between line and staff are a matter of authority. Line has authority for direct supervision of employees, whereas staff provides advice and counsel. There may be line authority within a staff section. Management is responsible for defining these positions clearly.

Functional authority takes place when an individual or department is delegated authority over functions in one or more additional departments. This has occurred in the development of infection control and quality-assurance systems in which professional nurses have line authority to hospital management and staff authority to nursing management, or line authority to nursing management and staff authority to other divisions. The functional staff does this through delegated authority to consult and prescribe procedures, and sometimes policies, for the function as it is to be carried out in the other departments. These delegated authority functions are clearly defined and carefully restricted. They are usually limited to procedures and time frames and do not include personnel or context. They should not weaken or destroy the authority and thus the effectiveness of line managers. For example, staff personnel might be assigned authority to recruit nurses, with line managers retaining final authority over hiring. The nurse administrator should ensure effective use of staff functions by line managers so as to make effective use of the advice of experts and reduce duplication of effort of line managers. Staff gives information that will facilitate the solution of problems. Line managers in an effective and cooperative relationship seek such information.

Service departments are not necessarily staff in their authority relationships. Usually, they are a grouping of activities that facilitate the work of other departments through their operating functions. An example of this is the hospital's maintenance department, which provides the service of a functioning plant in which patient services are provided. It has the authority for performing its functions and may provide some staff advice and counsel. Within a hospital, as in any business, there may be many service departments, such as word processing centers, learning resource centers, and others.

Activities are grouped together to provide for economical specialization. There may be service units for labor relations, contracts, legal matters, purchasing, and others. They may have functional authority, but care must be taken to keep them from causing divided loyalties, from delaying performance, and from displaying arrogance. They should provide for uniformity of procedures, policies, and standards for skilled service and a smooth operation. Exhibit 6-8 shows a set of standards for evaluation of the effectiveness of line and staff relationships within a nursing division, department, or unit in a hierarchical organization.

Matrix Structure

A matrix management structure superimposes a horizontal program management over the traditional vertical hierarchy. Personnel from various functional departments are assigned to a specific program or project and become responsible to two bosses—a program manager and their functional department head. Thus an interdisciplinary team is created with core and extended team members. A longitudinal study of geriatrics matrix team program showed initial increased costs offset after a year by decreased acute care readmission rates, emergency room use, and nursing home placement. Mortality was significantly decreased and the functional ability of patients increased.[96]

The matrix organization design enables timely response to external competition and facilitates efficiency and effectiveness internally through cooperation among disciplines.

A matrix organization has the following characteristics:[97]

1. Maintenance of old-line authority structures.
2. Specialist resources obtained from functional areas.
3. Promotion of formation of new organizational units.
4. Decision making at the organizational level of group consensus, the first-line management level.
5. The exercise of authority by the matrix manager over the functional manager.
6. Cooperative planning, program development, and allocation of resources to accomplish program objectives.
7. Assignment of functional managers to teams that respond to the chief of the functional discipline and matrix manager.

Matrix nursing organizational structures have the following advantages:[98]

1. Improved communication through vertical and horizontal control and coordination of interdisciplinary patient care teams.
2. Increased organizational adaptability and fluidity to respond to environmental changes.
3. Increased efficiency of resource use with fewer organizational levels and decision making closer to primary care operations.
4. Improved human resource management because of increased job satisfaction with achievement and fulfillment, improved communication, improved interpersonal skills, and improved collegial relationships.

Matrix nursing organizational structures have the following disadvantages:[99]

1. Potential conflict because of dual or multiple lines of authority, responsibility, and accountability relationships.
2. Role ambiguity.
3. Loss of control over functional discipline as a result of a multidisciplinary team approach.

Decentralization (Flat, Horizontal, Participatory) Structure

Flat organizational structures are characteristic of decentralized management. Decentralization refers to the degree to which authority is shifted downward within an organization to its divisions, services, and units. Decentralization is delegating decision-making responsibilities to the ones doing the work—participatory management. Implementation of a philosophy of decentralized decision making by top management sets the stage for involving more people—perhaps even the entire staff—in making decisions at the level at which an action occurs. Both decentralized management and participatory management delegate authority from top managers downward to the people who report to them. In doing so, objectives or duties are assigned, authority is granted, and an obligation or responsibility is created by acceptance. The employee is accountable for results.[100]

In nursing, as in other organizations, delegation fosters participation, teamwork, and accountability. A first-line manager with delegated authority will contact another department to solve a problem in providing a service. The first-line manager does not need to go to his or her department head, who in turn would contact the department head of the other service, creating a communication bottleneck. The people closest to the problem solve it, resulting in efficient and cost-effective management. Research conducted on Magnet hospitals found that most of the hospitals have a decentralized structure in which nurses had a feeling of control over their unit work environment.[101] Porter O'Grady identified the following conditions as essential for effective decentralization:[102]

1. Freedom to function effectively
2. Support from peers and leaders
3. Concise and clear expectations of the work environment
4. Appropriate resources

Participatory Management

Structure of Decentralized and Participatory Organizations

Traditional hierarchical structures with increasingly authoritative levels of management frighten employees, threaten their need for security, and make them uncomfortable. Economic events of the 1990s made way for horizontal organizational structures with no rank, no boss, and no seniority. Flat organizational structures are flourishing. They are increasing management and employee association and commitment and reducing the number of managers and manuals, titles, and executive suites.[103] In nursing, there are reports of the elimination of nurse manager positions, with committees of professional nurses elected by unit staff to manage unit activities. These nurses' efforts are facilitated by the new breed of leaders, who are democratic, participative, and laissez-faire (or free rein) and who involve their followers in making decisions, setting objectives, establishing strategies, and determining job assignments. These nurse leaders place emphasis on people, employees, and followers and their participation in the management process. These nurses are employee-centered and relationship-centered.

Decentralized organizational structures are compatible with primary nursing. Decisions are made, goals are set, peer review and evaluation take place, schedules are made, and primary nurses resolve conflicts. Levels of practice are built into staffing.[104] Exhibit 6-9 outlines standards for evaluating decentralization of authority in a nursing division, department, service, or unit.

EXHIBIT 6-9

Standards for Evaluating Decentralization of Authority in a Nursing Division, Department, Service, or Unit

STANDARDS

1. Authority for decision making is delegated to the lowest operating level consistent with:
   a. Competence of subordinate managers
   b. Responsibility and accountability
   c. Economic management of enterprise
   d. Costs involved
   e. Need for uniformity and innovation of policy
   f. Management philosophy
   g. Subordinate managers' desires for independence
   h. Development of subordinate managers
   i. Need for evaluation and control
   j. Physical location of subordinate managers
   k. Organizational dynamics
2. Delegated authority is clear, specific, certain, and written. It is known by each subordinate manager.
3. Delegated authority supports the organizational, departmental, service, and unit goals, policies, standards, and plans.
4. Delegated authority is consistent with requirements of regulatory agencies, private and governmental.

Trust

Participatory management is based on a philosophy of trust. The employee is trusted to complete the task, with periodic progress reports and a final review with management. The time and rate of participation should be managed to control stress. Managers who empower and facilitate employee performance communicate trust. This process will demonstrate the employee's capabilities and reveal shortcomings.

Motorola has had a participatory management program in effect since 1968, with almost all of its thousands of US employees involved in it at some stage. These three basic ideas of their program embody trust:[105]

1. Every worker knows his or her job better than anybody else.
2. People can and will accept responsibility for managing their own work if that responsibility is given to them in the proper way.
3. Intelligence, perspective, and creativity exist among people at all levels of the organization.

Commitment

Personal involvement in managing a nursing service requires commitment from the chief nurse and other nurse managers. Managers should be highly visible to the staff, supporting and nurturing them. In turn, the staff should also be committed, a characteristic they will develop from association with the committed managers. They gain this commitment from seeing their bosses out at the production level where patients are being treated, from cooperating with their colleagues and managers in a spirit of teamwork, and from acquiring feelings of accomplishment.

Nursing commitment comes from knowing that the purpose of the organization is patient care and that the managers are working with the nurses to produce that care. Staff shares in making decisions and in coming to consensus with the bosses. This experience in participation "turns them on and tunes them in" so that they do not want to be lazy or mediocre or to featherbed. Commitment inspires staff to be industrious, outstanding, and productive. Under participatory management, commitment is elicited, not imposed.

Professional nurses are motivated to develop their human skills, resulting in increased self-esteem. They have a sense of accomplishment and feel that management has supported their accomplishments. They feel they are expanding their worth through their work.

Goals and Objectives

Conflict resolution is a major requirement or goal of participatory management. Conflict is inevitable when human beings work together, but it is not productive to process or outcomes. In nursing, as in other occupations, conflict produces stress and results in turnover and absenteeism. Employees can be sensitized to deal with potential and real conflict and to take action to reduce its destructive consequences: fear, anger, distrust, jealousy, and resentment. Reducing the destructiveness of conflict can be accomplished by establishing a climate of openness with procedures for problem solving, persuasion, bargaining, and dealing with organizational politics. The goal is to reduce adversarial relations, which is accomplished through joint planning and problem solving and facilitating employee consultation[106]

A key goal for a nursing organization is to keep itself healthy. Participatory management encourages a healthy work environment. Participation will make maximum use of employees' abilities without relinquishing the ultimate authority and responsibility of management. Professional nurses want to have input into decisions but do not want to do the job of managers. They want the support of managers, to be able to talk with them and to be informed. Without this support, nurses develop anger and hostility, which results in absenteeism and lower productivity.

Goal-setting activities can occur with reasonably frequent performance review and feedback. Nursing personnel bring their goals and objectives to conferences with managers. The process is reciprocal, with the manager and employee together developing goals and objectives that are challenging, clear, consistent, and specific. Nurses and managers will both be motivated, healthy stress will be increased, and undesirable stress will be reduced.

Career development programs for professional nurses help to reduce conflict and inspire loyalty to an organization. Provided with job information, nurses can set goals for themselves that relate to promotion, tenure, and job security. Differences in work attitudes and personal aspirations are recognized. There is less professional role conflict. New employees, who are young and fresh out of college, should be given information about the nature of the organization, current and future availability of jobs, career opportunities and career ladders, and management goals and responsibilities. Managers learn about the professional nurse employees' aspirations and expectations and should help them set a course and monitor it.[107]

Autonomy

Autonomy is the state of being independent, of having responsibility, authority, and accountability for one's work and personal time. Professional employees indicate they want autonomy for practicing their profession and in making decisions about their work. They do not want their decisions made for them by hospital administrators, physicians, or others. They want to be treated as equal partners and colleagues in the health care delivery system. This desire for autonomy has increased as nurses have developed increasingly sophisticated knowledge and skills and have used them with effective results.

Professional nurses want autonomous control over conditions under which they work, including pace and content. Such decisions are often in conflict with management's coordination role, a conflict that can be mitigated by involving professional nurses in delegating coordination of activities.[108]

Professional nurses are willing to assume and accept responsibility and to be held accountable for a charge. They want authority, the rightful and legitimate power to fulfill the charge. This authority comes from their expert knowledge and skill, their license, their position, and their peers.[109]

The autonomy of professional nurses is evident in an organization in which management trusts nurses by giving them freedom to make decisions and take actions within the scope of their knowledge. Nurses are thus free to exercise their authority. This freedom is legitimized in the bylaws of their departments and in job descriptions, performance appraisals, and management support of their decisions. Nurses' independent behavior includes acknowledging mistakes, taking action to correct them, and preventing them from happening again.

The professional nurse is accountable for the consequences of his or her actions. Relationships exist between responsibility, authority, autonomy, and accountability.

To have autonomy, nursing employees should be involved in setting their own goals and be allowed to determine how to accomplish their goals. This principle applies to all nursing employees. When professional nurses work with other nursing employees, they should facilitate participation and input from these groups. This approach promotes interest, trust, and commitment.[110]

A study of nurse autonomy found variations in perceptions of whether the nurses were expected to exhibit autonomy and of whether they were supported in exhibiting it. The typical nurse exhibiting the highest level of autonomy was a female with a master's degree practicing in a clinical administrative role in the emergency room who perceived an expectation to function autonomously to a high degree. The typical nurse exhibiting the lowest level of autonomy was a male staff nurse in the operating room or post-anesthesia with less than a master's degree who perceived an expectation to practice autonomously to a low extent or was unsure of the expectation for autonomy. No change was found in the perceived levels of autonomy from studies done 15 years before. Highest scores were found among nurses practicing in the emergency room, psychiatry, and critical care, areas in which institutions and physicians grant the greatest autonomy. Nurses at the master's level had the highest scores in autonomy. Below that level, poor role definition, role confusion, and poor role modeling contribute to a socialization process that encourages all nurses to act the same. Conversely, nurses in administrative roles have clearer role expectations and correspondingly higher scores on autonomy. Apparently, they are not empowering their practice staff to have the same level of autonomy. The authors found from the results of their study that their findings may indicate that autonomy is not expected or supported by hospitals.

To foster greater autonomy, nurses need to be included in decision making, policy setting and financial decisions. They need to have role clarity and to be educated at a higher level for autonomous practice. Greater attention needs to be paid to role modeling to facilitate understanding of nursing independent, dependent, and interdependent aspects. When elements are identified within one area of practice that promote autonomy, they need to be incorporated into other areas as well.[111]

A study of graduating students at one university indicated that the students ranked high on individual autonomy. It would appear that lack of professional status is not due to lack of autonomy in individual nurses. Therefore, consideration must be given to the denial of autonomy by employing institutions as the root cause. Nurses probably arrive at their first job with more autonomous attitudes than do women in other industries. Serious consideration should be given to the role that institutions play in blocking nurses' efforts at achieving professional autonomy. Nursing education should address this issue by looking critically at existing programs and working to educate nurses who will be able to claim their rightful professional status.[112]

Top Management

What is the role of top management under a decentralized system with participatory management? Its role is directed toward results. Top management shares in planning and implementing the program. Because effective controls are needed to monitor performance of lower-level units, top managers use computers to assist in making decisions and developing controlling techniques for decentralization.

In one research study, 18 of 20 hospitals had some decentralization; 77% had some decentralization down to the unit level. The overriding purpose of decentralization was to increase worker satisfaction. Decentralization resulted in increased morale and job satisfaction and greater motivation among managers and workers. Personnel development, flexibility, and effective decision making all increased; conflict decreased, along with operational costs, negative attitudes, and underuse of managers. The work force stabilized and became more effective and efficient. The study indicated that most managers do not understand the concept of delegation, are not effective communicators, do not concentrate on goals, and do not delegate according to the abilities and interests of their employees.[113] With the dynamics of decentralization, each unit works with its own budget; job descriptions are clear, concise, flexible, and current; in-service training is effective; performance standards are clear; employee recognition occurs; and accountability is enforced at all times.

Vertical Versus Horizontal Integration

Vertical integration combines decentralization with integration. When businesses and industries decentralize operations into product lines and subsidiaries, each unit maintains its partnership and identity within the corporate structure. Before the advent of the prospective payment system and competition among hospitals, the industry was largely characterized by horizontal integration of departments within divisions. Some examples are nursing; operations related to patient care services, such as pharmacy, physical therapy, and occupational therapy; operations related to plant management, including housekeeping; and finance.

As competition increased, hospitals began the quest to diversify into new markets. New corporate structures that included umbrella corporate management with subsidiary companies were formed. As hospitals struggle for survival, many choose vertical integration as a means of capturing lost revenues through control of input and output. Whether all efforts at vertical integration will be successful depends on the market share of products and services captured. Moderate effects on operating costs as a result of hospital mergers have been reported.

Among the objectives of vertical integration are the following:[114]

1. Conversion of internal cost centers into revenue producers. An example is medical supply and durable medical equipment. Heretofore, hospitals would refer discharged patients to hospital or medical equipment companies to purchase dressings, wheelchairs, and the like. Some hospitals have formed their own companies to sell and rent medical supplies and equipment to ambulatory patients and to other subsidiaries within the corporate structure. Profits go to the hospital subsidiary instead of to the medical supply company.
2. Development of new and expanding markets for hospitals. These include home health care, which was formerly referred to a public health agency or private home health care agency. Referrals have increased dramatically with early discharge of patients. Hospital corporations have also formed health insurance companies such as preferred provider and health maintenance organizations.

From the viewpoint of function rather than of structure, organizations have focused on the vertical dimension of decentralized decision making. This vertical dimension aims for representation by levels of employees, thereby restricting decentralization to a single function or issue considered to be of primary importance to the organization. Health care has sometimes focused on issues of marketing and quality control, in which decisions are made up or down the hierarchy.

Horizontal integration is also important to the success of participatory management. Integration of the decentralized decision-making process horizontally or laterally links traditionally separate functional hierarchies. The objective is to improve communication across functions, with mutually influential inputs from different interest groups whose individual values, objectives, and loyalties have previously been compartmentalized into obstructions to lateral integration. The organizational structure and functions require adaptation to models that will support participatory processes.[115] Organizational integration requires a merger of information technology that reports results for all organizational entities.[116] Health care systems are sometimes horizontally and vertically integrated for maximum service integration, service delivery, patient capture, and medical education.[117]

Training

Managers at all levels of nursing should subscribe to the philosophy of participatory management if it is to be successful. All managers and employees must unfreeze the present system of attitudes and values. This unfreezing process will require a comprehensive, well-planned training program. Training will promote a sense of job security by preparing everyone for changed roles. Staff members at every level learn the reasons for participatory management, the advantages and disadvantages, and the roles they will play.

Managers might be threatened by the concept of participatory management if they perceive that their authority is being diminished. Their training program will require that their competencies be assessed. This training will include developing managers' abilities to be frank with employees, to be willing to admit to past failures, and to encourage contributions from their workers and be influenced by them. Managers need to learn to deal with justifying the existence of their jobs.[118]

More than 1,000 businesses in the United States are involved in some form of participatory management. Many nursing organizations subscribe to the notion of participatory management to some degree. Centralized management and authority are becoming history in the development of the science of human behavior.[119] Because they have been subjected to centralized, authoritarian management for so long, nursing personnel will need to be schooled in the process of participatory management. This will include training to make input into collaborative decision making.

In participatory management a complementary relationship exists between managers and practitioners, rather than a hierarchical one. Training is done to prepare staff and prevent insecurity. Availability of managers qualified to function in participatory management increases decentralization. Training of supervisors will focus on changes in their needs as well as their functions. Supervisors will learn to gain self-fulfillment from delegating and team building.[120]

Management training of supervisors will include group dynamics, problem solving, planning, and decision making. Such training can occur through conferences, workshops, and seminars. It should be rewarding and continuous to be successful. It will relieve the threats supervisors feel from challenges by employees, from exposure of their weaknesses, from perceived loss of prestige and power, and from "digging in" to keep control.[121]

Changed Roles of Supervisors

Decentralization with participative management means that roles must be redefined and coordinated to prevent conflict. Nurse managers and primary nurses have increased management responsibility. For some, this will mean decreased hands-on clinical responsibility. Supervisors of nurse managers have decreased responsibility for unit management and become mentors, role models, and facilitators. With a flattened organizational structure, some may lose jobs while others have the overall scope of their responsibility increased.[122]

In one experiment in decentralized patient education, all clinical nurses caring for patients became the teachers. The assistant head nurse became the facilitator, that is, the person responsible for planning and developing objectives for patient education programs and for promoting staff interest and participation in all phases. The education department became the resource available to coordinate teaching programs in support of the primary nurse. The advantages of decentralized versus centralized patient education include using all nursing and health personnel for education, providing education to a maximum number of patients and families, and having each nurse assume professional responsibility for patient education.[123]

As supervisors learn to delegate authority, they modify the climate that promotes deviant behavior by giving professional nurses what they want: the authority to manage themselves. Because authority gives the supervisors initiative in performing their jobs and freedom to question managers, managers should expect loyalty in return. The profession of nursing does not employ nurses; organizations do. Participatory management is a process in which there must be an ongoing dialogue with constraints: nurses will control their profession, and management uses its input to set objectives and priorities and to review output. Nurse employees cannot control the enterprise, and management cannot compromise the professional or ethical standards of professional nurses.[124]

In participatory management, the supervisor facilitates rather than directs the work force. Traditional supervising functions are delegated downward. There must be clear delineation of a manager's basic responsibilities, distinct from behavioral or management style. Managers can gain satisfaction from their ability to make clinical nurses successful and satisfied. The interpersonal skills and conceptual abilities demanded of supervisors will increase. Supervisors should be challenged and should have a future. Supervisors promote implementation of committee decisions, listen, and offer assistance.[125]

Because fewer supervisors will be needed, career development programs for college-educated nurses must provide them promotional opportunities as clinical practitioners, managers, teachers, or researchers. Supervisors are important to the success of decentralized decision making and employee involvement in the management of nursing and the health care system. They should be taught to manage under employee involvement programs. They need to learn that they will have more time to plan and organize work and to be creative. Their jobs can be expanded upward, but they should keep in contact with employees and encourage participation by everyone.

Communication

Good communication within the nursing organization is essential to an effective employee participation program. Good communication is effective communication; it is evident in employees who are informed about the business of nursing. Such employees know what management is saying and what management's intentions are. Management knows what employees are saying and how that squares with the perceptions that management is working to develop. Broken communication contributes to stress and leads to direct economic losses through low productivity, grievances, absenteeism, turnover, and work slowdowns or strikes.

Flat organizational structures promote effective communication. Managers plan the vehicles, content, and intent of effective communication, and they monitor the process. Supervisors are important to effective communication and (as another aspect of their changed roles) work to ensure its openness. Management attitudes should promote truth, frankness, and openness.

Participation enhances commitment and interdepartmental and intradepartmental communication. In medium-sized and large organizations, a communication center will operate 24 hours a day. Message delivery will be facilitated. Computers will be used to communicate instantly, nurse to nurse, nurse to manager, manager to nurse, and nurse to others. Messages will be hand-delivered when necessary.

Decentralization requires a movement away from mainframe information processing toward distributed systems of smaller computers. This change increases flexibility and control at lower organizational levels, giving users heightened feelings of ownership of the system. Packaged software then offers fast relief for specific application needs. End user involvement with computer applications increases.[126]

With direct communication, the middle person is eliminated and time is saved. The problem of missing medical laboratory or radiology reports is taken up between the primary nurse or the nurse manager and the manager of the department immediately responsible.[127] Increased representation of clinical nurses on hospital and departmental committees improves communication. The goal is to facilitate the flow of information, not to embody it in the authority of a management position. Objectives, group brainstorming, and self-directed work teams are vehicles of effective communication used in participatory management.

Advantages of Participatory Management

The following is a list of advantages of participatory management as cited by writers in business, industry, and health care, including nursing.[128]

1. High trust and mutual support
2. Increased accountability of managers and employees
3. Reduced ambiguity in work requirements for practitioners and employees as a result of improved communication
4. Enhanced role for the clinical nurse; self-supervision; active involvement of employees in identifying and solving problems; encouragement of employee contributions; career development
5. Increased independence of the nursing division
6. Legal clarity
7. Teamwork
8. Improved organizational communication, with nurses being briefed on all phases of the nursing business, including revenues, costs, and strategic plans, thereby increasing employees' understanding of the organization
9. Decreased absenteeism
10. Increased effectiveness and productivity; improved quality of work; higher level of mastery
11. Uplifted morale and motivation at work; increased excitement from fluctuating participation (participation makes work and values visible)
12. Increased job satisfaction
13. Recognition of contributions because participation increases individual and organizational capacities to learn, adapt, and develop toward higher levels of excellence

Practice and Research

In the Motorola participatory management program, factory-level employees in Plan I belong to groups of 50 to 250 people who set targets and valid standards that measure current cost, in-process quality, product deliveries, inventory levels, and housekeeping and safety. Representatives belong to working committees that review ideas, recommendations, and issues of waste and quality. The committees solve problems and send recommendations to a representative steering committee for review. Committee involvement of workers improves communication. Improved product quality or customer satisfaction is evident in increased sales and profits and results in financial bonuses to employees. In this process, each employee can see the effect of his or her contributions on the group and feel a sense of accomplishment. In one instance, as a result of the participatory management process at Motorola, a 4% loss of gold went to zero in 2 months. Production volume at one plant went up 33% with fewer employees. Team spirit and a sense of cooperation existed between management and employees, who worked with less supervision.[129]

Research studies have reported greater motivation and satisfaction when subordinates participate in performance appraisal. Research also indicates that mutual goal setting improves performance, increases productivity, satisfies employees' need for fulfillment and self-actualization, and thus contributes to the well being of the organization. Participatory management develops mature, healthy, self-directed personalities among employees.[130]

Disadvantages of Participatory Management

Some of the disadvantages of participatory management are as follows:[131]

1. Occasional failures will occur.
2. Initiation of programs takes time and money.
3. Policies and procedures must be changed.
4. It is sometimes difficult to determine which responsibilities are whose, even though other ambiguities are reduced.
5. There is a lacking of knowledge of the process and individuals' responsibility in the process.
6. Employees having too little attachment to the organization, not being interested in work, and having a weak commitment to the work ethic; employees and managers not getting along; employees having a poor assessment of their supervisors; and employees having low regard for organization-wide openness are some of the reasons managers cite for failure of participatory management.
7. It is difficult to change management style to true participation.
8. Employees who view management as being autocratic perceive participatory performance appraisal as being insincere, patronizing, and manipulative. The person who initiates it has gone "soft."
9. Self-evaluation is threatening because the employee feels exposed to the views of others.

All of these disadvantages will be overcome by a committed chief nurse executive who prepares and implements a plan with supervisors and educators who are prepared psychologically, politically, and technically. The chief nurse executive selects and develops key people (the human beings developing human beings), works toward a long-term future, and is accessible.

Activities Involving Nurses in Participatory Management

Some of the programs and structures that can be used to involve nurses in participatory management are job enrichment, personalization, primary nursing, shared governance, entrepreneurship, gain sharing, and pay equity.

Job Enrichment

Job enrichment satisfies the motivation to fulfill higher-order needs, including variety within and among jobs and a strategy that challenges by emphasizing performance output over job processes. Job enrichment creates jobs with greater responsibility and more flexibility and promotes personal development.

Enrichment requires preparation and careful implementation. By focusing on the whole job, it makes maximum use of and expands employee skills. It includes decision-making authority. Growth from job enrichment prevents apathy, burnout, and alienation. Employees can choose to assume more responsibility for particular assignments. Lateral transfers are supported with job postings and project assignments. Output, not the process used to produce it, is evaluated. Professionals respond to orders from other professionals, an indication that professional nurses will respond best to enrichment programs developed by competent professional nurse managers whose management styles promote participation and involvement. Enrichment works best with hard workers who like to work best with friendly people.[132]

Job enrichment and redesign are related to the employee's needs for learning, challenge, variety, increased responsibility, and achievement. Herzberg's two-factor theory (hygiene factors vs motivation factors) is one approach to job enrichment: growth and motivation factors are achievement, recognition, work, responsibility, and advancement. Increasing hygiene factors such as salary, job security, and working conditions does reduce dissatisfaction among employees but *does not motivate them*.

A job characteristics model structures work for effective performance, personal rewards, and job satisfaction. Job characteristics are variety, task entity, task significance, autonomy, and job-based feedback. Research indicates that increased job enrichment and increased quality of communication predict the development of greater self-efficacy of employees.[133]

Personalization

Personalization is a strategy that focuses on people and knowledge, not numbers and politics. Those who use personalization stress empathy and involve professionals in making critical decisions that affect them. Career development opportunities are facilitated by advertising jobs, allowing transfers, giving feedback to job applicants, allowing and providing liberal training and development, and promoting based on objective measures.[134]

Primary Nursing

Primary nursing as a modality of nursing care delivery makes nursing worthwhile work, enhances nurses' self-esteem through performing a complete function, produces results of a personal endeavor, and realizes collegial and collaborative relationships.[135] In a hospital setting where primary nursing is practiced, decentralization of patient care delivery systems provides the most efficient nursing care. Primary nurses are accountable. The ideal environment for self-governance is primary nursing with a stable, mature, self-directed, skilled, and committed staff trained in leadership skills.[136] Other nursing modalities that are compatible with participatory management are modular nursing, team nursing, case management, and collaborative practice models.

Shared Governance

Shared governance is defined as the allocation of control, power, or authority among mutually interested parties. Data supporting reduction in turnover and increases in levels of nursing satisfaction are evidence of successful outcomes of shared governance processes. The principles of shared governance are more consistent with the principles of professionalism than are the principles of participatory management. The following are the main principles of shared governance:[137]

1. Shared governance is not a form of participatory management. Participatory management means allowing others to participate in decisions over which a line manager has control.
2. Shared governance is not management driven. All activities that are neither direct caregiving nor related to that process are in support of it.
3. Shared management has no locus of control. Accountabilities of a role are attributed to the role from within the role; they can never be assigned, nor can they be given away.
4. Models should be based on a clinical rather than an administrative organization.
5. Governance should be representative in nature, not democratic.
6. Representatives should be elected, not selected.
7. Bylaws should provide a system of checks and balances, and they should be passed by a majority vote of the entire nursing staff.

Three models of shared governance are the congressional model, the unit-based model, and the councilor model. All three models delineate four broad areas of accountability: practice, quality, education, and management. Accountabilities of practice include practice standards, job descriptions, care delivery systems, and nursing representation in hospital-wide committees. Additional quality issues include practice standards, job descriptions, the care delivery system, and nursing representation in hospital-wide committees. Accountabilities for quality include delineation of data sources, evaluation criteria, evaluation processes, and mechanisms for quality improvement, credentialing, peer review, and research.

Education accountabilities include needs assessment, incorporation of new standards of research, and evaluation of educational endeavors. Accountabilities of management include provision of resources, including human and financial resources; implementation of council or committee decisions; interdepartmental problem solving; and facilitation of staff problem solving, decision making, and leadership.[138]

Under collaborative governance, managers become integrators, facilitators, and coordinators. Clinical managers are educated in decision making, team building, group dynamics, goals and objectives development, interviewing skills, budgeting, disciplining, and rewarding. Unit personnel develop policy. Structure is kept informal except for areas governed by law, regulations, and efficiency, in which representative central committees operate. Unit personnel decide whether their unit will be "open," in which case personnel float in and out, or "closed." For the system to work, all unit employees must buy into it. It takes years to build successful collaborative governance. A successful system is in a constant state of flux and chaos. This system is based on shared beliefs including such assumptions as knowledge is power; risk-taking, with or without success, is growth; individuals are unique in their contributions; and maximum productivity results when organizational and personal values are congruent.[139]

To prepare for self-management, there must be a committed administration, a prepared staff, time, a willingness to make mistakes and move on, and managers who are able to relinquish decision-making power over daily operations. Those responsible for fostering self-management must prepare for a fundamental change in the perception of "self as manager" and "subordinate" roles and responsibilities. In self-management, it is more important than ever for management to set and communicate clear expectations. Without a safe environment, self-management will fail because people will avoid changing or taking risks. Ongoing training and information sessions, with feedback and practice, are fundamental to the success of the new model. Gaining trust of staff and first-line supervisors and managers is made possible through modeling self-management principles and practices in the administrative structure of the organization.[140]

Although it appears that shared governance is expanding, a persistent question relates to whether its benefits are being objectively evaluated. Research studies show that nurses gain job satisfaction and growth satisfaction from working in a nurse-managed special care unit with a shared governance management model.[141] Surveys of nurses involved in horizontal integration through hospital acquisition indicate that nurses value shared governance and professional nursing autonomy.[142] Descriptive reports of shared governance organizations report the following:

- Shared governance decentralizes decision making, disperses power, increases participatory management, and enlarges the span of control. It can be unit based, department-based, or organization-based.[143]
- Shared government involves staff in management, education, quality, and practice issues that support changes in skill-mix and patient-focused care systems.[144]
- Shared governance as an organizational structure supports vertical integration, product line development, and an organizational culture with strong relationships.[145]

Entrepreneurship

As decentralization and vertical integration strategies are implemented in health care organizations, a great opportunity exists for professional nurses to be involved in entrepreneurship. Nurses can form small companies with the support of government agencies and private businesses. Such companies require venture capital, which can, with sufficient preparation, be obtained from the government and the private health care industry. As an example, in the face of greater professional nurse shortages, health care agencies might find it advantageous to contract with corporate nurse personnel agencies or vertical integration spin-offs that become nurse staffing subsidiaries, durable medical goods subsidiaries, and clinical nursing care subsidiaries.

The following five strategies promote entrepreneurship:[146]

1. Decentralize.
2. Give actual responsibility and authority to key executives.
3. Let executives express their managerial skills, and give them a chance to make their own business mistakes on the road to excellence.
4. Monitor these executives and encourage them to make business decisions on their own, so that they can measure the results of these decisions not only in dollars and cents, but also in terms of the effects on the people involved.
5. Establish a basic corporate policy that people are the biggest asset of the company, and make it clear that the development of these people will contribute greatly to the company's strength.

Entrepreneurship in nursing will be good for professional nurses and the health care industry because it will create independent thinkers who are motivated to be productive, creative, and more competitive in the marketplace. They will become like other business people who have a strong desire to control their own careers.

Gain Sharing

Gain sharing is a group incentive program in which employees share in the financial benefits of improved performance. It has many of the same advantages and disadvantages as other methods of participatory management. Top management is sensitive to the employees' goals, and employees identify with the organization through greater involvement.

Initiation of gain sharing takes a long-term plan that includes application of these three phases of the change process:[147]

1. Unfreezing: Do an organizational diagnosis, a management questionnaire on gain sharing, a bonus calculation, and an employee attitude survey.
2. Moving: Establish employee ownership with a task force of employees, meetings, and training of employees and managers. Involve everyone at once.
3. Refreezing: Institutionalize the plan, continued training, improved motivation and communication, goals, periodic reviews, periodic elections to task forces or committees, and annual reviews.

The results of gain sharing are measurable: savings, improved labor-management relations, fewer grievances, less absenteeism, and reduced turnover. Gain sharing adds money to intrinsic rewards. Stock ownership and profit sharing are economic rewards similar to gain sharing. Gain sharing, stock ownership, and profit sharing may not be legally possible in not-for-profit organizations. However, increased financial benefits can be made available through legal means such as merit pay, certification pay, and clinical promotions. Also, vertically integrated corporations have profit-making ventures under their corporate umbrellas.

All gain-sharing programs must be appropriately installed by employers to achieve maximum employee motivation, participation, and trust in management.

Pay Equity

Pay equity between management and employees is an issue of participatory management. Incentive programs for employees are a part of participatory management programs. Employees receive intrinsic satisfaction from public recognition and praise, but they also obtain extrinsic rewards from financial bonuses, stock options, and profit sharing.[148]

Professional nurses, like other professional workers, frequently respond negatively to the strategy of linking financial benefits to promotion into management. They want financial reward for accomplishing personal and organizational objectives that increase productivity and reduce turnover and absenteeism. These rewards can be in the form of nonmanagerial advancement of salary, status, recognition, autonomy, and responsibility. This can be accomplished through dual ladders, that is, clinical promotions that match management promotions. Such promotions preserve nurses' professional career opportunities with financial rewards based on graduated pay scales that can be objectively measured through levels of achievement culminating in mastery.

Restructuring Nursing Organizations

The survival of many hospitals is threatened as they compete for growth and a competitive edge in the marketplace. Consumers and payers are searching for organizations that are efficient in producing positive, cost-effective health care. For this reason, Flarey indicates that the governing boards may need to be reconstituted. Members of governing bodies should focus on patient care. Many hospitals include the chief nurse executives in governing board meetings as active participants.[149] Exhibit 6-10 provides questions through which to evaluate organizational function.

Kanter defines synergies as "interactions of businesses that would provide benefits above and beyond what the units could do separately."[150] Synergies are a positive consequence of restructuring in which organizations are downsized (employees cut), demassed (middle management cut), and decentralized. The aim of restructuring is to achieve synergies from the value of adding up the parts to create a whole.[151] One of the elements of restructuring would be to build a synergistic model of a governing body. A synergistic model for the governing body as suggested by Flarey considers governing body functions such as defining mission, quality of care, strategic planning, financial viability, community relations, policy development, and decision making.

Old organizational forms do not work in today's health care environment. Sovie recommends development of special project teams to design the required structure and system change. She gives the following as the first five steps of restructuring:

1. Create an organizational culture marked by commitment to high-quality care and superior, responsive service to all users including patients, families, physicians, nurses, and other staff.
2. Redesign the organizational structure to flatten it and eliminate or reduce barriers among departments, disciplines, and services.
3. Empower the staff, invest in employee education and training, and create mechanisms to ensure information flow.
4. Develop special project teams to design the required system changes; nurture and promote innovation and pilots of new approaches.
5. Celebrate accomplishments and innovators, and champion care for the caregivers; support, recognize, and reward.

EXHIBIT 6-10

Evaluating Organizational Function

Answer the following questions as a final evaluation of your organizing function within a department or unit. For those checked No, plan changes so that they will result in effective organizing. Then implement the management plan.

	YES	NO
1. Is there evidence that organizing is an intentional and ongoing function of the division, department, service, or unit?	_____	_____
2. Is there evidence that organizing changes as plans, goals, or objectives change?	_____	_____
3. Is there evidence that managers are developed or replaced to fit organizational changes emerging from changed plans and objectives?	_____	_____
4. Are organizational managerial relationships clearly structured to give security to individual managers?	_____	_____
5. Has authority been delegated to appropriate levels of managers?	_____	_____
6. Is there evidence that delegation of authority has been balanced to retain control of appropriate administrative functions by the chief nurse executive?	_____	_____
7. Is information dissemination clearly separated from decision making?	_____	_____
8. Is the authority delegated commensurate with the responsibility?	_____	_____
9. Is there evidence of acceptance of responsibility and authority by subordinate managers?	_____	_____
10. Is there evidence that subordinate managers have the power to accomplish the results expected of them?	_____	_____
11. Is there evidence that authority and responsibility have been confined within divisional, departmental, service, or unit boundaries?	_____	_____
12. Is there evidence of balance in support and use of staff functions?	_____	_____
13. Is there evidence of balance in support and use of functional authority?	_____	_____
14. Is there evidence of maintenance of the principle of unity of command?	_____	_____
15. Is there evidence of efficient and effective use of service departments?	_____	_____
16. Is there evidence of too many levels of managers (overorganization)?	_____	_____
17. Is there evidence of unneeded line assistants to managers (overorganization)?	_____	_____
18. Is there evidence that the nursing division, department, service, or unit is organized to facilitate accomplishment of its specified objectives by its personnel?	_____	_____
19. Is there evidence that the nursing division, department, service, or unit structure has been modified to fit human factors after being organized to accomplish its specified objectives?	_____	_____
20. Is there evidence that the nursing division, department, service, or unit is organized to accomplish planning for recruiting and training to meet present and future personnel needs?	_____	_____
21. Is there evidence that the organizational process is flexible enough to adapt to changes in its external and internal environment?	_____	_____
22. Are changes in organization justified, based on deficiencies, experience, objectives, purpose, and plans?	_____	_____
23. Is there evidence that the organizing process is balanced between inertia and continual change?	_____	_____
24. Is there evidence that all nursing personnel know the organizational structure and understand their assignments and those of their co-workers?	_____	_____
25. Is there evidence that the nursing organizational charts are widely used?	_____	_____
26. Is there evidence that nursing organizational charts provide comprehensive information to all workers?	_____	_____
27. Is there evidence that there are job descriptions and job standards for every job and that they are widely used by nursing managers?	_____	_____
28. Is there evidence that nursing employees are all oriented to the nature of the nursing organizing process?	_____	_____
29. Is there evidence that the organizing process within the nursing division, department, service, or unit prevents waste or unplanned costs?	_____	_____
30. Is there evidence that the nursing organization has an effective span of control by managers?	_____	_____
31. Are the lines of authority within the nursing organization clear?	_____	_____
32. Is there evidence that the management information system is effective?	_____	_____
33. Is there evidence that each employee has only one supervisor?	_____	_____
34. Is there evidence that the CNE has absolute responsibility for subordinate nursing managers?	_____	_____
35. Is there evidence that all nursing managers are able to effect their leadership abilities?	_____	_____

The goals are improvement of patient care, organizational success, and staff satisfaction.[152]

Restructuring of organizations includes downsizing and elimination of middle managers. The hands-on workers are thus empowered to provide clients (customers, patients) what they need and want. Before they can be empowered, hands-on nursing workers need to have management training for their new roles. The span of control is greater when hands-on workers are educated, trained, motivated, stable, and empowered. Such workers neither want nor need micromanagement. The manager with a widened or expanded span of control now becomes mentor, guide, facilitator, and coach.

Small departments can be consolidated under one department head through empowerment. Examples are physical therapy, occupational therapy, endoscopy, neurodiagnostics, sleep disorders, social services, and respiratory therapy. Issues of loss of power and authority arise and must be resolved so that job shrinking and empowerment can occur. Managers who spend time protecting their turf decrease productivity of their workers. Nurse managers of their units can do all hiring, resolve patient complaints, budget authority associated with staffing and patient losses, and provide orientation to new managers. Clearly, the span of control for top managers can increase as first-line managers are empowered.

Downsizing is a common organizing activity in the corporate world, including health care organizations and institutions. The goals of downsizing are to decrease costs and increase profits. While decentralization and participatory management are identified with downsizing, the goals are not always the same. Decentralization and participatory management have increasing job satisfaction and increased productivity as primary goals.

Companies are now reporting that the hoped-for results of downsizing have not occurred. There have been huge emotional and financial costs to employees and significant costs to American corporations. Between 1983 and 1993, Fortune 500 companies eliminated 4.7 million people from their payrolls. Job cuts do not necessarily lead to improved productivity. Gains in production are frequently traced to firms with growing employment. Mass layoffs do not inspire worker loyalty; workers should be well prepared for restructuring.[153]

Business must adapt organizational structures because of marketplace demands related to greater rates of change, higher competitive intensity, and information technology. Health care organizations should do the same. What services should a business offer, and what should it divest? Hospitals are high cost producers. The excessive vertical integration since diagnosis-related groups (DRGs) may be to blame. The emerging organizational structure is messy: some resources need to be centralized to improve productivity by responding to customers' needs. A good organization will have key aspects of both consistency and inconsistency.[154]

When reengineering organizations, leaders should use key strategies such as emotional management, professional empowerment, and empowerment by values. Staff members are given room to grow and to learn from their mistakes.[155]

Excessive organizational structures are inhibitors to quick responses to change. Get staff out into the field. This includes accounting, purchasing, personnel, and others. There should be only three to five layers of management in the total organization. Every CEO should look at the corporate structure from the perspective of increasing the span of control through reduction of layers of management. Matrix organization brought about de facto centralization as groups were connected to groups by dotted lines on organization charts. The most effective management structure is supervisor, department head, and boss. In health care organizations, this would be nurse manager, nurse executive, and hospital administrator.

Winning companies have three to nine fewer levels of management. Winning companies have workers doing their own maintenance, self-inspection, direct costing, and just-in-time inventory management. Winning companies have few people at headquarters level. They decentralize database management, eliminate approval signatures, retrain middle managers, and increase spending authority at unit level.[156]

Mergers and acquisitions result in unified management teams with single executive managers. As examples, one CEO replaces two to several, one assistant administrator for nursing replaces two to several, and one department head replaces two to several. Desirable characteristics include a highly visible chief nurse executive, a professional practice model of patient care, nursing diagnosis as the basis for nursing care delivery, and collaborative practice among professions.

An organizational analysis should be done to gain the theory and skills needed to intervene in complex organizational systems. Areas analyzed include formal organizational structure, power bases, leadership, communication system, and organizational climate (see Exhibit 6-10). Used to prepare clinical nurse specialists, it could be used by nurse managers and practicing CNSs.[157]

The Organization of Work

Work is organized according to the stages in the process. In some areas, the work moves to the skills and tools; examples are coronary care nursing and operating room nursing. Sometimes a team moves different skills and different tools to the work—for example, when an operating room team moves to a delivery room to perform a caesarean section. We certainly find combinations in nursing.

Much of the work in nursing is accomplished by a functionally structured organization. Clarity is an advantage of the functional structure, because the individuals know where they stand, and they understand their tasks. Functional structures are usually stable. A disadvantage is that sometimes the task neither relates to the whole structure nor contributes to the common purpose. Functional structures are rigid, and frequently they neither prepare nurses for the future nor train nor test them. Functional organizations become costly when friction builds up and requires coordinators, committees, meetings, troubleshooters, and special dispatchers. Functional organizations make low psychological demands on people; people in such organizations tend to focus on their efforts only. Small functional organizations are economical and foster good communications. These organizations are good when one kind of work is done. Usually they require that decisions be made at the top. Nurses within them have narrow visions, skills, and loyalties. Employees of such organizations focus on function rather than on results and performance. The functional process does not usually apply to top management positions or to performance of innovative work by employees.

Nursing Care Delivery Systems

Managed care and case management appear to be leading innovations in health care delivery. Benefits are controlled costs, improved outcome monitoring, reduced bureaucracy, less travel time for patients, and fewer people to sort out or confront. Patient care needs and outcomes should be assessed and evaluated by nurses. Nurses who refer needs to others should determine priority of patient care tasks. This is the essence of work redesign that will retain nursing autonomy and influence.[158]

Some health care institutions integrate standards of practice into their nursing care delivery systems. Structure and process standards are stated as outcome standards and are used to measure the overall effectiveness of the nursing division. The integration is accomplished throughout the core committees of the nursing division, including quality assessment, policy and procedure, job description, and other committees. This is done through nursing care plans and the computer system. The nursing care plans may be generic or individual and include nursing diagnosis/problems, intervention/discharge plans, and goals.[159] Five examples of nursing care delivery systems are presented below.

Example 1: Nursing Practice Model

Valley Baptist Medical Center (VBMC) in Harlingen, Texas, built a nursing practice model that included unit action committees on each nursing unit, a comprehensive integrated tool called the restorative care path, variance analysis, permanent care teams with clinical managers, assistant clinical managers, licensed vocational nurses, nursing assistants, and collaborative nurse physician practice with a physician-nurse liaison committee. As credentialing and recredentialing of physicians is considered the ultimate form of peer review, it should be considered for peer review of nurses.[160]

Example 2: Group Practice

Nursing group practice at Catherine McAuley Health System "is a formal membership of professional nurses who contract to provide nursing care for a specific patient population." Nurses may contract privately or as employees of an organization. They provide 24-hour coverage 365 days a year. The group's staffing for cardiothoracic surgery includes 16 nurses, 2 certified surgical technologists, and one clinical nurse manager who reports to the clinical director of operating room services. The group eliminated the first-line manager, making the clinical nurse manager a resource facilitator, liaison, and mentor. A supportive climate emphasizes trust, accountability, and responsibility. The criteria for group practice membership include clinical competence and leadership ability. Evaluating peers use a clinical ladder with described behaviors. The practice model is shared governance: practice, education, and performance improvement assurance councils.

The following are suggested activities to implement a group practice:

- Define roles and organization structure.
- Determine program costs.
- Decide on membership criteria and staffing mix.
- Set salary guidelines (e.g., hourly or salaried status).
- Work with the hospital administration in writing policies and planning for implementation.
- Plan to evaluate the success of the program using specific, predetermined instruments.

Staff satisfaction, cost, and quality assurance all improved. Turnover rate decreased. Problems such as surgical complications and poor communications were prevented. Products and techniques were changed to reduce costs. Turnaround times were faster. Financial recognition was made quarterly. Incorrect sponge and instrument counts were reduced 25%.[161]

Example 3: Helper Model

The helper model of health care delivery is widespread. It matches RNs with nurse aides. To work efficiently, the helper model requires the following:[162]

1. Experienced RNs at the competent or proficient levels of practice.
2. Permanent RN-nurse aide pairs.
3. Enhanced primary nursing.

4. Support for agency and float nurses.
5. Policy for attendance that targets incentive and reward programs.
6. Thoroughly prepared RNs/nurse aides.
7. Support systems.
8. Follow-up in-services.

Example 4: Differentiated Practice

Role theory underlies the concept of differentiated practice, which defines the levels of competence within which two categories of RNs will practice: nurses with bachelor's degrees and those with associate degrees.

The BSN (bachelor of science in nursing) level is the professional practice level; the ADN (associate degree in nursing) is the associate or technical practice level. These practice levels can function within a variety of different delivery systems, including team and primary systems. The premise for differentiated practice is that professional practice exercises the nurse's autonomous decisions, including personal acceptance of risks and responsibilities in making professional judgments. Extended education at a BSN level or higher is required preparation for this role at the professional practice level.[163] The differentiated group professional practice (DGPP) model has three major components, of which differentiated care delivery is one:[164]

1. Group governance.
2. Differentiated care delivery.
3. Shared values.

A differentiated practice system or delivery model has the following components:

1. Differentiated RN practice.
2. Use of nurse extenders.
3. Primary case management.

Differentiated care delivery is designed so that nurses with varying educational preparation and work experience can most efficiently use their knowledge and skills, while delegating nonnursing tasks to assistive personnel. Nurse extenders are delegated tasks rather than patient assignments.[165]

The differentiated practice role has three basic components:

1. Provision of direct care.
2. Communication with and on behalf of patients.
3. Management of patient care.

A differentiated practice maximizes available registered nurse resources for efficiency and effectiveness. "Differentiated practice is a strategy that calls for licensed and practicing nurses to be used in accord with their respective experience, ability, and formal and continuing education. Further, differentiated practice is defined as both a human resource deployment model and an alternative to primary nursing and case management." It is role differentiation. More education and experience are needed for cognitive skills.[166]

In an ethnographic study of differentiated practice in an operating room, it was found that introduction of a new role requires insight into setting and an emphasis on staging and orientation of employees to the new role.[167] Otherwise, introduction of a new role can create turmoil and job insecurity. To use the differentiated practice mode, the nurse's knowledge and skills are assessed (see Exhibit 6-11).

Styles and others advocate differentiated credentialing. What are the goals of differentiated credentialing and what would it accomplish? In the practice environment, cost effectiveness often calls for varied nursing personnel. It is essential that the professional level be designated. To gain public respect and rights of self-determination, nursing must adhere to the professional norm. Role-delineated relationships with other health professionals and incentives for improvement are dependent on identification of professional status. In brief, higher standards of care; clear public recognition and specificity in authority, accountability, roles, and responsibilities; and rewards for the professional nurse are the goals of the entry effort.

The proposed solution might work like this: BSN education, RN licensure, followed with national generalist

EXHIBIT 6-11

Differentiated Practice Assessment

RN PROFESSIONAL

BSN prepared
Makes complex decisions and interactions
Cost management of supplies, clinical alternatives, flexible scheduling of personnel, and case loads
Structures the unstructured
Cognitive role and highly skilled tasks
Care manager
Independent judgments, initiative, problem solving
Coaches self-managed work team
Manages all resources, fiscal and material
Consults with other disciplines
Discharges patients

RN ASSOCIATE OR TECHNICIAN

Non-BSN RN
Assists the professional nurse
Performs high-skill tasks such as chemotherapy
Special tests and procedures
May lead self-managed work team coached by professional nurse
Direct care provider
Uses common, well-defined diagnoses
Works in structured settings and situations

certification with the title CPN (certified professional nurse), and then a differentiated practice with recognition/reimbursement.[168]

Example 5: Relationship-Based Care Model

Creative Health Care Management consultants developed a nursing practice model called the Relationship-Based Care.[169] The model is based on theories of caring and relationships, relationships between the health care employee and the patient and family; the health care employee's relationship with self, and his or her relationship with peers.[170] The model is structured on the following dimensions:[171]

1. Teamwork
2. Professional nursing
3. Leadership
4. Care delivery
5. Resources
6. Outcomes

Analyzing Organizational Structures in a Division of Nursing

Analyzing the organizational structure of a division of nursing entails six main steps, which should be used when major organizational problems occur, such as friction among department heads over authority, staffing problems, and the like. These steps also apply to organizing a new corporation, division, or unit and to reorganizing. They are as follows:

Step 1

Compile a list of the key activities determined by the mission and objectives of patient care. The written philosophy and vision statements will help by indicating important values to be considered. Once this list is completed, it must be analyzed. Group similar activities together. What are the central load-carrying elements? Most will be related to primary care, and philosophy will usually dictate that excellence of patient care is a requirement for the accomplishment of objectives.

Whenever the strategy changes, the organizational structure should be reviewed and analyzed. This includes changes in mission, philosophy, vision, objectives, and the operational plan for accomplishing the objectives. The analysis of key activities can be done according to the kinds of contributions made. These will include the following:

1. Results-producing activities related to direct patient care, such as training, recruiting, and employment.
2. Support activities, which may include those related to vision or future, values and standards, audit, advice, and teaching.
3. Hygiene and housekeeping activities.
4. Top management activities to include "conscience" activities such as vision, values, standards, and audit as well as managing people, marketing, and innovation.

Service staffs such as those performing advisory and training support should be limited. They should be required to abandon an old activity before starting a new one. Prevent them from building empires as a career. Informational activities are the responsibility of top management though they stem from support such as controller and treasurer. There must be a system for disseminating information. Hygiene and housekeeping need the attention of nurses if they are to be done well and cheaply. This does not mean that nurses will do these tasks, but rather that nurses will recognize their importance and support and facilitate their being done by the appropriate departments. Contract services are the answer in some instances.

Consider whether the groups of key activities should be rank-ordered in the sequence in which they will occur.

Step 2

Based on the work functions to be performed, decide on the units of the organization. Decision analysis will be important here, since it must be decided which kinds of decisions will be required and who will make them. Decisions involving functions of future commitments may have to be a top management function, depending on the degree of futurity of a decision and the speed with which it can be reversed. It will be necessary to analyze the impact of decisions on other functions; the number of functions involved will be an important factor. Qualitative factors such as decisions involving ethical values, principles of conduct, and social and political beliefs will have to be analyzed. The frequency of the decision will influence its placement: Is it recurrent or is it rare? In principle, all decisions should be placed at the lowest level and as close to the operational scene as possible.

Step 3

Decide which units or components will be joined and which separated. Join activities that make the same kind of contribution. This will require relations analysis and will be related to the sequence of key activities or functions.

Step 4

Decide on the size and shape of the units or components.

Step 5

Decide on appropriate placement and relationships of different units or components. This will result from the relations analysis (Step 3). There should be the smallest possible number of relationships, with each made to count.

Step 6
Draw or diagram the design and put it into operation. This will result in an organizational chart or schema.

Departmentation
These steps should be used when major organizational problems occur, such as friction among department heads over authority and staffing problems. They also apply to organizing a new corporation, division, or unit and to reorganizing an established entity. Steps 3, 4, and 5 involve departmentation, the grouping of personnel according to some characteristic.

Departmentation is an organizing process. For departmentation purposes, functional specialties are formed from clusters of units with similar goals. In most of our health care institutions, the functions of nursing are grouped into a division or department. Within that division or department are further groupings of nursing personnel by specialization, such as medical, surgical, pediatric, and obstetric. Sometimes the grouping is further broken down into areas of subspecialization. This process is termed functional departmentation. Clients may also be grouped according to degree of illness, such as minimal, intermediate, or intensive care.

There are advantages and disadvantages of functional departmentation. Among the advantages are focus on the basic activities of the enterprise through a logical and time-proven method of organizing, efficient use of specialized personnel, simplified training, and tight control by top administration. A big disadvantage for nursing is that people tend to develop tunnel vision about their specialty and the service or unit within which they work.

Time departmentation is common within health care organizations. Personnel are grouped by shift. This has important implications for administration as the activities of shifts have to be grouped according to qualifications and numbers of personnel on any shift.

Territorial departmentation involves grouping of activities according to geography or physical plant. This is more common in merged organizations with geographically separated units. Some activities, such as staff development, may be assigned by territory and specialization as well as being grouped by function.

Territorial departmentation should encourage participation in decision making in provision of health services to a wider population base and be of a nature that will prevent illnesses and injuries. There may be justification for the exploration and formation of consortiums using the principle of territorial departmentation. For example, several small hospitals in an area could contract for consultant services in research, clinical nurse specialist services, or nursing education services.

In addition to functional, time, and territorial departmentation, there is the fourth option, product departmentation. This approach has implications for health care, although its ultimate achievement may not always be immediately practical. Increasingly, the products of nursing care are focused on the health needs of populations and those who need not only the illness care but also the care that keeps aging populations healthy; that maintains health and prevents injury and disease in the large group who take voluntary risks such as smoking, reckless driving, poor eating, poor exercising, or using artificial mood changers; that promotes a clean environment; that modifies the health risks associated with human reproduction; and that decreases the need for illness care. In the vertically integrated organization, product line departmentation is common.

Departmentation could be done on the basis of consumer needs or demands. There is a distinct possibility that health care institutions will offer people a choice of services in the future, thereby giving them the opportunity to select those services that will be covered by third-party payers and those that will be paid for out-of-pocket. Also, the times the services will be given and who will be giving them may well be part of the choice.

There may be no pure form of departmentation that will work in the health care institution. It may be more important to look at all the variables in order to group people to facilitate successful production of health care services. In the matrix organization, product and functional forms of departmentation are combined. Projects have managers who move products through production stages in coordination with managers of each production stage. We will see more use of matrix organizations in nursing as health care takes on new dimensions.

At the present, nursing services are usually organized using a mix of departmentations. So long as the system is based on logic, it will provide a viable and efficient organization. Use Exhibit 6-12 to evaluate departmentation of nursing service activities and personnel.

The Informal Organization

Every formal organization has an informal one. The informal organization meets the needs of individuals with similar backgrounds, values, hobbies, interests, and physical proximity. It meets their needs for sharing experiences and feelings. Some administrators try to hinder the effects of informal organizations because they facilitate the passing of information. The information may be rumor, but the best way to combat rumor is by free flow of truthful information. Only information that might violate individual privacy or the survival and health of the enterprise should be kept from subordinates. The informal organization can help to serve the goals of the formal organization if it is not made the servant of administration. It should not be controlled. A

EXHIBIT 6-12
Standards for Evaluation of Departmentation

1. Nursing activities have been grouped to attain goals and sustain the enterprise.
2. Nursing activities have been grouped for intradepartmental and interdepartmental coordination.
3. Personnel roles have been designed to fit the capabilities and motivation of persons available to fill them.
4. Personnel roles have been designed to help employees contribute to departmental or unit objectives.
5. Personnel roles provide optimum and economic job enlargement.
6. Nursing activities have been grouped for full use of resources, people, and material.
7. Nursing activities have been grouped for optimum cost benefits.
8. Nursing activities have been grouped to match special skills to special needs.
9. Nursing activities have been grouped to achieve an optimum management span.
10. Nursing activities and personnel have been grouped for optimum correlation for decision making and problem solving.
11. Nursing activities have been grouped to achieve minimal levels of management by providing for delegation of responsibility and authority to the lowest competent operational level.
12. Nursing activities and personnel have been grouped to eliminate duplication of staff services and centralized services of specialists.
13. Nursing activities and personnel have been grouped to facilitate production of products and services that will promote health of individuals and groups.
14. Nursing activities and personnel have been grouped to promote soundness of industrial relations programs and fiscal policies and procedures.
15. Nursing activities have been grouped to fulfill time demands of shifts.
16. Nursing activities have been grouped to achieve priorities and allow for change and flexibility in achievement of objectives.
17. Nursing activities have been grouped to facilitate training of employees.
18. Nursing activities have been grouped to facilitate communication.

major shortcoming in its use is that not all employees are part of the informal organization.

Nurse managers should encourage and nurture informal organizations that do the following:

1. Provide a sense of belonging, security, and recognition.
2. Provide methods for friendly and open discussion of concern.
3. Maintain feelings of personal integrity, self-respect, and independent choice.
4. Provide an informal and accurate communication link.
5. Provide opportunities for social interaction.
6. Provide a source of practical information for managerial decision making.
7. Are sources of future leaders.

Problems can include creation of conflicting loyalties, restricted productivity, and resistance to change and management's plans.[172]

Minimum Requirements of an Organizational Structure

1. *Clarity:* Nurses need to know where they belong, where they stand in relation to the quality and quantity of their performances, and where to go for assistance.
2. *Economy:* Nurses need as much self-control of their work as they can possibly be given. They need to be self-motivating. There should be the smallest possible number of overhead personnel necessary to keep the division and units operating and well maintained.
3. *Direction of vision:* Nurse managers must direct their vision and that of their employees toward performance, toward the future, and toward strength. Nurses must understand their own tasks and the common tasks of the organization. They should see that their tasks fit the common tasks so that the structure helps communication.
4. *Decision making:* Nurses should be organized to make decisions on the right issues and at the right levels. They should be organized to convert their decisions into work and accomplishments. The chair of the department of nursing and the staff make all nursing decisions and see that nursing work is done.
5. *Stability and accountability:* Nurses should be organized to feel community belonging. They can adapt to show objectives requiring changes in their functions and productivity.
6. *Perception and self-renewal:* Nursing services should be organized to produce future leaders. The organizational structure should produce continuous learning for the job each nurse holds and for promotion.

To apply design principles that are appropriate, the nurse manager uses a mixture of all that are productive, including the following:

- Organizational needs derive from the statements of mission and objectives and from observation of work performed.
- Organizational design and structure develop to fit organizational needs, so that people perform and

contribute to achieving the work of the division of nursing.

- A formal organization should be flexible and based on policy that promotes individual contributions to the achievement of organizational objectives.
- A formal organization is efficient when it promotes achievement of objectives with a minimum of unplanned costs or outcomes. Most results should be planned for, should give satisfaction to supervisors and employees, and should not occasion waste and carelessness. When grouping activities for organizing purposes, the supervisor or administrator should examine the benefits and disadvantages of alternate groupings.
- A formal organization should build the least possible number of management levels and forge the shortest possible chain of command. This eliminates stresses and levels of friction, slack, and inertia.

Exhibit 6-12 outlines standards for evaluating departmentation of authority in a nursing division, department, service, or unit.

Organizational Effectiveness

The product or output of an organization is termed *organizational effectiveness* (OE). There should be a relationship between organizational effectiveness and *organizational performance* (OP). Nurse managers define the goals and provide the resources for both organizational effectiveness and organizational performance. The goals have many dimensions, which can include the following:

1. Patient satisfaction with care.
2. Family satisfaction with care.
3. Staff satisfaction with work.
4. Staff satisfaction with rewards, intrinsic and extrinsic.
5. Staff satisfaction with professional development: career, personal, and educational.
6. Staff satisfaction with organization.
7. Management satisfaction with staff.
8. Community relationships.
9. Organizational health.

Nurse administrators control these dimensions of organizational effectiveness. Proactivity is more successful in developing them than is reactivity.[173] The organizational effectiveness of hospitals could be improved if administrators would enter into general or limited partnerships with nurses. Hospitals have moved to vertical integration to capture the lost revenues of retrospective reimbursement. General hospitals have entered into services such as home care, long-term care, psychiatric care, rehabilitation, hospice care, rental and sale of durable medical supplies, and many other profit-making services. Although they call for general or limited partnerships with physicians, they ignore nurses as a potential source of partnerships for profit. Instead, the not-for-profit status of hospital inpatient beds is reputed to be maintained by policies that tie nursing to charity and idealism rather than to viability and profitability. Such statements as the following validate this tie: "Keeping nursing care in the not-for-profit hospital corporation preserves the oldest tradition of hospitals and their role in serving the needy."[174]

Nurses can overcome this attitude by themselves becoming proactive. As an example, nurses could plan a limited partnership that would provide contract nurses through a staffing agency owned by them. They could offer a hospital a contract to provide needed personnel on a first priority basis, with surplus personnel provided for other institutions. The contract could provide for up-to-date continuing education of the agency nurses through cooperative arrangements with the contracting hospital. Profits would be shared, and nurses would perceive that the hospital supported nursing entrepreneurship, thus contributing to their morale and professional esteem. Other ventures could be added to improve OP as well as OE and to give nurses a sense of ownership.

Vertical integration, mergers, linkages, and multihospital systems have created more and new corporate nurse roles. The corporate nurse is physically and organizationally removed from daily nursing service operations. As such, the corporate nurse reviews data from a number of hospitals and organizations, comparing outcomes. Having access to much data and many specialties, and serving on corporate committees, the corporate nurse creates a personal power base. She or he can develop systems for member organizations in such areas as management education, nursing division policy, search and selection of nurse executives, research, quality assurance, risk management, and others.[175]

Symptoms of Malorganization

Recurring problems signal malorganization. They indicate that the focus is on the wrong elements of the business when it should emphasize key activities, major business decisions, performance, and results rather than secondary problems. Another symptom of malorganization is too many meetings attended by too many people. Such meetings are poor tools for accomplishing work. An alternative is to give individual assignments, to meet only to report, and to avoid duplication. Committees are instruments of participation and communication and must be made productive. Too many management levels are another symptom of malorganization.

Build the least possible number of management levels and forge the shortest possible chain of command. This eliminates stresses and levels of friction, slack, and inertia.

If people always have to worry about other people's feelings, there will be overstaffing. If the organization is put together to get the job done, layers of coordinators will not be needed. Fit the chart to the organization and its needs rather than drawing a chart and building the organization to support it.

Summary

There is no best design for a nursing organization, nor are there universal design principles. Nurse managers need to work for an ideal organizational structure, and they need to be pragmatic. They should build, test, concede, compromise, and accept. They should design the simplest organization for getting the job done. They should focus on key activities to produce key results. The organization is productive when the people are performing care that meets clients' needs and for which employees have a sense of accomplishment.

An organization can be shaped through the following:

1. Enacting job enlargement that is qualitative and meaningful, interesting, and intellectually rewarding.
2. Making the structure more manageable. Increasing clinical nurses' autonomy reduces the organization's size.
3. Increasing the span of control of the manager.
4. Shortening the hierarchy.
5. Involving the employees in participation.
6. Decentralization.
7. Increasing the employee's stake in his or her own performance.
8. Increasing creativity while maintaining fiscal responsibility.
9. Replacing direction and control with advice.
10. Meeting employees' needs.

One main way to get employees involved in the shape of the organization is through committee work. Committees provide employees with a representative voice in the management of organizations. A standing committee has continuity as an organizational entity, whereas an ad hoc committee is formed for a purpose and disbanded when that purpose is fulfilled. Committees can facilitate communication, promote loyalty, pool special human resources, reduce resistance to change, and give people opportunities to work together. They should have purposes, objectives, and operational procedures. Committees can waste time if they make a premature decision or do not accomplish their objectives. They can be made effective by application of the management functions of planning, organizing, directing (leading), and controlling (evaluating).

Chairs of committees need knowledge and skills of group dynamics, which can be provided through staff development programs for all nurses desiring it. Groups work in five phases:

1. Forming or orientation phase.
2. Conflict or storming phase.
3. Cohesion or norming phase.
4. Working or performing phase.
5. Termination phase.

Group techniques include the Delphi technique, brainstorming, the nominal group techniques, and focus groups, among others. Group leaders either are appointed (formal leaders) or emerge from the group (informal leaders).

Self-directed work teams increase participatory management by broadening jobs and increasing employee cohesiveness. Self-directed work teams enable the employees to have more decision-making abilities, thereby improving employee satisfaction, productivity, and commitment to the organization.

Decentralization disburses authority and power downward to the operational units of an organization. Increased productivity, improved morale, increased favorable attitudes, and decreased absenteeism are the products of decentralized decision making. Decentralization supports participatory management, the characteristics of which are trust, commitment, involvement of employees in setting goals and objectives, autonomy, inclusion of employees in decision making, change and growth, originality, and creativity.

Decentralized and participatory organizations are usually flat or horizontal, employee- and relationship-centered. They are vertically integrated to enhance revenue production by developing new markets for health care organizations.

Training is essential to the success of participatory management because managers are often threatened by loss of authority. They have to be prepared for their new roles. Practicing nurses need to be able to perform as collaborators in the management of nursing organization and the health care institution. With their new roles comes increased accountability for practicing nurses. Managers become facilitators.

Although participatory management has numerous benefits or advantages, it also has some disadvantages. Among those disadvantages are occasional failures, occasional difficulty fixing responsibilities, and difficulty in changing employee perceptions of previously authoritarian management.

The nursing management function of organizing is an evolving one. It evolves as nurse managers learn and apply the knowledge gained from research and experience in business and industry. They further develop the organizing function through nursing research and experience in nursing management.

APPLICATION EXERCISES

EXERCISE 6-1

Use the list entitled "activities that promote a positive organizational climate" in this chapter as a point of discussion for a group of your peers. Assess the organizational climate in the organization in which you are a student or an employee. Compare this with the list of activities that promote a positive organizational climate. Add activities missing from this list.

EXERCISE 6-2

Read the following articles:

Bruhn, J. G. (1996). Creating an organizational climate for multiculturalism. *Health Care Supervision, 1*, 11–18.

Butcher, A. H. (1994). Supervisors matter more than you think: Components of a mission-centered organizational climate. *Hospital Health Services Administration, 6*, 505–520.

Counte, M. A., Glandon, G. L., Oleske, D. M., & Hill, J. P. (1992). Total quality management in a health care organization: How are employees affected? *Hospital Health Services Administration, 6*, 503–518.

DeLellis, A. J. (1997). Creating a climate of mutual respect among employees: A workshop design. *Health Care Supervision, 1*, 48–56.

Gibson, J. M. (1998). Using the Delphi Technique to identify the content and context of nurses' continuing professional development needs. *Journal of Clinical Nursing, 7*, 451–459.

Jones, L. C., Guberski, T. D., & Soeken, K. L. (1990). Nurse practitioners: Leadership behaviors and organizational climate. *Journal of Professional Nursing, 5*, 327–333.

Keuter, K., Byrne, E., Voell, J., & Larson, E. (2000). Nurses' job satisfaction and organizational climate in a dynamic work environment. *Applied Nursing Research, 1*, 46–49.

Mattiasson, A. C. & Andersson, L. (1995). Organizational environment and the support of patient autonomy in nursing home care. *Journal of Advanced Nursing, 10*, 1149–1157.

Piscopo, B. (1995). Organizational climate, communication, and role strain in clinical nursing faculty. *Journal of Professional Nursing, 3*, 113–119.

Answer the following questions:

- What characteristics of organizational climate were evident in these articles?
- How did these characteristics impact negatively or positively on professional nurses?
- What actions could be taken to improve any negative impacts on professional nurses' performance?

EXERCISE 6-3

Use Exhibit 6-8, Standards for Evaluating the Effectiveness of Line and Staff Relationships in a Hierarchical Organization, to evaluate the nursing division, department, service, or unit in which you work as a student or an employee. Involve your colleagues.

EXERCISE 6-4 Explore the concept of the high-tech home care nurse who can bring critical care nursing and medical services directly into the home care environment. Make a business plan to develop high-tech home care as a new product.

Carruth, A. K., Steele, S., Moffett, B., Rehmeyer, T., Cooper, C., & Burroughs, R. (1999). The impact of primary and modular nursing delivery systems on perceptions of caring behavior. *Oncology Nursing Forum*, *1*, 95–100.

McNeal, G. J. (1998a). Care of the critically ill client at home. *Nursing Clinics of North America*, *2*, 267–278.

McNeal, G. J. (1998b). Telecommunication technologies in high-tech homecare. *Nursing Clinics of North America*, *2*, 279–286.

EXERCISE 6-5 Organize a team to study the concepts of circular organizational charts and organigraphs. Draft a circular organizational chart for a department or unit of the organization in which you work or are a student. Outline a process for doing an organigraph of a nursing unit and implement it.

EXERCISE 6-6 Describe the form of the organizational structure of the nursing division and unit in which you work as a student or employee. Discuss the changes that could be made to make it more functional.

EXERCISE 6-7 Use Exhibit 6-10, Evaluating Organizational Function, to evaluate the nursing organization chart of the organization in which you work as a student or employee.

EXERCISE 6-8 Attend meetings of several committees for the purpose of identifying behavior of members in group task roles. Identify the role each member is playing. Write a brief summary of your observations. Do the same for members in group-building and maintenance roles and members in individual roles.

EXERCISE 6-9 Examine the collective minutes of an ad hoc committee. Identify the phases of the committee and link each phase with recorded behaviors. Summarize your findings.

EXERCISE 6-10

1. Use Exhibit 6-3, Checklist for Evaluating Meeting Effectiveness, and Exhibit 6-2, Standards for Evaluating Nursing Committees, to evaluate a nursing meeting in the organization in which you work as a student or as an employee.
2. When the minutes of the same meeting have been distributed, use Exhibit 6-3 to evaluate them. Is there a difference between the actual meeting and the minutes? What is it? How can the process be improved? Make a management plan (using the following format) to improve the committee's meetings and/or the minutes. Be tactful and use a positive approach in your planning.

MANAGEMENT PLAN

OBJECTIVE:

ACTIONS	TARGET DATES	ASSIGNED TO	ACCOMPLISHMENTS

EXERCISE 6-11 This is a group exercise.

1. Form groups of six to eight persons each.
2. Select group leaders and recorders.
3. List characteristics of decentralization and participatory management evident in your organization. (15 minutes)
4. List characteristics of centralized management evident in your organization. (15 minutes)
5. List changes you would like to see implemented to increase decentralization of decision making in your organization. (20 minutes)
6. Report. (20 minutes)

NOTES

1. Liebler, J. G. & McConnell, C. R. (2004). *Management principles for health professionals.* Sudbury, MA: Jones and Bartlett Publishers, 166.
2. Argyris, C. (1973). Personality and organization theory revisited. *Administrative Science Quarterly, 18*, 141–167.
3. Fayol, H. (1949). *General and industrial management* (C. Storrs, Trans.). London: Sir Isaac Pittman & Sons, 53–61.
4. Urwick, L. (1944). *The elements of administration*. New York: Harper & Row, pp. 37–39.
5. Peters, T. (1987). *Thriving on chaos*. New York: Harper & Row.
6. Gilles, D. (1994) Organization structure. In D. Gilles (Ed.), *Nursing management: A systems approach* (3rd ed.). Philadelphia: W.B. Saunders, 129.
7. Gibson, J. L. Ivancevich, J. M., & Donnelly, J. H., Jr. (1994). *Organizations: Behavior, structures, processes* (8th ed.). Burr Ridge, IL: Richard D. Irwin, Inc., 539–541.
8. Hall, R. H. (1963). The concept of bureaucracy: An empirical assessment. *The American Journal of Sociology*, 32–40.
9. Ibid.
10. Hall, R. H. (1968). Professionalization and bureaucratization. *American Sociological Review*, 92–104.
11. Sofarelli, D. & Brown, D. (1998). The need for nursing leadership in uncertain times. *Journal of Nursing Management*, 201–207.
12. Rizzo, J. R., House, R. J., & Lirtzman, S. I. (1970). Role conflict and ambiguity in complex organizations. *Administrative Science Quarterly, 15*, 150–162.
13. Warda, M. (1992). The family and chronic sorrow: Role theory approach. *Journal of Pediatric Nursing*, 205–210.
14. MacLeod, J. A. & Sella, S. (2002). One year later: Using role theory to evaluate a new delivery system. *Nursing Forum*, 20–28.
15. Miller, J. O. & Carey, S. J. (1993). Work role inventory: A guide to job satisfaction. *Nursing Management*, 54–62.
16. Dunphy, D. (1983). Personal and organizational change—Status and future direction. *Work and People*, 3–6.
17. Johnson, J. & Luciano, K. (1983). Managing by behavior and results—Linking supervisory accountability to effective organizational control. *The Journal of Nursing Administration*, 19–26.
18. Dayani, E. C. (1983). Professional and economic self-goverance in nursing. *Nursing Economic$*, 20–23.
19. Argyris, 1973.
20. Ridderheim, D. S. (1986). The anatomy of change. *Hospital & Health Services Administration*, 7–21.
21. del Bueno, D. J. & Vincent, P. M. (1986). Organizational culture: How important is it? *Journal of Nursing Administration*, 15–20.
22. Moore, W. W. (1991). Corporate culture: Modern day rites and rituals. *Healthcare Trends and Transitions*, 8–13, 32–33.
23. Dyer, W. G. & Dyer, W. G., Jr. (1986). Organizational development system change or culture change? *Personnel*, 14–22.
24. Desatnick, R. L. (1986). Management climate surveys: A way to uncover an organization's culture. *Personnel*, 49–54, 14–22.
25. Sovie, M. D. (1993). Hospital culture—Why create one? *Nursing Economic$*, 69–75.
26. Ray, M. A. (1989). The theory of bureaucratic caring for nursing practice in the organizational culture. *Nursing Administration Quarterly*, 31–42.
27. Fleeger, M. E. (1993). Assessing organizational culture: A planning strategy. *Nursing Management*, 39–41.
28. Thomas, C., Ward, M., Chorba, C., & Kumiega, A. (1990). Measuring and interpreting organizational culture. *Journal of Nursing Administration*, 17–24.
29. Kramer, M. & Schmalenberg, C. (2002). Staff nurses identify essentials of magnetism. In M. McClure & A. Hinshaw (Eds.), *Magnet hospitals revisited: Attraction and retention of professsional nurses.* Washington: American Nurses Publishing, 52.
30. Ibid.
31. Peters, T. (1991, September 24). Experts' strengths can be a weakness. *San Antonio Light*, p. B3.
32. Munn, H. E., Jr. (1984). Organizational climate in the health care setting. *The Health Care Supervisor*, 19–29.
33. Desatnick, 1986.
34. Holt Ashley, M. (1985). Motivation: Getting the medical units going again. *Nursing Management*, 28–30.
35. Knaus, W., et al. (1986). An evaluation of outcome from intensive care in major medical centers. Annuals of Internal Medicine, 104, 410–418.
36. ANA, 2004, pp. 15, 16, 17, 19, 20.
37. Ibid., p. 28.
38. Ibid.
39. Ibid., p. 3.
40. Kowalski, K. (1995). Teambuilding. In P. Yoder-Wise, *Leading and managing in nursing*. Missouri: Mosby-Year Book, Inc., 286–288.
41. Ibid., in Dyer, W. (1987). *Team building issues and alternatives*. Boston: Addison-Wesley.
42. Schaffner, T. & Bermingham, M. (1993). Creating and maintaining a high-performance team. In *Nursing Leadership: Preparing for the 21st Century*. Washington, DC: American Hospital Publishing, Inc., American Organization of Nurse Executives, 80.
43. Ibid.

44. Ibid.
45. Russell-Babin, K. (1992). Team building for the staff development department. *Journal of Nursing Staff Development*, 231–234; San Juan, S. P. (1998). Team building: A leadership strategy. *Journal of the Phillippine Dental Association*, 49–55.
46. Nave, J. L. & Thomas, B. (1983). How companies boost morale. *Supervisory Management*, 29–33.
47. Drucker, P. F. (1973). *Management: Tasks, responsibilities, practice*. New York: Harper & Row, 564.
48. McClure, M., Poulin, M., Sovie, M., & Wandelt, M. (2002). Magnet hospitals: Attraction and retention of professional nurses (the original study). In M. McClure & A. Hinshaw (Eds.), *Magnet hospitals revisited: Attraction and retention of professional nurses*. Washington: American Nurses Publishing, 12.
49. Mayo, E. (1946). *The human problems of industrial civilization*. Boston: Harvard Business School.
50. Stevens, B. J. (1975). Use of groups for management. *Journal of Nursing Administration*, 14–22.
51. Benne, K. D. & Sheats, P. (1948). Functional roles of group members. *Journal of Social Studies*, 41–49.
52. Ibid.
53. Ibid.
54. Dixon, N. (1984). Participative management: It's not as simple as it seems. *Supervisory Management*, 2–8.
55. Caramanica, L. (1984). What? Another committee? *Nursing Management*, 12–14; Jay, A. (1982). How to run a meeting. *Journal of Nursing Administration*, 22–28.
56. Northouse, L. L. & Northouse, P. G. (1985). *Health communication: A handbook for health professionals*. Englewood Cliffs, NJ: Prentice Hall; Brightman, H. J. & Verhowen, P. (1986). Running successful problem solving group. *Business*, 15–23.
57. Beeber, L. S. & Schmitt, M. H. (1986). Cohesiveness in groups: A concept in search of a definition. *Advances in Nursing Science*, 1–11.
58. Tipping, J., Freeman, R. F., & Rachlis, A. R. (1995). Using faculty and student perceptions of group dynamics to develop recommendations for PBL training. *Academic Medicine*, 1050–1052; Cook, S. H. & Matheson, H. (1997). Teaching group dynamics: A critical evaluation of an experiential programme. *Nursing Education Today*, 31–38; Krejci, J. W. & Malin, S. (1997). Impact of leadership development on competencies. *Nursing Economic$*, 235–241; Abusabha, R., Peacock, J., & Achterberg, C. (1999). How to make nutrition education more meaningful through facilitated group discussion. *Journal of the American Dietetic Association,* 72–76.
59. Hodgetts, R. M. (1990). *Management theory, process and practice* (5th ed.). Orlando, FL: Harcourt Brace, 286.
60. Mosley, D. C., Pietri, P. W., Jr., & Megginson, L. C. (1996). *Management: Leadership in action* (5th ed.). New York: Harper Collins, 456.
61. Northouse & Northouse, 1985, 240–241.
62. Lloyd-Jones, G., Fowell, S., & Bligh, J. G. (1999). The use of the nominal group technique as an evaluative tool in medical undergraduate education. *Medical Education*, 8–13; Swansburg, R. C. (1995). Nominal group technique. In B. Fuszard (Ed.), *Innovative Strategies in Nursing* (2nd ed., pp. 93–100). Gaithersburg, MD: Aspen.
63. Ekblad, S., Marttila, A., & Emilsson, M. (2002). Cultural challenges in end-of-life care: Reflections from focus groups' interviews with hospital staff in Stockholm. *Journal of Advanced Nursing*, 623–630; Corring, D. J. & Cook, J. V. (1999). Client-Centered care means that I am a valued human being. *Canadian Journal of Occupational Therapy*, 71–82; Hind, M., Jacjson, D., Andrewes, C., Fulbrook, P., Galvin, K., & Frost, S. (1999). Exploring the expanded role of nurses in critical care. *Intensive Critical Care Nursing*, 147–153; Dewar, B. J. & Walker, E. (1999). Experiential learning: Issues in supervision. *Journal of Advanced Nursing*, 1459–1467; Dreachslin, J. L. (1998). Conducting effective focus groups in the context of diversity: Theoretical underpinnings and practical implications. *Qualitative Health Research*, 813–820; Jinks, A. M. & Daniels, R. (1999). Workplace health concerns: A focus group study. *Journal of Management in Medicine, 13*(2–3), 95–104; Hildebrandt, E. (1999). Focus groups and vulnerable populations. Insight into client strengths and needs in complex community health care environments. *Nursing Health Care Perspectives*, 256–259; Reiskin, H., Gendrop, S., Bowen, A., Wright, P., & Walsh, E. (1999). Collaboration between community nurses and nursing faculty using substance abuse prevention focus groups. *Nursing Connections*, 31–36; Hirst, S. P. (2000). Resident abuse: An insider's perspective. *Geriatric Nursing*, 38–42; Lowry, R. J. & Craven, M. A. (1999). Smokers' and drinkers' awareness of oral cancer: A qualitative study using focus groups. *British Dental Journal*, 668–670.
64. DesRosier, M. B. & Zellers, K. C. (1989). Focus groups: A program planning technique. *Journal of Nursing Administration*, 20–25.
65. Ibid.
66. Rosenblum, E. H. (1982). Groupthink: The peril of group cohesiveness. *Journal of Nursing Administration*, 27–31; Rowland, H. S. & Rowland, B. L. (2002). *Handbook for nurse administrators*. Philadelphia, PA: Lippincott; Leo, M. (1984). Avoiding the pitfalls of management think. *Business Horizons*, 44–47.
67. Ibid.
68. Dumaine, B. (1994, September 5). The trouble with teams. *Fortune*, 86–88, 90, 92.
69. Caudron, S. (1993). Teamwork takes work. *Personnel Journal*, 76–84.
70. Manz, C. C., Keating, D. E., & Donellon, A. (1990). Preparing for an organizational change to employee self-management: The managerial transition. *Organizational Dynamics*, 15–26.
71. Seelhoff, K. L. (1992). Six steps to team problem solving. *Hotels*, 26.
72. Brandon, G. M. (1996). Flattening the organization: Implementing self-directed work groups. *Radiology Management*, 35–42; Yeatts, D. E. & Schultz, E. (1998). Self-managed work teams: What works? *Clinical Laboratory Management Review*, 16–26.
73. Stevens, 1975.
74. Dixon, 1984.
75. Mohrman, S. A. & Ledford, G. E., Jr. (1985). The design and use of effective employee participation groups: Implication for human resource management. *Human Resource Management*, 413–428.
76. Fried, B. & Rundall, T. (1994). Managing groups and teams. In S. Shortell & A. Kaluzny, *Health care management: Organization design and behavior* (3rd ed., pp. 144–147). New York: Delmar.
77. Jay, 1982; Auger, B. Y. (1967). How to run an effective meeting. Commerce; Swansburg, R. C. (1976). *Management of patient care services*. St. Louis: Mosby; Kanter, R. (1989). *When giants learn to dance*. New York: Simon & Schuster; Stevens,1975, Stevens, B. J. (1997). *The nurse as executive* (4th ed.). Gaithersburg, MD: Aspen.
78. Pugh, D. S., Hickson, D. J., Hinings, C. R., & Turner, C. (1969). The context of organization stuctures. *Administrative Science Quarterly*, 91–114; Leatt, P. & Schneck, R. (1982). Technology, size, environment, and structure in nursing subunits. *Organizational Studies*, *3*(3), 221–242.

79. Institute of Medicine (IOM). (2000). *To err is human: Building a safer health system for the 21st century*. Washington, DC: National Academy Press.
80. Institute of Medicine (IOM). (2004). Transforming the work environment of nurses. *Quality Chasm Series*. Washington, DC: National Academy Press, 2.
81. Ibid., 8, 9, 12, 13.
82. Marquis, B. & Huston, C. (1996). Roles and functions in organizing. *Leadership Roles and Management Functions in Nursing: Theory and Application*. Philadelphia: Lippincott-Raven, 144–149.
83. Ibid.
84. Ibid.
85. Fanning, M. M. (1997). A circular organization chart promotes a hospital-wide focus on teams. *Hospital Health Services Administration*, 243–254.
86. Ibid.
87. Mintzberg, H. & Van der Heyden, L. (1999). Organigraphs: Drawing how companies really work. *Harvard Business Review*, 87–94, 184.
88. Pugh, Hickson, Hinings, & Turner, 1969.
89. Roznowski, M. & Hulin, C. L. (1985). Influences of functional specialty and job technology on employees' perceptual and affective responses to their jobs. *Organizational Behavior and Human Decision Processes*, 186–208.
90. Leatt & Schneck, 1982.
91. Pugh et al., 1969.
92. Ibid.
93. Leatt & Schnek, 1982.
94. Ibid.
95. Roznowski & Hulin, 1985.
96. Newman, J. G. & Boisoneau, R. (1987). Team care and matrix organization in geriatrics. *Hospital Topics*, 10–15.
97. McClure, M. L. (1984). Managing the professional nurse: Part I. The organizational theories. *The Journal of Nursing Administration*, 15–21; Timm, M. M. & Wavetik, M. G. (1983). Matrix organization: Design and development for a hospital organization. *Hospital & Health Services Administration*, 46–58; American Organization of Nurse Executives (AONE). (1984). *Organizational models for nursing practice.* Chicago: American Hospital Association.
98. Ibid.
99. Ibid.
100. Mosley, Pietri, & Megginson, 1996, 274–277, 346, 582.
101. McClure, Poulin, Sovie, & Wandelt, 2002.
102. Koloroutis, M. (2004). *Relationship-based care: A model for transforming practice*. Minneapolis, MN: Creative Health Care Management, 75.
103. Klaus, J. (1983). Corporate pyramids will tumble when horizontal organizations become the new global standard. *Personnel Administrator*, 56–59.
104. Elpern, E. A., White, P. M., & Donahue, A. F. (1984). Staff governance: The experience of the nursing unit. *The Journal of Nursing Administration,* 9–15.
105. Weisz, W. J. (1985). Employee involvement: How it works at Motorola. *Personnel,* 29–33; Poteet, G. W. (1984). Delegation strategies: A must for the nurse executive. *Journal of Nursing Administration*, 18–27.
106. Fine, R. B. & Walton, R. E. (1985). From control to commitment in the workplace. *Harvard Business Review*, 77–84.
107. Raelin, J. A., Sholl, C., & Leonard, D. (2002). Professional work environment. *Nursing Administration Quarterly*, 82–88.
108. Ibid.
109. Batey, M. V. & Lewis, F. M. (1982). Clarifying autonomy and accountability in nursing services: Part I. *Journal of Nursing Administration*, 13–17.
110. Bragg, J. E. & Andrews, I. R. (1984). Participative decision making: An experimental study in a hospital. In B. Fuszard, *Self-Actualization for nurses* (pp. 102–110). Rockville, MD: Aspen.
111. Collins, S. S. & Henderson, M. C. (1991). Autonomy: Part of the nursing role? *Nursing Forum*, 26(2), 23–29.
112. Bough, S. (1992). Nursing students rank high in autonomy at the exit level. *Journal of Nursing Education*, 58–64.
113. Shoemaker, H. & El-Ahraf, A. (1983). Decentralization of nursing service management and its impact on job satisfaction. *Nursing Administration Quarterly,* 69–76.
114. Snail, T. S. (1998). Organizational diversification in the American hospital. *Annual Review of Public Health, 19*, 417–453.
115. Clegg, C. W. & Wall, T. D. (1984). The lateral dimension to employee participation. *Journal of Management Studies*, 429–442.
116. Friedman, B. A. (1997). Orchestrating a unified approach to information management. *Radiology Management*, 30–36.
117. James, D. M. (1998). An integrated model for inner-city healthcare delivery: The Deaconess center. *Journal of the National Medical Association*, 35–39.
118. Weisz, 1985.
119. Walton, 1985.
120. Simons, B. J. (2002). Particpatory management strategies. *Journal of Nursing Administration*, *2*, 72–78.
121. Schuster, M. H. & Miller, C. S. (1985). Employee involvement: Making supervisors believers. *Personnel,* 24–28.
122. Simons, B. J., 2002.
123. Malkin, S. & Lauteri, P. (1980). A community hospital's approach: Decentralized patient education. *Nursing Administration Quarterly*, 101–106.
124. Raelin, Sholl, & Leonard, 2002.
125. Walton, 1985.
126. Robinson, M. A. (1991). Decentralize and outsource: Dial's approach to MIS improvement. *Management Accounting*, 27–31.
127. Cox, C. L. (1980). Decentralization uniting authority and responsibility. *Supervisor Nurse*, 28, 32.
128. Gordon, G. K. (1982). Developing a motivating environment. *The Journal of Nursing Administration*, 11–16.
129. Weisz, 1985.
130. Lovrich, M. P. (2000). Managing employees through participatory management. *Nursing Management*, 56–62; Schuster & Miller, 1985.
131. Shoemaker & El-Ahraf, 1983; Lovrich, Weisz, 1985; Cox,1980.
132. Raelin, Sholl, & Leonard, 2002; Shoemaker & El-Ahraf, 1985; Walton, 1985.
133. Parker, S. K. (1985). Enhancing role breadth self-efficacy: The roles of job enrichment and other organizational interventions. *Journal of Applied Psychology*, 835–852.
134. Raelin, Sholl, & Leonard, 2002.
135. Bragg & Andrews, 1984.
136. Probst, M. R. & Noga, J. M. (1980). A decentralized nursing care delivery system. *Supervisor Nurse*, 57–60; Elpern, White, & Donahue,1984.
137. Porter-O'Grady, T. (1992). *Implementing Shared Governance*. St. Louis, MO: Mosby.
138. Ibid.
139. Jacoby, J. & Terpstra, M. (1990). Collaborative governance: Model of professional autonomy. *Nursing Management*, 42–44.
140. T. Maldonado, T. (1992). Lecture, senior management class. San Antonio, TX: Incarnate Word College.
141. Pugh, Hickson, Hinings, & Turner, 1969.
142. George, V. M., Burke, L. J., & Rodgers, B. L. (1997). Research-based planning for change: Assessing nurses' attitudes toward governance and professional practice autonomy after hospital acquisition. *Journal of Nursing Administration*, 53–61.

143. Prince, S. B. (1997). Shared governance. Sharing power and opportunity. *Journal of Nursing Administration*, 28–35.
144. Joiner, G. & Wessman, J. (1997). Expanding shared governance beyond practice issues. *Recruitment, Retention, Restructuring Research*, 4–7.
145. Aikman, P., Andress, I., Goodfellow, C., LaBelle, N. & Porter-O'Grady, T. (1998). System integration: A necessity. *Journal of Nursing Administration*, 28–34.
146. Levinson, R. E. (1985). Why decentralize? *Management Review*, 50–53.
147. Hatcher, L. L. & Ross, T. L. (1985). Organizational development through productivity gainsharing. *Personnel*, 42, 44–50; Walton, 1985.
148. Walton, 1985.
149. Flarey, D. L. (1991).The nurse executive and the governing body. *Journal of Nursing Administration*, 11–17.
150. Kanter, 1989, 36.
151. Ibid., 57–67.
152. Sovie, M. D. (1990). Redesigning our future: Whose responsibility is it? *Nursing Economics$*, 21–26.
153. Genasci, L. (1994, July 24). Downsizing not always effective, experts say. *San Antonio Express-News*, p. H3.
154. Kaestle, P. (1990). A new rationale for organizational structure. *Planning Review*, 20–22, 27.
155. Staring, S. & Taylor, C. (1997). A guide to managing workforce transitions. *Nursing Management*, 31–32.
156. Peters, T. (1987). *Thriving on Chaos*. New York: Harper & Row, 424–438.
157. Reddecliff, M., Smith, E. L., & Ryan-Merritt, M. (1989). Organizational analysis: Tool for the clinical nurse specialist. *Clinical Nurse Specialist*, 133–136.
158. del Bueno, D. L. (1993). Paradigm shifts—What's good and not so good for health care. *Nursing & Health Care*, 100–101.
159. McAllister, M. (1990). A nursing integration framework based on standards of practice. *Nursing Management*, 28–31.
160. Adams, R. A. & Rentfro, A. R. (1988). Strengthening hospital nursing: An approach to restructuring care delivery. *Journal of Nursing Administration*, 12–19.
161. Schmekel, C. E. (1991). Nursing/Group practice. *AORN Journal*, 1223–1226, 1228.
162. Metcalf, K. M. (1992). The helper model: Nine ways to make it work. *Nursing Management*, 40–43.
163. Manthey, M. (1991). Delivery systems and practice models: A dynamic balance. *Nursing Management*, 28–30.
164. Milton, D., Verren, J., Murdaugh, C., & Gerber, R. (1992). Differentiated group professional practice in nursing: A demonstration model. *Nursing Clinics of North America*, 23–29.
165. Ibid.
166. Ehrat, K. S. (1991). The value of differentiated practice. *JONA*, 9–10.
167. Graph, C., Roberts, K., & Thorton, K. (1999). An ethnographic study of differentiated practice in an operating room. *Journal of Professional Nursing*, 364–371; Smith-Blair, N., Smith, B. L., Bradley, K. J., & Gaskamp, C. (1999). Making sense of a new nursing role: A phenomenological study of an organizational change. *Journal of Professional Nursing*, 340–348.
168. Styles, M., Allen, S., Armstrong, S., Matsurra, M., Stannard, D., & Ordway, J. S. (1991). Entry: A new approach. *Nursing Outlook*, 200–203.
169. Koloroutis, 2004, 11.
170. Ibid., 4.
171. Ibid.
172. Han, P. E. (1983). The informal organization you've got to live with. *Supervisory Management*, 25–28.
173. Cameron, K. (1986). A study of organizational effectiveness and its predictors. *Management Science*, 87–112.
174. Ibid.
175. Beyers, M. (1984). Getting on top of organizational change: Part 3. The corporate nurse executive. *Journal of Nursing Administration*, 32–37.

REFERENCES

American Nurses Association (ANA). (1991). *Standards of clinical nursing practice*. Washington, DC: Author.

American Nurses Association (ANA). (1995). *Scope and standards for nurse administrators*. Washington, DC: Author.

Antrobus, S. & Kitson, A. (1999). Nursing leadership: Influencing and shaping health policy and nursing practice. *Journal of Advanced Nursing*, *8*, 746–753.

Badovanic, C. C., Wilson, S., & Woodhouse, D. (1999). The use of unlicensed assistive personnel and selected outcome indications. *Nursing Economic$*, *3*, 194–200.

Bailey, K. L. (1998). Establishing private duty in a Medicare world. Caring, *1*, 29–31.

Bichan, M. S., Hegge, M. J., & Stenvig, T. E. (2004). A tiger by the tail: Tackling barriers to differentiated practice. *The Journal of Continuing Education in Nursing, 22*(3), 109–112.

Bigelow, B. & Arndt, M. (2000). The more things change, the more they stay the same. *Health Care Management Review*, 65–72.

Bowen, M., Lyons, K. J., & Young, B. E. (2000). Nursing and health care reform: Implications for curriculum development. *Journal of Nursing Education*, 27–33.

Call, A. (1992). Building bridges. *Nursing Times*, 44–45.

Clark, D. A., Clark, P. F., Day, D., & Shea, D. (2000). The relationship between health care reform and nurses' interest in union representation: The role of workplace climate. *Journal of Professional Nursing*, 92–96.

Cody, M. (1996). Vertical integration strategies: Revenue effects in hospital and Medicare markets. *Hospital Health Services Administration*, 343–357.

Collins, C. & Green, A. (1999). Public sector hospitals and organizational change: An agenda for policy analysis. *International Journal of Health Planning Management*, 107–128.

Coluccio, M. & Havlick, K. (1998). Shared leadership in a newly merged medical center. *Nursing Administration Quarterly,* 36–39.

Dawkins, C., Oakley, D., Davis, J., & Erwin, N. (1991). Collaboration as an organizational process. *Journal of Nursing Education,* 189–191.

Dennis, K. E. (1983). Nursing's power in the organization: What research has shown. *Nursing Administration Quarterly*, 47–60.

Dienemann, J. & Glazner, T. (1992). Restructuring nursing care delivery systems. *Nursing Economic$*, 253–258, 310.

Galvin, K., Andrewes, C., Jackson, D., Cheesman, S., Fudge, T., Ferris, R., et al. (1999). Investigating and implementing change within the primary health care nursing team. *Journal of Advanced Nursing*, 238–247.

Gardner, D. L. (1991). Assessing career commitment: The role of staff development. *Journal of Nursing Staff Development*, *7*(6), 263–266.

George, J. R. & Bishop, L. K. (1971). Relationship of organizational structure and teacher personality characteristics to organizational climate. *Administrative Science Quarterly*, 467–475.

Glazner, L. (1992). Understanding corporate cultures: Use of systems theory and situational analysis. *AAOHN Journal*, 383–387.

Glover, D. (1993, July 21). Everett hospitals to unify management. *Seattle Post-Intellegencer*, p. B2.

Hansten, R. I. & Washburn, M. J. (1999). Individual and organizational accountability for development of critical thinking. *Journal of Nursing Administration*, 39–45.

Hart, S. K. & Moore, M. N. (1989). The relationship among organizational climate variables and nurse stability in critical care units. *Journal of Professional Nursing*, 124–131.

Haynie, L. & Garrett, B. (1999). Developing a customer-service and cost-effectiveness team. *Journal of Healthcare Quality*, 28–29, 32–34.

Heilriegel, D. & Slocum, J. W. (1972) Organizational climate: Measures research and contingencies. *Academy of Management Journal*, 255–280.

Hirsch, J. (1987). Organizational structure and philosophy. *Nursing Administration Quarterly*, 47–51.

Hodgetts, R. M. (1990). Management: Theory, process, and practice (5th ed.). Orlando, FL: Harcourt, Brace, 138–231.

Ingersoll, G. L., Kirsch, J. C., Merk, S. E., & Lightfoot, J. (2000). Relationship of organizational culture and readiness for change to employee commitment to the organization. *Journal of Nursing Administration*, 11–20.

Jablin, F. M. (1982). Formal structural characteristics of organizations and superior-subordinate communication. *Human Communication Research*, 338–347.

Jones, L. C., Guberski, T. D., & Soeken, K. L. (1990). Nurse practitioners: Leadership behaviors and organizational climate. *Journal of Professional Nursing*, 327–333.

Joyce, W. F. & Slocum, J. (1982). Climate discrepancy: Refining the concepts of psychological and organizational climate. *Human Relations, 11*, 951–972.

Kerfoot, K. (1999). The culture of courage. *Nursing Economic$*, 238–239.

King, C. & Koliner, A. (1999). Understanding the impact of power in organizations. *Seminars in Nursing Management*, 39–46.

Koloroutis, M. & Moe, J. K. (2000). Assessment: The first step in creating a more system-wide approach to nursing practice. *Journal of Nursing Administration*, 97–103.

Krampitz, S. D. & Williams, M. (1983). Organizational climates: A measure of faculty and nurse administrator perception. *Journal of Nursing Education*, 200–206.

Laschinger, H. K., Wong, C., McMahon, L., & Kaufmann, C. (1999). Leader behavior impact on staff nurse empowerment, job tension, and work effectiveness. *Journal of Nursing Administration*, 28–39.

Lehrman, S. & Shore, K. K. (1998). Hospitals' vertical integration into skilled nursing: A rational approach to controlling transaction costs. *Inquiry*, 303–314.

Miller, E. (1999). Reengineering the role of the nurse manager in a patient-centered care organization. *Journal of Nursing Care Quality*, 47–56.

Mills, P. K. & Posner, B. Z. (1982). The relationships among self-supervision, structure, and technology in professional service organizations. *Academy of Management Journal*, 437–443.

Payne, R. L. & Mansfield, R. (1973). Relationships of perceptions of organizational climate to organizational structure, context, and hierarchical position. *Administrative Science Quarterly*, 18, 515–526.

Perryman-Starkey, M., Rivers, P. A., & Munchus, G. (1999). The effects of organizational structure on hospital performance. *Health Services Management Research*, 232–245.

Peters, T. (1992, November 12). McKenzie exemplifies structureless corporation of future. *San Antonio Light*, pp. B1, B8.

Pillar, B. & Jarjoura, D. (1999). Assessing the impact of reengineering on nursing. *Journal of Nursing Administration*, 57–64.

Poulton, B. C. (1999). User involvement in identifying health needs and shaping and evaluating services: Is it being realized? *Journal of Advanced Nursing*, 1289–1296.

Pritchard, R. D. & Karasick, B. W. (1973). The effects of organizational climate on managerial job performance and job satisfaction. *Organizational Behavior and Human Performance, 9*,126–143.

Schaffner, J. W., Alleman, S., Ludwig-Beymer, P., Muzynski, J., King, D. J., & Pacura, L. J. (1999). Developing a patient care model for an integrated delivery system. *Journal of Nursing Administration*, 43–50.

Seago, J. A. (1999). Evaluation of a hospital work redesign: Patient-focused care. *Journal of Nursing Administration*, 31–38.

Shortell, S. M., Jones, R. H., Rademaker, A. W., Gillies, R. R., Dranove, D. S., Hughes, E. F., et al. (2000). Assessing the impact of total quality management and organizational culture on multiple outcomes of care for coronary artery bypass graft surgery patients. *Medical Care*, 207–217.

Spitzer-Lehman, R. & Yahn, K. J. (1992). Patient needs drive an integrated approach to care. *Nursing Management*, 30–32.

Swansburg, R. C. (1976). Management of patient care services. St. Louis: Mosby.

Swansburg, R. C. (1977). *Self-Study Module-27-77: The organizing function of nursing service administration.* Hattiesburg, MS: University of Southern Mississippi.

Swansburg, R. C. (1978). *Nurses & patients: An introduction to nursing management.* Hattiesburg, MS: Impact III.

Theile, J. R. (1983). The anatomy of an organization. *Nursing Administration Quarterly*, 42–45.

Tushman, M. & Nadler, D. (1986). Organizing for innovation. *California Management Review*, 74–92.

Valanis, B. (2000). Professional nursing practice in an HMO: The future is now. *Journal of Nursing Education*, 13–20.

Van Mullem, C., Burke, L. J., Dohmeyer, K., Farrell, M., Harvey, S. John, L., et al. (1999). Strategic planning for research use in nursing practice. *Journal of Nursing Administration*, 38–45.

Walston, S. L. & Bogue, R. J. (1999). The effects of reengineering: Fad or competitive factor. *Journal of Healthcare Management*, 456–476.

Wong, F. K. (1998). The nurse manager as a professional-managerial class: A case study. *Journal of Nursing Management*, 343–350.

APPENDIX 6-1

Nursing Council By-Laws

ARTICLE I
NAME

1.1 The name of this Committee shall be the Nursing Council.

ARTICLE II

The purpose of this Council shall be:

2.1 To ensure excellence in nursing care which will return patients to their best possible state of health or will enable them to die with dignity.
2.2 To provide a climate which will promote and support the practice of professional nursing.
2.3 To provide a forum for the discussion of management and patient care concerns.

The function of the Council shall be:

2.4 To ensure excellence in nursing care.
  a. Through the development and support of ad hoc committees.
  b. Through the support of XYZ Standards of Care.
2.5 To develop nursing service employees to their fullest potential.
  a. Through the development and support of ad hoc committees.
  b. Through the support of XYZ Standards of Care.

ARTICLE III
MEMBER

The members of this Council shall be:

3.1 All members of Nurse Manager Council Group, Clinical Council, Executive Council, committee chairs, and representatives from the XYZ College of Nursing.

ARTICLE IV
OFFICERS

The officers shall consist of:

4.1 Chair, Vice-Chair, and Parliamentarian
  a. All officers shall be elected by secret ballot.
  b. A majority of votes cast will be required to be elected.
  c. In the event a majority of votes is not achieved by the first ballot, a run-off between two candidates having the most votes shall be required.
  d. Ballots shall be counted by the Administrative Secretary and RTN I.
  e. Officers shall serve for one year and are eligible for reelection for one consecutive term.
4.2 Officers, together with the Assistant Administrator of Nursing, shall constitute a governing board.
4.3 In the event of a vacancy:
  a. The Vice-Chair replaces the Chair.
  b. The Parliamentarian shall replace Vice-Chair.
  c. The new Parliamentarian will be appointed by the governing body.
4.4 Duties of the officers:
  a. The Chair shall work closely with the other officers of the Council. The Chair and other officers shall meet one week prior to each regular meeting for the purpose of developing and distributing the agenda and establishing time limits for discussion. The Chair is responsible to the Council for the smooth and effective functioning of its committees. The Chair is a voting member of the Executive Council and is responsible to the Council for communicating recommendations to the Executive Council. The Chair shall function according to the guidelines established in *Robert's Rules of Order.*
  b. The Vice-Chair shall assume the duties of the Chair in his or her absence and shall serve as Chair of the nominating committee.
  c. The Parliamentarian shall oversee that the Business of Nursing Council is conducted according to *Robert's Rules of Order.*
4.5 Qualifications for office—Must be members of Nursing Council.

ARTICLE V
MEETINGS

5.1 Regular meetings shall be held quarterly.
5.2 The annual meeting shall be held in November, at which time annual reports of officers and Chair shall be read and officers elected.
5.3 Special meetings shall be called by the Chair. The purpose of the meeting shall be stated in the call and at least two days notice will be given.

ARTICLE VI
QUORUM

A quorum of the Council shall be one-third of the membership. The presence of a quorum shall be documented in the minutes.

ARTICLE VII
COMMITTEES

7.1 Policy and Procedures Committee
  a. Purpose
    1. To establish guidelines, policies, and instructions for performance of procedures in accordance with the current standards of nursing practice for personnel of the Department of Nursing. The guidelines are specific and prescribe the precise action to be taken under a set of circumstances.
    2. To annually appraise policies and procedures followed by nurses, and to develop new policies to meet present and future needs.

(continued)

APPENDIX 6-1 *(continued)*

3. To assure compliance between nursing policy and hospital policy.

b. Membership
   1. Members shall be appointed from each of the divisions within the Department of Nursing and from the XYZ College of Nursing. One member shall be appointed from each of the following: Executive Council, Staff Development, and Nursing Resources. Two members shall be appointed from the USA College of Nursing. Three members (one Nurse Manager or Clinical Specialist, one staff RN, and one LPN) shall be appointed from each of the following divisions: Medical Surgical, Maternal Child, Critical Care, and Special Services.
   2. Each member shall have an alternate appointed to attend in the member's absence.
   3. Members are to be appointed to serve a two-year term, beginning January 1 of each year.
   4. Each representative may be reappointed for one consecutive term. Only one-half of the membership shall turn over annually.

c. Meetings
   1. The policy and procedures committee shall meet at least six times annually.
   2. The time, date, and place of meetings shall be determined by the Chair.
   3. Minutes of the meeting shall be recorded and kept on file in Nursing Service.
   4. The Chair of this committee shall be elected by its membership.

d. Duties
   1. To accept written recommendations from an individual or committee regarding the need for a policy or procedure.
   2. Identify independently the need for a policy or procedure.
   3. To research the literature and other resources to determine common, accepted nursing practice.
   4. To develop policy and procedures statements.
   5. To annually review and revise as necessary all current policies and procedures.
   6. To report to Nursing Council at each regular meeting.
   7. To prepare a written annual report outlining the accomplishments of the committee. The report shall be prepared by the Chair of the committee and submitted to the Chair of the Nursing Council.

7.2 Nominating Committee will meet during the last quarter prior to the annual meeting as called by the Chair. The slate of nominees shall be presented to Council for consideration one month prior to the annual meeting.

7.3 By-Laws

a. Purpose—To review the by-laws of the Nursing Council and make recommendations to the Council for by-laws revision.

b. Membership
   1. A Chair shall be elected from Nursing Council following the annual meeting.
   2. Members shall be volunteers from Nursing Council.

c. Meetings
   1. The Chair shall determine the frequency, time, date, and place of meetings.
   2. Minutes of the meeting shall be recorded and kept on file in Nursing Service.

7.4 Ad Hoc Committees

a. Purpose—To provide a vehicle by which specific tasks or programs can be assumed by a committee.

b. Membership
   1. Membership shall follow the same format as for standing committees, unless the council decides that a smaller, more specific group, will be more appropriate.
   2. Members can be appointed by Nursing Council or the committee may elect its Chair during its first meeting.

c. Meetings
   1. During the first meeting, the committee shall:
      a. Define its purpose.
      b. Outline the necessary steps to achieve the purpose.
      c. Establish a tentative timetable.
   2. Minutes of the meetings shall be recorded and kept on file in Nursing Service.

d. Duties
   1. The committee Chair shall report to Nursing Council during regular meetings.
   2. When the committee has completed its task, a final recommendation is made to Nursing Council for approval. Upon acceptance of this final recommendation, the Ad Hoc Committee is dissolved.

7.5 RTN-I

a. Purpose—To provide a forum for the discussion of topics relating to the practice of professional nursing at USAMC.

b. Membership
   1. RTN from each unit or area and float pool for term of one year.
   2. Any RTN may attend as an observer.

APPENDIX 6-1

3. Adviser chosen by the committee and approved by administration. The adviser is a non-voting member.
4. Officers are chosen by the committee.

c. Duties
1. To identify problems related to professional nursing and recommend solutions to Nursing Council.
2. To disseminate information to coworkers.
3. To review at monthly meetings all approved new and/or revised policies and procedures.
4. To accept and assume responsibility for projects delegated by Nursing Council.
5. To report to Nursing Council at each regular meeting. The report shall include:
    a. Problems identified concerning professional nursing.
    b. Recommendations for the solution of the identified problems.
    c. Progress on delegated projects.
    d. Summary of monthly committee activities.
6. To prepare an annual written report outlining the accomplishments of the committee. This report shall be prepared by the committee Chair and submitted to the Chair of Nursing Council.

7.6 Nurse Practice Committee

a. Purpose
1. To assist in identifying potential or actual problems related to quality of care, recommend corrective action, develop and plan for corrective action, and review effectiveness of corrective actions until an acceptable level of compliance is obtained. An additional charge of the committee is to develop and/or revise Nursing Standards of Care and Practice.

b. Membership
1. The Clinical Administrator for Nursing Practice shall assume position of Chair.
2. The Nurse Practice Committee is comprised of a Registered Nurse from each nursing unit within the hospital.

c. Duties
1. To review and evaluate Quality Assurance monitoring.
2. To evaluate the effectiveness of previous actions taken to improve care based on follow-up and tracking.
3. To plan appropriate actions that will improve the delivery of nursing care and affect patient outcomes.
4. To communicate and implement the planned action and follow-up at the unit level.
5. To identify trends for potential monitoring and evaluation.
6. To report Quality Assurance analysis to Nursing Council at each regular meeting.

d. Meetings
1. The committee will meet at least monthly or as called by the Chair.
2. Each committee member will receive written notice prior to meetings for attendance.
3. An annual written report summarizing the accomplishments of the committee shall be prepared by the Chair and shall be presented to Nursing and Executive Council.

ARTICLE VIII
PARLIAMENTARY AUTHORITY

The business of this group shall be conducted according to *Robert's Rules of Order.*

ARTICLE IX
AMENDMENTS

The by-laws may be amended at any regular meeting by a majority vote. Any member of Council may present an amendment for vote.

The proposed amendment must be presented to the Committee in writing one month prior to voting.

CHAPTER 7

Leadership and Evidence-Based Management

Linda Roussel, RN, DSN

Do not seek to follow in the footsteps of the wise. Seek what they sought.
Basho

LEARNING OBJECTIVES AND ACTIVITIES

- Describe *transformational leadership* and *evidence-based management*.
- Define *leadership*.
- Explain trait theories of leadership.
- Match examples to Gardner's nine tasks to be performed by leaders.
- Match examples to individual leadership behavioral theorists.
- Match examples to the theory of transformational leadership.
- Discuss similarities between leadership and management.
- Match examples to interpersonal bases of power.
- Describe quantum leadership in a new age of health care.

CONCEPTS: Transformational leadership, evidence-based management, trait theories of leadership, behavioral theories of leadership, leadership styles, gender issues of leadership, buffering, quantum leadership.

NURSE MANAGER BEHAVIORS: Facilitates involvement of registered nurses, other staff members, and patients/clients/residents in interdisciplinary identification of desired outcomes; emphasizes problem solving, results, analysis of failure, tasks, control, and decision making; collaborates with appropriate departments in promoting integrated systems to support nursing service delivery; and decision analysis.

NURSE EXECUTIVE BEHAVIORS: Facilitates the establishment and continuous improvement of clinical guidelines related to outcomes that provide direction for continuity of care and that are attainable with available resources; focuses on creating spirit and commitment, seeking advice and feedback, empowering constituents, and modeling appropriate behavior as symbols of values and norms.

Introduction

Leadership is critical to successful organizational outcomes. Leadership is central to safety in a variety of industries as well as to an organization's competitive cost position after a change initiative.[1–3] Transformational leadership has been specifically identified by the Institute of Medicine (IOM) in its work on medical error and patient safety.[4] Changes in nursing leadership have been underscored in creating safe environments for patients and staff, particularly as the weakening of clinical leadership has been cited as a cause of organizational concerns and issues.[5] The IOM described factors of problematic leadership, including the following:[6]

- Increased emphasis on production efficiency (bottom-line management)
- Weakened trust (reengineering initiatives, poor communication patterns)
- Poor change management (inadequate communication, insufficient worker training, lack of measurement and feedback, short-lived attention, limited worker involvement in developing change initiatives)
- Limited involvement in decision making pertaining to workdesign and workflow (hierarchical structures, limited voice on councils, committees)
- Limited knowledge management (process failures, limited second-order attention)

In order to address these challenges, the following recommendations were made by the IOM for health care organizations (HCOs), particularly related to acquiring nurse leaders for all levels of management (e.g., at the organization-wide and patient care unit levels). Nurse leaders should do the following:[7]

- Participate in executive decision within the HCOs.
- Represent nursing staff to organization management and facilitate their mutual trust.
- Achieve effective communication between nursing and other clinical leadership.
- Facilitate input of direct-care nursing staff into operational decision making and design of work processes and workflow.
- Be provided with organizational resources to support the acquisition, management, and dissemination to nursing staff of the knowledge needed to support their clinical decision making and actions.

While no one particular organizational structure for locating nursing leadership across all HCOs was identified, the focus of the recommendations was on well-prepared clinical nurse leaders at the most senior level of management. Magnet hospitals have found some positive outcomes related to staff and patient satisfaction that correlated with participatory and transformational leadership. Clearly, transformational leadership is called for to address these challenges, to improve quality outcomes for patients and staff, and to heighten overall organizational effectiveness.[8]

History

Florence Nightingale, after leaving the Crimea, exercised extraordinary leadership in health care for decades with no organization under her command.[9]

One of the purest examples of the leader as agenda-setter was Florence Nightingale. Her public image is that of the lady of mercy, but under her gentle, soft-spoken manner, she was a rugged spirit, a fighter, and a tough-minded system changer. In mid-19th century England a woman had no place in public life, least of all in the fiercely masculine world of the military establishment. Nightingale took on the establishment and revolutionized health care in the British military services. Yet she never made public appearances or speeches and, except for her two years in the Crimea, held no public position. She was a formidable authority on the evils to be remedied, she knew exactly what to do about them, and she used public opinion to goad top officials into adopting her agenda.

Florence Nightingale was both leader and manager.[10]

Leadership Defined

Researchers have studied leadership for decades, but experts still do not agree on exactly what it is. Many persons use the term leadership as if it were a magic quality, something one is born with or for which one simply has a talent. However, like talent for music and art, talent for leadership involves much knowledge and disciplined practice. Many definitions of leadership have been written, including that of Stogdill, who defines it as "the process of influencing the activities of an organized group in its efforts toward goal setting and goal achievement."[11] A difference in responsibilities exists among group members, and each member influences the group's activities. A leader is one others follow willingly and voluntarily.[12]

Stogdill's definition of leadership can be applied to nursing. In nursing practice, goals of patient care are set. Each patient has a nursing care plan that lists the problems that interfere with achieving physical, emotional, and social needs. For each problem, a goal is set and an approach or nursing prescription is written. An interdisciplinary team may identify problems, set goals, and write prescriptions. The team is influenced by the most highly skilled nurse available, the registered nurse who coordinates the care. Each interdisciplinary team member assumes different responsibilities in performing the total team functions.

The same principles may be applied to the entire division of nursing. Usually, the title of the head of the division is assistant administrator, vice president, chair, or director of nursing services. The division head is responsible for influencing all nursing employees toward achieving the stated purpose and objectives of the division of nursing. The nurse administrator is influenced by a stated philosophy or statement of beliefs about the kinds of services to be rendered by the personnel of the division of nursing. The total staff includes personnel in different job categories, including nurse managers, nursing case managers of shifts, and clinical nursing personnel, each with different responsibilities.

Gardner defines leadership as "the process of persuasion and example by which an individual (or leadership team) induces a group to take action that is in accord with the leader's purposes or the shared purposes of all."[13] Numerous other definitions of leadership exist. These definitions include the terms leader, follower or constituent, group, process, and goals. One can conclude that leadership is a process in which a person inspires a group of constituents to work together using appropriate means to achieve a common mission and common goals. Constituents are influenced to work together willingly and cooperatively with zeal and confidence and to their greatest potential.[14]

Leadership is a social transaction in which one person influences others. People in authority do not necessarily exert leadership. Rather, effective people in authoritative positions combine authority and leadership to assist an organization to achieve its goals. Effective leadership satisfies four primary conditions:[15] (1) a person receiving a communication understands it, (2) this person has the resources to do what is being asked of him or her, (3) the person believes the behavior being asked of him or her is consistent with personal interests and values, and (4) the person believes the request is consistent with the purposes and values of the organization.

According to McGregor,[16] There are at least four major variables now known to be involved in leadership: (1) the characteristics of the leader; (2) the attitudes, needs, and other personal characteristics of the followers; (3) the characteristics of the organization, such as its purpose, its structure, the nature of the task to be performed; and (4) the social, economic, and political milieu.

Leadership is a highly complex relationship that changes with the times. Such changes are brought about by management, unions, or outside forces. In nursing, changes in leadership are wrought by nursing management, nursing educators, nursing organizations, unions, and the expectations of the clientele (patients and their families).

Talbott said, "Leadership is the vital ingredient that transforms a crowd into a functioning, useful organization."[17] The theme in these definitions seems always to be the same: "Leadership is the process of sustaining an initiated action. It is certainly not a matter of pointing in a direction and just letting things happen. Leadership is the conception of a goal and a method of achieving it; the mobilization of the means necessary for attainment; and the adjustment of values and environmental factors in the light of the desired end."[18]

In all of the definitions, leadership is viewed as a dynamic, interactive process that involves three dimensions: the leader, the followers, and the situation. Each dimension influences the others. For instance, the accomplishment of goals depends not only on the personal attributes of the leader but also on the follower's needs and the type of situation.[19]

Leadership Theories

Trait Theory

Much of the early work on leadership focused on the leader. This research was directed toward identifying intellectual, emotional, physical, and other personal traits of effective leaders. The underlying assumption was that leaders are born, not made.

After many years of research, no particular set of traits has been found that predicts leadership potential. There are several possible reasons for this failure. According to McGregor, "Research findings to date suggest that it is more fruitful to consider leadership as a relationship between the leader and the situation than as a universal pattern of characteristics possessed by certain people."[20] This statement implies that leadership is a human relations function and that different situations may require quite different characteristics from a leader. It is generally accepted in nursing that authoritarian power is effective in times of crisis but that otherwise it promotes instability.

Despite the shortcomings of the trait theory, some traits have been identified that are common to all good leaders. Such traits as honesty, trustworthiness, integrity, fair, skilled communicator, goal-oriented, dedicated, committed, and hard working continue to surface in the literature.

Gardner's Leadership Studies

Two major treatises of Gardner's writings that relate to the traits of leadership are *The Tasks of Leadership* and *Leader-Constituent Interaction*.[21] Gardner identifies nine tasks to be performed by leaders:[22]

1. Envisioning goals. These include envisioning the best a group can be, solving problems, and unifying constituencies. Goals may involve extensive research. They may be shared, and they come from many sources. Long-term goals lend greater stability than do short-term goals.
2. Affirming values. Communities have "shared assumptions, beliefs, customs, ideas that give meaning, ideas that motivate." These include norms or values. Values embody religious beliefs and secular philosophy. Society celebrates its values in art, song, ritual, historic documents, and textbooks. People will strive to meet standards that affirm their values and motivate them. Values must be continually rebuilt or regenerated, with leaders assisting to rediscover and adapt traditions to the present. Leaders reaffirm values through words, policy decisions, and conduct.
3. Motivating. Leaders stimulate people to serve society and solve its problems. They balance positive attitudes and acts with reality. They look toward the future with confidence, hope, and energy. Loss of confidence breeds rigidity, fatalism, and passivity. Poverty negatively affects morale, learning, and performance. Leaders correct the circumstances of negative attitudes and defeat. Involving employees in decisions gives them a sense of power and ownership. Leaders resolve failure, frustration, and doubt and use intuition and empathy to solve problems.
4. Managing. Leadership and management overlap. Leaders set goals, plan, fix priorities, choose means, and formulate policy. They also build organizations and institutions that outlast them. Leaders keep the

system functioning by setting agendas and making decisions. Leaders mold public opinion and exercise political judgments.

5. Achieving workable unity. Leaders function in a pluralistic society in which conflict is necessary if there are grievances to be settled. Conflict is also necessary in competing commercially, settling civil suits, and bringing justice to the oppressed. Conflict must be resolved to achieve cohesion and mutual tolerance, internally and externally. Society is fragmented and must not be polarized. Conflict resolution requires political skills: brokering, forming coalitions, mediating conflicting views, de-escalating rhetoric and posturing, saving face, and seeking common ground. People must trust each other most of the time to prevent or resolve conflict. Leaders raise the level of trust.
6. Explaining. Leaders must communicate effectively. They teach.
7. Serving as a symbol. Leaders speak for others. They represent unity, collective identity, and continuity.
8. Representing the group. All human systems are interdependent. Leaders take a broad view of events.
9. Renewing. Leaders blend continuity with change. They are innovators who awaken the potential of others. They visit the front lines and keep in touch. Leaders sustain diversity and dissent, and they change the social order.

Leader-Constituent Interaction

Charismatic Leaders

Gardner defines *charisma* as the quality that sets one person apart from others: supernatural, superhuman, endowed with exceptional qualities or powers. Charismatic leadership can be good or evil. Charismatic leaders emerge in troubled times and in relation to the state of mind of constituents. They eventually run out of miracles and "white horses," even though the leaders are magnetic, persuasive, and spellbinding.

Masses of people will often follow the charismatic leader. Such masses have historically been labeled unstable. Worry about mob rule and instability still exists. Social disorder is embodied in the Constitution of the United States.

Influence of Constituents on Leaders

Constituents and leaders have an equal influence on each other. Constituents confer the leadership role. Good constituents select good leaders and make them better. In politics, constituents may follow any leader unless they are bureaucratic constituents (such as government employees) who feel constrained to mute their support. Loyal constituents support leaders who help them meet their needs and solve problems.

Influence of Leaders on Constituents

Leaders choose to be leaders. They must adapt their leadership style to the situation and their constituents. In doing so, they weigh the following considerations: the degree of structure they want in relationships with constituents; the degree or hierarchy of authority, formality, discipline, constraint, and control; and the degree of focus on task versus that on people.

Leaders influence their superiors and their subordinates and have the courage to defy their constituents. Sam Houston was a leader of this type. He opposed the secession of Texas from the United States, going against his constituents. A leader may show different faces to pluralistic groups of constituents, including special interest groups.

Transforming Leaders

Transforming leaders respond to people's basic needs, wants, hopes, and expectations. They may transcend the political system or even attempt to construct it in order to operate within it. Transforming leadership is innovative, and it evolves.

The best leadership may be that which focuses on self-development and self-actualization. Leaders should develop the strengths of constituents and make them independent.[23]

Behavioral Theories

Behavioral theories include Douglas McGregor's Theory X and Theory Y, Rensis Likert's Michigan studies, Blake and Mouton's Managerial Grid and Kurt Lewin's studies. Each of these is described here in more detail.

McGregor's Theory X and Theory Y

McGregor related his theories to the motivation theories of Maslow. McGregor states that each person is a whole individual living and interacting within a world of other individuals. What happens to this person happens as a result of the behavior of other people. The attitudes and emotions of others affect this person. The constituent is dependent on the leader and desires to be treated fairly. A successful relationship is desired by both and depends on the action taken by the leader.

Security is a condition of leadership. Constituents need security and will fight to protect themselves against real or imagined threats to these needs in the work situation. Leaders must act to give constituents this security through avenues such as fair pay and fringe benefits. Unions act to solidify job security.

An effective leader creates an atmosphere of approval for constituents. Such an atmosphere is created through the leader's manner and attitude. Given the genuine approval of their leader, constituents will be secure. Otherwise, they will feel threatened, fearful, and insecure.

Knowledge is another condition of effective leadership espoused by McGregor. Employees have security when they know what is expected of them, including the following:[24]

- Knowledge of overall company policy and management philosophy.
- Knowledge of procedures, rules, and regulations.
- Knowledge of the requirements of the subordinate's job duties, responsibilities, and place in the organization.
- Knowledge of the personal peculiarities of the constituent's immediate leader.
- Knowledge by the constituent of the leader's opinion of his or her performance.
- Advance knowledge of changes that may affect the constituent.

Consistent discipline is another condition for effective leadership. People are met with approval when they do their jobs according to expectations. They should know what to expect in terms of disapproval when they do not meet expectations. Leaders should be consistent in setting standards and expecting constituents to meet them. Even discipline must occur in an atmosphere of approval.

Security encourages independence, another condition for effective leadership. Insecurity causes a reactive fight for freedom. Security that stimulates independence is desired. Constituents need to become actively independent by being involved in contributing ideas and suggestions concerning activities that affect them. When workers are secure and encouraged to participate in solving the problems of work, they provide new approaches to solutions. They work to achieve the goals of the organization and feel they are a part of it.

With security and independence, constituents develop a desire to accept responsibility. The level of responsibility can be increased at a pace commensurate with preservation of constituents' security. Having security gives constituents pleasure and pride. Leaders need security before they can delegate responsibility to constituents.

All constituents need a provision for appeal, that is, an adequate grievance procedure by which they can take their differences with their superiors to a higher level in the organization. Leaders who do the jobs expected of them and who treat constituents in ways that meet their needs and give them security achieve self-realization and self-development.[25]

Likert's Michigan Studies

Likert and his associates at the Institute for Social Research at the University of Michigan conducted extensive leadership research. They identified four basic styles or systems of leadership: System I, exploitative-authoritative; System II, benevolent-authoritative; System III, consultative-democratic; and System IV, participative-democratic.

A measuring instrument for evaluating an organization's leadership style was developed by Likert's group. It contains 51 items and encompasses variables of the concepts of "leadership, motivation, communication, interaction-influence, decision making, goal setting, control, and performance goals."[26]

It is generally conceded that leadership behavior improves in effectiveness as it approaches System IV.

Blake and Mouton's Managerial Grid

The Managerial Grid is a two-dimensional leadership model. Dimensions of this model are tasks or production and the employee or people orientations of managers.[27]

Two key dimensions of managerial thinking are depicted on the Grid: concern for production on the horizontal axis, and concern for people on the vertical axis. They are shown as 9-point scales; 1 represents low concern, 5 represents an average amount of concern, and 9 is high concern.

These two concerns are interdependent; that is, although concern for one or the other may be high or low, they are integrated in the manager's thinking. Thus, both concerns are present to some degree in any management style. Study of the Grid enables one to sort out various possibilities and the attitudes, values, beliefs, and assumptions that underlie each approach. When one is able to objectively see one's own behavior compared to the soundest approach, it provides motivation to change in order to more closely approximate the soundest management. When group members come to share 9, 9 values, beliefs, attitudes, and assumptions, they develop personal commitment to achieving group goals as well as their individual goals. In doing so they develop standards of mutual trust and respect that cause them to elevate cooperation and communication.

Blake and Mouton contend that the 9, 9 style is the one most likely to achieve highest quality results over an extended period of time. The 9, 9 style, unlike the others, is based on the assumption that there is no inherent conflict between the needs of the organization for performance and the needs of people for job satisfaction.

Finally, as an orienting framework, the Grid serves as a map to more effective ways of working with and through others. When group members have this common frame of reference for what constitutes effective and ineffective approaches to issues of mutual concern, they are able to take corrective action based on common understanding and agreement about the soundest approach and an objectivity when actions taken are less than fully sound.

Kurt Lewin's Studies

Lewin's leadership studies were done in the 1930s. Lewin examined three leadership styles related to forces within the leader, within the group members, and within the situation. From Lewin's studies, the leadership styles emerging were autocratic, democratic, and laissez-faire. The autocratic leader makes decisions alone, and tends to be more concerned with task accomplishment than with concern for people. In contrast, the democratic leader involves followers in the decision-making process and is people-oriented, focusing on human relations and teamwork. The laissez-faire leader is permissive and generally abstains from leading the staff, which often results in low productivity and employee frustration.

Other behavioral studies include the Ohio State studies, which use a quadrant structure that relates leadership effectiveness to initiating structure (with emphasis on the task or production) and consideration (with emphasis on the employee). These studies identified four primary leadership styles relating to those leaders with high initiating structure to low initiating structure and those with low consideration to high consideration.

The Ohio State Researchers used the Leader Behavior Description Questionnaire. Items related to initiating structure and to consideration describe how leaders carry out their activities. Both factors are considered simultaneously rather than on a continuum. As to which combination works best, the situation determines the style.[28]

Problems with Leadership Questionnaires

According to Phillips and Lord, the accuracy of leadership questionnaires is debatable. Yet they are often the only feasible way to measure leadership in real-world settings. Some researchers consider reliable questionnaires accurate. However, these authors contend that any systematic sources of variance, such as leniency error, halo, or implicit theories, can produce high internal consistency. Factor structures produced solely on the basis of implicit leadership theories do not tell users of these questionnaires anything about accuracy.

The Leader Behavior Description Questionnaire was flawed because its subjects form an overall leadership impression before completing it. Questionnaires can be improved by requiring "observers to distinguish between the presence and absence of specific, conceptually equivalent behaviors in videotaped stimulus materials."[29]

Most questionnaire-based leadership research has been conducted in laboratory settings. The results are biased by the fact that some conditions do not exist in typical field settings. Research participants do not know or have contact with the target leader; thus the behavioral-level accuracy of their responses is limited. Phillips and Lord make the following suggestions to improve research techniques of existing behavioral description questionnaires:[30]

1. Assess whether the level of accuracy required for the purpose is classification or behavioral.
2. Assess whether the level of accuracy produced by the chosen measurement technique is classification or behavioral.
3. Evaluate the research setting for potential biases "such as rote knowledge of performance, leniency in describing superiors, or other relevant rater characteristics."
4. If biases exist, judge whether they are likely to be confounded with substantive variables of interest to the user.
5. Collect global measures of leadership and leniency during the measurement process.

Leadership Style

Other studies of leadership focus on style, including contingency-situational leadership models that focus on a combination of factors, such as the people, the task, the situation, the organization, and environmental factors. These models combine theories of Fred F. Fiedler; Paul Hersey, Kenneth H. Blanchard, and D. E. Johnson; and William J. Reddin.

Fiedler's Contingency Model of Leadership Effectiveness

There must be a group before there can be a leader. Fiedler describes three classifications that measure the kind of power and influence the group gives its leader. The first and most important of these is the relationship between the leader and the group members. Personality is a factor, but its influence depends on the group's perception of the leader. Second is the task structure, the degree to which details of the group's assignment are programmed. If the assignment is highly structured, the leader will have less power. If the assignment requires planning and thinking, the leader will be in a position to exert greater power. Third is the positional power of the leader: great power does not always yield better group performance. The best leader has been found to be one who has a task-oriented leadership style. This style works best when the leader has great influence and power over group members. When the leader has moderate influence over group members, a relationship-oriented style works best.

The organization shares responsibility for a leader's success or failure. Leaders can be trained to learn in which situations they do well and in which they fail. The job can be fitted to the leader. The appointee can be given a higher rank or can be assigned constituents who are nearly equal in rank and status. Most appointees can be given sole authority or can be required to consult with the group. The appointee can be given detailed instructions or independence. A highly successful and effective leader avoids situations in which failure is likely. That leader seeks out situations that fit his or her leadership style. Knowledge of strengths and weaknesses helps in choosing this style.[31]

Fiedler's theory is one of situations: leadership style will be effective or ineffective depending on the situation.

Life Cycle Theory of Hersey, Blanchard, and Johnson

Hersey, Blanchard, and Johnson follow a situational approach to leadership. A person's leadership style focuses on a combination of task behaviors and relationship behaviors. Focus on task behaviors is "characterized by endeavoring to establish well-defined patterns of organization, channels of communication, and ways of getting jobs accomplished." Focus on relationship behavior relates to "opening up channels of communication, providing socio-emotional support, actively listening, 'psychological strokes,' and facilitating behaviors."[32]

Reddin's Three-Dimensional Theory of Management

Reddin combined Blake and Mouton's Managerial Grid with Fiedler's contingency leadership model. The outcome was a three-dimensional theory of management; the dimensions are adapted from Managerial Grid theory, contingency leadership style theory, and effectiveness theory. These possible combinations result in four basic leadership styles as described below:

1. Separated, in which both task orientation and relationship orientation are minimal.
2. Dedicated, in which task orientation is high and relationship orientation is low. Dedicated leaders are dedicated only to the job.
3. Related, in which relationship orientation is high and task orientation is low. Related leaders relate primarily to their constituents.
4. Integrated, in which both task orientation and relationship orientations are high. Integrated leaders focus on managerial behavior, combining task orientation and relationship orientation.

These management styles are identified below:

- Executive leaders are integrated and more effective than are compromiser leaders, who are less effective integrated leaders.
- Developer leaders are related and more effective than missionary leaders, who are less effective related leaders.
- Bureaucrat leaders are separated and more effective than deserter leaders, who are less effective separated leaders.
- Benevolent autocrat leaders are dedicated and more effective than autocrat leaders, who are less effective dedicated leaders.

The range of effectiveness is a continuum. As in other theories of leadership, the effective behavior of the leader is relative to the situation. Effective leaders apply leadership styles after assessing situations.[33]

Transformational Leadership

The health care system is experiencing tremendous change and chaos, and the problems of organizations are increasingly complex. Health care organizations are restructuring and redesigning the way patient care is delivered to meet the challenges of these changes. In addition, health care is prohibitively expensive for many Americans. Hospitals and emergency rooms are financially burdened by the uninsured who suffer from violence, drug overdose, and HIV infection. Many people, especially in rural areas and inner cities, do not have access to health care because hospitals are downsizing and a shortage of health care personnel exists. Leaders must find ways to keep staff motivated in this chaotic, unstable environment. Therefore, effective leaders in this atmosphere of rapid change will acknowledge uncertainty, be flexible, and consider the values and needs of constituents.[34]

Bennis and Nanus describe a theory of leadership called transformational leadership. They define a transformational leader as one who "commits people to action, who converts followers into leaders, and who may convert leaders into agents of change."[35] These authors believe that the nucleus of leadership is power, which they define as the "basic energy to initiate and sustain action translating intention into reality."[36] Transformational leaders do not use power to control and repress constituents. These leaders instead empower constituents to have a vision about the organization and trust the leaders so they work for goals that benefit the organization and themselves.

Leadership is thus not so much the exercise of power itself as it is the empowerment of others. This does not mean that leaders must relinquish power, but rather that reciprocity, an exchange between leaders and constituents, exists. The goal is change in which the purpose of the leader and that of the constituent become enmeshed, creating a collective purpose. Empowered staff become critical thinkers and are active in their roles within the organization. A creative and committed staff is the most important asset that an administrator can develop.[37]

Transformational leaders will mobilize their staff by focusing on the welfare of the individual and humanizing the high-tech work environment. Experts favor a leadership style that empowers others and values collaboration instead of competition.[38] People are empowered when they share in decision making and when they are rewarded for quality and excellence rather than punished and manipulated. When the environment is humanized, people are empowered, feel part of the team, and believe they are contributing to the success of the organization. Leaders who share power motivate people to excel by inspiring them to be part of a vision rather than punishing them for mistakes.[39] In nursing, empowerment can result in improved patient care, fewer staff sick days, and decreased attrition. Nurses who are transformational leaders have staff with higher job satisfaction and who stay in the organization for longer periods.[40]

Nurse executives who like to feel in charge may feel threatened by the concept of sharing power with staff. So they need to be personally empowered to assist in the empowerment of others. They will have a sense of self-worth and self-respect and confidence in their own abilities. Bennis and Nanus believe the most important trait of successful leaders is having positive self-regard.[41] Self-regard is not, however, self-centeredness or self-importance; rather, leaders with positive self-esteem recognize their strengths and do not emphasize their weaknesses. A leader who has positive self-regard seems to create in others a sense of confidence and high expectations. Techniques used to increase self-worth include visualization, affirmations, and letting go of the need to be perfect.[42]

Through research and observations, Bennis defined four competencies for dynamic and effective transformational leadership: (1) management of attention, (2) management of meaning, (3) management of trust, and (4) management of self.[43] The first competency is the management of attention, achieved by having a vision or sense of outcomes or goals. Vision is the image of a realistic, attainable, credible, and attractive future state for an organization.[44] Vision statements are written to define where the health care organization is headed and how it will serve society. They differ from mission and philosophy statements in that they are more futuristic and describe where energies are to be focused.[45]

The second leadership competency is management of meaning. To inspire commitment, leaders must communicate their vision and create a culture that sustains the vision. A culture or social architecture as described by Bennis and Nanus is "intangible, but it governs the way people act, the values and norms that are subtly transmitted to groups and individuals, and the construct of binding and bonding within a company."[46] Barker believes that "social architecture provides meaning and shared experience of organizational events so that people know the expectations of how they are to act."[47]

People are committed to visions that are mutually developed, are based on a sense of quality, appeal to their values and emotions, and are feasible yet challenging.

Nursing leaders transform the social architecture or culture of health care organizations by using group discussion, agreement, and consensus building, and they support individual creativity and innovation. To do this, Barker believes that the nurse transformational leader will pay attention to the internal consistency of the vision, goals, and objectives; selection and placement of personnel; feedback; appraisal; rewards; support; and development.[48] For example, rewards and appraisals must relate to the goals, and the vision must be consistent with the goals and objectives. Most importantly, all the elements must enhance the self-worth of individuals, allow creativity, and appeal to the values of nurses. For many nurse leaders, these are new skills that will take time and support from mentors to develop.

Because vision statements are a new concept to many, nursing leaders should provide opportunities for staff to openly explore feelings, criticize, and articulate negative reactions. Face-to-face meetings between nursing leaders and staff are desirable because in reactions involving trust and clarity, memorandums and suggestion boxes are not adequate substitutes for direct communication.[49]

The third competency is the management of trust, which is associated with reliability. Nurses respect leaders whose judgment is sound and consistent and whose decisions are based on fairness, equity, and honesty. Staff can be heard to comment about leaders they trust with statements such as "I don't always agree with her decision, but I know she wants the best for the patients." Bennis believes that "people would much rather follow individuals they can count on, even when they disagree with their viewpoint, than people they agree with but who shift positions frequently."[50]

The fourth competency is management of self, which is knowing one's skills and using them effectively. It is critical that nurses in leadership positions recognize when they lack management skills and then take responsibility for their own continuing education. Incompetent leaders can demoralize a nursing unit and contribute to poor patient care. When leadership skills are mastered by nurse leaders, stress and burnout are reduced. Nurse leaders thus need to master the skills of leadership.[51]

Although effective leaders support shared power and decision making, they continue to accept responsibility for making decisions even when their decisions are not popular. Constituents like to have their wishes considered, but there are times when they want prompt and clear decisions from a leader. This is especially true in times of crisis.[52]

Transformational leaders are flexible and able to adapt leadership styles to the chaos and rapid change occurring in the current health care environment.

Differences Between Leadership and Management

Managers come from the "headship" (power from position) category. They hold appointive or directive posts in formal organizations. They can be appointed for both technical and leadership competencies, usually needing both to be accepted. Managers are delegated authority, including the power to reward or punish. A manager is expected to perform functions such as planning, organizing, directing (leading), and controlling (evaluating). Informal leaders, by contrast, are not always managers performing those functions required by the organization. Leaders often are not even part of the organization. Florence Nightingale, after leaving the Crimea, was not connected with an organization but was still a leader.

Zaleznik indicates that the manager is a problem solver who succeeds because of "persistence, tough-mindedness, hard work, intelligence, analytical ability, and, perhaps most important, tolerance and good will."[53]

Managers focus on results, analysis of failure, and tasks—management characteristics that are desirable for nurse managers. Effective managers also need to be good leaders. Managers who are leaders choose and limit goals. They focus on creating spirit and in doing so, they develop committed constituents. Manager-leaders do this by seeking advice and solutions to problems. They ask for information and provide positive feedback. Leaders understand the power of groups. They empower their constituents, making their subordinates strong—the chosen ones, a team infused with purpose. Mistakes are tolerated by manager-leaders who challenge constituents to realize their potential.

Managers emphasize control, decision making, and decision analysis. As manager-leaders, they are concerned with modeling appropriate behavior as symbols of values and norms. Effective manager-leaders are technically capable and provide assurance in crises.

Managers focus inward but add the leadership dimension of connecting their group to the outside world, focusing intense attention on important issues. They escalate issues and complaints up the organization to be handled quickly and appropriately, rather than try to control them.[54]

Although managers are sometimes described in less glowing terms than leaders, successful managers are usually successful leaders. Leadership is a desirable and prominent feature of the directing function of nursing management.

Similarities Between Leadership and Management

Gardner asserts that first-class managers are usually first-class leaders. Leaders and leader-managers distinguish themselves beyond run-of-the-mill managers in six respects:[55]

1. They think longer term—beyond the day's crises, beyond the quarterly report, beyond the horizon.
2. They look beyond the unit they head and grasp its relationship to larger realities—the larger organization of which they are a part, conditions external to the organization, global trends.
3. They reach and influence constituents beyond their jurisdiction, beyond boundaries. Thomas Jefferson influenced people all over Europe. Gandhi influenced people all over the world. In an organization, leaders overflow bureaucratic boundaries—often a distinct advantage in a world too complex and tumultuous to be handled "through channels." Their capacity to rise above jurisdictions may enable them to bind together the fragmented constituencies that must work together to solve a problem.
4. They put heavy emphasis on the intangibles of vision, values, and motivation and understand intuitively the nonrational and unconscious elements in the leader-constituent interaction.
5. They have the political skill to cope with the conflicting requirements of multiple constituencies.
6. They think in terms of renewal. The routine manager tends to accept the structure and processes as they exist. The leader or leader-manager seeks the revisions of process and structure required by changing reality.

Good leaders, like good managers, provide visionary inspiration, motivation, and direction. Good managers, like good leaders, attract and inspire. People want to be led rather than managed. They want to pursue goals and values they consider worthwhile. Therefore, they want leaders who respect the dignity, autonomy, and self-esteem of constituents.[56]

Effective nurse executives combine leadership and management.

Mitchell describes five major requirements for every executive, implying that being an effective executive requires the attributes of a leader:[57]

1. Adjustment to a complex social environment of several or many units
2. Ability to influence and guide subordinates
3. Emotional and intellectual maturity as a preparation for leadership
4. Ability to think through and make decisions, and to translate decisions into effective action
5. Capacity to see beyond the immediate or surface indications and, with experience, to acquire perspective

Effective nurse leader-managers will work to achieve these same requisites.

Leadership is a subsystem within the management system. It is included as an element of management science in management textbooks and other publications. In some, the term *leading* has replaced the term *directing* as a major function of management. In such a context, communication and motivation are elements of leadership (a concept that could be debated according to management theorists' philosophical bent).

Management includes written plans, clear organizational charts, well-documented annual objectives, frequent reports, detailed and precise job descriptions, regular evaluations of performance against objectives, and the administrative ordering of theory.[58] Nurse managers who are leaders can use these tools of management without making them a bureaucratic roadblock to autonomy, participatory management, maximum performance, and productivity by employees.

Leadership Versus Headship

A job title does not make a person a leader, nor does it cause a person to exercise leadership behavior over subordinates. This is as true of nurses as it is of personnel in industry or the military services. It is a mistake to refer to the dean of a college, a professor of nursing, a nurse administrator, a supervisor, a nurse manager, or any nurse as a leader by virtue of position. That person is in a headship position rather than a leadership one, because "leadership is more a function of the group or situation than a quality which adheres to a person appointed to a formal position of headship."[59] A person's behavior will indicate whether that person also occupies a functional leadership position.

Gardner writes that not all people in positions of high status are leaders. Some are chief bureaucrats or custodians. Their high status does have "symbolic values and traditions that enhance the possibility of leadership" as people have higher expectations of people in headship positions.[60] Authority embodied in a title or position of headship is legitimized power; it is not leadership.[61]

Appointed heads are not selected by persons they will direct. Appointed heads frequently work toward organizational goals while ignoring the personal goals of employees. Their authority comes from high in the organization and not from their influence within the group.

Leadership is an attempt to influence groups or individuals without the coercive form of power.

In cases in which heads are elected by the group, they keep their positions only as long as they satisfy the members' needs for affiliating with the organization. They are responsible only to the group, whereas the appointed head is usually responsible to both the appointive authority and the group. Nurses who are elected to chair committees or who preside over professional organizations will not be reelected unless they satisfy the members' needs.

Appointed heads may lack the freedom to choose relationships with subordinates because their supervisors do not allow it. They will have authority and power without being accepted by the group. If appointed nurse managers are allowed to and can exercise their leadership abilities, they can be accorded leadership status by the group. The nurse managers will understand and motivate employees in order to be trusted by them.[62]

Preparation of Nursing Leaders

Gardner believes that 90% of leadership can be taught.[63] Education begins in basic nursing education programs. To develop risk-taking behaviors and self-confidence, students should be encouraged to create new solutions and to disagree and debate and should be allowed to make mistakes without fear of reprisal. Faculty should encourage and support students who exercise their leadership abilities in projects and organizations on campus and in the community.

When nurses graduate and enter the work force, most are not ready to assume a leadership role. They require opportunities for self-discovery to understand their strengths and for skill building. This skill building occurs through on-the-job training, along with support from peers and mentorship from effective leaders. These mentors must be dynamic, not status-quo-seeking role models who teach nurses how to preserve sameness. Tack writes that in order to be prepared for the future, leaders must be mentored by "those who see the world differently and project a dramatically different future, those who tend to shake things up rather than follow established precedents."[64]

Organizational managers, including nurse executives, will teach managers the nature of leadership. They will train nurse managers in leadership skills and put managers in the proper environment to learn leadership. This will include "starting up an operation, turning around a troubled division, moving from staff to line, working under a wise mentor, serving on a high-level task force and getting promoted to a more senior level of the organization."[65]

Nurse executives and managers should be trained to coach their constituents on leadership skills. Constituents can be trained to help managers in leadership. Leaders can listen and articulate, persuade and be persuaded, use collective wisdom to make decisions, and teach constituents to relate or communicate upward.

Gender Issues

Because the majority of nurses are women, it is essential to understand gender issues. Research indicates that gender differences do exist in leadership styles and competencies.[66] Masculinity has been associated with being task oriented and using a direct approach for solving problems. Femininity has been characterized as being people-oriented and supportive, sharing feelings, and caring for others. Desjardins and Brown conducted 2-hour interviews of 72 college presidents that included questions concerning, power, conflict resolution, and learning style. The findings indicated that the majority of women practiced leadership in a care-connected style.[67] This orientation, first described by Gilligan, values intimacy and nurturing in interactions with others.[68] The majority of decisions made by men are in the justice and rights mode, first described by Kohlberg in his work on moral reasoning.[69] This style of decision making values autonomy, objectivity, and fairness.

Research is needed on gender issues related to nursing leadership.

Rosener's research supports the thesis that leadership style is connected to gender issues. Rosener describes four major areas of difference in the women leaders whom she studied. First, these women tend to encourage participation; second, they share power and information more readily; third, they attempt to enhance the self-worth of others; and fourth, they energize others.[70]

It is important to remember that the modes and traits described by both researchers are gender-related but not gender-specific. Women and men fall into both modes, but more men are found in the justice and rights mode.[71] Rosener's work also indicates that men operate more often through management transactions, exchanging rewards for services rendered or punishments for poor performance. Men, she found, also work more out of the power of their positions.[72]

Gender issues as they relate to leadership in health care organizations have not been well studied. Dunham and Klahefn found that male and female nurse executives are not more likely to exhibit transformational leadership rather than transactional leadership, which focuses more on day-to-day operations.[73] Borman's research on executives in health care organizations indicates that women, more than men, identify connections to others and flexibility as important characteristics of leaders.[74] The literature points out that flexibility may be a desirable attribute in a rapidly changing or restructured organization; therefore, women may have an advantage over men.[75]

Gender differences in leadership style and competencies do not translate into one style being better than the other. However, if nurses are sensitized to gender differences, they will accept individuals for their unique leadership strengths instead of resisting them. This accepting atmosphere will encourage nurses (both men and women) to develop self-confidence and become strong leaders.

Nursing and Leadership Health Care Policy

Nursing is conspicuous by its absence from lists of national leaders. National consumers do not perceive nurse leaders as having power. The health care system has failed to recognize nurses as professionals who have knowledge useful in creating solutions to complex problems. Cutler's perspective of nursing educators and nursing service personnel is that they have been the product of directive and authoritarian leadership.[76]

Historically, nurses have avoided opportunities to obtain power and political muscle. The profession now understands that power and political savvy will assist in achieving its goals to improve health care and to increase nurses' autonomy. Also, if the health care system is to be reformed, nurses must participate individually and collectively. Nurses need to find ways to influence health care policy making so that their voices are heard.[77] Milio believes that nurses have the capacity for power to influence public policy and recommends the following steps to prepare:[78]

1. Organize.
2. Do homework. Learn to understand the political process, interest groups, specific people, and events.
3. Frame arguments to suit the target audience by appealing to cost containment, political support, fairness and justice, and other data relevant to particular concerns.
4. Support and strengthen the position of converted policy-makers.

5. Concentrate energies.
6. Stimulate public debate.
7. Make the position of nurses visible in the mass media.
8. Choose the most effective strategy as the main one.
9. Act in a timely fashion.
10. Maintain activity.
11. Keep the organizational format decentralized.
12. Obtain and develop the best research data to support each position.
13. Learn from experience.
14. Never give up without trying.

Nurses in leadership positions are most influential.[79]

Buffering

Nursing leaders can act as buffers or advocates for nurses. In doing so, they protect constituents from internal and external pressures of work. Nurse managers can reduce barriers to clinical nurses completing their clinical work.

Buffering protects practicing clinical nurses from external health system factors, the health care organization, other supervisors and employees, top administrators, the medical staff, and themselves when their behavior jeopardizes their careers. Buffering is another facet of the theory of leadership related to management, and it requires leadership training.

The nurse practitioner, the extended-role nurse, staff nurses, and ancillary personnel can be protected by buffering action by nurse managers. Professional nurses do not want to have additional responsibilities delegated if they are already under severe pressure and stress. Delegation of decision making is power; delegation of work is drudgery. Professional nurses are there to motivate, not to dissatisfy.

Smith and Mitry suggest three methods of buffering, the benefits of which will be improved performance, better morale, increased loyalty, a healthier organization, and respect for leaders.[80]

1. Coordinating work—that is, support services and standardized records.
2. Insulating by intervening with pressure groups and creating unity of command.
3. Evaluating the impingement.

Management writers say there is a difference between leadership and managers, but their textbooks and writings on the subject all include leadership content. Professional nurses want to be led, not directed or controlled. Also, nurse managers can learn the concepts, principles, and laws that will assist them in becoming effective leader-managers.

Different situations require different leadership styles. The leader-manager assesses each situation and exercises the appropriate leadership style. Some employees want to be involved; others do not. There must be a fit between the leader and constituents. The leader demonstrates this by changing style and training others until a transition is made. A flexible leadership style is necessary and vital.

EXHIBIT 7-1
Conceptual Foundations

NEWTONIAN

- Mass production
- Compartmentalism
- Reductionism
- Analysis
- Discrete action

QUANTUM

- Envision the whole
- Integration
- Synthesis
- Relatedness
- Team action

Future Direction: Quantum Leadership

Porter-O'Grady and Malloch describe *quantum leadership* as new leadership for a new age. From a conceptual perspective, quantum theory considers the whole, integration, synthesis, relatedness, and team action. Exhibit 7-1 compares the Newtonian and the Quantum perspective. "Quantum theory has taught us that change is not a thing or an event but rather a dynamic that is constitutive of the universe."[81] Quantum leadership incorporates transformation, a dynamic flow that integrates transitions from work, rules, scripts, chaos, and loss. Adaptation considers such driving forces from sociopolitical, economic, and technical perspectives. The term *chaos* used in quantum leadership refers to the transitional period focused on relational and whole systems thinking as compared to separate components and linear thinking. Exhibits 7-2 and 7-3 provide a pictorial view of the conceptualization of transformation for quantum leadership. "New rules will apply in the new age."[82] Exhibit 7-4 outlines seven imperatives underscoring the need to consider quantum leadership for dramatic changes mandated in this new age.

Summary

The theory of nursing leadership is a part of the theory of nursing management. Leadership is a process of influencing a group to set and achieve goals. There are

EXHIBIT 7-2

The Universal Cycle of Transformation. This illustration shows the dynamic and interacting forces of transformation.

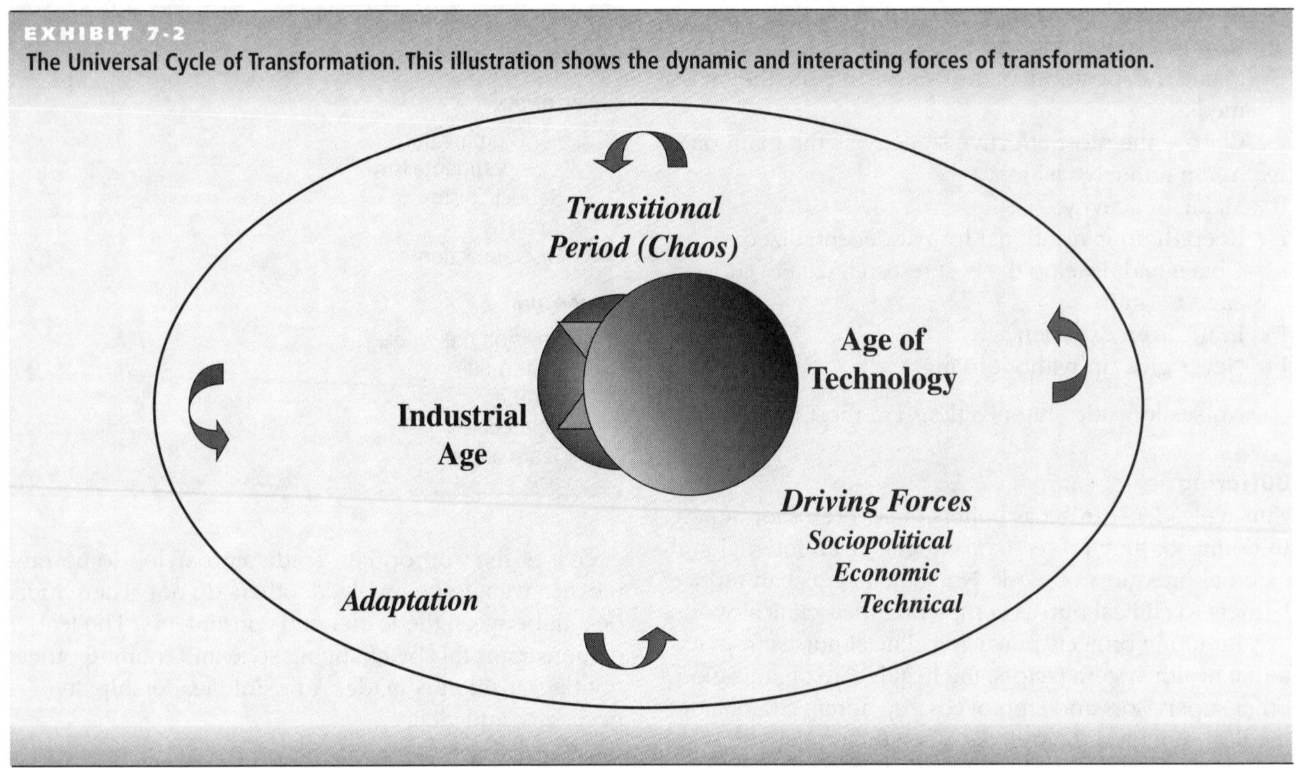

EXHIBIT 7-3

Universal Dynamics of Transformation. This illustration shows the continuous cycle of interacting processes that are the focus of the transforming work of leadership.

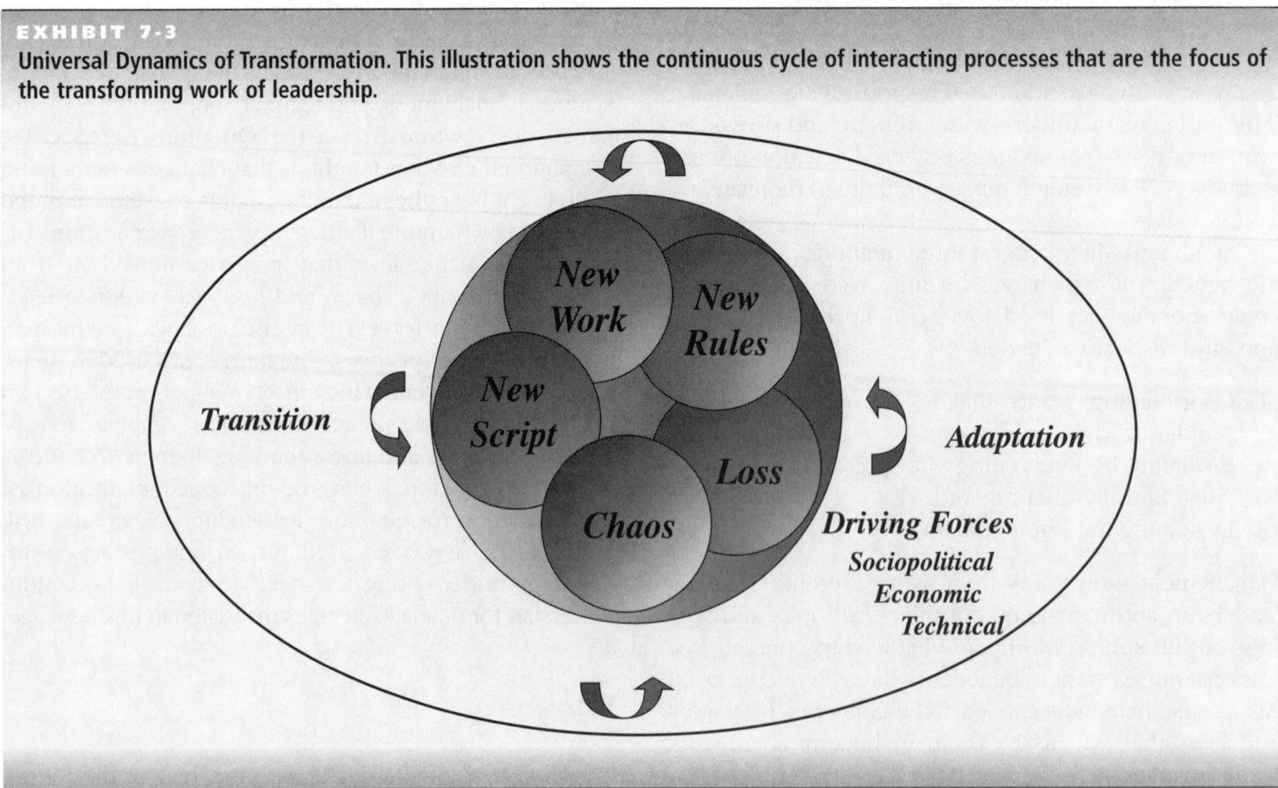

EXHIBIT 7-4
Seven New Age Imperatives

1. Open access to health information
2. Medicine/nursing based on genomics
3. Mass-customized diagnosis and treatment
4. User-specific insurance programs
5. Integration of allopathic and alternative therapies
6. Payment incentives tied to outcomes (quality)
7. Focused service settings for specific populations

several major theories of leadership. One of the earliest is the trait theory, which suggests that leaders have many intellect, personality, and ability traits. Trait theory has been succeeded by other leadership theories indicating that managers, including nurse managers, can learn the knowledge and skills requisite to leadership competencies.

Behavioral theories of leadership include McGregor's Theory X and Theory Y, Likert's Michigan studies, Blake and Mouton's Managerial Grid, and Lewin's studies.

Other studies of leadership focus on contingency-situational leadership styles and factors such as people, tasks, situations, organizations, and environment. Theorists include Fiedler; Hersey, Blanchard, and Johnson; Reddin, and Gardner. John W. Gardner's study of leadership includes the nature of leadership, identification of leadership tasks, leader-constituent interaction, and the relationship between leadership and power.

Bennis and Nanus define a theory of leadership they call transformational. This leadership method involves change in which the purposes of the leader and follower become intertwined. The effective leader creates a vision for the organization and then develops a commitment to the vision. Bennis and Nanus believe that the wise use of power is the energy needed to develop commitment and to sustain action.

Nurse managers should learn to practice leadership behaviors that stimulate motivation within their constituents, practicing professional nurses, and other nursing personnel. These behaviors include promotion of autonomy, decision making, and participatory management by professional nurses. These behaviors are facilitated by effective nurse manager-leaders.

Quantum leadership offers a new age perspective as one transforms and redesigns the workplace into a culture of greater safety and quality.

APPLICATION EXERCISES

EXERCISE 7-1

Name a nurse you consider to be an outstanding leader and state why you consider him or her outstanding.

EXERCISE 7-2

Brower describes the leader in politics as a person of stature who can rally the people, a person with outstanding ability and character. He says there is an emotional bond between the leader and the led, a "bond which must exist between a leader and his people if either is to confront greatness."[83] He thinks that the abrasive strains of television may have irreparably damaged the bond between leader and led. Television shows leaders in their weaknesses because it constantly focuses on them. It was once thought that a talent such as President Jefferson would freely rise to the top in a natural aristocracy. American leaders would be people of ability and morality; they would be wise and virtuous. According to Brower, "Leadership, a relationship, depends very much on the basis of current enthusiasm or negation. Indeed it cannot exist at all in this country without the consent of the governed. We may very well be short on leadership because we are short on ourselves."[84]

Assuming that the characteristics of leadership are applicable to occupations, government, business, industry, and service institutions and professions, list three characteristics described by Brower and apply them to nursing.

EXERCISE 7-3 Kurt Lewin suggests that there are three leadership styles: autocratic, democratic, and laissez-faire.

1. Which leadership style does your supervisor exhibit?
2. List three of his or her activities or decisions that illustrate the style.
3. How does your supervisor's leadership style affect your work and attitude?

EXERCISE 7-4 Gardner asserts that first-class managers are usually first-class leaders. He believes that leaders and leader-managers distinguish themselves beyond the general run of managers in six respects. Give brief examples of how nurses you know fit all or some of the six characteristics.

EXERCISE 7-5 From the theory of leadership described in this chapter, describe and discuss actual examples of leadership demonstrated by persons in your organization. Consider:

1. Gardner's nine tasks performed by leaders
2. A charismatic leader
3. A transforming leader
4. McGregor's Theory X and Theory Y
5. Likert's authoritative and democratic systems
6. Leadership style
7. The implications for staff development

NOTES

1. Baldridge National Quality Program. (2003). *Criteria for performance excellence*. Gaithersburg, MD: National Institute of Standards and Technology.
2. Davenport, T., Delong, D., & Beers, D. (1998). Successful knowledge management projects. *Sloan Management Review, 1*, 43–57.
3. Heifetz, R. & Laurie, D. (2001). The work of leadership. *Harvard Business Review, 79*(11), 131–140.
4. Page, A. (Ed.). (2004). *Keeping patients safe, transforming the work environment of nurses*. Washington, DC: The National Academies Press.
5. Ibid.
6. Ibid.
7. Ibid., p. 136.
8. Ibid.
9. Gardner, 1986a, 8.
10. Gardner, 1986b, 15; Huxley, E. (1975). *Florence Nightingale*. New York: G. P. Putnam's Sons.
11. Holloman, C. R. (1986). Leadership or headship: There is a difference. *Notes & Quotes*, 4; Holloman, C. R. (1986). "Headship" vs. leadership. *Business and Economic Review*, 35–37.
12. Lundborg, L. B. (1982). What is leadership? *Journal of Nursing Administration*, 32–33.
13. Gardner, 1986a, 6.
14. Holloman, 1986; Levenstein, A. (1985). So you want to be a leader? *Nursing Management*, 74–75; Jones, G. R. (1983). Forms of control and leader behavior. *Journal of Management*, 159–172; McGregor, D. (1966). *Leadership and motivation*. Cambridge, MA: MIT Press, 70–80.
15. Merton, R. K. (1969). The social nature of leadership. *American Journal of Nursing*, 2614–2618.
16. McGregor, 1966, 73.
17. Talbott, C. M. (1971). Leadership at the man-to-man level. Supplement to the *Air Force Policy Letter for Commanders*, 13.
18. Mitton, D. G. (1969). Leadership: One more time. *Industrial Management Review*, 77–83.
19. Kilpatrick, J. (1974, February). Conservative view. *Sun-Herald* (Biloxi, MS), , p. 4.
20. McGregor, 1966, 75.
21. Gardner, 1986b, 1986c, 1986d.
22. Gardner, 1986b, 7.
23. Gardner, 1986c.
24. McGregor, 1966, 55–57.
25. Ibid., 49–65.
26. Likert, R. (1967). *The human organization*. New York: McGraw-Hill, 4–10.
27. The Grid synopsis was furnished courtesy of Scientific Methods, Inc., Box 195, Austin, TX, 78747.
28. Megginson, L., Mosley, D., & Pietri, P., Jr. (1989). *Management: Concepts and applications* (3rd ed.). New York: Harper & Row, 346–347, 352–353.
29. Phillips, J. S. & Lord, R. G. (1986). Notes on the practical and theoretical consequences of implicit leadership theories for the future of leadership measurement. *Journal of Management*, 33.
30. Ibid.
31. Fiedler, F. E. (1969). Style or circumstance: The leadership enigma. *Notes & Quotes*, 3; Megginson, Mosley, & Pietri, 1989.
32. Hersey, P., Blanchard, K. H., & Johnson, D. E. (1996). *Management of organizational behavior: Utilizing human resources* (7th ed.). Englewood Cliffs, NJ: Prentice Hall, 134–135.
33. Reddin, W. J. (1970). *Managerial effectiveness*. New York: McGraw-Hill, 230; Hodgetts, R. M. (1986). *Management: Theory,*

process and practice (4th ed.). Orlando, FL: Academic Press, 319–320.
34. Barker, A. M. (1991). An emerging leadership paradigm. *Nursing and Health Care*, 204–207.
35. Bennis, W. & Nanus, B. (1985). *Leaders: The strategies for taking charge*. New York: Harper & Row, 3.
36. Ibid., p. 15.
37. Lundeen, S. P. (1992). Leadership strategies for organizational change: Applications in community nursing centers. *Nursing Administration Quarterly*, 60–68.
38. Tack, M. W. (1991). Future leaders in higher education: New demands and new responses. *Phi Kappa Phi Journal*, 29–31; Desjardins, C. & Brown, C. O. (1991). A new look at leadership styles. *Phi Kappa Phi Journal*, 18–20.
39. Bennis & Nanus, 1985.
40. Medley, F. & Larochelle, D. R. (1995). Transformational leadership and job satisfaction. *Nursing Management*, 64JJ–64NN.
41. Bennis & Nanus, 1985, 57.
42. Barker, 1991.
43. Bennis, W. (1991). Learning some basic truisms about leadership. *Phi Kappa Phi Journal*.
44. Bennis & Nanus, 1985.
45. Barker, A. M. (1990). *Transformational nursing leadership: A vision for the future*. Baltimore: Williams and Wilkins.
46. Bennis & Nanus, 1985.
47. Barker, 1991, 207.
48. Ibid.
49. Gardner, 1986c.
50. Bennis, 1991, 24.
51. Campbell, R. P. (1986). Does management style affect burnout? *Nursing Management*, 38A–38B, 38D, 38F, 38H.
52. Gardner, 1986c.
53. Zaleznik, A. (1977). Managers and leaders: Are they different? *Harvard Business Review*, 68.
54. Zenger, J. H. (1985). Leadership: Management's better half. *Training*, 44–53.
55. Gardner, 1986a, 12.
56. Zenger, 1985.
57. Mitchell, W. N. (1968). What makes a business leader? *Notes & Quotes*, 2.
58. Zenger, 1985.
59. Holloman, 1969.
60. Gardner, 1986a, 6.
61. Ibid.
62. Holloman, 1986.
63. Gardner, 1986a.
64. Tack, 1991, 30.
65. Zenger, 1985.
66. Desjardins & Brown, 1991.
67. Ibid.
68. Gilligan, C. (1982). *In a different voice: Psychological theory and women's development*. Cambridge, MA: Harvard University Press.
69. Kohlberg, L. (1981). *The philosophy of moral development, moral stages and the idea of justice*. San Francisco, CA: Harper and Row.
70. Rosener, J. (1990). Ways women lead. *Harvard Business Review*, *1*, 19–24.
71. Desjardins & Brown, 1991.
72. Rosener, 1990.
73. Dunham, J. & Klahefn, K. A. (1990). Transformational leadership and the nurse executive. *Journal of Nursing Administration*, *1*, 28–34.
74. Borman, J. S. (1993). Women and nurse executives: Finally, some advantages. *Journal of Nursing Administration*, *1*, 34–40.
75. Helgesen, S. (1990). *The female advantage*. New York: Doubleday.
76. Cutler, M. J. (1976). Nursing leadership and management: An historical perspective. *Nursing Administration Quarterly*, *1*, 7–19.
77. Murphy, N. J. (1992). Nursing leadership in health policy decision making. *Nursing Outlook*, 158–161.
78. Milio, N. (1984). The realities of policy making: Can nurses have an impact? *Journal of Nursing Administration*, *1*, 18–23.
79. Ibid.
80. Smith, H. L. & Mitry, N. W. (1984). Nursing leadership: A buffering perspective. *Nursing Administration Quarterly*, *1*, 45–52.
81. Porter-O'Grady, T. & Malloch, K. (2004). *Quantum leadership: A textbook of new leadership*. Sudbury, MA: Jones and Barlett Publishers.
82. Ibid., 61.
83. Brower, B. (1971, October 8). Where have all the leaders gone? *Life*, 708.
84. Ibid.

REFERENCES

Aiken, L. (2002). Superior outcomes for magnet hospitals: The evidence base. In McClure, M., Hinshaw, A. (Eds.), *Magnet hospitals revisited: Attraction and retention of professional nurses*. Washington, DC: American Nurses Publishing.

Aroskar, M. (1994). The challenge of ethical leadership in nursing. *Journal of Professional Nursing*, 270.

Bennis, W. (1994). *On becoming a leader*. Reading, MA: Addison Wesley.

Blanchard, K. H. & Sargent, A. B. (1986). The one minute manager is an androgynous manager. *Nursing Management*, 43–45.

Buhler, P. (1993). Managing in the 90s. *Supervision*, 17–19.

Catton, J. J. (1971). Applying leadership to people problems. Supplement to the *Air Force Policy Letter for Commanders*, 30.

Davis, C. K., Oakley, D., & Sochalsk, J. A. (1982). Leadership for expanding nursing influence on health policy. *Journal of Nursing Administration*, 15–21.

Dixon, D. L. (1999). Achieving results through transformational leadership. *Journal of Nursing Administration*, 17–21.

Dunham-Taylor, J. (1995). Identifying the best in nurse executive leadership: Part 2, interview results. *Journal of Nursing Administration*, 24–31.

Dunning, H. F. (1963). Nobody can give you leadership. *Notes & Quotes*, 3.

Feinberg, M. R. (1965). *Effective psychology for management*. Englewood Cliffs, NJ: Prentice Hall.

French J. & Raven, B. (1959). The basis of social power. In D. Cartwright (Ed.), *Studies in power*. Ann Arbor: Institute for Social Research, University of Michigan.

Gardner, J. W. (1986a). *The nature of leadership: Introductory considerations*. Washington, DC: Independent Sector.

Gardner, J. W. (1986b). *The tasks of leadership*. Washington, DC: Independent Sector.

Gardner, J. W. (1986c). *The heart of the matter: Leader-Constituent interaction*. Washington, DC: Independent Sector.

Gardner, J. W. (1986d). *Leadership and power*. Washington, DC: Independent Sector.

Gevedon, S. (1992). Leadership behaviors of deans of top-ranked schools of nursing. *Nursing Education*, 221–224.

Glucksberg, S. (1968). Some ways to turn on new ideas. *Think*.

Goldberg, D. (1978, November 23). What makes a leader? *Mississippi Press*, p. D6.

Gunden, E. & Crissman, S. (1992). Leadership skills for empowerment. *Nursing Administration Quarterly*, 6–10.

Hodgetts, R. M. (1990). Management: Theory, process and practice (5th ed.). Orlando, FL: Harcourt, Brace, Jovanovich.

Jennings, E. E. (1962). The anatomy of leadership. *Notes & Quotes, 274*, 1, 4.

Jones, G. R. (1983). Forms of control and leader behavior. *Journal of Management*, 159–172.

Kaprowski, E. J. (1968). Toward innovative leadership. *Notes & Quotes, 351*, 2.

Keenan, M. J., Hoover, P. S., & Hoover, R. (1985). Leadership theory lets clinical instructors guide students toward autonomy. *Nursing and Health Care*, 83–86.

Kleinman, C. S., (2003). Leadership roles, competencies, and education, how prepared are our nurse managers, *Journal of Nursing Administration, 33*(9), 451–455.

Koontz, H. (1965). Challenges for intellectual leadership or management. *Notes & Quotes, 315*, 1, 4.

Levenstein, A. (1984a). Where nurses differ. *Nursing Management*, 64–65.

Levenstein, A. (1984b). Leadership under the microscope. *Nursing Management*, 68–69.

Lorentzon, M. (1992). Authority, leadership, and management in nursing. *Journal of Advanced Nursing*, 525–527.

Manthey, M. (1992). Leadership: A shifting paradigm. *Nurse Educator*, 5–14.

McDaniel, C. & Wolfe, G. A. (1992). Transformational leadership in nursing service: A test of theory. *Journal of Nursing Administration*, 60–65.

Pike, O. (1987, January). Rutan, Yeager showed what leadership is about. *Mobile Press Register*, p. A4.

Podsakoff, P. M., Todor, W. D., & Schuler, R. S. (1983). Leader expertise as a moderator of the effects of instrumental and supportive leader behaviors. *Journal of Management*, 173–185.

Smith, H. L., Reinow, F. D., & Reid, R. A. (1984). Japanese management: Implications for nursing administration. *Journal of Nursing Administration*, 33–39.

Upenieks, V. V. (2003). What constitutes effective leadership? Perceptions of magnet and nonmagnet nurse leaders. *Journal of Nursing Administration, 33*(9), 456–467.

Yanker, M. (1986). Flexible leadership styles: One supervisor's story. *Supervisory Management*, 2–6.

CHAPTER 8

Human Resource Development: Managing a Culturally Diverse Work Force

Susan Jacob, RN, MSN

The most exciting breakthroughs of the twenty-first century will occur not because of technology but because of an expanding concept of what it means to be human.

John Naisbitt and Patricia Aburdene[1]

LEARNING OBJECTIVES AND ACTIVITIES

- Develop a list of strategies to use in recruiting students into nursing education programs, considering the involved diversity issues.
- Develop an effective nurse recruitment advertisement.
- Conduct an effective simulated interview of a nurse applicant.
- Conduct an effective simulated interview as a nurse applicant.
- Discuss the nurse credentialing process of an employing agency.
- Describe the assessment center process.
- Determine turnover rates for an agency.
- Define the terms *human resource development, autonomy, empowerment,* and *andragogy*.
- Discuss the relevence of autonomy and empowerment in human resource development in nursing.
- Apply the concept of andragogy to human resource development in nursing.
- Discuss the promotion and termination policies of an employing organization.
- Analyze causes of conflict and its relationship to human resource issues.
- Make plans to manage conflict.
- Use techniques or skills for managing conflict.
- Discuss cultural diversity and its relationship to human resource issues.

CONCEPTS: Human resource management (HRM), recruiting, selecting, credentialing, assigning, assessment center, retaining, turnover, career planning, human resource development (HRD), autonomy, empowerment, andragogy, promoting and terminating, conflict, conflict management, cultural diversity, cultural sensitivity, cultural awareness, and cultural competence.

NURSE MANAGER BEHAVIORS: Plans, organizes, directs, and controls all aspects of the development of a human resource management program that meets all legal requirements governing personnel employment. Manages people. HRM policies and procedures reflect industry standards.

NURSE EXECUTIVE BEHAVIORS: Establishes direction, aligns persons, stimulates motivation, and inspires people to make useful change in performing their nursing roles. Uses input from employees to identify those factors that will recruit and retain the best personnel available. Promotes human resource management activities reflecting the cutting edge of advancements in the field. Uses research results to develop a model of HRD that leads people and makes them productive by putting to use their specific knowledge and strengths.

Introduction

The theory of human resource management in nursing includes knowledge of recruiting, selecting, credentialing, assigning, retaining, developing, promoting, and terminating nursing personnel. Recruiting has two facets: recruiting students into nursing programs and recruiting registered nurses (RNs) into health care institutions and agencies.

Recruiting

Recruiting Students into Nursing

The number of new entrants into baccalaureate nursing programs needs to be increased to keep pace with the demand for professional nurses. Consideration of a culturally diverse work force is essential given the culturally diverse population we serve.

The number of programs for registered nursing students in the United States increased from 1387 in 1980 to 1508 in 1997. Of these, baccalaureate programs increased from 377 to 523 and associate's degree programs from 697 to 876, while the number of diploma programs decreased from 311 to 109. Nursing enrollment in registered nursing preparation programs decreased from 270,228 in 1994 to 268,350 in 1995; 261,219 in 1996; and 238,244 in 1997. The number of graduates decreased from 97,052 in 1995 to 94,757 in 1996. Enrollment in all nursing programs, including baccalaureate, associate's degree, and diploma programs, decreased in 1997.[2] In 1998, approximately 9,904,000 persons were employed in the health services industry.[3] In 1996, there were 2,162,000 active RNs in the United States, up from 1,273,000 in 1980. The rate per 100,000 population increased from 560 to 815 during this period.[4]

Since 1995, enrollment in all basic nursing education programs (baccalaureate, associate's degree, or diploma) has fallen each year by approximately 5%. A study by Buerhaus predicts that by the year 2020, the RN workforce will be nearly 20% below projected requirements. The Bureau of Labor Statistics estimates the number of nurses needed by 2008 will increase by 450,864.[5]

The business of recruiting students into nursing requires long-term strategies for all educators and providers. Recruitment will be more effective if potential consumers of nursing services are involved. Professional nurses can work through community organizations to involve the community in changing the image of nursing and in the recruitment effort. The image of nursing should reflect the qualifications and credentials of caregivers that provide safe, effective care to individuals and communities.

Research Study

In a descriptive design survey, 641 college-bound high-school seniors were surveyed to determine why nursing is not selected more frequently as a career. The survey was taken to obtain data helpful to nurse educators in developing strategies to increase the number of high-school seniors who choose a career in nursing. A majority of those sampled had grade point averages between 3.00 and 3.99, and 92.3% did not choose nursing as a career.

Questions measuring knowledge regarding nursing education, hours, salaries, and work settings indicated that the overall knowledge of these areas of nursing among respondents was fairly accurate. Students were relatively uninformed, however, about the roles and tasks of nurses, and 91.8% were unaware that nurses worked with computers.

The overall opinion about nursing was favorable. A large percentage (86%) of students believed that nurses mainly followed doctors' orders, but many students (72.5%) believed that nurses make a lot of money and many (81.1%) also believed that nursing is a career only for smart people. Very few students believed that nurses do important work (5.4%); that nursing is challenging (9.4%), a real profession (9.3%), or an important profession (5.4%); or that it provides a good opportunity to help people (3%).

Neither knowledge nor opinion of nursing was significantly associated with students choosing or not choosing nursing as a career. Significant differences in gender, ethnicity, and age existed between students who chose nursing and those who did not. Students who chose nursing as a career were significantly more likely to be African-American, female, and 16 to 17 years of age. No significant differences in religion, socioeconomic status, or grade point average existed between those who chose nursing and those who did not. Knowing a nurse personally, caring for a seriously ill person, having a family member who is a nurse, and living with someone who is seriously ill were significantly associated with the decision to become a nurse. The reason cited most frequently for choosing nursing was the desire to help people. Those who did not choose nursing indicated a dislike for being near dying people and insufficient salary as the main reasons. These findings are important to nurse educators as they plan recruitment strategies aimed at increasing the enrollment of high-school students in baccalaureate nursing programs.[6]

Every major agency or institution employing nurses should have a committee that focuses on the recruitment of students into nursing education programs. Small organizations can form recruitment consortiums. Clinical nurses should be well represented because their ideas will give an authentic and positive image of professional nursing practice.[7]

Exhibit 8-1 lists activities to pursue in recruiting students into nursing education programs.

Recruiting Nurses into Employment

In 1980, there was a national shortage of 100,000 hospital nurses.[8] A flood of publicity on this shortage led to the formation of a National Commission on Nursing. This commission listed "eight top themes in descending order

EXHIBIT 8-1

Strategies for Recruiting Students into Nursing Education Programs

1. Form a committee to create a plan.
   a. Include clinical nurses
   b. Set goals
   c. Create a management plan for each goal
2. Obtain recruitment materials from organizations.
   a. National League for Nursing (NLN)
   b. American Nurses Association (ANA)
   c. American Organization of Nurse Executives (AONE)/American Hospital Association (AHA)
   d. National Student Nurses Association (NSNA)
   e. American Association of Colleges of Nursing (AACN)
   f. State
   g. Local
3. Prepare additional recruitment materials.
   a. News stories for newspapers, TV, and radio
   b. Posters for schools
   c. Speakers' bureau
   d. Model speeches
   e. Tours
4. Coordinate with other nurse education programs and prospective employers of nurses.
   a. Associate degree programs
   b. Diploma programs
   c. BSN programs
   d. Hospitals
   e. Public health
   f. Staffing agencies
   g. Ambulatory care facilities
   h. Nursing homes
   i. LPN programs
   j. Other
5. Prepare and offer consultation programs for junior and senior high schools.
   a. Administrators
   b. Teachers
   c. Guidance counselors
   d. Students, including potential dropouts
   e. Financial advisers
   f. Language and cultural resource advisers
6. Coordinate activities of recruiters in schools of nursing.
   a. Sources of information by telephone and mail
   b. Target adults seeking second careers, men, minorities, and immigrants
7. Involve community agencies in recruitment efforts.
   a. Professional organizations
   b. Social organizations
   c. Service organizations
   d. Others
8. Evaluate results accomplished.
   a. Number and locations of programs presented
   b. Number of students counseled
   c. Number of followups
   d. Number of applicants to local or other programs
   e. Homerooms visited
   f. Career days held by high schools, schools of nursing, and employers
   g. Inquiries to source persons by telephone or letter
9. Do work-study programs.
   a. High schools with employer
   b. High schools with schools of nursing
   c. Schools of nursing with employers
   d. Cooperative education

of importance" that it considered significant in reducing the shortage:[9]

1. Nursing leadership should be an integral part of senior management.
2. Nurses should be more involved in all levels of hospital decision making.
3. Nurses' management skills should be developed, and nurses should be provided more opportunities for leadership positions.
4. The organizational structure should be decentralized to facilitate communication and decision making.
5. Collaborative or joint practice programs between nurses and physicians should be established.
6. The nursing educational system needs to be rationalized in terms of entry-level requirements and clinical practice preparation.
7. Career development programs for clinical practice and administrative positions should continue to be developed and implemented.
8. Nursing leaders should be appointed to key committees to foster and strengthen nurses' interaction with medical staff and the board of directors of the agency.

During the next 20 years the supply of nurses ebbed and flowed with changes in reimbursement systems and restructuring of the entire health care system.

Today, more than 10 million people, almost 10% of employed Americans, work in the health care system. Further increasing the demand for health care are a growing US population and baby boomers becoming eligible for Medicare. The work force of nurses also is aging.[10]

EXHIBIT 8-2

Criteria for Developing an Effective Nurse Recruitment Advertisement

1. Target the population.
2. Catch the reader's attention.
3. Consider a picture that depicts a professional nurse in action, the kind of action nurses say they want.
4. List several factors that attract nurses. These may include:
   a. Opportunity for self-fulfillment
   b. Knowledge of helping others
   c. Intellectual stimulation
   d. Educational opportunity
   e. Fellowship with colleagues
   f. Adequate income
   g. Opportunity for innovation
   h. Opportunity to choose hours
   i. Opportunity for advancement
   j. Chance to be a leader
   k. Adequate support systems
   l. Child-care facilities
   m. Good fringe benefits
   n. Entrepreneural opportunities
5. Involve clinical nurses in developing the advertisement.
6. Test the advertisement on the clinical nurse staff.
7. Run the ad in the Sunday newspapers, selecting those that are read by the target population.
8. Run the ad in nursing journals that are read by the target population.
9. Establish a web site.
10. Provide for telephone and mail replies from applicants.
    a. Free telephone numbers
    b. Specific address
    c. Fax number and e-mail address
11. Provide for effective telephone and mail replies to be returned from the organization.
    a. The phone should be answered with positive responses that elicit interviews. Clinical nurses making immediate follow-up calls to prospective applicants can be effective.
    b. Effective packages of recruitment materials mailed to prospective applicants. (Depict and detail factors listed under number 4.)
12. Arrange for interview, including a visit to the organization.
    a. Contact person and sponsor
    b. Travel reimbursement
    c. Paid room and meals
    d. Interviews with person doing hiring; personnel specialists, including recruiter; and clinical nurses
13. Make a follow-up offer in writing.
14. Form a cadre of retired nurses (over 65 years of age)
    a. Establish with an appealing name
    b. Use a specific identification (a uniform or patch)
    c. Identify specialties needed
    d. Identify shifts needed
    e. Reward with good pay and continuing education

Job Sharing

One option for nursing is job sharing, that is, two persons filling one full-time equivalent job at a ratio of work agreed on by them. This option is convenient for nurses who want and can afford to work part-time and need the personal time off. Less acceptable to nurses has been mandatory sharing of work in organizations in which technology and restructuring have reduced the amount of available labor for pay.[11] One outcome of this dissatisfaction has been lower enrollments in registered nurse programs.

The Recruiter

Many large organizations employ a nursing recruiter, who may be a professional nurse or a personnel recruitment specialist. Either employee should work from a management plan that includes input from clinical nurses working within the organization.

The objective of the recruiter is to attract qualified professional nurses to apply for jobs. First, information about the organization's job openings is made known to the target population through advertisements in Sunday newspapers, in nursing journals, and on the Internet. The ads should be broad enough to give potential applicants knowledge of particular positions, salaries, and fringe benefits and the organizational climate. Results of studies of factors that attract nurses can be used as a basis for developing job ads. Exhibit 8-2 lists criteria for developing an effective newspaper, nursing journal, or Internet advertisement.

In 1983, an American Academy of Nursing study described both nurse administrators and staff nurses as agreeing on which factors attracted nurses to become and remain employees of hospitals. Among those factors were "adequate and competent colleagues, flexibility in scheduling, educational programs that allow for professional growth, and recognition as individuals."[12] Institutions that met these criteria were labeled *magnet hospitals*.

Today, magnet hospitals lure nurses like no other professional practice environments. They not only retain nurses, but they also benefit patient care as well as the organization. They provide multidimensional value including the following:[13]

1. Quality of nursing leadership
2. Organizational structure
3. Management style
4. Personnel policies and programs
5. Quality of care
6. Professional models of care
7. Level of autonomy
8. Quality assurance
9. Consultation and resources
10. Community and the hospital
11. Nurses as teachers
12. Image of nursing

13. Nurse-physician relationships
14. Professional career development

A formal nurse recruitment plan is suggested for each fiscal year, because objectives will be influenced by factors such as structural reorganization, turnover and retention, and vacant positions. The following are six steps of a formal plan:[14]

1. Gathering a database through situational scanning, forecasting, and variance audits comparing demand with supply data.
2. Setting objectives.
3. Designing strategies to accomplish the objectives.
4. Establishing the annual nurse recruitment budget.
5. Implementing the strategies through operational plans.
6. Evaluating and using feedback to take corrective action.

Marketing

Several authors recommend a marketing approach to recruitment of nurses. Such an approach would focus on the nurse as the consumer of employment. Connelly and Strauser advocate a marketing audit of the nursing environment. Exhibit 8-3 presents a scheme for a marketing

EXHIBIT 8-3

Marketing Survey for Recruiting and Retaining Nurses

1. Number of vacant positions.
   a. Current
   b. Previous month
   c. Percentage increase (or decrease)
2. Turnover rate by month and unit.
3. Exit interview results.
   a. Number of interviews performed
   b. Number of negative comments (list separately) (See Appendix 8–3)
4. New hire demographics.
   a. Diploma graduates
   b. AD graduates
   c. BSN graduates
   d. MSN graduates
   e. Doctoral graduates
   f. Average years of experience
   g. Males
   h. Females
   i. Average age
   j. Percent married
   k. Percent with children of preschool age
   l. Percent with children in school
   m. Percent minorities
   n. Other
5. Demographics of employed nurses. Profile the "stayers" and target similar recruits.
   a. Diploma graduates
   b. AD graduates
   c. BSN graduates
   d. MSN graduates
   e. Doctoral graduates
   f. Average years of experience
   g. Males
   h. Females
   i. Average age
   j. Percent married
   k. Percent with children of preschool age
   l. Percent with children in school
   m. Percent minorities
   n. Other
6. Attitude survey (list results separately).
7. Audit of meeting minutes.
   a. Staff nurses
   b. Others (list results separately)
8. Audit of performance evaluations (list results separately). Include variations by education, specialty, and longevity.
9. Salary levels (list by clinical level and longevity).
10. Overtime.
    a. Hours by month and unit
    b. Costs
    c. Include variations by education, specialty, and longevity
11. Absenteeism data.
    a. Daily average
    b. Cause
    c. Monthly total
    d. Include variations by education, specialty, and longevity
12. Agency nurse use.
    a. Hours by month and unit
    b. Costs
    c. Include variations by education, specialty, and longevity
13. Monthly budget variances by unit.
14. Utilization of productivity reports (refer to Chapter 7).
15. Acuity data by category and unit.
16. Average daily census by day of week and by month (report trends).
17. Recruiting expenses.
18. Major competitors for prospective hires.
19. Analysis of professional literature on recruitment and availability.
20. Analysis of patient relations reports.
21. Reputation and visibility of the organization and division.
    a. Community
    b. Employees
    c. Organizational culture
    d. Location of employment
22. Factors causing nurses to avoid organization.
23. Factors that would attract nurses to organization because it is a superior place to work.
24. Sources for recruiting nurses.

survey for recruiting and retaining nurses that includes some of these ideas. The marketing plan would be a management plan that would determine what needs to be done to sell employment to prospective professional nurses. Data would be analyzed, objectives set and evaluated, and a plan made and promoted.[15]

The primary focus of the selling approach to nurse recruitment is the needs of the employer. This approach is more effective when nurses are plentiful. Marketing focuses on many things: the needs of the prospective employee as customer; factors such as job profile, organizational culture, working location and conditions, the reputation of the institution, and compensation; and the institution as a superior place to work.[16]

Selecting, Credentialing, and Assigning

Selecting, credentialing, and assigning are all part of the hiring process.

Selecting

Selecting includes the interviewing, the employer's offer, the applicant's acceptance, and the signing of a contract or written offer. Although the chief nurse executive may interview and hire prospective applicants, it is best for the nurse manager who will directly supervise the employee to do the hiring. The manager should elicit the input and support of clinical nurses with whom the prospective employee will be working.

The Interview

Thompson defines an interview as "an equal level, face-to-face discussion between a job seeker and a person with full authority to fill the position under discussion."[17] Nurses, as the job seekers, want a face-to-face discussion with the person who has hiring authority. They may be considering several jobs, having narrowed the field down to those that specifically fit their career goals.

The nurse recruiter or an HR specialist will have completed a personnel file that contains a completed application form; a resume or curriculum vitae; references; and any documents that are required by policy or law, such as a current, valid license to practice nursing and school transcripts. The interviewer should prepare for the interview by reading the information in the applicant's file. Exhibit 8-4 is a checklist to use in reviewing the file. The interviewer should make notes of questions to ask about the information contained in the file. Adequate time should be set aside for the interview, which should take place in a private office where there will be no interruptions. An interview guide will be helpful in conducting an interview satisfactory to both the nurse manager and the applicant (see Exhibit 8-5).

EXHIBIT 8-4

Checklist for Reviewing Job Applicant's Folder

1. The application form
   a. Completed as directed
   b. Written statements are positive
   c. Contains no blanks
   d. Contains no gaps in employment data
2. References
   a. Listed
   b. Have been checked
   c. Are satisfactory
   d. Need further checking
3. Registered Nurse licensure
   a. Has been verified
   b. Is current and valid
   c. No legal suits pending
4. Transcripts
   a. Have been verified
   b. Are available
5. Forms signed
6. Curriculum vitae or resume
   a. Up to date
   b. Lists career goals
7. Job description provided, including blank performance contract
   a. Clinical level established as__________
   b. Years of longevity established as__________
8. Salary information available
   a. Base salary: $__________
   b. Clinical level pay: $__________
   c. Longevity pay: $__________
   d. Differential: $__________
   e. Credentialing (certification): $__________
   f. Total pay: $__________
   g. Paydays made known

All candidates for nurse jobs should be treated as professionals. It is illegal to ask them certain questions, such as those listed in Exhibit 8-6. Because information about age and date of birth may be necessary for insurance or other benefits, it can be obtained after the candidate is hired. Candidates will have questions they want answered. When complete information cannot be given, the interviewer should make a note, get the information, and communicate it to the candidate as quickly as possible. Exhibit 8-7 lists questions that candidates may ask and that the interviewer should be prepared to answer. Eye contact, rapport, and followup after the interview are important strategies to incorporate into the interview

EXHIBIT 8-5
Interview Guide

CANDIDATE:
DATE AND TIME OF INTERVIEW:

1. Arrange seating.
2. Make introductions and establish rapport.
3. Ask prepared questions.
   a. Tell me about yourself.
   b. What is your present job?
   c. What are your three most outstanding accomplishments?
   d. What is the extent of your formal education?
   e. What three things are most important to you in your job?
   f. What is your strongest qualification for this job?
   g. What other jobs have you held in this or a similar field?
   h. What were your responsibilities?
   i. Do you mind irregular working hours? Explain.
   j. Would you be willing to relocate? To travel?
   k. What minimum salary are you willing to accept?
   l. Are you more comfortable working alone or with other people?
4. Answer candidate's questions.
5. Note the following: Candidate was
   a. On time
   b. Well-dressed
   c. Well-mannered
   d. Positive about self
6. Maintain eye contact.
7. Note candidate's personal values.
8. Close the interview.
   a. Make an offer
   b. Obtain acceptance
   c. Set timetable for making offer or receiving response to offer

EXHIBIT 8-6
Questions That Are Illegal

Employment interviewers are forbidden by law to ask the following questions:

1. Age
2. Date of birth
3. The length of time residing at present address
4. Previous address
5. Religion; church attended; spiritual adviser's name
6. Father's surname
7. Maiden name (of women)
8. Marital status
9. Residence mates
10. Number and ages of children; who will care for them while applicant works
11. Transportation to work, unless a car is a job requirement
12. Residence of spouse or parent
13. Whether residence is owned or rented
14. Name of bank; information on outstanding loans
15. Whether wages were ever garnished
16. Whether bankruptcy was ever declared
17. Whether ever arrested
18. Hobbies, off-duty interests, clubs

process. Exhibit 8-8 outlines the hiring executive's responsibilities as well as those of the candidate.

The Assessment Center Process

Hiring is an investment in the right and best-qualified person. Interviewing techniques are often cursory and do not result in hiring the right person. Assessment center techniques should be considered for the hiring of all categories of nursing personnel. DelBueno, Weeks, and Brown-Stewart define the assessment center as "a comprehensive, standardized process by which multiple sampling techniques are used to determine an individual's actual or potential ability to perform skills and activities vital to success on the job." The assessment center process pools information from total sources and for noted performance dimensions. It may be used to plan orientation programs, for promotions, and for placement in clinical and career ladders. It is a cost-effective process because it avoids the unneeded orientation and turnover costs of hiring the wrong applicant.[18]

Sullivan, Decker, and Hailstone describe an assessment center for the selection of a nurse manager that has the following 17 job dimensions, each of which is subdivided into abilities that are observed and scored:[19]

1. Clinical nursing background
2. Development of subordinates
3. Delegation/management control
4. Planning and organization
5. Perception/sensitivity
6. Problem analysis
7. Problem solving/decision making
8. Risk taking
9. Initiation/leadership
10. Communication skills
11. Listening skills
12. Energy level
13. Stress tolerance
14. Resilience
15. Assertiveness
16. Behavioral flexibility
17. Accessibility

EXHIBIT 8-7

Possible Questions from Candidates and Tips for Interviewing

QUESTIONS

1. How much job security does this job have?
2. What previous experience does this type of job require?
3. What is the future of this type of job?
4. What is the growth potential for this particular job?
5. Where will the most significant growth for this type of job in the health care industry occur?
6. What is the starting salary for this job?
7. How do pay raises occur?
8. How does one find out when other job openings occur?
9. What are the fringe benefits of this job?
10. What are the requirements for working shifts and weekends?
11. What is the floating policy?
12. What are the opportunities for continuing education?
13. What are the opportunities for promotion?
14. What child care facilities are available?
15. What are the staffing and scheduling policies?

TIPS

1. Keep the atmosphere positive, pleasant, and businesslike.
2. Focus on the essential goals.
3. Provide answers in a brief, factual, and friendly manner; use a soft and clear tone of voice; maintain a relaxed posture; and keep hands still.
4. Do not attempt to bluff answers to questions.
5. Review information sent to you before the interview.
6. Be prepared for questions related to personal philosophy and style, community relations, professional goals, clinical and administrative style, decision-making ability, flexibility in working with diverse groups, fiscal issues, personnel management, and group relationships.
7. Avoid controversial issues of religion, abortion, and politics; do not discuss confidential matters.
8. Do not identify problems or offer solutions unless asked, and then indicate the need to have more information and time to study the issue.

The following are some other characteristics of this process:[20]

1. Exercises are developed to measure job dimensions.
2. Assessors from the supervisor group are selected and trained to rate the candidates.
3. The Head Nurse Assessment Center (HNAC) is conducted for one day. Each candidate is assessed by at least two persons.
4. Reliability and validity of assessment centers are high. The HNAC has many benefits, including selection of competent nurse managers, objectivity,

EXHIBIT 8-8

What Happens During an Interview

THE HIRING EXECUTIVE

1. Gives information about job and institution.
2. Assesses the competencies the candidate possesses in relation to the job opening.
3. Evaluates the candidate's personal characteristics in relation to the staff members with whom candidate will work (fit to staff).
4. Assesses candidate's potential to move organization toward its goals.
5. Assesses candidate's enthusiasm and state of health.
6. Forms impressions about candidate based on behavior, appearance, ability to communicate, confidence, intelligence, personality.
7. Assesses candidate's ability to do the job.
8. Determines facts about candidate.

THE CANDIDATE

1. Gives information about self.
2. Assesses the opportunity for developing and using competencies on the job.
3. Assesses ability to relate to the employees with whom candidate will work.
4. Assesses potential for achieving personal career goals.
5. Assesses the institution's climate and the morale of the employees.
6. Assesses opportunities for promotion and success.
7. Assesses own ability to do the job.
8. Determines facts about the organization and working conditions.

broader applicant support, consistency, selection of qualified applicants, nurse manager development, and improved management reputation.
5. Among the drawbacks of the HNAC are that it is stressful, time-consuming, and tiring for assessors; it favors outsiders; and it causes intimidation.
6. The process is job-specific.
7. The process is equitable to minorities and women.
8. Supervisors who will work with applicants select them.
9. The process has self-development value for participants.
10. The process is expensive, is stressful, may favor conformists, and may create self-fulfilling prophecies.
11. The process diminishes the risk for hiring or promoting inappropriate candidates.
12. The process is used in more than 2000 companies.

In a similar process, a master interview tool has been developed that categorizes content such as documented clinical and administrative expertise, research, education, and other significant factors. Points are assigned according to the weight of each rating category for various positions. A pool of interview questions is developed to determine the applicant's ability to communicate, organize thoughts, solve problems, and relate to others; to assess the applicant's knowledge, philosophy, experience, and personality traits; and to reveal the applicant's frame of reference, level of expectation, attitudes, feelings, and management style. Interview panels consist of three members, the chair being appointed by the chief nurse executive. The tool is claimed to have fairly high interrater reliability, to decrease interview time, and to assist in selecting the most qualified applicant.[21]

The Search Committee

A job opportunity that has a large impact on the organization will result in the appointment of a search committee. The objective is to obtain input into the hiring process from the people who will be affected by the appointment. Such committees are widely used in higher education, as faculty members expect to share in the governance of the institution and particularly in the area of curriculum. The following is an outline of search committee procedures:

1. A search committee is appointed by the chief executive officer (CEO) with input from the population to be affected.
2. A chair will be appointed by administration or elected by the search committee to serve as the liaison between the two.
3. The search committee's responsibilities will be clearly laid out by policy or by the committee itself. Most committees will recruit, screen, interview, and recommend applicants. Administrators generally make final decisions about appointments. Members of search committees are committed to their tasks and responsibilities. They may be committing themselves to five or six months of arduous work. The search committee usually agrees at the outset to consider all information about applicants confidential. It will not discuss any individual candidate outside the committee, except in general terms of progress reports to staff or faculty.
4. The search committee decides on a strategy for recruiting candidates and implements it.
5. Applications are screened after references and credentials have been obtained.
6. Applicants are scheduled for interviews and visits to the institution. Exhibit 8-9 contains a list of possible search committee interview questions.
7. After all applicants have been interviewed, the committee meets to analyze the information and rank the candidates.
8. A list of recommended applicants is sent to the CEO.
9. The CEO invites an applicant for a return visit and decides whether to make a job offer.

EXHIBIT 8-9

Preparatory Questions for Search Committee

1. What style of management do you follow?
2. What are your personal weaknesses and strengths?
3. What are your perceptions of the role the person in this job will perform?
4. How can this organization benefit your career?
5. What are your ideas of what the relationship should be between nurses and physicians?
6. What job in nursing would you like most to have?
7. What do you view as the role of nursing in this organization?
8. What do you view as the role of nursing in the community?
9. What do you think of collective bargaining?
10. How would you go about determining that your department operates efficiently and effectively?
11. Why should I (we) hire you?
12. How would you go about meeting the goals of the organization?
13. How would your family adapt to this area?
14. What are your career goals?

Credentialing

Credentialing is the process by which selected professionals are granted privileges to practice within an organization. In health care organizations this process has been largely confined to physicians. Limited privileges have been granted to psychologists, social workers, and selected categories of nurses such as nurse anesthetists, surgical nurses, and midwives. These categories generally have been restricted by physician credentialing policies and fall into the category of allied professional staff. The purpose of credentialing is to provide one mechanism by which nurses and other health care professionals can ensure that they possess the level of knowledge and skill required to perform the advanced activities required of them and consequently avoid negative legal repercussions. This process is considered especially relevant to advanced practice nurses.[22]

The Joint Commission on Accreditation of Healthcare Organizations (JCAHO) requires that hospitals investigate, develop recommendations, reach conclusions, and be responsible for their actions in credentialing the medical staff. Licensing and certification provide data to consider in the process.

Components

The components of a credentialing system for nurses would be as follows:

- Appointment. Evaluation and selection for nursing staff membership.
- Clinical privileges. Delineation of the specific nursing specialties that may be performed and the types of illnesses or patients that may be managed within the institution for each member of the nursing staff.
- Periodic reappraisal. Continuing review and evaluation of each member of the nursing staff to ensure that competence is maintained and is consistent with privileges.[23]

Criteria for Appointment

Criteria for appointments include proof of licensure, education and training, specialty board certification, previous experience, and recommendations. Clinical privileges criteria include proof of specialty training and of performance of nursing procedures or specialty care during training and previous appointments.

Professional nurses have mostly been hired through HR departments, but nurse managers should give consideration to increasing the professional status of nursing through the credentialing process.

The American Nurses Association (ANA)

A 1979 report of the Committee for the Study of Credentialing in Nursing included 14 principles of credentialing related to the following:[24]

1. Those credentialed
2. Legitimate interests of involved occupation, institution, and the general public
3. Accountability
4. A system of checks and balances
5. Periodic assessments
6. Objective standards and criteria and persons competent in their use
7. Representation of the community of interests
8. Professional identity and responsibility
9. An effective system of role delineation
10. An effective system of program identification
11. Coordination of credentialing mechanisms
12. Geographic mobility
13. Definitions and terminology
14. Communications and understanding

Credentialing in a hospital relates to appointing health professionals to the staff. Credentialing by professional organizations, such as ANA certification–recertification programs, can be a qualification for such appointments.[25]

The American Nurses Association, Inc. established the ANA Certification Program in 1973 to provide tangible recognition of professional achievement in a defined functional or clinical area of nursing. The American Nurses Credentialing Center (ANCC) became its own corporation, a subsidiary of ANA in 1991. More than 150,000 nurses throughout the U.S. and its territories in 40 speciality and advanced practice areas of nursing carry ANCC certification. While the role for nurses continues to evolve, ANCC has responded positively by the reconceptualization of certification and Open Door 2000, a program that enables all qualified registered nurses, regardless of their educational preparation, to become certified in any of five speciality areas: Gerontology, Medical-Surgical, Pediatrics, Perinatal, and Psychiatric and Mental Health Nursing.

Credentialing at Carondelet St. Mary's Hospital and Health Center in Tucson, Arizona, focuses on patient care, leadership, and education. Benefits to the nurses include clinical ladder promotions, compensation, paid education time, tuition reimbursement, and a paid day monthly for meetings and research. Patients benefit from improved infection control, reduced numbers and increased healing of pressure ulcers, new product introduction, and improved teaching. The employer benefits from retention of satisfied customers, nurses, and patients.[26]

Assigning

Assigning professional nurses to jobs is the third part of the hiring process. During the assignment period the new nurse is oriented to the job description and its use. Although assignment to a specific position may not be possible during the selecting and credentialing processes, candidates should have a choice of the possible units to which they will be assigned.

Where can a candidate who wants to work in the operating room (OR) be assigned when there are no vacancies in the OR? The candidate can be offered a choice of vacant positions. Make a verbal or written contract to transfer the individual to a vacated OR position when one becomes available. If others are waiting for a similar assignment, indicate the order in which they will be assigned to the OR.

Candidates should not receive assignment surprises when they arrive for orientation. When assignment policies are fair, reasonable, and acceptable, candidates will start work with a positive attitude. A principle for a nurse manager to follow is to provide necessary orientation and training to nursing employees to ensure competency, job satisfaction, and high productivity in the particular assignments they are accepting.

Leadership requires that nurse managers be absolutely truthful in dealing with assignment of personnel, including reassignment by floating to other units.

Retention

The retention of competent professional nurses in jobs is a major problem of the US health care industry, particularly for hospitals and long-term care facilities. Most Americans change jobs about 15 times by the age of 35, and nurses are no exception. Nurses change and achieve major career goals four or five times in their lifetime, including changing their specialty or the role they play in the profession.[27] Many do both. Some even retire from two or more systems.

Spitzer-Lehmann indicates that it is better to retain nurses than to recruit them. The advantages include cost benefits, high morale, and high-quality care. A study indicated that nurses stayed in their jobs when they received peer support, participated in a professional practice model, received tuition reimbursement, and had input into decision making; when communication was open; and when medical staff was supportive.[28] The policy of floating to other units should be discontinued or modified to provide nurses with confidence and comfort in the workplace. Other retention strategies include providing for assistance when needed, recognizing the private lives of employees, and matching skills and abilities to jobs. Employees want meaningful work assignments; equal, not subordinate, treatment; opportunities for development and use of knowledge and skills; and flexibility and independence on the job. Employees' perceptions of the work environment should be evaluated frequently. Feedback should be frequent and include the institution's financial position, strategy, market position, and future plans.[29]

Because 70% of families are headed by a single working parent or by two wage earners, vanguard companies are changing their corporate culture to accomplish goals of work force dedication, focus, and productivity. Vanguard companies consider it good business to make coming to work easier for employees; the outcomes have been loyalty, dedication, and team spirit. Vanguard companies are changing corporate culture to do the following:[30]

- Make it family-friendly.
- Provide child care around the clock.
- Foster candor, assertiveness, and commitment.
- Focus on managers bringing about cultural change through a common collaborative management style and an HR philosophy, the bedrocks of which are equity and flexibility.
- Provide elder care referral.
- Provide professional counseling for coping with stress.
- Provide paid days off for taking care of personal obligations.
- Empower managers and the work force.
- Provide resources.
- Tailor the culture to the individual's needs.

An insurance company adopted a service strategy to retain its employees and its customers. Through a problem-solving process called DOME (diagnosis, objectives, method, and evaluation), the company determined that service was a commodity as well as a product line. The service strategy was identified as "an organizing principle that directs people to provide services that benefit the customers." To accomplish this end, the fragile elements of motivation and staff commitment require that a motivational environment be created and maintained. This environment should address quality of work life, morale, energy levels, and optimism. This kind of environment creates new promotional and training opportunities.[31]

Turnover

The annual national turnover rate among hospital nurses is between 20% and 70%. An organization should determine its turnover rate by unit and by organization. Such determinations should be done monthly to keep abreast of trends. Nurses who leave should be profiled and classified by average age, marital status, type of program from which they graduated, additional education, years of experience, specialty, sex, race, and any other characteristic that will give clues that could decrease turnover and increase retention of competent nurses. Nurse managers should also review the performance of nurses who leave and should conduct exit interviews.

The crude turnover rate depicts the volume of turnover and is not a very selective index. Other data that provide information about turnover and retention are the mean and median service of nurses who stay. These data provide the average tenure of employees.[32] The sum of the number of months of employment of each nurse as well as other data can be determined by having a good nursing management information system (NMIS), which will accumulate the data on electronic spread sheets.

Turnover includes both replacement and transfer employees. The direct costs of turnover are attributed to recruitment of replacements. The costs of turnover range from $1280 to $50,000 per RN turnover. Turnover benefits include savings on salaries and benefits and the infusion of new knowledge and ideas. Incentives for retention include financial ones, flexible scheduling, participative management, job expansion, job enrichment, job reframing (looking at a job in a new way), and preventive career maintenance.[33]

The Leadership, Evaluation, and Awareness Process (LEAP) was developed by DeBerry. The outcome of LEAP has been an 80% reduction in turnover of first-line managers at an average turnover cost of $125,000 each and a positive cost-benefit analysis. LEAP is a common preselection process for first-line managers. It consists of the following steps:[34]

- A one-day program called "Is Management for Me?" covering the realities of management; 60% of attendees self-selected out of competition.
- A developmental session with current managers covering skills such as charisma, individual consideration, intellectual stimulation, courage, dependability, flexibility, integrity, judgment, and respect for others.
- An evaluation of the attendee by coach, by peers, and by self-profile on nine leadership skills.
- A panel of executives using "in-basket" exercises and oral and written tests on nine skills; 75% of candidates were endorsed.
- Application.

Job Expectations and Satisfaction

Ginsberg and coauthors contend that the high turnover rate in nursing is a result of job dissatisfaction. In a study of nurse job and career satisfaction and dissatisfaction, 6277 surveys were mailed to nurses in a five-county area around Jacksonville, Florida. There were 1921 responses, with the following rank-order results:[35]

1. Money was the number one concern and the preferred remedy for dissatisfaction.
2. Recognition.
3. Hours and scheduling.
4. Too much responsibility for money.
5. Stress.

A study surveyed 279 nursing seniors in five schools in northern Alabama to determine why new graduates select particular settings and why many leave in a short time. The new graduates had the following expectations:[36]

1. Full-time work.
2. Day work or a desired shift (46% of single nurses and 36.5% of married nurses would work evenings).
3. Work in a medium-sized to large hospital.
4. Good salary.
5. Pleasant working conditions.
6. Self-fulfillment and a sense of achievement from giving adequate and complete care.
7. Educational opportunities, intellectual stimulation, and opportunity to develop new skills.
8. Satisfactory supervision by nurse managers.
9. Recognition and encouragement.
10. Professional autonomy and power.
11. Work in a community that offers higher education opportunities and a good place to raise a family. Factors considered important included good schools, a low crime rate, an economically stable region, a low tax structure, and a low cost of living.

Many would not consider working in small hospitals (17.2%), veteran's administration or federally owned hospitals (19.5%), investor-owned hospitals (18.8 percent), nursing homes (65.7%), doctor's offices or clinics (18.6%), temporary or private-duty agencies (41%), or psychiatric or mental health clinic (45.5%).[37] In addition, more baccalaureate degree nurses expected to become head nurses, supervisors, and public health nurses than did associate's degree nurses.

Drucker states that salaries are not the basic problem with nurse retention and recruitment, a position in opposition to the results of most surveys. He states, "The basic problem is that nurses aren't allowed to do nursing. I've been saying that now for 20 years. The doctors still treat nurses as if they were scullery maids, and that's just not going to work any longer." Drucker believes that hospital administrators must change the attitudes of doctors and that focusing nurses' responsibilities on their professional role and increasing their salaries will improve retention.[38]

A study of nurse manager satisfaction in Massachusetts hospitals indicated that nurse managers were dissatisfied with educational reimbursements received (50%), inadequate role orientation (52%), support from other hospital departments (59%), the lack of control over budget process (12%), salary (53%), added duties of expanded role (60%), staffing issues (73%), information received (40%), and negative effects of stress (67%). A plan developed to alleviate these dissatisfactions was to be implemented by nurse executives.[39]

Career Planning

Nurse managers must recognize the results of nurse satisfaction surveys. They must learn to manage professional nurses so that they will achieve career and job satisfaction. The first step is to establish a career plan for professional nurses within the nursing organization.

To be successful in their careers, professional nurses need a sense of personal fulfillment and job significance. Nurse managers create these conditions by determining and correcting the causes of the following:[40]

- Anxiety and uncertainty
- Inability to meet personal and organizational goals
- Lack of clarity about roles played
- Contradictory demands
- Dissatisfaction with human relations
- Rebellion against rules, policies, and regulations
- Inherent complexity of the nature of the tasks of the job
- Competition
- Overwork and underutilization
- Lack of personal and professional growth
- Dissatisfaction with the quality of associates

Nurse managers should restructure nursing services to link assignments and responsibilities to education, experience, and competence. This connection should be a part of a career program for professional nurses that achieves the following goals:[41]

- Provides more promotions and pay for clinical nurses.
- Provides higher pay for increased competence and increased participation.
- Provides for continuing education to upgrade knowledge and skills.
- Provides clinical rotation policies that prevent burnout.
- Meets scheduling and salary preferences.

Career Counselor

A career counselor should be part of the grand strategy for establishing a nursing career program. Even though an organization may not have a career counselor, every nurse should have one in the person of a superior. The counselor should be able to help nurses advance their careers in nursing and not just within the organization. At least one counselor should be available to help nurses assess their interests, skills, and values; to assist with analyzing all the open options; and to aid in making the career plans that will lead to achieving career goals. The plan also includes work experiences related to off-duty time, such as courses, workshops, community service, professional activities, and other activities specifically related to goals. It is a total plan that develops individuals professionally to meet their career aspirations.

Staff Development Career Counselor

One group to contact about career opportunities is the staff development department. Because counselors in such departments traditionally serve in an organizational relationship that provides a staff service to line management of the nursing hierarchy, nursing administration should identify their role. Traditionally, the staff development department fulfills functions of initial orientation and conducts classes in cardiopulmonary resuscitation, intravenous therapy, and the like. In contrast, some departments are moving toward a career development orientation by becoming involved in functions such as specialty orientation and training and in implementing the process of planning, organizing, directing, and evaluating the development of nurses through levels of competency in clinical practice, management, teaching, and research.

Sovie labels the career development functions of the staff development department as professional identification, professional maturation, and professional mastery. These areas can be related to a career ladder program in which competencies have been identified for the nurse practicing at several rungs of the ladder. The competencies are stated in the form of job descriptions, and they increase in complexity. Policies and procedures exist for the process of climbing the ladder. A program of staff development for career advancement facilitates the process.

Sovie's model could educate nurses to gain advanced specialized knowledge and skills through individual plans, with staff development educators acting as counselors and teachers. Nurses could learn to provide the leadership in solving the health care problems of patients and families. They could develop materials for patient and family education. They could learn how to be a primary nurse in practicing the nursing process, not just within the nursing modality. They could learn how to engage in professional nursing dialogue with colleagues. Training for nurses could include the competencies of consulting, participation in quality assurance activities, processing and applying reports of research findings, participation in research, and involvement in committee functions. This learning could be part of a personal career plan.[42]

Career Ladders

Clinical nursing offers the most diverse kinds of opportunities. Clinical nursing was largely a nonpromotable area until recent years. Numerous interesting clinical areas had been expanded with advanced technology, but nurses seldom could be promoted within a clinical area. This is changing fast with the development of clinical career ladders and levels of increasing competence to mastery. A career ladder requires individual effort, assisted by organizational support and reward. When appropriately conceived and implemented, a career ladder program results in career satisfaction for the nurse and increased productivity for the employer.

A clinical ladder is a horizontal development system based on specific criteria used to develop, evaluate, and promote nurses who intend to remain at the bedside. Clinical ladders apply to nurses who want to remain in the clinical setting, whereas career ladders are for those who leave the clinical realm in pursuit of a future in administration, teaching, or research.

A clinical career ladder should do the following:

1. Improve the quality of patient care.
2. Motivate staff in the following areas:
   a. Job proficiency and expertise, that is, motivate nurses to reach their highest level of professional competence.
   b. Pursuit of education, which is an important factor in mobility.
   c. Development of career goals.

EXHIBIT 8-10
Basic Clinical Ladder Model

A. CLINICAL/STAFF NURSE I (BEGINNER/NOVICE)

1. Experience and Education
   Current state licensure with less than one year of experience.
2. Description
   a. Needs close supervision.
   b. Performs basic nursing skills/routine patient care.
   c. Begins to develop patient assessment skills/communication skills.

B. CLINICAL/STAFF NURSE II (ADVANCED BEGINNER)

1. Experience and Education
   a. Current state licensure with more than one year of experience.
   b. BSN with more than 6 months of experience.
   c. MSN without experience.
2. Description
   a. Demonstrates adequate/acceptable performance.
   b. Can differentiate importance of situations and set priorities.
   c. Requires less supervision.
   d. Demonstrates interest in continuing education.

C. CLINICAL/STAFF NURSE III (COMPETENT)

1. Experience and Education
   a. Current licensure with two or more years of experience.
   b. BSN with more than one year of experience.
   c. MSN with more than 6 months of experience.
2. Description
   a. Demonstrates unsupervised competency using the nursing process.
   b. Is able to plan and organize in terms of short-range and long-range goals.
   c. Demonstrates direction in actions.
   d. Accepts leadership responsibility readily.
   e. Demonstrates well-developed communication skills.
   f. Shares ideas and knowledge with peers.

D. CLINICAL/STAFF NURSE IV (PROFICIENT)

1. Experience and Education
   a. Current licensure with 3 years of clinical experience and pursuit of BSN.
   b. BSN with more than 2 years of experience.
   c. MSN with more than one year of experience.
2. Description
   a. Demonstrates specialized knowledge and skills.
   b. Continues professional education.
   c. Assumes leadership/supervisory responsibility.
   d. Recognizes and adjusts to situations that vary from the norm.
   e. Delegates responsibility appropriately; uses wide range of alternatives in solving problems.

E. CLINICAL/STAFF NURSE V (EXPERT)

1. Experience and Education
   a. MSN with more than 2 years of appropriate clinical experience.
   b. BSN required with more than 3 years of experience; pursuing MSN.
2. Description
   a. Demonstrates expertise in clinical practice.
   b. Assumes/delegates personnel and management responsibility.

3. Provide methods of objective and measurable performance evaluation, and reward clinical competence for the purpose of advancement.
4. Promote retention within the clinical area and reduce the turnover rate.

Performance criteria in any clinical ladder system should be clearly differentiated and specific at each level. The evaluation process must be measurable. Salary differentials must be significant enough to provide motivation. Any system should involve evaluation of educational and leadership criteria as well as skill performance. Exhibit 8-10 is a basic clinical ladder model that can be added to or fleshed out by management.

Spitzer and Bolton report the results of a staff survey of 956 career-track RNs. There were 583 respondents who strongly agreed to the following statements about salary and salary equity:[43]

- "When first hired, staff nurses should be paid according to years of experience, acute care experience, and education."
- "Salary adjustments (raises) should be based on clinical performance, additional acquired education, and additional clinical experience (regardless of specialty)."

Human Resource Development

Definition

Human resource development (HRD) is the process by which corporate management stimulates the motivation of employees to perform productively. HRD provides the stimuli that motivate nursing personnel to provide nursing care services to clients at quality and quantity standards that keep the health care organization reputable and financially solvent, the nurses satisfied with their professional accomplishments and quality of work life, and the clients treated successfully.[44]

Human resource development practices the concepts of democracy. In HRD, people grow and prosper from learning to use the skills of problem solving, logic, inquiry, critical thinking, and decision making. HRD is a lifelong process. It is also a process of helping and sharing that leads to competence and satisfaction with both the process and outcomes. The HRD process facilitates self-direction, self-discipline, focus on immediate problems, and satisfaction related to employee participation in problem solving and decision making.[45]

Obviously, nurse administrators and managers of today's work force must be well schooled in HRD. HRD theory includes the theory of change, problem solving and decision making, leadership, motivation, communication, participatory management, decentralization, and adult education. In nursing, HRD should be a proactive program as well as a part of strategic planning.

In recent years, HRD in many health care organizations has been strongly influenced by the following:

- A change in reimbursement systems from retrospective to prospective. These systems are cost-driven.
- A change in the structuring of health care organizations with the development of product lines, especially outpatient or ambulatory surgical centers, wellness programs, women's health programs, free-standing rehabilitation facilities, and many more.
- The decentralization of nursing organizations, which has made unit nurse managers department heads and eliminated intermediate levels of nursing management. Nursing staff governance and differentiated nursing practice are emerging. Case management and managed care are evident.

Health care organization administrators and nurse managers at all levels are learning that efficiency and effectiveness result from advanced HRD programs. These advanced programs facilitate human relationships, reliability, initiative, autonomy, and talents. They do so through policies, procedures and leadership that are fair, promote trust, reduce stress, communicate through feedback, and increase productivity without undue emphasis on costs. Keeping employees satisfied with the work environment decreases turnover, an expensive aspect of human resource management (HRM). Good HRD programs are therefore cost-effective.

Autonomy and Empowerment

As part of HRD, health care corporations should increasingly develop programs to enlarge the authority of professional nurses, increase their say in management of their clinical practice discipline, and improve their career development possibilities. The organization's administration and its employees want control over HRD events. As stakeholders in the health care system, clinical nurses and managers both have an obligation to keep the enterprise healthy. As economic stakeholders, nurses need security of income through wages and benefits, whereas management's stake is profits and, in some cases, dividends for shareholders. Nurses have a psychological stake in their need for dignity. Nurses and managers have potential stakes related to rights and obligations, efficiency and controls, and the trend toward greater employee influence in decisions and subsequent outcomes. These stakes should be spelled out in policies. The leader who balances motivation with control will manage effectively as "human beings strive to be involved and to gain influence over their lives to the extent that they are psychologically ready to do so and to the extent that economic organizational conditions allow them to do so."[46]

People want to work hard, perform well, learn new skills, and be involved in decisions about their work. They want to have input into placement and promotion. Managers who support the professional autonomy of nurses support empowerment of this group. Professional nurses thus gain control of their lives through feeling and using their own strength and power. Empowerment is therapeutic and spiritual; it is healthy for both employees and the organization.[47]

Empowerment seeks to increase the power and influence of professional nurses.[48]

Self-Help

A goal of HRD is the development of a self-reliant learner who remains a knowledgeable and skilled worker in the future. Another goal is the development of workers who learn and use the skills of self-help and of diagnosing their learning needs, being able to explore options in learning, thinking divergently, making decisions, and evaluating their roles in cooperation at work and in the world.[49] The HRD program uses leadership, staff development, and the theory of adult education to accomplish these goals.

Andragogy

In HRD and staff development, learners are adults, and educational programs are based on theories of adult education. *Andragogy* is a concept and theory of adult education based on assumptions about adults as learners. According to Knowles, the concept is a behavioral one and incorporates the following beliefs:[50]

1. The adult learner needs to be self-directing and treated with respect.
2. An environment needs to be established that allows adults to participate in making decisions that affect their lives.
3. Because adults have experiences to share with others, experiential techniques should be a part of adult education. Because adults are more closed to new concepts, they need to be "unfrozen."
4. Adults should be able to immediately apply what they have learned. Learning should relate to doing something or learning a skill.
5. Social role development determines an adult's readiness to learn.
6. Adults go through a sequence of learning from being dependent personalities to being self-directing, accumulating a reservoir of experience and shifting their orientation toward learning from subject-centered to performance-centered.

Adult education reflects lifelong learning and is well established in nursing. Because staff development in nursing relates to adults, it should follow the precepts of adult learning, a humanistic educational process that values the individual. In nursing education, andragogy creates a horizontal power relationship between teacher and student.[51]

Adult education enriches one's life because more education leads to better employment. To pursue higher education is a personal decision that can be advanced by management. An example is completion of the bachelor of science (BSN) by associates degree in nursing (ADN) or diploma graduates. Research has validated that increased productivity comes from investing in people and their education.

Sanderson focuses on the midcareer group (individuals 35 to 55 years of age) as the largest group in the organization. He indicates that the group has grief and confusion that lead to reassessment, which leads to further redefinition of values and goals and on to future commitment. It is during this period that self-fulfillment and self-actualization needs emerge.[52] An effective HRD program at this phase (or these phases) of work life could include the following:

- Providing mentorship activities.
- Assisting leaders to help employees to balance work, family, and self-development through programs promoting and supporting positive growth orientation.
- Assisting employees in making a fit with jobs within the organization by moving up, across, down, or out.
- Creating opportunities for staff to gain satisfaction from work.
- Providing variety and challenges in the job.
- Creating an aggressive organizational development program that values people; balances work, leisure, and learning; provides a climate for the whole person; redesigns positions to promote flexible hours, job sharing, pairing (teams), and permanent part-time positions; institutes self-managing work teams; emphasizes innovation; provides strong rewards and recognition; and creates a peer support program.
- Creating an aggressive staff development program that accomplishes all of the foregoing. It would include training in the skills of coaching, counseling, and mentoring; managing life transitions; retraining; expanded sabbaticals; providing opportunities for job exchanges outside the organization and in new fields; and creating a career subsidization fund.[53]

Typology for Human Resource Development of Personnel

Odiorne suggests a four-category typology for HRD of personnel: stars, workhorses, problems, and deadwood. He suggests training each group separately as follows:[54]

1. **Stars.** Stars are a small group of personnel with high potential whose performance lives up to that potential. Managers should educate stars to increase performance and develop their potential once they have been identified by the assessment center method, review board method, or staff analysis method.

   Top managers still pick successors like themselves with perceived star qualities, such as adaptability to change, company and career orientation, ability to manage self-expression, lateral and upward mobility, dedication, loyalty, adaptivity, quiet differentiation, early achievement, ability to work in a web of tensions, gamesmanship, flexibility, and ability to generalize.

   Stars of the future will be surrounded by technology, be comfortable with high-level decision making and problem analysis, do less traveling, have more span of control over work, and be collaborative group leaders. Future stars will also be innovative. On their way to stardom, they will acquire a master's degree in business administration (MBA) or nursing administration (MSN); use skills; be creative; create new jobs; and be technology entrepreneurs, engineers, and scientists. Stars will appreciate the liberal arts as the accumulated knowledge of civilization. Future stars will have skills of rational thought, decision making, problem solving, ethical evaluation, communication; knowledge of government; and special education and experiences. Future stars will be trained by stars as mentors who are goal oriented, are superior performers, behave to be imitated, support and help, delegate responsibility, give feedback, exhibit a positive attitude, mentor women and minorities, are sponsors, and provide support groups. Some nurses are stars inculcated with the success ethic. Nursing leaders can develop HRD programs that will provide the ingredients.
2. **Workhorses.** These persons can be trained to improve their performance. They can be motivated using theories of Maslow, McGregor, and Herzberg, among others. They should be well paid for their work, participate in decision making by merging personal and organizational goals, and be provided with opportunities for job enrichment. Organizational development will motivate workhorses through job design, working conditions, increased variety of tools, development of higher skills, assignment of increased responsibility, job rotation, content change, and team competition. Workhorses thrive on HRD programs that provide for personal growth, self-fulfillment, and use of abilities to perform meaningful work in a pleasant workplace.
3. **Problems.** Problem employees exhibit undesirable behavior that can be corrected by remedial training. They may exhibit emotional outbursts or immaturity, ignore important things, be overcome by trivia, be slow to respond to change, retain obsolete ideas and procedures, treat people unfairly, enforce rules too rigidly, retain authority, fail to communicate, be too lax, or lack a sense of timing and the ability to anticipate. To avoid or remedy their poor performance, training should be preceded by specifying performance standards, removing obstacles to success, providing the needed training, providing favorable consequences for doing right, providing feedback, encouraging self-control, and helping with personal problems.
4. **Deadwood.** Deadwood is a term used to describe workers who do not respond to training or developmental discipline. They should be fired, using appropriate HR procedures. Not only are they nonproductive, but they also negatively influence workhorses and problems.

Nurse managers may want to turn workhorses into stars, which requires need and drive on the part of the workhorse. Bell Laboratories and Dupont Company have had considerable success in doing this. Stars say the most important skills include technical competence and taking initiative to go beyond basic job duties.[55]

Promoting

One way for nurse managers to ensure that all professional nurses have promotion opportunities is to develop a promotion system that indicates all promotion categories within the organization.

Nurse managers should develop specific promotion policies with input from all categories of professional nurses and the HR department. These policies should include the following:[56]

1. All vacant positions will be posted even if change in pay and rank does not occur. Some nurses will want to change units, specialty, shifts, and so on.
2. All interested applicants should file applications for promotion in the HR department.
3. Personnel in the HR department should prepare promotion rosters that rank all candidates by education,

experience, and performance. The best-qualified candidate should be at the top of the list.

4. Applicants should be interviewed and rated by the same set of criteria, a process described previously in this chapter in the section titled Selecting.
5. The best-qualified candidates should be selected for promotion.
6. The results of the promotion process should be announced. Those not selected should be notified and counseled individually rather than learn that they were passed over from a third party or by seeing the list of those promoted.
7. The promotion system must be fair and be perceived as fair by professional nurses.

An effective promotion policy provides the same opportunity for people of equal ability to apply and treats such people equitably during interviews. Employees who are not promoted should be allowed to discuss their disappointment. Managers may expect a temporary decrease in performance from them.[57]

Darling and McGrath write that nurses experience much trauma when moving upward from clinical to managerial nursing. They are unaware of the transition process involved in a promotion, including the fact that their social and professional ties with other clinical nurses are cut. They take on more responsibilities and burdens and soon feel isolated and alone. They gain visibility and prestige but also receive complaints instead of appreciation from their staff.[58]

To prevent promotion trauma, supervisors of promotees can plan a transition program that will alert promotees to the changes in relationships that will occur. Such a program will help keep them from blaming their difficulties on personal failings. A transition program should include clear role descriptions and expectations, clear job descriptions, and classes in management to help them gain the needed knowledge and skills. Staff development is as essential for nurses promoted to management as it is for those who stay in the clinical domain. They should know what to expect and how to deal with Darling and McGrath's five stages of promotion: uninformed optimism, informed pessimism, hopeful realism, informed optimism, and rewarding completion. A management development program will keep clinical nurses who are promoted to manager positions from bailing out at the second stage.[59]

Terminating

Employees cannot be terminated at will. They are protected by public policy set forth in the National Labor Relations Act, the Civil Rights Act of 1964, the Age Discrimination in Employment Act, the Vocational Rehabilitation Act, and the Occupational Safety and Health Act. Laws also protect whistle-blowers.

Employees should be terminated only after all efforts to retain them have been exhausted. The theory of management includes concepts and principles that, when learned and applied by nurse managers, will assist employees to be competent and productive. Punishment or disciplinary action should be a last resort and should be progressive, moving from verbal conference, to a recorded conference, to suspension, to discharge. Such action should be covered by written policies and procedures.

First-line nurse managers should have authority to fire employees. They should consult with superior managers and HR personnel when terminating staff to make sure the action will stand up in court. All policies must be legal, and they must be consistently and correctly enforced. All employees are entitled to a fair hearing and review. The process allows for appropriate representatives for employees at investigating interviews. Terminated employees should be paid all benefits they have accrued.[60]

Firing an employee is an unpleasant job. It is done for the following reasons:

- Economic downturns when employees are in surplus.
- Personality mismatches occur, that is, everything has been tried, including transfers, but the employee does not fit anywhere.
- Progressive discipline in which the employee fails to meet previously agreed on performance expectations.
- Incorrigibility, that is, the employee has made serious mistakes, stolen, or has other gross failures.

The nurse manager needs to plan the session well ahead and be prepared to do the following:

- Coordinate with the personnel office, superiors, unions, outplacement people, and others.
- Keep the firing from the grapevine.
- Time the session for the end of the day and middle of the week to keep it confidential and to rebuild the organization.
- Be straightforward and up-front.
- Have all documentation ready.
- Deal with four stages of employee reaction: shock with physical symptoms, rejection, emotion, and withdrawal. Be quiet during the shock and emotion stages. Confirm the message during rejection. Provide information during the withdrawal stage and terminate the meeting.[61]

Cultural Competence

"Culturally competent individuals value diversity and respect individual differences regardless of one's race, religious beliefs, or ethnocultural background."[62] Culture can be described as the sum total of socially transmitted behavioral patterns, including the arts, beliefs, values, customs, and lifeways and other products of human work and thought of a population of people that focus on their worldview and decision making.[63] Just as the expectation is that health care professionals will be sensitive to the cultural influences of those for whom they care, the nurse administrator must also be culturally sensitive in recruitment, hiring, and retention strategies. It is important to increase one's cultural awareness and sensitivity, as culture is largely unconscious and can be powerfully influential in communication, decision making, and handling conflict.

Terms such as *cultural awareness, cultural sensitivity,* and *cultural competence* are often included in discussions of cultural diversity and are at times used interchangeably. Purnell and Paulanka distinguish these definitions, describing cultural awareness as a greater appreciation of the external signs of diversity, including arts, music, outward appearance, and physical features. Personal attitudes and increasing awareness of one's own communication patterns so as not to offend someone from a different cultural background are hallmarks of cultural sensitivity. When one increases cultural sensitivity, it is with the expectation that this will facilitate cultural competence. The following outlines characteristics of cultural competence as described by Purnell and Paulanka. Though these indicators are applied to clients, they may also be applied to health care providers.

1. Developing an awareness of one's own existence, sensations, thoughts, and environment without letting them have an undue influence on those from other backgrounds.
2. Demonstrating knowledge and understanding of the client's culture, health-related needs, and culturally specific meanings of health and illness.
3. Accepting and respecting cultural differences.
4. Not assuming that the health care provider's beliefs and values are the same as the client's.
5. Resisting judgmental attitudes such as "different is not as good."
6. Being open to cultural encounters.
7. Being comfortable with cultural encounters.
8. Adapting care (communication, decision making, conflict resolution) to be congruent with the client's culture.
9. Cultural competence is a conscious process and not necessarily linear.[64]

Cultural competence becomes increasingly important given the diversity of our work force and consumers. For example, the 2000 US census recorded the following population statistics:

1. 75.1% Whites,
2. 12.5% Hispanic/Latino (of any race),
3. 12.3% Black/African American,
4. 0.9% American Indian or Alaska Native,
5. 3.6% Asian,
6. 0.1% Native Hawaiian or other Pacific Islanders,
7. 5.5% some other race, and
8. 2.4% two or more races.[65]

Dealing with conflict can be particularly challenging in the management of a culturally diverse work force. Conflict management serves to improve communication, work relationships, and productivity outcomes.

Conflict Management

Creating a healthy work environment is critical to a culture of quality and safe health care delivery systems. The American Organization of Nurse Executives (AONE), the professional association for nurse executives and nurse leaders, strongly supports the identification and adoption of evidence-based management practices, which include attention to work redesign. An education and research priority of AONE is creating positive and healthy work environments in nursing and health care. This is a challenge at best, requiring understanding of the organization's culture in handling conflict, costs of conflict, the impact of organizational complexity, barriers to managing conflict, and strategies for effective conflict resolution.[66]

Rapid changes in health care, including dismantling of the traditional structure in health care organization, have resulted in an atmosphere of the unknown. Additionally, uncertainties caused by changes in roles and role relationships and uncharted and evolving relationships with new categories of health care workers have added to the perplexing work environment. These factors often lead to conflict in the workplace. Symptoms such as high levels of negativity and passivity; poor leadership; ineffective problem-solving skills; strangled communication flow; volatile emotions, with anger surfacing; difficulty accepting changes; and recruitment and retention difficulties further create conflicting individual and organizational goals.[67]

> Conflict is defined as: An expressed struggle between at least two interdependent parties, who perceive incompatible goals, scarce rewards, and interference from the other party in achieving their goals. They are in a position of opposition in conjunction with cooperation.[68]

Conflict relates to feelings, including feelings of neglect, of being viewed as taken for granted, of being treated like a servant, of not being appreciated, of being ignored, of being overloaded, and other instances of perceived unfairness. Conflict relates to ignoring an individual's self-esteem and worth. The individual's feelings may build from anger to rage. During this time, overt negative behaviors such as brooding, withdrawing, arguing, instigating unrest among staff, or fighting can be observed. The individual can let feelings and behavior interfere with job performance, resulting in carelessness, mistakes in areas of responsibility, and reduced productivity for the unit of service.

Characteristics of Conflict

The characteristics of a conflict situation are as follows:[69]

- At least two parties (individuals or groups) are involved in some kind of interaction.
- Mutually exclusive goals or mutually exclusive values exist, either in fact or as perceived by the parties involved.
- Interaction is characterized by behavior destined to defeat, reduce, or oppress the opponent or to gain a mutually designated victory.
- The parties face each other with mutually opposing actions and counteractions.
- Each party attempts to create an imbalance or relatively favored position of power vis-á-vis the other.

Conflict in health care organizations can be viewed from a structural or political perspective. From the structural perspective, conflict interferes with the accomplishment of organizational purposes. Bolman and Deal note that hierarchical conflict raises the posibility that the lower the level of employee the more likely that management directives may be subverted. Conflict among major partisan groups can undermine an organization's effectiveness and the ability of its leadership to function.[70]

Assessing Conflict

Hawkins and Kratsch describe different aspects of assessing a conflict situation, noting symptoms, underlying issues, and incorrect assumptions that can influence how the problem is defined. How this is handled may facilitate or hinder resolution of the true issue.[71]

Symptoms of conflict may include negative body language such as eye-rolling, turning away, repetition of story or request, disruptive behaviors (throwing objects, slamming doors), avoidance behaviors, turnover, compensation claims, and disability. Underlying needs and interest driving conflict may include needs not being met: resource needs (time, staff, space, information); psychological needs (recognition, respect, control, power, safety); emotional needs (fear, shame, sadness, loss, disappointment, support); and values in conflict (autonomy, dignity, honor, fairness or justice). Labels or inaccurate assumptions can also block resolution and are important to understand in assessing conflict. For example, labels such as "difficult family," "passive-aggressive coworker," "not a team player," "intellectual snob," "bully," "incompetent," and "uncooperative" may get in the way of true understanding of the issue and resolution.[72]

Causes of Conflict

Organizational Conflict

Conflict can be destructive or useful, depending on how it is handled by the leader. Conflict derives from misinformation and misperception: one party has information that the other does not have, or the parties have different information.

Stevens indicates that the three most often cited potential sources of conflict are human shortcomings, interpersonal failure, and the nature of an organization (not the people in it). Also, individuals as well as departments often oppose one another to gain prestige, power, or resources, or to show dominance.[73]

Marriner states that conflict arises because individuals have divergent views of their own power and authority and ambiguous jurisdictions. Conflict increases with the need for consensus, the number of organizational levels, the number of specialties, the degree of associations, and the degree of dependence of some parties on others. When separation in time and space exists, factionalism is fostered and communication barriers impede understanding. Even though policies, procedures, and rules regulate behavior; make relationships more predictable; and decrease arbitrary decisions; they impose controls over individuals that are likely to be resisted by those who value autonomy.[74]

Antecedent Sources of Conflict

Conflict may develop from a number of antecedent sources, including the following:[75]

- Incompatible goals.
- Distribution of scarce resources, when individuals have high expectations of rewards.
- Regulations, when an individual's need for autonomy conflicts with another's need for regulating mechanisms.
- Personality traits, attitudes, and behaviors.
- Interest in outcomes.
- Values.
- Roles, when two individuals have equal responsibilities but actual boundaries are unclear, or when

they are required to fill simultaneously two or more roles that present inconsistent or contradictory expectations.
- Tasks, when outputs of one individual or group become inputs for another individual or group, or outputs are shared by several individuals or groups.

Intraterritorial and Interterritorial Conflicts

Conflicts that originate within one person, group, or territory are called, respectively, intrapersonal, intragroup, or intraterritorial conflict.[76] In some instances, these categories overlap, and some types of conflict cross levels. These levels of conflict tend to increase in complexity and interdependence. There is less chance for conflict between people who have their own resources and perform entirely different tasks directed toward completely separate goals.[77] Nurse managers have limited resources, and those of health care organizations are diminishing, thus adding to existing stressors.

Intraterritorial Conflict

Evidence of conflict within hospitals is increasing. Nurses and nonprofessional personnel have gone on strike, conflicts between administrators and medical staff are portrayed in the media, and hospital–client conflicts are increasing as consumers level charges of inefficiency and inattention. Managers at all levels face increased interpersonal and departmental conflicts. Hospital administrators are demanding more accountability and pressuring managers to think in terms of cost-benefit ratios, cost accounting, and marketing strategies. Reviews and audits by external agencies are more frequent and exacting.[78] The contemporary professional expects collegiality, cooperation, and participatory management. Authoritarian management results in worker defiance, undermines employment relationships, and reduces work force capability.[79]

Interterritorial Conflict

Physicians view the physician–patient relationship as primary and all other care as secondary. With advanced practice registered nurses and physician assistants providing primary care in some areas, conflict is not unusual. However, in settings where roles have been defined, conflict has been reduced.

Physician–government conflict was stimulated with the enactment of the Medicare–Medicaid legislation of 1965. The government and other payers insist that care can be provided under certain conditions for a certain price, which challenges the physician's decision-making power in approaching patient care.[80] Strong leadership is needed to clearly establish the boundaries of the payers for care and the providers of care and to define the factors related to the compensation of providers. Changes in the marketplace have increased competition among health care providers, requiring increased productivity, improved service, and conflict resolution to maintain a market advantage. Increased competition has increased the need for research and new methods of patient treatment and management and has increased professionalization.[81]

Patient–physician conflict increases as patients move from submissive acceptance of care to questioning and challenging recommendations. Patients are asking questions about ordered tests and the need for a second opinion. Business and industry—as payers concerned with the economics of providing care—contribute to this conflict by encouraging employees to examine their bills to see that they accurately reflect tests and treatments ordered by physicians and received by patients.

Nurses and Conflict

Nurses experience some of the same categories of intragroup conflict as do physicians. There can be conflict between the following:

- Nurses and the hospital as employer (as attested to by nurses going on strike).
- Nurses and physicians, because of overlapping roles, nurses' desire for collegiality, and changing role relationships as nurses achieve increased levels of education.
- Nurses and lawyers, as nurses act as expert witnesses and are increasingly named as defendants in malpractice litigation.
- Nurses and patients, as patients seek more participation in care decisions.
- Nurses and families, as families buy into the concept of family-centered care.
- Nurses and those in other disciplines during efforts to establish collaborative role relationships.
- Nurses and government, because of governmental resistance to paying nurse-providers directly.
- Nurses and assistive personnel, as roles are being defined and identities of care providers become less clear.
- Nurses and nurses, because of differences in educational levels and philosophies about care delivery models.

Nurses and Intradisciplinary Conflict

Intradisciplinary conflict has the potential to be a serious problem for nurse administrators. The overriding cause of conflict among nurses stems from their major knowledge-assessing modes:

1. The empirical mode, which uses the senses and inductive reasoning.

2. The noetic mode, which uses intuitive feelings and abductive reasoning.
3. The rational mode, which uses defined standards or rules and deductive reasoning.

Each individual has a predisposition to use a particular style or a combination of the three. One research study shows a resulting dissimilar interpretation of reality that may lead to conflict between nurse managers and clinical nurses.

Intrapersonal Conflict and Redesign of Delivery Systems

Nurses are expected to experience intrapersonal conflict as delivery systems are restructured. Their education or employment experiences may cause them to have a preference for a particular nursing delivery modality. For example, nurses may have learned primary nursing in school and used that modality in the work setting. Acceding to the use of another modality challenges their values and comfort level. Research studies evaluating outcomes using functional, team, primary, and modular models are inconclusive and often contradictory.[82]

Nurses are involved in project management, also referred to as product-line management, service-line management, or program management. This decentralized organizational approach uses teams of specialists to achieve specific objectives in a specific time, especially when rapid change is needed. Team membership may cross vertical and horizontal lines. With multiple disciplines, specialists, treatments, and types of cancer, oncology is appropriate as a product line.[83] As rapid changes in health care delivery continue, the incidences of project management will increase. Other models, such as case management, in which nurses use critical paths to direct the care of hospitalized patients, will continue to evolve.

Interdisciplinary Conflict and Organizational Complexity

Guy studied the interdisciplinary concept as it relates to organizational complexity. She compared the amounts of conflict among professionals at a less complex psychiatric hospital and at a more complex psychiatric hospital. She concluded that complexity increases conflict even within homogenous disciplines. Guy suggests that assigning professional staff to interdisciplinary hospital committees should be recognized as the representation of groups rather than one representative view of each discipline. The complexity of the practice, discipline, or interaction is foundational to the conflict.[84]

Conflict Between the Patient's Family and Hospital Staff

Abramson, Donnelly, King, and Mallick have discussed the conflict that may arise within families during the course of discharge planning. They indicate that the impact of illness on the lives of patients and families is a major factor in the development of disagreements. Responses depend on life stage, the patient's age, and factors related to the family, such as degree of change required in the social situation, capacity for role flexibility, and problem-solving skills. Citing the research of Donnelly and King, they note the disagreements among family members but that 7.9% of the disagreements were among hospital staff only rather than between staff and patients and/or family members.[85]

Early attention to staff input for discharge planning is especially important in a climate in which the minimum length of stay for hospitalized patients is encouraged. According to Lowenstein and Hoff, nurse administrators confront major challenges in establishing care delivery systems that stress and promote creative nursing approaches to discharge planning.[86] In Lowenstein's and Hoff's study of registered nurses' involvement in discharge planning in eight hospitals, nurses were divided in their perception of whether nurses or social workers had primary responsibility for discharge planning. Only 88 nurses (39%) had attended an interdisciplinary team meeting. In this situation, nurses are probably experiencing role ambiguity and confusion. The potential for conflict within nursing and between nursing and other disciplines is inherent in this situation.

Nursing Dislocation and Redesign

According to Porter-O'Grady, many hospitals and nursing leaders are indifferent about the centrality of nursing and strongly advocate a decreased nursing leadership role in favor of a multidisciplinary integrated approach. He reports that there appears to be a tacit embarrassment regarding any concerted effort to delineate the critical role of nursing and nurses in leading change in institutional settings. There has been dialogue among health care providers suggesting that the creation of a universal, nonaligned caregiver might be in the best interest of the health care system. He believes that this is flawed thinking and that there must be someone who is concerned with the integration and continuum of patient services.[87] This would include attention to continuous quality improvement, cost containment, and patient-focused care.

Clearly, the role of the nurse will continue to change, as will the various modalities for restructuring patient care. However, the lack of role clarity will continue to be a major source of conflict as health care personnel establish different roles and relationships. Because resistance is a definitive part of the change process, it may become a major tactic for nurses if they perceive their influence diminishing within the developing interdisciplinary framework.

Defiant Behavior

Defiant behavior can create conflict. It produces guilt feelings in the person to whom it is directed. The nurse manager should take the position that the person expressing defiance is responsible for the conflict. Defiance is a threat to rational dialogue; it violates the acceptable protocols for adult interaction.

The defiant person challenges the authority of the nurse manager through obstinate and intransigent behavior. This behavior may be both verbal and nonverbal. Murphy describes three versions of the defier. The first is the competitive bomber, who simply refuses to work. Such people mutter statements that translate into "Go to the devil." They scowl and will walk away from the nurse manager or even walk off the job.[88] Competitive defiers can aggressively undermine the workplace environment and may plan deliberate assaults. They comment about unfair and terrible working conditions, manipulation, and lousy schedules. These behaviors are done to provoke managerial response. When a response to these behaviors is not elicited from the nurse manager, defiers sulk and pout to win the pity of peers or even higher management. The second defier is the martyred accommodator, who uses malicious obedience. Such persons work and cooperate but do so mockingly and contemptuously. They complain and criticize to enlist the support of others. A third category of defier is the avoider. These defiers avoid commitment and participation. They do not respond to the nurse manager. When conditions change, they avoid participation.[89]

Stress

Conflict leads to stress, fear, anxiety, and disruption in professional relationships. These conditions can, in turn, increase the potential for conflict. Stressors include having too little responsibility, lack of participation in decision making, lack of managerial support, having to keep up with increasing standards of performance, and coping with rapid technological change. The costs of stress in 1973 were estimated at 1% to 3% of the US Gross National Product. It is likely, given the current climate in organizations, these costs have risen.

Confrontations, disagreements, and anger are evidence of stress and conflict. Stress and conflict are caused by poorly expressed relationships among people, including unfilled expectations. Stress in patients leads to iatrogenic ailments, complications, and delayed recovery. It may be created by depression and anxiety. Stressed staff members cannot cope with stressed patients. Stressed staff display inefficiency, job dissatisfaction, and insensitive care. Staff, like patients, can develop iatrogenic ailments. Families, like patients, can add to stress when they are not managed appropriately. Increased stress for patients and staff members decreases effective use of staff time. These problems increase patient care costs because they increase the length of the illness and decrease nursing efficiency and effectiveness. In the future, these patients may go somewhere else for care, whether on their own initiative or the recommendations of physicians, relatives, friends, or acquaintances.[90]

Space

When nurses work in crowded spaces they must constantly interact with other staff members, visitors, and physicians. This is particularly true in crowded critical care units. Such conditions cause stress that leads to burnout and high turnover rates.

Physician Authority

Physicians are trained to be the major decision makers in patient care. Nurses want to be independent and to have professional responsibility and accountability for patient care. Nurses spend more time with patients than physicians do and often have valid proposals for altering therapeutic measures. Physicians sometimes ignore nurses' suggestions or indicate that they do not want feedback. Nurses become angry as their self-worth diminishes. Communication fails, particularly two-way communication.[91]

Gender

Gender is another source of interpersonal conflict in that men and women negotiate differently. According to Tannen, men are concerned with higher or lower hierarchical order as determined by indicators of status, such as privilege, income, or reputation. Women place more emphasis on how well they can relate to others.[92] Marcus says that when the importance of status is changed in a profession with a history of hierarchical ordering and expectations (such as men presuming that all women are their subordinates and women believing that all men are superficial), the environment is ripe for conflict. According to Marcus, when a man seeks to "interact relationally, men find him suspicious and women find him clumsy. And when a woman plays the hierarchical game, women see her as disloyal and men find her disingenuous."[93] Astute managers must be aware of the potential influence of gender when they seek to resolve conflict.

Beliefs, Values, and Goals

Incompatible perceptions or activities create conflict. This is particularly evident when nurses hold beliefs, values, and personal goals different from those of nurse managers, physicians, patients, visitors, families, administrators, and so on. Nurses' values may boil over into conflicts related to ethical issues involving do not resuscitate orders, callous statements that belittle human worth, abortion, abuse, acquired immune deficiency syndrome, and other problems. Personal goals may conflict with organizational goals, particularly with regard to staffing, scheduling, and the climate within which nurses work. Nurses who must violate their personal standards will lash out at the system. Violating personal standards is demeaning to nurses and causes loss of self-esteem and emotional stress. Nurses must know that they are valued and that their beliefs, values, and personal goals are respected. Like other people, nurses act to protect their personal or public image when confronted. They respond in terms of others' expectations of them because they want approval. They will defend their rights and their professional judgments. The ego is easily bruised and becomes a big problem in conflict. Defense becomes more heated when one or both parties to a conflict are uninformed or manipulated. When nurses are not recognized or respected, they feel helpless. They feel hopeless when they are unable to control the situation.[94]

Other Causes[95]

Change creates conflict that, in turn, impedes change. People who are not prepared for change feel threatened. They respond by fighting or failing to support the change.

Organizational climate and leadership style can create conflict when different managers set conflicting rules. Disciplinary problems can result from inadequate orientation and training and poor communication.

Off-the-job problems affect work performance, which leads to disciplinary problems and conflict. These problems include marital discord, drug use, alcoholism, mental stress, and financial concerns.

Age can create stress and conflict. As employees age they increasingly resent scrutiny of their work. Clinical nurses cannot always keep up with the physical demands of work as they grow older. They become fearful of not being able to compete with younger nurses and build up resentment that can lead to conflict.

Nurse managers are professional managers and directors of clinical nursing practice. They must cope with forces internal and external to the nursing organization. Pressures include cost containment, effectiveness of patient care, collective bargaining, consumer awareness and involvement, regulating agencies, entry-level qualifications, scope of practice, and mandated continuing education.

Computers are programmed to perform many of the management activities in business and industry. Hospitals are implementing nursing management information systems. Centrally controlled departments are being replaced with ad hoc task forces, project teams, and small autonomous business units. Downsizing of the organization is the result, with decentralization and fewer levels of management, thus increasing the pressures to increase the output without increasing the number of managers. Managers face increased accountability and more demanding performance evaluations. The remaining managers become anxious, insecure, and doubtful about the future, resulting in malaise and conflict. As hospitals implement nursing management information systems, nurse managers are affected.

People who have been discriminated against, such as members of racial minorities, may be especially sensitive to real or imagined slights. They may respond with confrontation, defensiveness, anger, and other conflict-producing behaviors.

Conflict Management

Discipline

In using discipline to manage or prevent conflict or to correct undesirable employee behavior, the nurse manager must know and understand the organization's rules and regulations on discipline. Rules and regulations must be clear, reasonable, and work related. Rules that are unreasonable or reflect personal bias invite infractions.

The following rules will help in managing discipline:[96]

1. Discipline should be progressive.
2. The punishment should fit the offense, be reasonable, and increase in severity for violation of the same rule.
3. Assistance should be offered to resolve on-the-job problems.
4. Tact should be used in administering discipline.
5. The best approach for each employee should be determined. Managers should be consistent and should not show favoritism.
6. The individual should be confronted and not the group. Disciplining a group for a member's violation of rules and regulations makes the other members angry and defensive, increasing conflict.
7. Discipline should be clear and specific.
8. Discipline should be objective; stick to facts.
9. Discipline should be firm; stick to the decision.
10. Discipline produces varied reactions. When emotions run high, conclude the session and schedule a second meeting.
11. The nurse manager performing the discipline should consult with the employee's immediate supervisor. Sometimes a manager's decision will be overruled. When managers work within the boundaries of official authority, however, the instances of being overruled should be minimal.
12. Nurse managers should build respect, trust, and confidence in their ability to handle discipline.

Consider Life Stages

Most organizations will have nurses at all life stages in their employ. Conflict can be managed by supporting individual nurses in attaining goals that pertain to their life stages. Three developmental stages are as follows:[97]

1. In general, in the young adult stage, nurses are establishing careers. Nurses at this stage may be pursuing knowledge, skills, and upward mobility. Conflict may be prevented or managed by facilitating career advancement.
2. In general, during middle age, nurses become reconciled with achievement of their life goals. These nurses often help develop the careers of younger nurses.
3. In general, after age 55 years, nurses think in terms of completing their work and retiring. Egos and ideals are integrated with accomplishments.

Communication

Communication is an art that is essential to maintaining a therapeutic environment. It is necessary in accomplishing work and resolving emotional and social issues. Supervisors prevent conflict with effective communication and should make it a way of life. To promote communication that prevents conflict, do the following:[98]

1. Teach nursing staff members their role in effective communication.
2. Provide factual information to everyone: be inclusive, not exclusive.
3. Consider all the aspects of situations: emotions, environmental considerations, and verbal and nonverbal messages.
4. Develop these basic skills:
    a. Reality orientation, by direct involvement and acceptance of responsibility in resolving conflict.
    b. Physical and emotional composure.
    c. Positive expectations that generate positive responses.
    d. Active listening.
    e. Giving and receiving information.

Active Listening

Active or assertive listening is essential to managing conflict. In order to be sure that their perceptions are correct, nurse managers can paraphrase what the angry or defiant employee is saying. Paraphrasing clarifies the message for both. Paraphrasing can help cool off the situation because it gives the employee time and the opportunity to hear the supervisor's perceptions of the emotions expressed.

Active assertive listening is sometimes called stress listening. Powell suggests these techniques for stress listening:[99]

1. Do not share anger; it adds to the problem. Remain calm and matter-of-fact.
2. Respond constructively in both verbal and nonverbal language. Be cheerful but sober. Maintain eye contact. Prevent interruptions. Bring problems into the open. Make the employee comfortable. Act serious. Always be courteous and respectful.
3. Ask questions and listen to the answers. Determine the reasons for the anger.
4. Separate fact from opinion, including your own.
5. Do not respond hastily. Plan a response.
6. Consider the employee's perspective first.
7. Help the employee find the solution. Ask questions and listen to responses. Do not be paternalistic.

Assertiveness Training

Assertive nurses, including managers, will stand up for their rights while recognizing the rights of others. They are straightforward and know that they are responsible for their thoughts, feelings, and actions. Assertive nurses also know their strengths and limitations. Rather than attack or defend, assertive nurses assess, collaborate, support, and remain neutral and nonthreatening. They can accept challenges and prevent conflict by helping others deal with their own anger.

Assertiveness can be taught through staff development programs. In these programs nurses are taught to make learned, thoughtful responses and to know when to say no, even to the boss. They learn to hold people to a standard and to know when to accept responsibility rather than to blame others. When they are dissatisfied, they do something to increase their satisfaction. Most assertive behaviors can be learned with the use of case studies, role playing, and group discussion.

When they finish their training, assertive nurses will use positive comments to reinforce expectations that others do their jobs. They will use praise and consideration to promote wellness and positive individual behavior. Nurse managers learn that direct communication of support to staff members increases staff job satisfaction.

Assertive nurses focus on data and issues when offering constructive criticism to the boss or constructive feedback to the staff, which encourages dialogue and produces solutions to problems rather than conflict. They ask for assistance or delay when it is needed.

People generally respond positively to assertion and negatively to aggression; however, some people respond negatively to assertion.[100]

Assessing the Dimensions of the Conflict

Greenhalgh has developed a system for assessing the dimensions of conflict. He views conflict as having been managed when it does not interfere with ongoing functional relationships. Participants in a conflict must be persuaded to rethink their views. A third party must understand the situation empathetically from the participants' viewpoints. The conflict may be the result of a deeply rooted antagonistic relationship.

Greenhalgh's Conflict Diagnostic Model has seven dimensions, each with a continuum from "difficult to resolve to "easy to resolve." Once the dimensions of the conflict have been assessed, those viewpoints that fall in the "difficult to resolve" domain should be shifted to the "easy to resolve" domain.[101] Although this model is presented from the perspective of managing conflict in organizations, it can be used in diagnosing conflict inherent in other situations, such as family violence.

Issue in Question

It has been stated previously that values, beliefs, and goals are difficult issues to bring to a reasonable compromise. Principles fall into the same category because they involve integrity and ethical imperatives. The third party must persuade the conflicting parties to acknowledge each other's legitimate point of view. The question is *How can principles be maintained while saving the organization and its employees?*

Size of the Stakes

The size of the stakes can make conflict hard to manage. When change threatens somebody's job or income, the stakes are high. The third party must try to keep egos from being hurt and gain some idea of what will be a satisfactory settlement to the parties. The parties ask: "If I give in now, what will I have to give up in the future?" Action may be postponed, if necessary, if solutions will create precedents that have the potential for causing future conflicts.

Interdependence of the Parties

People must view resources in terms of interdependence. However, if one group sees no benefits from the way resources are distributed, the members will be antagonistic. A positive-sum interdependence of mutual gain is needed.

Continuity of Interaction

Conflict is reduced in long-term relationships. Managers should opt for continuous, not episodic, interaction.

Structure of the Parties

Strong leaders who unify constituents to accept and implement agreements reduce conflict. When informal coalitions occur, their representatives should be involved in finding and implementing agreements.

Involvement of Third Parties

Conflicts are difficult to resolve when participants are highly emotional and resort to distorted irrational arguments, unreasonable stances, impaired communication, or personal attacks. Such conflicts can be resolved with a prestigious, powerful, trusted, and neutral third party. The third party can be an outside consultant, mediator, or arbitrator. The inside manager who acts as a judge or arbitrator causes polarization; inviting a third party makes the resolution public. Third parties must be involved, when the nurse manager, as party to a conflict, cannot resolve it.

Techniques or Skills for Managing Conflict

Aims

When involved in managing and resolving conflict, the nurse manager should aim to broaden the staff's understanding of the problem. Staff members should be helped to see the big picture rather than the limited perspective of each party and to voice their opinions about any number of acceptable alternative solutions to the conflict. The manager should then work on a compromise to stimulate the interaction and involvement of the parties, another aim of conflict management. Other aims include better decisions and commitment to decisions that have been made.

Strategies[102]

Avoidance

Avoidance is a strategy that allows conflicting parties to calm down. The nurse manager involved in a conflict can sidestep the issue by saying, "Let's both take time to think about this and set up a time for a future talk." This approach allows both parties to cool down and gather information. Avoidance can be used when the issue is not critical. Avoidance also can be used when the potential damage of immediate confrontation outweighs the benefits, in which case a third party may be involved. Certainly, the nurse manager as a third party can tell the parties to a conflict: "I want you both to go on with your work while I take time to determine the facts and analyze them." A future meeting should then be set, with a not-too-distant date.

Accommodation

The nurse manager who is party to a conflict can accommodate the other person by yielding and placing the other's needs first. This strategy is particularly effective when the issue is more important to the other person. Accommodation maintains cooperation and harmony and develops subordinates by allowing them to make decisions.

Competition

Nurse managers as supervisors can exert the power of their position at a subordinate's expense. Doing so enforces the rule of discipline. It is an assertive position that does not foster commitment to conflict resolution on the part of the subordinate.

Compromise

Taking a middle ground may resolve a conflict. This temporary strategy should be used when time is needed to work out a permanent satisfactory position. A compromise that leaves both parties dissatisfied is not a good one.

Collaboration

When both parties collaborate to solve conflict, they will both be satisfied. This is especially true of important issues in which integration of insights is needed. Collaboration takes time and energy. A consensual solution wins full commitment.

One of the areas in which collaboration could resolve conflict is that of physician–nurse relationships. The findings of one study undertaken to "examine the personal, organizational, and managerial factors that contribute to nurse–physician collaboration on patient care units," are as follows:[103]

1. There was a weak inverse relationship between collaboration and length of employment (personal factor).
2. There was no significant relationship between collaboration and education (personal factor).
3. Although turnover was low due to the system's rewards, productivity was low also (organizational factor).
4. There was low physician involvement in hospital affairs (organizational factor).
5. There was a significant positive relationship between primary nursing and collaboration (organizational factor).
6. There was greater collaboration on critical care units (organizational factor).
7. Collaboration and trust were increased by open communication, managed conflict, and meetings (managerial factor).
8. Collaboration increased with control of organizational stress (managerial factor).
9. Orientation, in-service education, and discussion with all groups produced positive collaboration (managerial factor).
10. Positive collaboration was related to standardization of work and skills, supervision, mutual adjustment, and group methods, including rounds (managerial factor).

One could conclude that collaboration contributes to satisfaction among nurses.

Resolving Conflict Through Negotiation

Negotiation is probably the most rapidly growing technique for handling conflict. According to Hampton, Summer, and Webber, negotiation includes bargaining power, distributive bargaining, integrative bargaining, and mediation. They are defined as follows:[104]

- Bargaining power. Refers to another person's inducement to agree to your terms.
- Distributive bargaining. What either side gains at the expense of the other. Most labor management bargaining falls into this category.
- Integrative bargaining. Negotiators reach a solution that enhances both parties and produces high joint benefits. Each party looks out for its own interests, with the focus shifting to problem solving, that is, from reducing demands to expanding the pool of resources.
- Mediation. Mediators attempt to eliminate surrender as a demand. They encourage each party to acknowledge that it has injured the other but is also dependent on the other.

Mediation

Mediation is a part of negotiation, but it also is a more intense strategy in its own right. The mediator is often brought into the process when the parties are locked in a positional posture. According to Marcus, the mediator must determine whether it is possible to get the parties to talk and to construct an adaptive process that will move them from confrontation, to cooperation, to resolution.[105] Marcus says mediation includes "premeditation appropriateness, premeeting investigation and party buy-in, party meeting, issue clarification, option building, option assessment, movement toward mutually acceptable solutions, and resolution and implementation."[106] In each phase, the mediator simultaneously engages in investigation, empathy, neutrality, managing the interaction, inventiveness, and persuasion. Because mediation is voluntary, either party can suspend or postpone the mediation. The mediator is without authority to impose a resolution. When a decision has been imposed on one or both parties as a function of legal, moral, organizational, or clinical considerations and there is no room for negotiation, then mediation is improper and it is fraudulent to suggest that there is room for discussion.[107]

Specific Skills

The following is a list of skills that are useful in managing or preventing conflict. Some ideas were mentioned earlier in this chapter. The manager should do the following:[108]

1. Establish clear rules or guidelines and make them known to all.
2. Create a supportive climate with a variety of options. This makes people feel comfortable about making suggestions. It energizes them, promoting

creative thinking and leading to better solutions. It strengthens relationships.

3. Tell people they are appreciated. Praise and confirmation of worth are important to everyone for job satisfaction.
4. Stress peaceful resolution rather than confrontation. Build a bridge of understanding.
5. Confront when necessary to preserve peace. Do so by educating people about their behavior. Tell them the behavior you perceive, what is wrong with it, and how it needs to be corrected.
6. Play a role that does not create stress or conflict. Do not play an ambiguous and fluctuating role that creates confusion among employees.
7. Judge timing that is best for all. Do not postpone an action indefinitely.
8. Keep the focus on issues and off personalities.
9. Keep communication two-way. Tune in to the message, to correct interpretation, and to the feeling level of the employee. Reassure people by listening to them vent. Listen for the real or underlying problem.
10. Emphasize shared interests.
11. Separate issues and confront those that are important to both parties.
12. Examine all solutions and accept the one that is most acceptable to both parties.
13. Avoid overriding your better judgment, becoming defensive, reprimanding the individual, cutting off further expressions of feelings, and monopolizing the conversation. These responses increase frustration and are ineffective management techniques.
14. When conflict is evident at decision-making or implementation stages, work to reach an agreement. Commit to a course of action that serves some interests of all parties. Seek agreement rather than power.
15. Understand barriers to cooperation or resolution and focus on the dynamics of conflict to resolve it.
16. Distinguish between defiant behavior and normal on-the-job mistakes. Defiance is usually an individual behavior. Determine who the defier is, and prepare for the confrontation emotionally and intellectually. Deal with one defiant person at a time. Establish authority and competence. Interview privately; teach, evaluate, resolve, guide, and deal with the defier. Do this immediately, and follow up in two days. Discuss behavior and consequences, including possible termination, keeping calm and steady. Assume adults have a sense of courtesy and cooperation. When challenged, respond on the spot and stand your ground. Then move to a private area or remove yourself from the scene.
17. Be a sponge to a verbal charge by an angry person.
18. Determine who owns the problem. Take responsibility for it as if you own it, and say thanks.
19. Determine needs that are being ignored or frustrations that require recognition and nurturing.
20. Help distinguish demands from dreams.
21. Build trust by listening, clarifying, and allowing the challenges to unwind completely. Give feedback to make sure you understand. Let people know you care and that you trust them. Indicate recognition of other viewpoints and willingness to work to improve the relationship. Be factual. Ask for feedback. Work out a common bridge of "must" items. When an employee has a valid point, recognize it, apologize if need be, and be genuine.
22. Renegotiate problem-solving procedures to forestall further anger, distrust, and defensiveness.

Results of Conflict Management

If attention is given to the role of the nurse manager in creating a climate for productive work by nurses, many of the causes of conflict will be eliminated. Knowledge and skills related to managing conflict when it occurs are essential to the role of nurse manager.

Conflict can be a constructive and positive source of energy and creativity when properly managed. Otherwise, conflict can cause an environment to become dysfunctional and destructive, draining energy and reducing both personal and organizational effectiveness. It can destroy initiative or creativity. Conflict can cause hostile and disruptive behavior, loss of team spirit, and loss of desire to work toward common goals. It can result in deadlock and stalemate. Managed conflicts do not escalate.[109]

Summary

Managing a diverse health care work force challenges the nurse administrator, particularly when considering recruitment, managing work relationships, and dealing with conflict.

A major focus of a theory of human resource management is that personnel should be managed for productivity, that is, for achieving the mission and objectives of the organization. Nursing management not only involves recruiting, selecting, credentialing, and assigning but also developing, retaining, promoting, and terminating nursing personnel.

The population from which all occupations will recruit will change greatly in the first decade of the 21st century. The demographic makeup of this population will shift, causing recruitment goals to change. Nurse managers should plan student recruitment at early stages of the secondary education process. Each nurse manager should work with other health care system managers and with secondary school teachers and counselors to prepare young men and women for careers in nursing.

Nurse managers should create conditions of work that will be attractive, including competitive salaries and fringe benefits, optional schedules, and satisfying conditions of work such as autonomy and recognition. Once nurses are recruited, selected, credentialed, and assigned, nurse managers should develop strategies to retain them.

For high-level positions, search committees are frequently used for recruiting. The implication is that professional workers will have input into selecting those with whom they will work and who will provide leadership. Nurse managers should consider a credentialing process for professional nurses similar to that used for physicians. It is essential that career planning be a major program within each nursing organization.

As the clinical practice discipline of nursing evolves, so will the concept of wholeness. Staff development thus becomes a component of the larger domain of HRD. Business and industry leaders have found that productivity is positively influenced by a focus on development of personnel to their fullest potential. As a consequence, the assembly lines in factories have given way to self-directed work teams. Given responsibility for making decisions and accomplishing the organization's mission, employees rise to fulfill expectations.

Adult education, or andragogy, is the process by which employees are kept updated to achieve both the goals of the organization and their own personal goals. Andragogy is also the process by which they develop their roles as citizens, with benefit to themselves, society, and the organization for which they work. Satisfied employees achieve organizational and personal objectives, satisfy customers, and make an organization successful.

Personnel who do not meet acceptable standards of performance should be counseled, warned in writing, and suspended without pay. When all else fails, they should be terminated.

The relationships among nurses and other personnel, patients, and families offer the potential for conflict. Therefore, nurse managers should know how to manage conflict.

Causes of conflict include defiant behavior, stress, crowded space, physician authority, and incompatibility of values and goals.

Conflict can be prevented or managed by discipline; consideration of people's life stages; purposive communication, including active listening; use of quality circles; provision of assertiveness training for nurse managers; and assessment of the dimensions of conflict.

Aims of conflict management include broadening understanding about problems, increasing alternative solutions, achieving a working consensus on decisions, and genuine commitment to the decisions that are made. Specific strategies include avoidance, accommodation, competition, compromise, collaboration, negotiation, and mediation. In addition, nurse managers can learn and use specific skills to prevent and manage conflict.

Conflict management keeps conflict from escalating, makes for a productive work environment, and can make conflict a positive or constructive force.

APPLICATION EXERCISES

The following exercises can be done in groups of students or employees. Form groups of five to eight persons. Select a leader to keep the group moving and a recorder to write the plan or report. Refer to the chapter text for techniques and skills for assessing and managing conflict.

EXERCISE 8-1

Case Study. You are called to a unit to resolve a conflict between an RN and LPN. They are shouting at each other in the hallway. The RN is the supervisor of the LPN. As you approach them you hear the following dialogue:

RN: I asked you to get Mr. W ready to go to x-ray, and you ignored me. The transport person was here and left because you would not help him.

LPN: I was busy with Mrs. L and could not leave her. Why didn't you get Mr. W ready? You apparently knew about it.

RN: It was your job. I assigned Mr. W to you.

LPN: I do my own work and part of yours. You are the RN. You are supposed to be the leader on this floor.

RN: Don't get sarcastic with me. I don't have to put up with it. I'm going to call the supervisor and report you for your insolence.

LPN: My insolence! Go ahead and report me! I'll tell the supervisor what a lazy bitch you are!

Outline a plan to deal with this conflict. You may use the following format:

1. What is (are) the cause(s) of the conflict?
2. Assess the dimensions of the conflict using Greenhalgh's Conflict Diagnostic Model.
3. List aims, strategies, and specific skills for resolving the conflict.

EXERCISE 8-2

Case Study. During the P.M. change-of-shift report an RN calls in ill and the staffing office says she cannot be replaced. This leaves only one RN, Mrs. K, for 26 patients. Mrs. K says, "If you do not get another RN for this unit, I am going to quit this job. I will not do it this shift, but I will not put up with this constant shortage of help. I don't care if it is an RN, but I should have people with some skills to get the patients cared for. The reason everyone quits around here is because they are over-worked, underpaid, and the hospital management does not give a damn. The place needs to be investigated."

Outline a plan to deal with this conflict. You may use the following format:

1. What is (are) the cause(s) of the conflict?
2. Assess the dimensions of the conflict using Greenhalgh's Conflict Diagnostic Model.
3. List aims, strategies, and specific skills for resolving the conflict.

EXERCISE 8-3

Case Study. A surgeon and a scrub nurse get into an argument during an operation. The surgeon tells the scrub nurse that she is stupid and that he does not want her to scrub for him again. The scrub nurse says that she is totally competent but that he expects her to read his mind. She says, "If you don't quit badgering me, I'm going to sue you and this hospital!" The argument escalates into a shouting match.

Outline a plan to deal with this conflict. You may use the following format:

1. What is (are) the cause(s) of the conflict?
2. Assess the dimensions of the conflict using Greenhalgh's Conflict Diagnostic Model.
3. List aims, strategies, and specific skills for resolving the conflict.

EXERCISE 8-4

Describe a recent instance of a conflict in which you were involved. Was it resolved satisfactorily? Can the group help in finding a better solution? Discuss.

EXERCISE 8-5

Do a library computer search on conflict management. Look at indices of nursing, business, and management periodicals. Prepare an abstract on two recent publications. The abstract should describe the value of the publication to the performance of the nurse manager.

NOTES

1. Naisbitt, J. & Aburdene, J. (1990). *Megatrends 2000*. New York: William Morrow and Company, 16.
2. US Census Bureau. (1999). *Statistical Abstract of the United States*, 132.
3. Ibid., 131.
4. Ibid.
5. State of the nursing shortage. (2000). *American Journal of Nursing*; Buerhous, P. I., Staiger, D. O., & Auerbach, D. I. (2000). Policy responses to an aging registered nurse workforce. *Nursing Economics*, 278–284.
6. Stevens, K. A. & Walker, E. A. (1993). Choosing a career: Why not nursing for more high school seniors? *Journal of Nursing Education*, 13–17.
7. Hodgkinson, H. L. (1986). Reform? Higher education? Don't be absurd! *Phi Delta Kappan*, 271–274.
8. American Hospital Association (AHA). (1980). Background on the national nursing shortage. In *Hospital nurse recruitment and retention: A source book for executive management*. Chicago: Author.
9. National Commission on Nursing. (1982). *Nursing in transition: Models for successful organizational change*. Chicago: American Hospital Association, Hospital Research and Educational Trust and American Hospital Supply Corporation, 41–42.
10. Gray, B. B. (1997, May 5). Another shortage? Bet on it, *HealthWeek*, 20.
11. Editorial. (1993, July 12). *Times-Colonist* (Victoria, British Columbia, Canada), p. A4.
12. American Academy of Nursing Task Force on Nursing Practice In Hospitals. (1983). *Magnet hospitals: Attraction and retention of professional nurses*. Kansas City, MO: American Nurses

Association, 99; Stein, T. (2000, May 1). Respect breeds contentment. *HealthWeek*, 10.

13. Jones-Schenk, J. (2001). How magnets attract nurses. *Nursing Management*, 41–42.
14. Pattan, J. E. (1992). Developing a nurse recruitment plan. *Journal of Nursing Administration*, 33–39.
15. Connelly, J. A. & Strauser, K. S. (1983). Managing recruitment and retention problems: An application of the marketing process. *Journal of Nursing Administration*, 17–22.
16. Pattan, J. E. (1991). Nurse recruitment: From selling to marketing. *Journal of Nursing Administration*, 16–20.
17. Thompson, M. R. (1975). *Why should I hire you?* New York: Jove Publications, 94.
18. delBueno, D. J., Weeks, L., & Brown-Stewart, P. (1987). Clinical assessment centers: A cost-effective alternative for competency development. *Nursing Economics*, 21–26.
19. Sullivan, E. J., Decker, P. J., & Hailstone, S. (1985). Assessment center technology: Selecting head nurses. *Journal of Nursing Administration*, 14.
20. Ibid.
21. Battle, E. H ., Bragg, S., Delaney, J., Gilbert, S., & Roesler, D. (1985). Developing a rating interview guide. *Journal of Nursing Administration*, 39–45.
22. Chaboyer, W., Forrester, K., & Harris, D. (1999). The expanded role of acute care nurses: The issue of liability. *Australian Health Review*, *22*(3), 110–117; Kamajian, M. F., Mitchell, S. A., & Fruth, R. A. (1999). Credentialing and privileging of advanced practice nurses. *AACN Clinical Issues*, 316–336.
23. Rowland, H. S. & Rowland, B. L. (1987). *Hospital legal forms, checklists, & guidelines*. Rockville, MD: Aspen, 17:1.
24. Committee for the Study of Credentialing in Nursing. (1979). Credentialing in nursing: A new approach. *American Journal of Nursing*, 674–683.
25. American Nurses Credentialing Center. (2004). Credentialing and Recertification. Retrieved on July 31, 2004 from http://www.nursingworld.org/ancc/inside.html.
26. Richelson, C. (1991). Update on credentialing. *Nursing Management*, 101–102.
27. Norris, P. E. (1982). *How to find a job*. Fairhope, AL: National Job Search Training Laboratories, 1.
28. Spitzer-Lehmann, R. (1990). Recruitment and retention of our greatest asset. *Nursing Administration Quarterly*, 66–69.
29. Ibid.
30. Berns, P. & Berns, J. (1992). Good for business: Corporations adopt the family. *Management Review*, *81*(9), 34–38.
31. Osler, W. (1992). Retention through a service strategy. *Manager's Magazine*, 18–23.
32. Duxbury, M. L. & Armstrong, G. D. (1982). Calculating nurse turnover indices. *Journal of Nursing Administration*, 18–24.
33. Jones, C. B. (1990). Staff nurse turnover costs: Part 1, a conceptual model. *Journal of Nursing Administration*, 18–23; Butler, T. & Waldroop, J. (1999). Job sculpting: The art of retaining your best people. *Harvard Business Review*, 144–152, 186; Mass, D. (1999). Staff retention: A major key to management's success. *Clinical Laboratory Management Review*, 266–274; Federwisch, A. (1999, September 13). Designer genes: How genomics could change your life. *HealthWeek*, 1; Gray, B. B. (1998, August 31). Get a tuneup. *HealthWeek*, 4.
34. DeBerry, L. (1992). Preselection process for first line managers cuts turnover. *Training*, 80.
35. Ginsberg, E., Patray, J., Ostow, M., & Brann, E. A. (1982). Nurse discontent: The search for realistic solutions. *Journal of Nursing Administration*, 7–11.
36. Burton, C. E. & Burton, D. T. (1982). Job expectations of senior nursing students. *Journal of Nursing Administration*, 11–17.
37. Ibid.
38. P. F. Drucker and D. Karl Bays discuss the toughest job: Running a hospital, Part 2. (1982). *HMQ*, 2–5.
39. Stengrevics, S. S., Kirby, K. K., & Ollis, E. R. (1991). Nurse manager job satisfaction: The Massachusetts perspective. *Nursing Management*, 60–64.
40. Levenstein, A. (1985). Career dissatisfaction. *Nursing Management*, 61–62.
41. Ginsberg, Patray, Ostow, & Brann, 1982; Crose, P. S. (1999). Job characteristics related to job satisfaction in rehabilitation nursing. *Rehabilitation Nursing*, 95–102.
42. Sovie, M. D. (1982). Fostering professional nursing careers in hospitals: The role of staff development, Part 1. *Journal of Nursing Administration*, 5–10.
43. Spitzer, R. B. & Bolton, L. B. (1984). Attitudes toward equitable pay. *Nursing Management*, 32, 36–38.
44. Beer, M., Spector, B., Lawrence, P. R., Mills, D. Q., & Walton, R. E. (1984). *Managing human assets*. New York: The Free Press.
45. Carter, P. D. (1988). Revitalizing society: Practicing human resource development through the life span. *Lifelong Learning: An Omnibus of Practice and Research*, *11*(6), 27–31.
46. Beer et al., 1984, p. 43.
47. Hammerman, M. L. (1988). Adult learning in self-help mutual/aid support groups. *Lifelong Learning: An Omnibus of Practice and Research*, *12*(1), 25–27, 30.
48. Kuokkanen, L. & Leino-Kilpi, H. (2000). Power and empowerment in nursing: Three theoretical approaches. *Journal of Advanced Nursing*, 235–241.
49. Cassivi, D. (1989). The education of adults: Maintaining a legacy. *Lifelong Learning: An Omnibus of Practice and Research*, *12*(5), 8–10.
50. Knowles, M. S. (1970). Gearing adult education for the seventies. *The Journal of Continuing Education in Nursing*, 11–17; Nielsen, B. B. (1992). Applying andragogy in nursing continuing education. *The Journal of Continuing Education in Nursing*, 148–151.
51. Milligan, F. (1997). In defense of andragogy. Part 2: An educational process consistent with modern nursing's aims. *Nurse Education Today*, 487–493.
52. Sanderson, D. R. (1989). Mid-career support: An approach to lifelong learning in an organization. *Lifelong Learning: An Omnibus of Practice and Research*, *12*(7), 7–10.
53. Ibid.
54. Odiorne, G. S. (1984). *Strategic management of human resources*. San Francisco: Jossey-Bass, 5.
55. Rigdon, J. E. (1993, May 3). Using new kinds of corporate alchemy, some firms turn lesser lights into stars. *The Wall Street Journal*, pp. B1, B13.
56. Who gets the promotion? (1992). *Small Business Reports*, *17*(10), 28; Pfister, B. (1999, March 28). Good timing, attitude, key to pay boost. *San Antonio Express-News*, pp. 25K, 31K.
57. Ibid.
58. Darling, L. A. W. & McGrath, L. G. (1983). The causes and costs of promotion trauma. *Journal of Nursing Administration*, 29–33.
59. Ibid.
60. Rutkowski, B. C. & Rutkowski, A. D. (1984). Employee discharge: It depends . *Nursing Management,* 39–42.
61. Dumville, J. C. (1993). Delivering the mortal blow. *Supervision*, *54*(4), 6–7.

62. Pernell, L. D. & Paulanka, B. J. (2005). *Guide to culturally competent health care*. Philadelphia: F. A. Davis, xvi.
63. Ibid.
64. Ibid., p. 4.
65. US Census Bureau. (2000). Retreived on October 1, 2004 from http://www.census.gov.
66. Hawkins, A. L. & Kratsch, L. S. (2004). Troubled units: Creating change. *AACN Clinical Issues*, *15*(2), 215–221.
67. Ibid.
68. Frost, J. H. & Wilmot, W. W. (1944). Making conflict work for you. In E. C. Hein & M. J. Nicholson (Eds.), *Contemporary leadership behaviors: Selected readings*. Philadelphia: J. B. Lippincott, 338.
69. Filley, A. C. (1980). Types and sources of conflict. In M.S. Berger, D. Elhart, S. C. Firsich, S. B. Jordan, and S. Stone, (Eds.), *Management for nurses: A multidisciplinary approach*. St. Louis: C. V. Mosby, 154–65.
70. Bolman, L. G. & Deal, T. E. (1991). *Reframing organizations: Artistry, choice, and leadership*. San Francisco: Jossey-Bass, 199.
71. Ibid.
72. Ibid.
73. Richardson, J. M. (1991). Management of conflict in organizations. *Physician Executive*, 41.
74. Marriner, A. (1984). *A guide to nursing management*. St. Louis: Mosby, 177–178.
75. Decker, P. J. & Sullivan, E. J. (1992). *Nursing administration: A micro/macro approach for effective nurse executives*. Norwalk, CT: Appleton & Lange, 551.
76. Ibid.
77. Hampton, D. R., Summer, C. E., & Webber, R. A. (1987). *Organizational behavior and the practice of management*. Glenview, IL: Scott, Foresman, 620–622.
78. Bertinasco, L. G. (1990). Strategies for resolving conflict. *The Health Care Supervisor*, 35–37.
79. Mauer, G. W. & Cramer, K. M. (1987). Unresolved conflicts entail opportunity costs. *Physician Executive*, 7–10.
80. Wenzel, F. J. (1986). Conflict: An imperative for success. *The Journal of Medical Practice Management*, 252–259.
81. Mauer & Cramer, 1987.
82. Anderson, C. L. & Hughes, E. (1993). Implementing modular nursing in a long-term care facility. *Journal of Nursing Administration*, 29–35.
83. Hermann, M. K., Alexander, J., & Kiely, J. T. (1992). Leadership and project management. In Decker & Sullivan, 1992, 571.
84. Guy, M. E. (1986). Interdisciplinary conflict and organizational complexity. *Hospital & Health Services Administration*, 111–121.
85. Abramson, J. S., Donnelly, J., King, M. A., & Mallick, M. D. (1993). Disagreements in discharge planning: A normative phenomenon. *Health and Social Work*, 58–59; Donnelly, J. & King, M. (1994). Extent and type of disagreement about discharge planning. *Health and Social Work*, 61.
86. Lowenstein, A. & Hoff, P. S. (1994). Discharge planning: A study of nursing staff involvement. *Journal of Nursing Administration*, 45–50.
87. Porter-O'Grady, T. (1994). The real value of partnership: Preventing professional amorphism. *Journal of Nursing Administration*, *24* (2), 11–15.
88. Murphy, E. C. (1984a). Managing defiance. *Nursing Management*, 67–69.
89. Ibid.
90. Murphy, E. C. (1984b). Communication and wellness: Managing patient/staff relationships. *Nursing Management*, 64–68.
91. Wlody, G. S. (1984). Communicating in the ICU: Do you read me loud and clear? *Nursing Management*, 54, 56–58.
92. Tannen, D. (1990). *You just don't understand: Women and men in conversation*. New York: Ballantine, 155–156.
93. Marcus, L. J., Dorn, B. C., Kritek, P. B., Miller, V. C., & Wyatt, J. B. (1995). *Renegotiating health care: Resolving conflict to build cooperation*. San Francisco: Jossey-Bass, 247.
94. Silber, M. B. (1984). Managing confrontations: Once more into the breach. *Nursing Management*, 54, 56–58.
95. Murphy, E. C. (1987). Practical management course. *Nursing Management*, 76–77; American Hospital Association (AHA). (1978). *Role, functions, and qualifications of the nursing service administrator in a health care institution*. Chicago: Author; Zemke, R. (1985). The case of the missing managerial malaise. *Training*, 30–33; Palich, M. A. (1983). What supervisors should know about discipline. *Supervisory Management*, 21–24; Greenhalgh, L. (1986). SMR Forum: Managing conflict. *Sloan Management Review*, 45–51.
96. Palich, 1983.
97. Murphy, 1987.
98. Murphy, 1984b.
99. Powell, J. T. (1986). Stress listening: Coping with angry confrontations. *Personnel Journal*, 27–29.
100. Clark, C. C. (1979). Assertiveness issues for nursing administrators and managers. *Journal of Nursing Administration*, 20–24.
101. Greenhalgh, 1986.
102. Baker, H. K. & Morgan, P. I. (1986a). Building a professional image: Handling conflict. *Supervisory Management*, 24–29.
103. Alt-White, A. C., Charns, M., & Strayer, R. (1983). Personal, organizational, and managerial factors related to nurse–physician collaboration. *Nursing Administration Quarterly*, 8–18.
104. Hampton, D. R., Summer, C. E., & Webber, R. A. (1987). Organizational behavior and the practice of management. Glenview, IL: Scott, Foresman, 635–639.
105. Marcus et al., 1995.
106. Ibid., pp. 341–342.
107. Ibid., p. 361.
108. Baker & Morgan, 1986a; Murphy, E. C. Practical management course. In R. Lamkin. (1984). Communicating effectively. *B & E Review*, 16; Baker, H. K. & Morgan, P. (1986b). Building a professional image: Using "feeling level" communication. *Supervisory Management*, 20–25; Murphy, 1984a; Greenhalgh, 1986; Silber, 1984.
109. Baker & Morgan, 1986a.

REFERENCES

American Hospital Association (AHA). (2002). *Hospital statistics 2002*. Chicago, IL: Author.

AHA Commission on Workforce for Hospitals and Health Systems. (2002). *In our hands: How hospital leaders can build a thriving workforce*. Chicago, IL: Author.

American Health Care Association (AHCA). (2002). *Results of the 2001 AHCA nursing position vacancy and turnover survey*. Washington, DC: Author.

Aiken, L., Haven, D., & Sloane, D. (2000). The magnet nursing services recognition program: A comparison of two groups of magnet hospitals. *American Journal of Nursing*, *100*(3), 26–36.

Bradley, C. (2000, April 17). Building a workforce. *HealthWeek*, *4*, 4.

Bradley, C. (2000, June 12). Taking our data to the street. *HealthWeek*, *6*, 4.

Bolster, C. & Hawthorne, G. (2004). Big raises all around. *Hospitals and health networks* [electronic version]. Retrieved September 12, 2004, from http://www.hospitalconnect.com/hhnmag/jsp/articledisplay.jsp?dcrpath=AHA/NewsStory-Article/data/httn0902Coverstory-salary&domain=HHNmag.

Buerhaus, P. I., Staiger, D. O., & Auerbach. D. I. (2000). Implications of an aging registered nurse workforce. *Journal of the American Medical Association*, *283*, 2948–2954.

Carpenter, J. E., Conway-Morana, P., Petersen, R., Dooley, B., Walters, B., & Wilder, M. (2004). Engaging staff in nursing recruitment and retention initiatives, a multihospital perspective. *Journal of Nursing Administration*, *34*(1), 4–5.

Chaudhuri, S. & Tabrizi, B. (1999). Capturing the real value in high-tech acquisitions. *Harvard Business Review*, 123–130, 185.

Chalfant, A. (1998, August 31). Money isn't everything. *HealthWeek*, 14.

Coffman, J. & Spetz, J. (1999). Maintaining an adequate supply of RNs in California. *Image*, 389–393.

Colavecchio, R. (1982). Direct patient care: A viable career choice. *Journal of Nursing Administration*, 17–22.

Cook, C. (2004). The many faces of diversity: Overview and summary. *Online Journal of Issues in Nursing*, *8*(1). Retreived from http://nursingworld.org/ojin/topic20/tpc20/tpc20ntr.htm.

Cooper, J. M. (1999). State of the nation: Therapeutic jurisprudence and the evolution of the right of self-determination in international law. *Behavioral Science Law*, *17*(5), 607–643.

Curtin, L. (2004). Adjusting to an aging workforce. Paper presented at the Conference on Solving the Nursing Shortage: Strategies for the Workplace and the Profession, June 1–4, 2004, Washington, DC: JCAHO.

Davenport, J., III. (1987). Is there any way out of the andragogy morass? *Lifelong Learning: An Omnibus of Practice and Research*, *11*(3), 17–20.

Derstine, J. B. (1995). Planning for career flexibility. *Gastroenterology Nursing*, *18*(6), 215–218.

Deutschendorf, A. (2003). From past paradigms to future frontiers: Unique care delivery models to facilitate nursing works and quality outcomes. *Journal of Nursing Administration*, *33*(1), 52–59.

Drucker, P. F. (1999). Management challenges for the 21st century. New York: HarperCollins.

Fabre, J. (2004). Improve patient safety and staff retention by mentoring your staff. *Nursing News*, *28*(1) 9, February 2004.

Fitzgerald, T. (2000, January 10). Nurse appeal. *HealthWeek*, 15.

Flaherty, M. (1999, August 16). Steps to success. *HealthWeek*, 20–21.

Flaherty, M. (1998, August 31). A nurse is a nurse. *HealthWeek*, 6–7.

Fuszard, B., Green, E., Kujala, E., & Talley, B. (1994). Rural nagnet hospitals of excellence: Part 1. *Journal of Nursing Administration*, 21–26.

Gray, B. B. (1998, August 31). Future work. *HealthWeek*, 10–11.

Hellinghausen, M. A. (1999, August 16). Looking good on paper. *HealthWeek*, 16–17.

Hellinghausen, M. A. (1999, December 6). Finding their way. *HealthWeek*, 1, 28.

Hensinger, B., Minerath, S., Parry, J., & Robertson, Kl. (2004). Asset protection: Maintaining and retaining your workforce. *Journal of Nursing Administration*, *34*(6), 268–272.

Hutchings, D. (1999). Partnership in education: An example of client and educator collaboration. *Journal of Continuing Education in Nursing*, 128–131.

Institute of Medicine (IOM). (2003). Unequal treatment: Confronting racial and ethnic disparities in health care. In B. Smedley, A. Stith, & A. Nelson (Eds.). Washington, DC: The National Academies Press.

Johns, C. (1999). Reflection as empowerment. *Nursing Inquiry*, 241–249.

Kiechel, W. (1994, April 4). A manager's career. *Fortune*, 68–72.

Kirsch, M. (2000). The myth of informed consent. *American Journal of Gastroenterology*, 588–589.

Kleinman, C. S. (2004). Leadership and retention, research needed. *Journal of Nursing Administration*, *34*(3), 111–113.

Kurec, A. S. (1999). Recruiting, interviewing, and hiring the right person. *Clinical Laboratory Management Review*, 251–261.

Kreitlow, B. W. (Ed.). (1981). *Examining controversies in adult education*. San Francisco: Jossey Bass.

Kress, K. (1999). Therapeutic jurisprudence and the resolution of value conflicts: What we can realistically expect, in practice, from theory. *Behavioral Science Law*, *17*(5), 555–588.

Landers, A. (1998, October 11). Nurses sick of long hours and paltry pay. *San Antonio Express-News*, p. 12H.

Lenz, R., Blaser, R., & Kuhn, K. A. (1999). Hospital information systems: Chances and obstacles on the way to integration. *Student Health Technology Information*, *68*, 25–30.

Lloyd, P., Braithwaite, J., & Southon, G. (1999). Empowerment and the performance of health services. *Journal of Managerial Medicine*, *13*(2–3), 83–94.

Mangan, K. S. (1999). Nursing schools perplexed by falling enrollments. *The Chronicle of Higher Education*, A41–A42.

McGinn, D. & McCormick, J. (1999, February 1). Your next job. *Newsweek*, 43–45, 48–51.

Mitchell, S. (2000, May 1). Raising the bar: Green light for accreditation agencies signals better nursing education. *HealthWeek*, 12.

Moore, A. (2004). Drive for diversity. *Nursing Standard*, *18*(39), 18–19.

Morgan, L. (1998, August 31). Look before you leap. *HealthWeek*, 15.

Netten, A. & Knight, J. (1999). Annuitizing the human capital investment costs of health care professionals. *Health Economics*, 245–255.

O'Brien-Pallas, Duffield, L. C., & Alksnis, C. (2004). Who will be there to nurse?: Retention of nurses nearing retirement. *Journal of Nursing Administration*, *34*(6), 298–302.

Page, A. (2004). *Keeping patients safe, transforming the work environment for nurses*. Washington, DC: The National Academies Press.

Parson, M. L. & Stonestreet, J. (2004). Staff retention: Laying the groundwork by listening. *Nursing Leadership Forum*, *8*(3), 107–113.

Pedersen, D. (1999, February 1). How we work now. *Newsweek*, 46–47.

Platzer, H., Blake, D. & Ashford, D. (2000). An evaluation of process and outcomes from learning through reflective practice groups on a post-registration nursing course. *Journal of Advanced Nursing*, 689–695.

Podeschi, R. L. (1987). Andragogy: Proofs or premises? *Lifelong Learning: An Omnibus of Practice and Research*, *11*(3), 14–16, 20.

Recruitment and retention: A positive approach. (1984). *Nursing Management*, 15–17.

Sloan, F. A., Conover, C. J., & Provenzale, D. (2000). Hospital credentialing and quality of care. *Social Science Medicine*, 77–88.

Snelgrove, S. & Hughes, D. (2000). Interprofessional relations between doctors and nurses: Perspectives from South Wales. *Journal of Advanced Nursing*, 661–667.

Strickland, D. & O'Connell, O. C. (1998). Saving your career in the 21st century. *Journal of Case Management*, 47–51.

Sturt, J. (1999). Placing empowerment research within an action research typology. *Journal of Advanced Nursing*, 1057–1063.

Swansburg, R. C. & Swansburg, P. W. (1984). *Strategic career planning and development for nurses*. Rockville, MD: Aspen.

Workplace trends: Who gets the promotion? (1992). *Small Business Reports*, *17*(10), 28.

Zairi, M. (1998a). Building human resources capability in health care: A global analysis of best practice—Part I. *Health Manpower Management*, *24*(2–3), 88–99.

Zairi, M. (1998b). Building human resources capability in health care: A global analysis of best practice—Part II. *Health Manpower Management*, *24*(4–5), 128–138.

Zairi, M. (1998c). Building human resources capability in health care: A global analysis of best practice—Part III. *Health Manpower Management*, *24*(4–5), 166–169.

CHAPTER 9

The Planning Process

Elizabeth Simms, RN, MSN

We shall not cease from our exploration and the end of all our exploring will be to arrive where we started and know the place for the first time.

T. S. Eliot

LEARNING OBJECTIVES AND ACTIVITIES

- Define the *mission* or *purpose statement* as it pertains to nursing services.
- Use a set of standards to evaluate a purpose or mission statement for a nursing agency.
- Write a purpose or mission statement for a nursing agency. Identify the vision and values to be imparted to customers.
- Define *philosophy* as it pertains to nursing services.
- Use a set of standards to evaluate the philosophy statement of a nursing agency.
- Write a philosophy statement for a nursing agency.
- Define *objectives* as they pertain to nursing services.
- Use a set of standards to evaluate the objectives statements of a nursing agency.
- Write objectives for a nursing agency.
- Define *planning*.
- Differentiate among examples of the purposes of planning.
- Differentiate among examples of the characteristics of planning.
- Differentiate among examples of the elements of planning.
- Describe strategy as it relates to the planning function of nursing services.
- Describe the strategic planning process.
- Describe operational planning.
- Define the *operational plan* (management plan) as it pertains to nursing services.
- Use a set of standards to evaluate an operational plan of a nursing agency.
- Differentiate among examples of strategic and tactical planning.
- Write a business plan.

CONCEPTS: Mission, purpose, vision, values, philosophy, objectives, planning, strategic planning, functional planning, venture planning, operational planning, divisional planning, unit planning, business plan.

NURSE MANAGER BEHAVIORS: Directs senior managers in developing statements of mission (purpose), vision, values, philosophy, and objectives. Authors strategic and operational planning with key management personnel and utilizes on a daily basis.

NURSE EXECUTIVE BEHAVIORS: Involves representatives of all units of the organization in developing and implementing statements of mission (purpose), vision, values, philosophy, objectives, and operational plans. Includes a system for evaluation, feedback, and update of these statements. Develops a strategic plan with inputs from representative personnel of the entire organization. Coaches management staff in developing and implementing operational plans that support the strategic plan. With management staff, performs periodic audits and identifies the potential for the need for change.

Introduction

This chapter discusses mission (or purpose), vision and values, philosophy (or beliefs) as the basic tools of management. Knowledge of their use is part of the theory of nursing management. These tools are part of the planning function of nursing management, and skill in using them successfully is part of the strategy of nursing management planning.

Written statements of purpose, vision and values, philosophy, objectives, and written strategic and operational plans are the blueprints for effective management of any enterprise, including a health care institution.

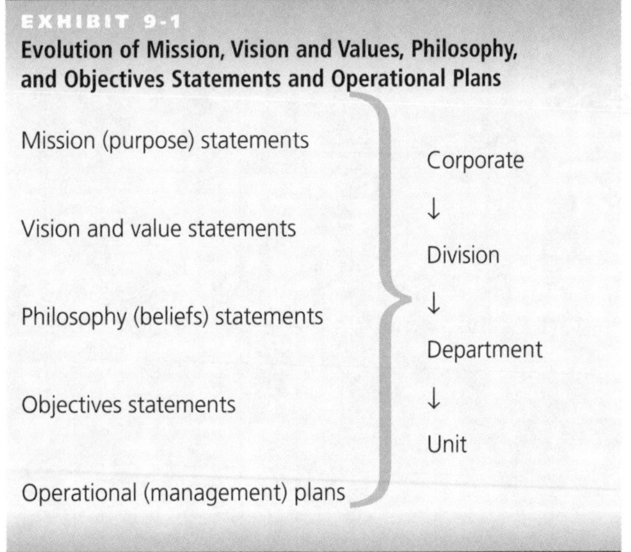
EXHIBIT 9-1
Evolution of Mission, Vision and Values, Philosophy, and Objectives Statements and Operational Plans

Statements	Level
Mission (purpose) statements	Corporate
Vision and value statements	↓ Division
Philosophy (beliefs) statements	↓ Department
Objectives statements	↓ Unit
Operational (management) plans	

These components of planning exist at each management level. Statements at the corporate level serve the top managers of the organization. Statements at the division level serve the managers and personnel of major divisions, such as nursing, operations, or finance. These statements evolve from and support those of the institution. Services, departments, and units each have written statements of purpose, vision and values, philosophy, objectives, and written operational plans that are developed from and support the documents at division and corporate levels (see Exhibit 9-1).[1]

Mission or Purpose, Vision, and Values

Mission or Purpose

The mission of an organization describes the purpose for which that organization exists. Mission statements provide information and inspiration that clearly and explicitly outline the way ahead for the organization. Mission statements provide vision.[2]

The purpose of any organization is to provide individuals with the means to lead productive and meaningful lives. Therefore, the purpose of the organization and each unit should be defined, a teamwork approach should prevail, constituents should be properly trained, and all individuals should be treated with respect.[3]

Every organization exists for specific purposes or missions and to fulfill specific social functions. For health care organizations, this means providing health care services to maintain health, cure illness, and allay pain and suffering.

A mission statement is the first step in the strategic planning process. Industry leaders have learned that customers are the most critical stakeholders and frequently note this fact in their mission statements.[4] Mission statements are used in successful business and industrial organizations to provide a clearly defined reason for being. These simple statements move the organization forward and are formulated for performance, products, and services. They contain statements of ethics, principles, and standards that are understood by workers. Workers who clearly perceive that they are pursuing meaningful and worthwhile goals through their individual efforts are more committed and dedicated than those who do not.[5]

The mission of an organization moves, guides, and delivers the organization to its perceived goal. It is widely held that the purpose or mission statement should be created from a vision statement that describes the things for which the company stands. The vision statement is created with the customer's needs in mind; to determine these needs, one must ask and listen to the customer. *External customers* are those who purchase the products or services of the organization. In nursing, external customers are prospective patients and families, accreditation and licensing officials, faculty and students, and even taxpayers and shareholders. *Internal customers* include employees, both departmental and intradepartmental. Appropriate current events should be noted through reading and meetings, highlighting those events that will enhance the mission of the organization and for which the clinical nurses will claim or share ownership.[6] The mission or purpose statement incorporates the culture of the organization, including strong leadership, rules and regulations, achievement of goals, and the notion that people are more important than work.[7]

Vision

The vision of an organization should be an image of the future the organization seeks to create; it is not an abstract tool, but a practical tool offering goals to be accomplished in terms that can ultimately be assessed. It is a mental prediction of the fulfillment of the organization's success. Employees who participate in developing the vision statement believe in their own abilities and are more committed to the organization than employees who do not participate. The vision statement is shared company-wide so that employees may live the vision. It is updated to keep pace with technology and trends.[8] A vision statement is sometimes considered more strategic than a mission statement.

Nurse managers must find both the vision and the courage to move nursing forward as a knowledge-intensive profession.

Vision, values, mission, or purpose statements are initially meaningful only to their creators.[9] Translated for the community, these statements place value on the way nurses care for people. Nursing education teaches the meaning of values such as tolerance and compromise. Diverse populations should be considered in developing vision and values statements for nursing organizations.

Values

Values are concepts of perceived worth or importance; examples of values are informality, creativity, honesty, quality, courtesy, and caring. Values are the moral rationale for business. Value statements make employees feel proud and managers feel committed. They give meaning to the right way to do things; they give employees enthusiasm and energy. Values bond people and set behavioral standards.[10] At least half of US corporations have a values statement. Agreement on values provides a mechanism for built-in quality; adherence to values makes organizations successful.[11]

Nursing Mission or Purpose

Defining a mission or purpose allows nursing organizations to be evaluated for performance. The mission describes what nursing should and will be; it describes the constituencies to be satisfied. The mission is the framework for the professional nurse manager's commitment to standards.

One of the major functions of a nursing entity is to provide nursing care to clients, which can include promotion of self-care concepts. Thus, the statement should include definitions of nursing and self-care as set by professional nurses.

Virginia Henderson has defined nursing as follows:[12]

> The unique function of the nurse is to assist the individual, sick or well, in the performance of those activities contributing to health or its recovery (or to peaceful death) that he would perform unaided if he had the necessary strength, will, or knowledge. And to do this in such a way as to help him gain independence as rapidly as possible.

Yura and Walsh describe the nursing process as follows:[13]

> . . . an orderly, systematic manner of determining the client's health status, specifying problems defined as alterations in human need fulfillment, making plans to solve them, initiating and implementing the plan, and evaluating the extent to which the plan was effective in promoting the optimum wellness and resolving the problems identified.

King defined nursing as:[14]

> . . . a process of action, reaction, interaction, and transaction whereby nurses assist individuals of any age group to meet their basic human needs in coping with their health status at some particular point in their life cycle. Nurses perform their functions within social institutions and they interact with individuals and groups. Therefore, three distinct levels of operation exist: (1) the individual; (2) the group; and (3) society.

Orem defined nursing as follows:[15]

> Nursing is an art through which the nurse, the practitioner of nursing, gives specialized assistance to persons with disabilities of such character that more than ordinary assistance is needed to meet daily needs for self-care and to intelligently participate in the medical care they are receiving from the physician. The art of nursing is practiced by "doing for" the person with the disability, by "helping him to do for himself," and/or by "helping him to learn how to do for himself." Nursing is also practiced by helping a capable person from the patient's family or a friend of the patient to learn how "to do for" the patient. Nursing is thus a practical and didactic art.

Kinlein suggested that "nursing is assisting the person in his self-care practices in regard to his state of health."[16]

Emerging from these and other theories of nursing are common terms central to the definition of nursing: nurse, patient or client, individual, group, society, nursing process, self-care, and health.

A further mission of nursing is to provide a public good. This purpose should be indicated in the mission statement of the nursing entity. Because it gives the reason for their employment, the mission statement is written so that all people working within the organizational entity can understand and abide by it. An ultimate strategy

EXHIBIT 9-2
Mission Statement of an Organization

SUBJECT: MISSION STATEMENT

It is the mission of the Metropolitan Medical Center to:

1. Provide a center of excellence in the provision of medical care to our patient population, regardless of age, race, religion, political beliefs, or sexual preference.
2. Provide a clinical setting in which physicians, nurses, and those of allied health services may experience enrichment of educational opportunities.
3. Create an atmosphere of innovation in practice and technology to benefit our clientele, internal and external.
4. Foster attitudes of creativity and compassion in care delivery in every person associated with the organization.
5. Develop and fund research opportunities to provide professional growth, and to seek improvements in evidence-based/best practice patient care.

EXHIBIT 9-3
Mission Statement of a Division

SUBJECT: PURPOSE STATEMENT OF THE DIVISION OF NURSING

The mission and purpose of the Division of Nursing supports the Mission statement of the Metropolitan Medical Center. It is the purpose of the Division of Nursing to:

1. Uphold the written standards of quality nursing care for our patient population.
2. Encourage an atmosphere that will foster continuing professional development of the nursing staff through educational opportunities and mentoring.
3. Promote nursing research activities, utilizing staff in cooperation with postgraduate nursing and faculty nursing.
4. Provide a framework for the evaluation of the quality of nursing care delivered.

is to have nursing personnel participate in developing mission statements and in keeping them updated so that they will be empowered to fully support them.

The mission should be known and understood by other health care practitioners, by clients and their families, and by the community. A statement of purpose must be dynamic, giving action and strength to evolving statements of philosophy, objectives, and management plans. Statements of purpose can be made dynamic by indicating the relationship between the nursing unit and patients, personnel, community, health, illness, and self-care. Exhibits 9-2, 9-3, and 9-4 are examples of mission statements of an organization, the division, and the unit, respectively. Exhibit 9-5 lists the standards for evaluation of the mission statements of an organization.

EXHIBIT 9-4
Purpose Statement of a Unit

SUBJECT: PURPOSE: ACUTE CARE UNIT

The purpose of the Acute Care Unit is consistent with and supports the purpose of the Division of Nursing. The purpose of the Acute Care Unit is to:

1. Provide excellence in nursing care through physical, emotional, and spiritual care for clients and their families; they will be afforded privacy, dignity, and respect.
2. Enable nursing staff to act as patient advocates, coordinating care across the disciplines to provide an optimal level of care.
3. Provide every client an individualized plan of care, taking into account cultural customs particular to each.
4. Monitor quality of care/performance of staff on a continuous basis, with monthly audits, peer review, and annual evaluations.

EXHIBIT 9-5
Standards for the Evaluation of Mission Statements of the Nursing Division and Its Departments, Services, and Units

1. The mission statement tells the reason for the existence of the nursing division, department, service, or unit in relation to the practice of nursing and of self-care as defined by the nursing staff and in relation to the service being provided to the community of clients. Once definitions of nursing and self-care have been developed by the nursing staff and ratified by the nursing administration, they may be quoted in the mission statement.
2. The nursing division mission statement supports the mission of the organization. Unit mission statements are customized by line personnel.
3. The statement indicates that the nursing organization exists to provide a public good.
4. The mission statement is developed by the people who will live by it.
5. It includes a set of core values held by the people who will live by it.
6. It is short, clear, and unambiguous; it has a clear meaning.
7. The mission statement describes the organization's uniqueness.

Proprietary changes have brought innovation and competition to the health care industry. They have also brought business techniques that have moved the hospital industry from being facilities-dominated to being market-driven. The corporate structures of for-profit hospitals consider product line and function and focus on mission. This focus has been adopted by not-for-profit hospitals that now look at mission statements in relation to new markets, market share, and diversification. The organization of these new not-for-profit corporate structures can be compared with a chain, with regionalization and integration as links. The leadership of these organizations is dynamic and future-oriented rather than being focused on maintenance.[17]

Good mission statements express the organization's vision and values, evoking passion in the employees. Good mission statements delineate the organization's uniqueness. Effective nurse leaders make sure that employees see, feel, and think the mission by following it themselves. They expect and accept resistance.[18]

Philosophy

A written statement of philosophy sets out values, concepts, and beliefs that pertain to nursing administration and nursing practice within the organization. It verbalizes the visions of both nurse managers and nurse practitioners regarding what they believe nursing management and practice to be. It states their beliefs as to how the mission or purpose will be achieved, giving direction toward this end. Statements of philosophy are abstract and contain value statements about human beings as clients or patients and as workers, about work that will be performed by nursing workers for clients or patients, about self-care, about nursing as a profession, about education as it pertains to competence of nursing workers, and about the setting or community in which nursing services are provided.

The character and tone of service are set by planning that evolves purpose and philosophy statements, one from the other, for the organization and each of its units.

Hodgetts states that "all managers bring a set of values to the workplace." Managers have economic, theoretical, political, religious, aesthetic, and social values. Values are inherent in a management philosophy.[19] Nurse managers must be involved and must reflect the values of the times in their statements of philosophy; their philosophy is crucial to the success of the organization, as a philosophy of caring from management pervades the patient care environment.[20]

Among the contents of a philosophy statement are the core values related to a nursing modality; the need for advanced preparation, continuing education, students, research, and nursing management; and nursing's role in the organization. Philosophy statements pertain to patients' involvement in their care and to their extended families. Philosophy statements also pertain to nurses' rights, including commitment to staff promotion, and nurses' responsibility to the profession.[21]

From a business aspect, the philosophy statement is an outgrowth of the culture. Most Fortune 500 companies have a philosophy statement; it is displayed on posters or plastic cards, in brochures, articles, annual reports, speeches, and books. People who believe in a company philosophy perform ethically, help employees make correct decisions, speak with one voice, have a sense of corporate purpose, and work more productively.[22]

Concerns prevalent in a business philosophy are customers and employees, quality, excellence, growth, profits, shareholders, and the society that the business will serve. The philosophy statement supports the mission statement as the glue that binds the separate parts together as a cohesive, productive whole. It motivates employees to accomplish complex tasks in an intimate, relatively simple work environment.[23]

A philosophy must be communicated zealously and totally supported by top management. As with the mission statement, the philosophy statement is most effective when developed by those who will live by it. Unlike mission and objectives statements, the philosophy statement remains constant.

Exhibits 9-6, 9-7, and 9-8 are examples of the philosophy statement of an organization, division, and unit, respectively.

EXHIBIT 9-6

Philosophy Statement of an Organization

SUBJECT: PHILOSOPHY OF THE METROPOLITAN MEDICAL CENTER

We believe that:

- The Metropolitan Medical Center is a center of excellence in care delivery, in educational opportunity, and in the development of research.
- We believe that we are the leaders in health care in our community; that health care entails prevention and wellness in addition to treatment of illness and injury.
- We strive to provide the most effective and innovative medical services to all clients.
- We must provide continual assessment of the quality of care provided by continuous evaluation of services; we will strive to improve performance based on Quality Assurance oversight.
- We will provide each patient with dignity, provide privacy and confidentiality, and permit the right to make choices in health care based on factual information provided by the medical/nursing staff.
- Metropolitan Medical Center employees are our major asset; they have the responsibility to perform their duties within the mission, vision and philosophy, and policies and procedures to strive toward the highest standard of care.
- Continued professional development of every employee, regardless of role served, is necessary to provide optimal patient care; it is a shared responsibility of the organization and each individual employee.
- Research is both necessary and beneficial to the continued growth of the health care professions; we will foster and fund research in conjunction with graduate nursing and medical personnel.
- We are committed to providing a safe environment to our clientele and to our employees through an active Risk Management department.
- It is the responsibility of the Metropolitan Medical Center to maintain fiscal integrity.

EXHIBIT 9-7
Philosophy Statement of a Division

SUBJECT: PHILOSOPHY OF THE DIVISION OF NURSING

We believe that:

- The philosophy of the Division of Nursing is and must be consistent with the philosophy of the Metropolitan Medical Center.
- Our function within the organization is to ensure the highest quality medical care is provided equally to each patient admitted for treatment.
- Health care begins with prevention and wellness, and must emphasize self-care. Nursing care delivery will be based on the work of nursing theorists and evidence-based practices.
- Our patients must be treated with dignity and care delivered on an individualized basis.
- A multidisciplinary approach to care is necessary to the physical, emotional, and spiritual well-being of our patients and their families.
- It is our responsibility to maintain qualified staff, in adequate numbers, to ensure the care needs of our clients and their families; "qualified" staff must be provided with the means of continuing professional development through mentoring and an active Education Department. The staff bears equal responsibility with the organization for continuing education.
- We must provide the framework, in conjunction with the Quality Assurance Department, for the continual evaluation of standards of care delivered.
- Research within our division is beneficial to patient care and staff development.

EXHIBIT 9-8
Philosophy Statement of a Unit

SUBJECT: PHILOSOPHY STATEMENT OF THE ACUTE CARE UNIT

- We believe that all patients deserve to be treated equally, with dignity and compassion, and provided with individualized plans of care.
- We believe that the goal of health care is the progression of the patient toward an optimal level of health, supported by education in self-care for the patients and their families.
- We believe that a multidisciplinary approach to care provides for complete services to our patients; it is the responsibility of the nursing staff to coordinate efforts among the disciplines.
- We believe that our staff is our greatest asset; preceptorships, mentoring, and organizational-based educational offerings give support toward continuing professional development.
- We believe that family is an extension of the patient and must be involved in the patient's progress. Information and education must be provided to allow optimal health care choices.

Exhibit 9-9 lists the standards for evaluation of philosophy statements of an organization.

Objectives

Objectives are specific statements of goals to be accomplished. They are action commitments through which the key elements of the mission will be achieved and the philosophy or beliefs sustained. Objectives are used to establish priorities. They are stated in terms of results to be achieved, and focus on the provision of health care services to clients. Like the statements of mission and philosophy, they must be meaningful, relevant, and functional. They must be alive. Moore states, "If objectives are presented in terms of what can be observed, they can serve as useful tools for evaluation of nursing care and personnel performance, and as a basis for planning educational programs, staffing, requisition of supplies and

EXHIBIT 9-9
Standards for Evaluation of Philosophy Statements of the Nursing Division, Department, Service, or Unit

1. A written statement of philosophy should exist for the nursing division and each of its units.
2. A written statement of philosophy should be developed in collaboration with nursing employees, the consumers, and other health care workers.
3. Nursing personnel should share in an annual (or more frequent) review and revision of the written statement of philosophy.
4. The written statement of philosophy should reflect these beliefs or values:
   (a) The meaning of the clinical practice of nursing.
   (b) Recognition of the rights of individuals and of the responsibility of nursing personnel to serve as advocates for those rights.
   (c) Selective other statements about humanity, society, health, nursing, nursing process, self-care relevant to external forces (community, laws, etc.) and internal forces (personnel, clients, material resources, etc.), research, education, and family as are deemed appropriate to accomplishing the mission of the division and each of its units.
5. The nursing philosophy should support the philosophy of the organization as expressed at all levels above the nursing division.
6. The statement of philosophy should give direction to the achievement of the mission.

equipment, and other functions associated with the nursing department."[24]

Drucker writes that mission and purpose, as well as the basic definition of a business, must be translated into objectives if they are to become more than insight, good intentions, and brilliant epigrams never to be achieved.[25]

Objectives are concrete statements that become the standards against which performance can be measured. According to Moore, nursing organizations should have objectives for evaluation of patient care, evaluation of personnel performance, planning of educational programs, staffing, and requisition of supplies and equipment. Objectives are the basic tactics of any business, including the business of nursing management. Objectives must be selective rather than global, multiple rather than single to balance a wide range of needs and goals related to nursing services for clients or patients. They must demand productive use of people, money, and material resources and be updated through innovation. Objectives direct the discharge of a social responsibility to the community. Objectives must be used, and one way to use them is to develop them into specific management and operational plans.

The nursing staff, and specifically the nurse manager, must decide where efforts will be concentrated to achieve results. Some areas of concentration have already been mentioned; others may be similar to those related to business and industry. These include marketing and the development of health care services in areas of need. Great potential exists in the area of prevention of disease and injury. Another area for objectives is innovation, which includes the introduction of new methods and particularly the application of new knowledge along with new technology.

Other areas for objectives are organization of and use of all resources: human, financial, and physical. Objectives address the need to develop managers as well as the needs of major groups within the division (such as nonmanagerial workers), labor relations, the development of positive employee attitudes, and maintenance and upgrading of employee skills. Objectives provide for attractive job and career opportunities and for activities to control worker assignment and productivity. They are the means by which productivity in nursing may be measured. (See Exhibit 9-10.)

Management balances objectives. There are short-term objectives, with their accomplishment in easy view or reach; long-term objectives; and some objectives in the "hope to accomplish" category. The budget is the mechanical expression of setting and balancing objectives. The nurse manager plans two budgets, one for operations and one for future capital expenditures. Some priorities will be set with the budget, as illustrated in Exhibit 9-11.

EXHIBIT 9-10

Examples of Categorical Areas for Writing Objectives

- *Evaluation of patient care.* To develop methods of measuring the quality of patient care.
- *Evaluation of personnel performance.* The patient benefits from close nursing supervision of all nonprofessional personnel who give patient care and from continuous appraisal of the nursing care given and the performance of all nursing personnel based on professional standards.
- *Planning educational programs.* The patient benefits from a continuous, flexible program of in-service education for all divisions of nursing personnel adapted to orientation, skill training, continuous education, and leadership development.
- *Staffing.* To establish a systematic staffing pattern for patient care so that all members of each department can function in accordance with their skill levels for the maintenance of continuity of nursing care and management of nursing service.
- *Requisition of supplies and equipment.* To supply nursing personnel with adequate resources to facilitate patient care; to anticipate future nursing needs and plan for the acquisition of needed resources.
- *Marketing.* To collaborate and consult with intradepartmental health team members for maximal effectiveness in promoting health care and disease prevention. New programs will be developed to meet identified needs.
- *Innovation.* To influence progressive nursing practices and research training programs in supporting changing trends that improve the quality of patient care.
- *Organization and use of all resources (human, financial, and physical).* To apply standards for decentralization of decision making and to increase efficiency and effectiveness of staffing and budgeting.
- *Social responsibility.* To support, publicize, and sustain service to the community in health endeavors.
- *Research and development.* To sustain the nursing profession and the organization.

EXHIBIT 9-11
Examples of Balanced Objectives

- *Long-term objective.* Write a plan to develop patient teaching guides for all areas.
- *Short-term objective.* Establish procedures for safe nursing care by having fire department personnel hold classes on fire evacuation procedures for all nursing personnel on all three shifts.
- *Future budget.* Plan with the budget director to have funds allocated to repaint patients' rooms and replace worn and torn furniture.
- *Current budget.* Implement the classes for expectant parents for which funds have been allocated.

Objectives are a fundamental strategy of nursing, as they specify the end product of all nursing activities. They must be capable of being converted into specific targets and specific assignments enabling nurses to understand the desired end point and the path toward that end; objectives become the basis and motivation for nursing achievement. They make possible the concentration of human and material resources and of human efforts. Objectives are needed in all areas on which the survival of nursing and health care services depends. In nursing, all objectives should be performance objectives that provide for existing nursing services. They should provide for abandonment of unneeded and outmoded nursing services and health care products and for new services and products; they should provide for existing patient populations, for new populations of patients, for the distributive organization, and for standards of nursing service. Last but not least, objectives should exist for research and development within the nursing arena.

Although concrete, objectives are not written in stone; they should be changed as necessary, particularly when evaluation proves them outmoded, when a change of mission occurs, or when the objectives no longer are functional.[26] Refer to Exhibit 9-12 for a breakdown of the elements of objectives.

Exhibits 9-13, 9-14, and 9-15 are examples of objectives for an organization, a nursing division, and a nursing unit, respectively. Exhibit 9-16 contains standards for evaluating the objectives of an organization.

Strategy

The theory of a business lies in its objectives, results, customers, and customer's values. Strategy converts theory into performance. In the 21st century, strategy is based on five certainties:[27]

1. The collapsing birthrate in the developed world.
2. Shifts in the distribution of disposable income.
3. Defining performance.
4. Global competitiveness.
5. The growing incongruence between economic globalization and political splintering.

"To create a future worth experiencing for nurses, strategic thinking and strategic planning are required of all nursing leaders. Strategy is the solution."[28]

EXHIBIT 9-12
The Elements of Objectives

- *A performance objective.* The patient receives individualized care in a safe environment to meet total therapeutic nursing needs—physical, emotional, spiritual, environmental, social, economic, and rehabilitative (also illustrates next provision).
- *Existing nursing services for existing patients.* Nurse consultants have been made available from medical nursing, surgical nursing, mental health nursing, and maternal and child health nursing. Their services can be requested by any professional nurse or physician.
- *Abandonment of outmoded nursing services and products.* Universal precautions have been implemented and the old handwashing basins have been discarded.
- *New nursing services for new groups of patients.* Plans are being made to offer consultative nursing services from the general hospital to nursing homes in the area. In the future this will be extended to retirement homes. Both actions are the result of market surveys.
- *Organization for new nursing services.* The nurse manager has evaluated the necessity of restructuring the organization of the division of nursing to provide new nursing services.
- *Standards of nursing service and performance.* The nurse manager has decided to use the *Standards of Nursing Practice* developed by the ANA Congress for Nursing Practice for all nurses within the division.

EXHIBIT 9-13

Goals of the Metropolitan Medical Center

GLOBAL GOALS

Increase patient population
Seek grants to provide funds for indigent population
Market hospital services to community
Create new markets
Expand upon services presently offered
Improve access to the hospital
Contract with medical schools for resident training
Contract with nursing schools for nursing clinicals
Capture maximum reimbursement
Initiate research
Improve efficiency

DEFINITIVE GOALS

A. Increase patient population
   1. Use incentives for MDs on staff
   2. Investigate joint ventures for specialized services
   3. Survey MDs within community
   4. Market HMO
B. Seek grants to provide funds for the indigent
   1. Division Administrators to write for grants
   2. Community-based volunteer funding
C. Market hospital services
   1. Public relations plan
   2. Increased effort for auxiliary volunteer base
   3. "Health awareness" presence at community events
   4. Management people in civic organizations
   5. Create user-friendly website
D. Expand services
   1. What new products can we sell?
   2. Private vendors for new equipment/training
   3. Feasibility study for clinics: prenatal, diabetes
E. Improve access to hospital
   1. New emergency room ramp
   2. Separate parking for emergency room clientele
   3. New main entrance
   4. Acquisition of adjoining land for increased parking
F. Contract with schools for professional training
   1. Contact University Medical school/incentives to students
   2. Contact University School of Nursing/stipends
   3. Contact Allied School of Health/stipends
G. Capture maximum reimbursement
   1. Training: Social Service Dept.–Medicare/Medicaid
   2. Case Management: Facilitate client flow
   3. Audit bills with charts
H. Initiate research
   1. Contact graduate schools/nursing organizations
   2. Contract with private industry/pharmaceutical companies
   3. Create website to publicize results

EXHIBIT 9-14

Objectives of the Division of Nursing

SUBJECT: OBJECTIVES OF THE DIVISION OF NURSING

The goals of the Division of Nursing are to provide the patient:

1. Physical, emotional, and spiritual individualized care within a safe environment.
2. Patient education to allow for optimal health care choices and participation in that health care.
3. Nursing staff who will act as patient advocates, coordinating care among all disciplines for the highest provision of services.
4. Benefits of a nursing staff supported by the Division of Nursing in educational endeavors meant to promote increased knowledge and skill.
5. Benefits of a positive working milieu in which nursing staff's job satisfaction is achieved.
6. Maximum nursing care presence at the bedside by providing ancillary staff to handle nonnursing functions.
7. Benefits from a supervisory staff able to monitor and evaluate care provided by nursing staff.
8. Benefits from implementation of nursing research results.

EXHIBIT 9-15

Objectives of a Nursing Unit

SUBJECT: OBJECTIVES OF THE ACUTE CARE UNIT

The Objectives of the Acute Care Unit are to provide the patient, family, and/or significant others:

1. Individualized care through assessment of the physical, emotional, and spiritual needs in a therapeutic, positive environment.
2. Care based upon the nursing process, with an adequate number of staff.
3. Cost-effective, quality care, with coordination of services by the primary nurse.
4. Adequate information to make the health care choices necessary to the attainment of an optimal level of functioning.
5. Nursing staff held to the highest standard of care, per hospital policy and procedure, with a framework for ongoing evaluation of performance.

EXHIBIT 9-16

Standards for Evaluation of Statements of Objectives for a Nursing Division, Department, Service, or Unit

1. The objectives for the nursing division, department, service, or unit should be in written form.
2. The objectives should be developed in collaboration with the nursing personnel who will assist in achieving them.
3. Nursing personnel should share in an annual (or more frequent) review and revision of the written statements of objectives.
4. The written statement of objectives should meet these qualitative and quantitative criteria:
   a. They operationalize the statements of mission and philosophy; they can be translated into actions.
   b. They can be measured or verified.
   c. They exist in a hierarchy or prioritized sequence.
   d. They are clearly stated.
   e. They are realistic in terms of human and physical resources and capabilities.
   f. They direct the use of resources.
   g. They are achievable (practical).
   h. They are specific.
   i. They indicate results expected from nursing efforts and activities; they are the ends of management programs.
   j. They show a network of desired events and results.
   k. They are flexible and allow for adjustment.
   l. They are known to the nursing personnel who will use them.
   m. They are quantified wherever possible.
   n. They exist for all positions.

Planning is the strategy of an organization and is essential to all businesses, including those providing health care. Planning techniques used in business and industry are increasingly being adopted by health care organizations. Strategy is the process by which an organization achieves success in a changing environment. Beckham states that "real strategy is a plan for getting from a point in the present to some point in the future in the face of uncertainty and resistance."[29] Nursing has only tapped the surface of a business strategy.[30] A myriad of services are available that can be offered to potential clients, such as telephone and e-mail access to information on drug prices, durable medical equipment prices, educational services, research briefs, and a host of therapeutic nursing products. A nursing strategy will outline how the firm achieves its strategic goals and objectives in a competitive marketplace.

Top management has to answer planning questions like these:

- Where do we go and what do we want to become? Such questions seek to define the organization's mission and objectives.
- What and where are we now? The purpose here is to examine and define the organization's philosophy and objectives.
- How can we best get there? The answer to this question will take the form of ongoing plans that include organizing, directing, and controlling concepts.

Such activities constitute the strategy of top management. They are developed into the strategy of the nursing division and subsequently into the strategy of nursing and other business units of the organization. Planning is neither a top-down nor bottom-up proposition. Each level must harmonize its strategies with those below and above.[31]

A focus on development and use of planning strategies gives direction, cohesion, and thrust to the nursing division. Nurse employees involved in achieving objectives and goals are motivated. These goals should be clearly defined and focus on the future without losing sight of the present. Successful implementation of management plans to achieve mission objectives and goals while sustaining philosophy results in productivity, profitability, and achievement. This process is managing, and managers perform it.[32]

Cavanaugh relates strategy to power, indicating that organizational power gives nurse managers the power to do their jobs better. Her suggestions for nurse managers to strategize are summarized as follows:[33]

1. Use the political system to turn personal power into organizational power.

2. Recognize the self-interests of others in the organization and use them in a win–win manner.
3. Diagnose, plan, and execute an effective political campaign to achieve a thoughtful, purposeful goal.
4. Define ways to achieve objectives while helping others. Know people and their goals.
5. Disengage from losing issues and from issues in which you have to defend yourself on someone else's turf. A technique for doing this is placing the issue at the end of an agenda or omitting it from the minutes.
6. Defend your territory.
7. Plan and carry out an offense on issues of your own choosing and commitment.
8. Build coalitions.
9. Exploit opportunities, using situations to your advantage. Go after winning issues.
10. Set up situations to benefit persons who can benefit you. Then deliver the goods at a cost-effective price.

A political climate exists in any organization, and its nature requires compromise, trade-offs, favors, and negotiation. Nurse managers must be political to gain their goals and objectives. Ehrat identifies four considerations of political strategy:[34]

1. Structural considerations. The first major political concept is to learn the history of the organization, including its past struggles and their outcomes. Budgets reflect one of these political outcomes. What is valued by the organization? The successful nurse manager identifies these valued data and operates within their constraints and boundaries.
2. Economic considerations. What are the costs versus the benefits? Give something in return for gaining something better. All departments expect to gain a fair share of an increased budget. To ensure that nursing has equity, nurse managers develop clientele, confidence, a meaningful network, administrative support, and effective platform skills. Nurse managers also exploit their opportunities. In gaining and sustaining this influence, they do not go beyond tolerated limits.
3. Procedural considerations. Timing is important and is learned from managerial experience and maturation. Resolution is needed to prepare for and carry out negotiation and compromise. Impact must be considered with respect to opposition, support, risks, price, and trade-offs, all of which require strategies.
4. Outcome-related considerations. The outcome must meet minimum standards of satisfaction and avoid problems. It must meet some needs of everyone. (Consensus means 70% to 80% approval, agreement, and support.)

Resources in the health care field are scarce, causing political conflicts and power struggles. Nurse managers should learn strategies associated with political knowledge and skills.[35]

The nurse manager moving into a new nursing management position plans strategies for success. From day one, this person arrives early, listens, is polite, and does not criticize his or her predecessor. This nurse manager makes friends with the boss, assumes authority, eliminates nonessentials, trains subordinates, and delegates decision making to them. He or she establishes a psychological distance, avoids gripers, treats all employees as adults, maintains an open mind, and follows good communication skills by keeping people informed and accepting their input.

When conflicts occur, the nurse manager does not take sides. This individual attends to actions that produce quick results, impact the organization, are favorable to employees, and require a small investment. Giving a sense of nursing's mission, its importance, its relevance, and the meaningfulness of nursing work provides vision. This is done by listening, sharing, developing mutual ideas, and enlisting the support of informal leaders.

A research study of the relationship between nursing department purpose, philosophy, and objectives and evidence of their implementation examined documents in 35 nursing departments. Specific indicators used were patient classification systems, staffing patterns, standards of patient care, and cost containment activity. Implementation rates of desired nursing activity varied from 9% to 25%, indicating that a "low rate of implementation negates a causal relationship between references in the documents to desired nursing activity and actual nursing activity." The researchers suggest that purpose statements are sometimes unrealistic and unachievable. The framework for this study should be used to expand the research in this area.[36]

What Is Planning?

Planning, a basic function of management, is a principal duty of all managers. It is a systematic process and requires knowledgeable activity based on sound managerial theory. The first element of management defined by Fayol is planning, which he defines as making a plan of action to provide for the foreseeable future. This plan of action must have unity, continuity, flexibility, and precision. Fayol outlines the contents of a plan of action for his business, a large mining and metallurgic firm. The plan included annual and 10-year forecasts, taking advantage of input from others. Planning improves with experience, gives sequence in activity, and protects a business against undesirable changes. Fayol's concept is that planning facilitates wise use of resources and selection of the best approaches to achieving objectives. Planning facilitates the art of handling people. Because planning can fail, it requires moral courage. Effective planning requires continuity of tenure. Good planning is a sign of competence.[37]

Urwick writes that research in administration provides needed information for forecasting. According to Urwick, investigations should be carried out and their results expressed in concrete terms. Planning should be based on objectives that should be framed in terms of making a product or providing a service for the community. Simplification and standardization are basic to sound planning procedures. The product or service should be of the right pattern. Planning provides information to coordinate work effectively and accurately. A good plan should be based on an objective; have standards; be simple, flexible, and balanced; and use available resources first.[38]

Planning is a continuous process, beginning with the setting of goals and objectives and then laying out a plan of action to accomplish them, put them into play, review the process and the outcomes, provide feedback to personnel, and modify as needed. As planning is put into action, the management functions of organizing, leading, and evaluating are implemented, making all management functions interdependent.

Planning is a mental process of decision making and forecasting. It is future-oriented and ensures desirable probable outcomes. Planning involves determining objectives and strategies, programs, procedures, and rules to accomplish the objectives.[39] In nursing, planning helps to ensure that clients or patients will receive the nursing services they want and need and that these services are delivered by satisfied nursing workers.[40]

Knowledge of the following factors relative to successful planning should be employed by successful managers:

- Characteristics of planning
- Elements of the planning process
- Strategic or long-term planning process
- Tactical or short-term planning process—functional versus operational planning
- Planning standards

Ackoff describes four orientations to planning: reactivism, inactivism, preactivism, and interactivism.[41]

1. *Reactivism.* Reactivism looks to the past and considers technology an enemy. It supports the old organizational forms of an authoritarian, paternalistic hierarchy. Control operates from the top, with plans submitted from the bottom. Problems are addressed separately, with immediate supervisors adjusting, editing, and adding to plans as they proceed through the hierarchy to the top. Reactive planning is ritualistic; in such systems, planning is considered a prerogative of management. Experience is considered the best teacher, and age gives knowledge, understanding, and wisdom. Technological advances of other organizations replace products and services of organizations oriented to reactive planning. Reactive organizations support the arts and humanities, people and values, a sense of history, feelings of continuity, and preservation of traditions. Reactivists do tactical (short-term or operational) planning.
2. *Inactivism.* Inactivism as a planning orientation prevents change; it operates by crisis management, in which the goal is to control discomfort without addressing its cause. Managers are kept busy with red tape and bureaucracy. The effective instrument is the committee, which operates to keep people busy until the work is outdated or success is thwarted by insufficient resources. Knowledge of current events plus connections is more important than is competence. Manners are valued. Inactivists do tactical or operational planning.
3. *Preactivism.* Dominant in US organizations, preactivist managers accelerate change to exploit the future. They believe technology causes change and is therefore a panacea. Values associated with preactivism include management by objectives, inventiveness, growth, permissiveness, decentralization, and informality. Planning is done from the top down, with objectives. The appeal of preactivism is that planning is associated with science, technology, and the future. Because preactivism is based mainly on long-term forecasting, it is often full of errors.
4. *Interactivism.* Interactivists believe the future can be created and therefore design a desirable future and invent ways to achieve it. In this view, technology is valued depending on how it is used; experience reveals problems, and experiment leads to their solutions. The focus is on development, learning, and adaptation. Interactivistic planners may establish a planning period for achieving goals, objectives, and ideals. Goals are considered ends to be attained within the planning period. Objectives are ends desired, with progress expected within the planning period. Ideals are ends that are not entirely attainable, but toward which progress is expected within and after the planning period. Interactivists emphasize normative planning.

The health care environment does not always support reactive planning by nurse managers. It is too competitive, both for patients and for scarce expert professional nurse providers. Nurse providers also resist authoritarianism and paternalism because they want to participate. Inactivism as a planning orientation is prevalent in subsidized government agencies, service departments of corporations, and universities. Nurse managers will participate in such planning in these institutions. Nurse managers fall into the technological traps of preactivism. Plans are frequently made; however, many never become operational. Preactivists concentrate on strategic (long-term) planning.

Ackoff's interactive planning–management model is a systems model that can be applied in nursing management to effect change. A planning board does interactive planning–management. In a decentralized organization the planning board is the nurse manager of a unit, his or her boss, and the employees of the unit.[42]

The following are the five phases of Ackoff's interactive planning–management model:[43]

1. *Formulation of the mess.* The "mess" is the future we are now creating. Formulation of the mess includes determination of the problems and opportunities facing the organization, how they interact, and factors that obstruct or constrain one from addressing them. The output of this phase is a scenario of the future the organization if its behavior and that of its environment do not change significantly.
2. *Ends planning* (idealized redesign) is the design of the desired future. The output of this phase is the idealized design. This design is focused on the present; it must be technologically feasible, operationally viable, capable of incorporating learning, and adaptable.
3. *Means planning* is inventing ways to close the gaps between the idealized present and the mess. It involves identifying potential means, evaluating the alternatives, and selecting the best ones.
4. *Resource planning* includes determining when, where, and what resources will be required and how they will be generated. Resources include facilities, equipment, personnel, information, money, and other inputs.
5. *Implementation and control* involve translating the decisions made in the previous phases into a set of assignments and schedules that specify responsible parties and realistic timeframes.

Exhibit 9-17 illustrates an interactive planning cycle.

Which type of planning is best for a nursing organization? Many nurse managers would opt for interactivism, because it is proactive. Some of the characteristics of reactivism, inactivism, and preactivism are also useful to nurse managers. One could assess the working environment, decide which orientation to planning is most productive, and attempt to move in that direction. A nurse manager could select a style of planning that blends reactivism, inactivism, preactivism, and interactivism. Ackoff and others opt for the interactive planning–management model.

Purposes

The following are some reasons for planning:[44]

- It increases the chances of success by focusing on results and not on activities.
- It forces analytic thinking and evaluation of alternatives, thereby improving decisions.
- It establishes a framework for decision making that is consistent with top management objectives.
- It orients people to action rather than reaction.
- It includes day-to-day and future-focused managing.
- It helps to avoid crisis management and provides decision-making flexibility.
- It provides a basis for managing organizational and individual performance.
- It increases employee involvement and improves communication.
- It is cost-effective.

Donovan wrote that planning has several benefits, among which are satisfactory outcomes of decisions; improved functions in emergencies; assurance of economy of time, space, and materials; and the highest use of personnel. She included decision making, philosophies, and objectives as key elements in planning.[45]

There is no purpose to the planning process unless there is a knowledge of and skill in applying those processes to the work situation; also necessary is skill in bringing the planning process up to the standard set when deficiencies exist.[46]

Characteristics

What is the nature of planning? What is so distinctive about it that requires a nurse administrator to have specialized knowledge and skills? In an environment of changing technology, mounting costs, and multiple activities, there is a need for the chief nurse administrator and subordinate managers to plan. The forecasting of events and the laying out of a system of activities or actions for accomplishing the work of nursing and of the organization are prerequisites to success. Koontz and Weihrich define planning as "selecting missions and objectives and the actions to achieve them; it requires decision making, that is, choosing future courses of action from among alternatives."[47] They see planning as an elementary function of management. In their view of

EXHIBIT 9-17

An Interactive Planning Cycle

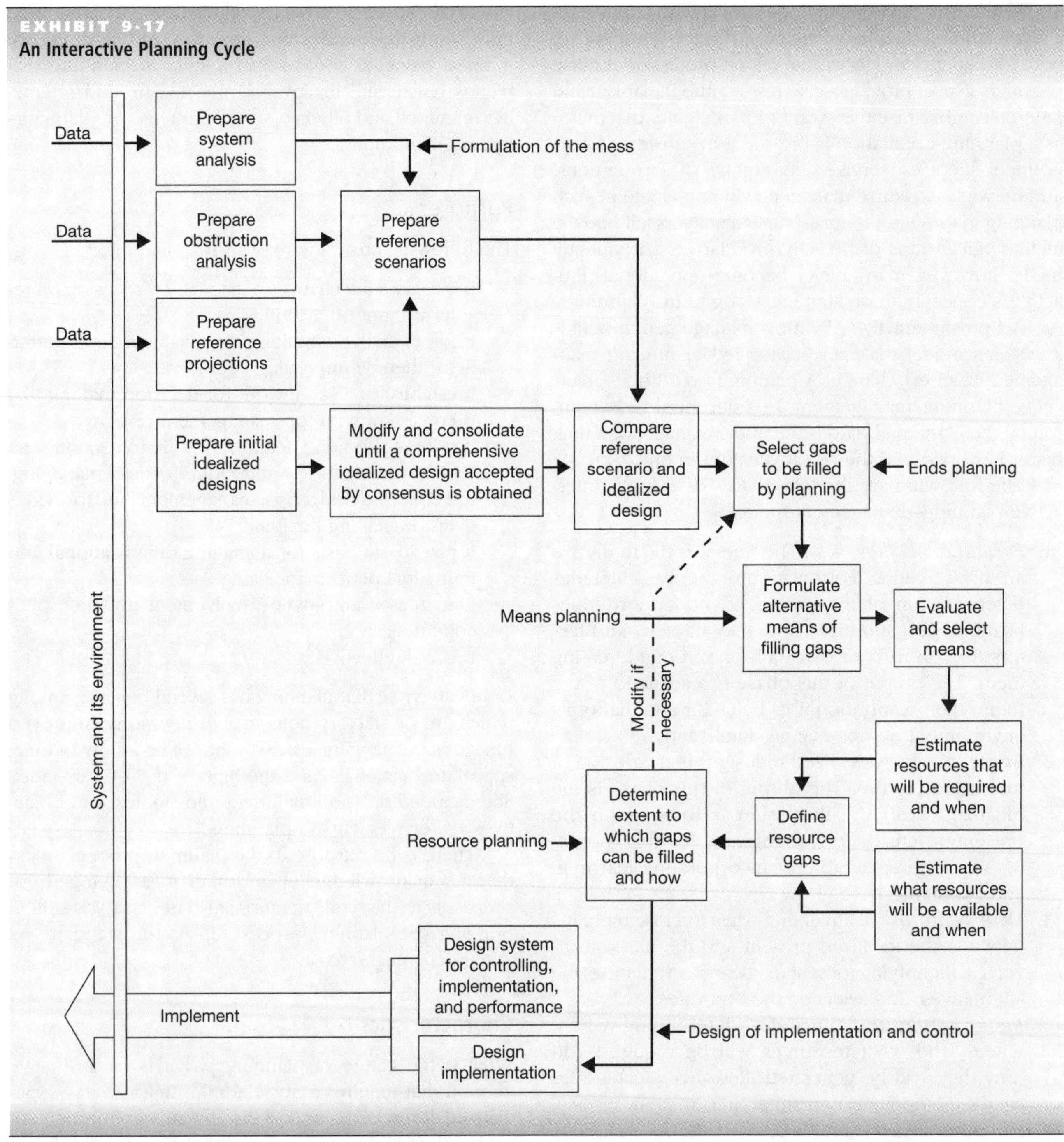

Source: Ackoff, R. L. (1981). An interactive planning cycle. In *Creating the Corporate Future* (p. 75.). Indianapolis, IN: John Wiley & Sons, Inc. Reprinted by permission of John Wiley & Sons, Inc.

planning, nurse administrators avoid leaving events to chance; instead, they apply an intellectual process to consciously determine the course of action to take to accomplish the work. Donovan states that the planning process must be deliberate and analytic to produce carefully detailed programs of action that will achieve objectives.[48]

The nurse manager plans effectively to create an environment in which nursing personnel will provide the nursing care desired and needed by clients. In such an environment, clinical nurses will make decisions about the modality of practice, and nurse managers will work with nursing personnel to establish and meet their personal objectives while meeting the objectives of the organization.

According to Hodgetts, planning forces a firm to forecast the environment, gives direction in the form of objectives, provides the basis for teamwork, and helps management learn to live with ambiguity.[49] Planning should be comprehensive, with nurse managers carefully determining objectives and making detailed plans to accomplish them.

It has generally been understood that top administrators in nursing focus on long-term or strategic planning, whereas operational nurse managers focus on short-term or tactical planning. This process is outmoded. All managers and representative clinical nurses should have input into strategic planning. There should be strategic plans for every unit.

Rowland and Rowland state that planning is largely a process of forecasting and decision making. It is future oriented, spanning time beginning in the present. These authors list the following phases of planning: determining objectives, collecting data, developing a plan of action, setting goals, and evaluating.[50]

Planning involves the collection, analysis, and organization of many kinds of data that will be used to determine both the nursing care needs of patients and the management plans that will provide the resources and processes to meet those needs. Accepting that nursing is a clinical practice discipline providing a human service, nurse managers plan to nurture the practitioners who provide the service.

The following are examples of data that need to be collected and analyzed for planning purposes:

1. Daily average patient census
2. Bed capacity and percentage of occupancy
3. Average length of stay
4. Number of births
5. Number of operations
6. Trends in patient populations
   a. Diagnoses
   b. Age groups
   c. Acuity of illness
   d. Physical dependency
7. Trends in technology
   a. Diagnostic procedures
   b. Therapeutic procedures
8. Environmental analysis
   a. Internal Forces impacting nursing: availability of nurses, turnover, other departments, delivery systems (including nursing modalities), theory-based practice, and physicians
   b. External Forces impacting nursing: government, education, accreditation bodies, third-party payers, and others
   c. Trends in health care and in nursing, including changes in characteristics
   d. Threats to the nursing profession
   e. Opportunities for the nursing profession

Exhibit 9-18 demonstrates examples of data that might be collected and analyzed for planning purposes by nursing managers.

Data on diagnostic and therapeutic procedures will be used to plan for new procedures, to revise old procedures, and to make new procedures known to nursing personnel; the preceding list is certainly not exhaustive.

Planning, a dynamic organizational process, has the characteristics of an open system. Planning does the following:

- Leads to success rather than failure.
- Prevents crisis and panic, which are costly and chaotic, distort achievement, and are dominated by a single person. Planning improves nursing division performance.
- Identifies future opportunities and expectations based on conditions through forecasting techniques that range from simple to complex.

EXHIBIT 9-18
Planning Data for Nurse Managers

- Live births have decreased 30% in the 3 years since the institution of a family planning program.
- Sixty-three percent of live births are discharged within a 24-hour period.
- The number of deliveries with complications has increased from 210 to 257 in 1 year.
- A new cardiac catheterization laboratory has been completed.
- The hospital planning board has decided to coordinate with other hospitals in the area to consolidate specialty services for newborn care, cardiovascular surgery, and neuroscience services.
- Enrollment of students for clinical nursing affiliation has increased from 450 to 792 in 1 year.
- Enrollment of students in the nursing cooperative education program has increased from 102 to 187 students.
- Medicare reimbursement pays $__ per patient for a day of home care.
- Early discharge has decreased average daily census from 381 to 304.
- Patient acuity has increased by 10.6 percentage points overall.

Simple forecasting techniques follow the process of gathering data and analyzing them to determine alternative decisions and the effects each decision will produce. Strengths, weaknesses, opportunities, and threats are part of this analysis, which leads to decision, choice, and implementation. In complex forecasting, computer-based mathematical models are available that are becoming less expensive, require a lot of time and specialized skills, and extend from 3 to 15 years. New simulation models are constantly improving and are essential to modern planning.

Planning rests on logical, reflective thinking that is neither cast in concrete nor all encompassing. If needed, leadership or top management will effect change to undertake effective planning. Leadership should obtain input from all levels to ensure success through format, procedures, time frames, maintenance, and input review.

Planning is the key element of nursing that gives it direction, cohesion, and thrust. It causes all nursing personnel to focus on goals and objectives and stimulates their motivation.

Through the planning process, nurse managers select and retain the elements of past and present plans that work. They focus on the future, and they implement and evaluate. Thus, they successfully manage nursing personnel and material resources to achieve the objectives of the nursing enterprise.

Elements

Although planning is characterized as a conceptual or thinking process, it produces readily identifiable specific elements, including written statements of mission or purpose, philosophy, objectives, and detailed management or operational plans. Operational plans are the blueprints by which the purpose, philosophy, and objectives are put into measurable actions. Management or operational plans include decision-making and problem-solving processes that include strategies, policies, and procedures.

The nursing division's strategic and operational plans are road maps that describe the business by name and location. Nurse managers will make them informative by including a summary of the work of the division. The summary describing the nursing division will include enough information to give outsiders a bird's-eye view of its totality, such as the nursing products and services provided (by quantity), admissions, discharges, patient days, number of patients by acuity categories, research projects, educational programs, students, outpatient visits, and other products and services. The description will summarize marketing activities of the nursing division, including total revenues and expenses, and will describe the managerial style of the division and its impact on employees, which will be related to the organizational plan of the division of nursing.

Planning is the assessment of the nursing division's strengths and weaknesses, covering factors that affect performance and facilitate or inhibit the achievement of objectives. This assessment process will have both long- and short-term objectives of its own. For example, if the clinical promotion ladder is a strength in nurse retention but is weakly applied by selective nurse managers, the problem will be addressed by written objectives.

Planning entails formulation of planning premises by extrapolating assumptions from the information analyzed.[51] If data indicate that nurses will be in increased supply because of increased enrollments in schools of nursing or in short supply as a result of increased opportunities in other fields, these findings should be translated into a premise. Other premises evolve related to increased salaries, benefits, and improved working conditions. These premises will lead to further premises for marketing a career in nursing to high-school students and persons changing careers.

Planning entails writing specific, useful, realistic objectives (the why) that will reflect both strategic and operational goals for the division of nursing and its personnel. Objectives become the reasons for an operational nursing management plan (the what), which will detail the activities to be performed, the time frames for their accomplishment (the when), the persons responsible for accomplishing the activities (the who), and strategies for dealing with technical, economic, social, and political aspects. These operational plans will have control systems for monitoring performance and providing feedback. They will address the budget.

In addition to the previous elements of planning, Meier indicates that good management begins "with a coordinated purposeful organization of people who collectively on a functional responsibility basis" do the following:[52]

- Plan the organization
- Provide personnel
- Provide facilities
- Provide capital
- Set performance standards
- Develop management information systems
- Activate people

Good management keeps the nursing agency successful, ensuring its growth, success, and direction and a return on investment in the future. It is the responsibility of the nurse manager to prepare a plan carefully. Beyers recommends that nurse executives be involved in the following elements of strategy planning:[53]

1. Product/market planning
2. Business unit planning
3. Shared resource planning
4. Shared concern planning
5. Corporate-level planning

Nursing in all areas, clinical and managerial, must consider competition. The patient will go where there is higher-quality nursing care, which results from effectively planned and managed change. Nurse educators should perform market surveys to determine the nursing products and services that consumers want.[54] This activity itself will constitute change and will result in changes.

Considering the theory of the business of the health care organization and of nursing, what practices or people need to be abandoned? This may include products, services, markets, distribution channels, and every end user who does not fit the theory of the business. End users do not need many organizations to get information; they use the Internet to obtain information on providers and services. Nursing's goal is to improve this information and these services in the interest of survival and progress; the opportunity is with maintaining physical and mental functioning of individuals and populations. Drucker suggests managers look at windows of opportunity:[55]

- The organization's own unexpected successes and failures, as well as the unexpected successes and failures of the organization's competitors.
- Incongruities, especially in the process, whether of production or distribution, or in customer behavior.
- Process needs.
- Changes in industry and market structures.
- Changes in demographics.
- Changes in meaning and perception.
- New knowledge.

Strategic Planning

Drucker defines strategic planning as "a continuous, systematic process of making risk-taking decisions today with the greatest possible knowledge of their effects on the future; organizing efforts necessary to carry out these decisions and evaluating results of these decisions against expected outcome through reliable feedback mechanisms."[56]

Nursing administrators can increase effectiveness through strategic planning, which can promote professional nursing practice and the long-term goals of the organization and the division of nursing. Clear, complete plans are developed in seven areas of key results, designed to include standards of performance which will challenge and inspire:[57]

1. Client satisfaction
2. Productivity
3. Innovation
4. Staff development
5. Budget goals
6. Quality
7. Organizational climate

Strategic planning in nursing is concerned with what nursing should be doing. Its purpose is to improve allocation of scarce resources, including time and money, and to manage the agency for performance. Strategic planning provides strategic forecasting from one to more than 20 years. It should involve top nurse managers and representatives of all levels of nursing management and practice; including input from clinical nursing personnel promotes professional satisfaction throughout the nursing department. It will include analysis of factors such as projected technological advances, the internal and external environments, the nursing and health care market and industry, the economics of nursing and health care, availability of human and material resources, and judgments of top management.[58]

The strategic planning process is used to acquire and develop new health care services and product lines, including new nursing services and products. Strategic planning is also used to divest outdated services and products. Both activities present moral and ethical dilemmas for the managers and practitioners of nursing. Strategic planning can foster better goals, better corporate values, and better communication about corporate direction. It can lead to changes in operation, management, and organization. Strategic planning can produce better management strategy and analysis and can forecast and mute external threats.

The process of strategic planning is more important than the plan itself. The process serves to give planners a sense of direction, involves everyone, and enables unexpected opportunities to be seized and unexpected crises to be dealt with.[59]

"Environmental scans" are tools of the strategic planning process. These scans include identification of future trends, risks, and opportunities. Environmental scans also identify projected governmental, demographic, and social changes that will affect nursing strategic planning in an era of health care reform, aging population, single parenthood, drug use, crime and violence, and problems in the education system.[60]

Odiorne recommends the following process for crafting strategic plans:[61]

1. Identify the major problems of your organization to determine where you are headed and where you want to be. This process is called *gap analysis*. This technique examines markets, products, customers, employees, finances, technology, and community relations. Cabinets or task forces from each area may be helpful in performing gap analysis and identifying major problems.
2. Examine outside influences that relate to the key problems of your organization. Focus on the few major issues.
3. List the critical issues, that is, those that affect the entire organization, have long-term impact, and are based on irrefutable evidence rather than media hype.
4. Rank the critical issues according to their importance to your organization, and plan accordingly: "must do," "to do," and "important, but not urgent." Then divide these critical issues into "success producers" and "failure preventers."
5. Decide the issues critical to all organization managers.
6. Include time in the budget.

Exhibit 9-19 lists ways in which strategic planning can be used to improve management. The process of strategic planning has several phases, as summarized in Exhibit 9-20.

Strategic planning includes both planning of the process and strategy for implementing the plan. During the strategic planning process, analysis of the business environment and the internal capabilities of the organization for producing a product or service suited to success in the business environment are analyzed. Goals and strategies are also set during the planning process.[62]

Peters believes that strategic planning should be a line exercise rather than a staff one. The focus should be on building a work force that is well trained, flexible, and quality conscious.[63] Strategic plans should be developed from the bottom up, the front line where business occurs. The written plan should be shared with everyone and should not be slavishly followed since it will be constantly affected by change and should be modified every year.[64]

Obviously, with constant, quick changes in markets and operations, time management is vital to strategic planning. Strategic plans should be capable of being quickly made and changed.

Implementation of strategic plans includes strategies related to proper activities, organizational structure, company resources, and support systems. The various strategic plans of the organization should be linked to avoid internal conflicts. These links include operations, finance, human relations, marketing, budgeting, and personal action. All the elements of a strategic plan make up a system, and these elements of a system need constant monitoring for their success.[65]

Strategic, or long-term, planning came into vogue after World War II and is widely used in business and industry. It is becoming prevalent in the health care world because of technological change, modernization of the industry, increased government roles, and increased complexity of nursing management. In strategic planning, nurse managers are required to manage in the future tense by defining the future of nursing in areas such as setting objectives, developing an organization to achieve those objectives, allocating resources, and implementing objectives through specific policies and plans. He or she must continually evaluate and provide feedback for accomplishing these objectives and developing new strategic plans with new objectives that include planning for research use in nursing practice.[66]

A strategic plan is coldly objective in evaluating what the nursing business is and what it will be. It does not leave success to chance, and it prevents the status quo from paralyzing nursing progress. Strategic planning leads to strategic management and becomes an integral

EXHIBIT 9-19
How Strategic Planning Can Be Used to Improve Nursing Management

- To provide accountability and monitoring of performance; to tie merit to performance.
- To set up more formal planning programs and require divisional and unit planning.
- To integrate strategic plans with operational and financial plans.
- To think and concentrate more on strategic issues.
- To improve knowledge of and training in strategic planning.
- To increase top management involvement and commitment.
- To improve focus on competition, market segments, and external factors.
- To improve communication from top administration and nursing management.
- To allow better execution of plans.
- To be more realistic and rationalize and vacillate less.
- To improve the development of nursing management strategies.
- To improve the development and communication of nursing management goals.
- To put less emphasis on raw numbers.
- To anticipate the future and plan for it.
- To develop the annual budget.
- To focus on quality outputs that will improve nurse performance and productivity, decrease losses, and increase return on equity.

EXHIBIT 9-20

Summary of Phases of Strategic Planning Process

PHASE 1
THE MISSION AND THE CREED

Develop statements that define the work, the aims, and the character of the division of nursing. These include idea statements of shared values and beliefs. They are called mission (or purpose) and creed (or philosophy) statements, and relate to personnel, patients, community, and all other potential customers.

PHASE 2
DATA COLLECTION AND ANALYSIS

Collect and analyze data about the health care industry and nursing. Such data should include internal forces that define the work and affect employees, clients, stockholders, and creditors; technological advances; threats; opportunities to improve growth and productivity; external forces such as competition, communities, governmental and political issues, and legal requirements; marketing and public relations or image; trends in the physical and social work environments; and communication. Use simple and complex forecasting techniques including trend lines, group consensus, nominal group process, and a qualitative decision matrix that uses probabilities based on conditions of certainty, risk, and uncertainty.

PHASE 3
ASSESS STRENGTHS AND WEAKNESSES

Define those factors from the data analysis that influence management of the division of nursing. List them as strengths/opportunities that will facilitate effectiveness and achievement of goals and objectives or as weaknesses/threats that will impede achieving goals and objectives. Define the current position and strength of the unit.

PHASE 4
GOALS AND OBJECTIVES

Write realistic and general statements of goals. Break the goals down into concrete written statements of objectives the division of nursing intends to accomplish in the next 3 to 5 years.

PHASE 5
STRATEGIES

Identify untoward conditions that could develop in achieving each objective. Note administrative actions to avoid or manage them. Use this information to modify goals and objectives, making contingency plans for alternative actions. Define the organization needed for implementing strategic plans. It should be interactive if cross-functional activities are involved—a matrix organization.

PHASE 6
TIMETABLE

Develop a timetable for accomplishing each objective. Identify by geographic units as well. This phase will produce or become part of the plans.

PHASE 7
OPERATIONAL AND FUNCTIONAL PLANS

Provide guidelines or general instructions that lead functional and operational nurse managers to develop action plans to implement the goals and objectives. These will include detailed actions, policies, practices, communication and feedback, controlling and evaluation plans, budgets, timetables, and persons to be held accountable.

PHASE 8
IMPLEMENTATION

Put the plans to work.

PHASE 9
EVALUATION

Provide for formative evaluation reports before, during, and after the implementation of operational plan. Provide for summative evaluation that is quantified. Report actual versus expected results. Evaluate the strategic mission, and plan frequently. Provide continuous feedback that can be used to modify and update the plan. Use people who implement the plan to evaluate it.

part of thinking in all management operations, including budgeting, information, compensation, organization, leadership development, patient education, and decision support systems.[67]

One of the benefits of strategic planning is that it gives a sense of direction to the managers and practitioners of nursing within the organization. The strategic plan becomes a flexible control mechanism that can be modified to deal with variables, conserve resources, and provide professional satisfaction. The strategic plan deals concretely with complex projects or programs in multistage time sequences.[68]

Conclusions About the Strategic Planning Process

Strategic planning is often considered to be a goal-setting process that is largely carried out by top management. There are many instances of long-term plans being made but fewer instances of their having been put to use. Operating nurse managers need to be trained in the strategic planning process; include techniques to involve operational managers and thereby commit them to decisions. Development of global goals and strategies broadens the identification and solution of problems, reducing threats to and unveiling opportunities for the organization.

The demonstrated usefulness of scientific planning will influence the behavior of operating managers. Rewards, in the form of both pay and praise, will motivate these operating managers.

Strategic planning has many benefits. It provides for objective consideration of strategic choices or options that are better matched with organizational goals and objectives. With strategic planning, the outlook becomes future-oriented, resources are allocated systematically, and rapid change is accommodated.[69] Strategic plans must be dynamic to take advantage of these benefits, projecting trends and directions. These plans are the blueprints that are to be updated as the environment changes the phases and stages in the process of strategic planning (summarized in Exhibit 9-20).

A cyclic model of strategic planning provides for continuous assessment of an organization's mission, values, vision, and primary strategies. This assessment is based on feedback from benchmark analysis, shareholder impact, and progress in implementation of strategies.[70]

If they are to survive, urban health care organizations will have to do strategic planning similar to that done by many rural hospitals. This will include the following:[71]

- Involvement of outside organizations in fostering community change.
- A high degree of community commitment and investment in all stages of the process.
- Comprehensive identification of problems in the health care system by outside consultants.
- The use of periodic meetings of communities confronting similar issues.
- Identification and development of local leadership.
- Enhancing teamwork among local health care providers.
- Development of conflict-resolution mechanisms within health care organizations.

Health care institutions have to make global competitiveness a strategic goal. With the world awash in "virtual money" in portfolios of investments, health care leaders have responsibility for institutional investments of endowment funds. For-profit institutions are a part of people's investment portfolios.[72] Nurse leaders should take advantage of this situation through the strategic planning process.

Functional and Operational Planning

Objectives must be converted into actions, that is, activities, assignments, and deadlines, all with clear accountability. The action level is where nurse managers eliminate the old and plan for the new. It is where time is put into perspective and new and different methods can be tried. The action level is where nurse managers answer these questions over and over again: What is it? What will it be? What should it be?

An *operational plan* is the written blueprint for achieving objectives; it is the organization and direction of the delivery of nursing care. It includes planning to create a budget; to create an effective organizational structure that will encompass a quality monitoring process; and to direct nurse leaders, an administrative staff, and new programs.[73]

The operational plan does the following:

- Specifies the activities and procedures that will be used.
- Sets timetables for the achievement of objectives.
- Tells who the responsible persons are for each activity and procedure.
- Describes ways of preparing personnel for jobs and procedures for evaluating patient care.
- Specifies the records that will be kept and the policies needed.
- Gives individual mangers freedom to accomplish their objectives and those of the institution, division, department, or unit.

The operational plan is sometimes called a *management plan* (see Exhibits 9-21 and 9-22).

Nursing planning performed at a service or departmental level is referred to as *functional planning*. It generally relates to a specialty service within a nursing division. For example, the staff development director would be included in development of the strategic plan but would develop operational plans for staff development as a whole and for specific services or units. Likewise, the director of a home health care agency would assist in developing the strategic plan for the company but would develop agency mission, philosophy, goals, objectives, and operational plans. With decentralization each nurse manager would develop a strategic plan for his or her unit to be integrated into the organization's strategic plan.

Operational plans are everyday working management plans developed from both long-term objectives and the strategic planning process and short-term or tactical plans. In development of operational objectives, new strategic objectives can emerge, or old ones can be modified or discarded. Strategic and tactical plans are made into operational plans and carried out at all levels of nursing management.

EXHIBIT 9-21

Operational Plan

OBJECTIVE

The clients receive skilled nursing services to meet their total individual needs as diagnosed by professional nurses. This process is systematic, beginning with the gathering of base data, and it is planned, implemented, evaluated, and revised on a continual basis. It covers physical, emotional, spiritual, environmental, social, economic, and rehabilitational needs and includes health teaching involved in the planning of total client care. Its ultimate goal is to assist clients to, or return them to, optimal health status and independence as quickly as possible.

ACTIONS	TARGET DATES	ACCOMPLISHMENTS
Institute primary care nursing	January 1–June 30	Assigned to Ms. Scott. Decision made to attempt to use self-care concepts of Orem: (1) definition, and (2) nursing systems.
1. Assign problem of overall development of a plan	January 31	
2. Assign development of a self-care concept for application using Orem and Kinlein as references	February 15	January 19: Assigned to Ms. Longez. In a discussion with Ms. Scott and Ms. Longez, the decision was made to investigate application of self-care using the nursing process as described by Kinlein. The nursing staff were particularly interested in the nursing history process described by Kinlein. Ms. Longez has added this dimension to her assignment. She has requested Mr. Jarmann be assigned to assist her, and he has agreed.
3. Organize resources	February 28	February 5: Ms. Scott has just updated me on the project. A good portion of her plan has been developed. They are now making a staffing plan, including job descriptions and job standards. February 27: The plan is completed and has been discussed with me. A few minor adjustments are being made.
4. Coordinate plan	March 31	
(a) Nursing personnel		Done. All want to participate.
(b) Administrator		Done.
(c) Public relations		Announcements made to community through news media.
(d) Physicians		Done and well received.
(e) Other as needed		Presented to board per request of administrator. They want progress reports.
5. Select and train staff	April 30	Assigned to Ms. Finch for training. Will be assisted by Ms. Scott and Ms. Longez. I will select staff with their recommendation.
6. Implement	June 30	Ms. Scott wants to direct implementation and I have concurred.

Operational managers develop goals, objectives, strategies, and targets to set the strategic plan in motion. They match each unit goal or objective to a strategic goal or objective; their objectives can be much more detailed and specific than the strategic objectives. Numerous operational objectives can support one strategic objective.

All aspects of an operational plan are based on goals and on their achievement. The individual leadership style determines whether goal setting will be top-down or bottom-up. Bottom-up goal setting is participatory, using guidelines from the operational manager.[74] Participatory goal setting is believed to increase workers' commitment and achievement. Increased participation leads to greater group cohesiveness, which in turn fosters increased morale, increased motivation, and increased achievement and productivity. Individuals, including nurse managers, can ensure greater relative success in achievement of goals by building additional resources and time into their plans. Nurse managers who reject the goals of participating staff should explain reasons for rejection. Participation in goal setting alone will not ensure success. Exhibit 9-23 suggests a timetable for strategic and operational planning. Like the plan itself, such planning should be flexible.

The concept of goals as global in nature and objectives as detailed is sometimes confusing to some participants in the planning process, particularly nurse managers. In nursing, written organizational goals have seldom been used and probably did not exist in many agencies. More attention is now being given to this aspect of management. External influences create the demand

EXHIBIT 9-22

Standards for Evaluation of Management Plan of Nursing Division, Department, Service, or Unit

1. The written management plan should operationalize the strategic goals of the organization as well as the objectives of the nursing division, department, service, or unit. It should specify activities or actions, persons responsible for accomplishing them, and target dates or time frames, as well as providing for evaluation of progress. Each activity or action should be listed in problem-solving or decision-making format, as appropriate.
2. The management plan is personal to the incumbent, who should select the standards for developing, maintaining, and evaluating it. The nurse manager should solicit desired input from appropriate nursing persons and others.
3. The actions listed should reflect planning for the following:
   a. Nursing care programs to ensure safe and competent nursing services to clients.
      i. The nursing process, including data gathering, assessment, diagnosis, goal setting and prescription, intervention and application, evaluation, feedback, change, and accountability to the consumer.
      ii. A process and outcome audit.
      iii. Promotion of self-care practices.
   b. Establishment of policies and procedures for employing competent nursing personnel: recruitment, selection, assignment, retention, and promotion based on individual qualifications and capabilities without regard to race, national origin, creed, color, sex, or age.
   c. Integration of nursing care programs into the total program of the health care organization and community through committee participation in professional and service activities, and credentialing of individuals in organizations, including nursing organizations.
   d. A budget that is evaluated and revised as necessary.
   e. Job descriptions that include standards stated as objectives, outcomes, or results, and that are known to the incumbents.
   f. Specific utilization of personnel. This part of the plan should:
      i. Conform to a staffing plan that is based on timing nursing activities and rating of patients.
      ii. Match competencies of people to total job requirements.
      iii. Place prepared people in practice.
      iv. Place prepared people in administration.
      v. Place prepared people in education.
      vi. Place prepared people in research.
      vii. Foster identification of non-nursing tasks and their assignment to appropriate other departments or non-nursing personnel.
      viii. Recognize excellence in all fields: administration, education, research, and practice.
   g. Provision of needed supplies and equipment for nursing activities.
   h. Provision of input into remodeling and establishing required physical facilities.
   i. Orientation and continuing education of all nursing personnel.
   j. Education of students in the health care field according to a written agreement and collaborative implementation between faculty of the educational institutions and personnel of the service organization.
   k. Development of nursing research staff, research activities, and application of the research findings of others.
   l. Evaluation of all objectives—organizational, divisional, departmental, and at the service and unit level, as well as those stated in the individual's job description and standards.
4. The management plans should have mileposts that are reasonable and attainable, with deadlines included.
5. Management plans should be based on complete information.

for a strategic plan, and more nurse managers have had management education and training.[75]

Some organizations do not develop separate goals and objectives. Instead, they develop objectives and from them create management plans. In actual practice, as organizational objectives are developed into operational plans, specific goals and objectives are written for each major activity. The goal is to plan, assess progress toward goals and objectives at all levels, and provide feedback to all levels of management.

Planning New Ventures

In an era of competitiveness, every nurse manager may be called on to develop ideas for new ventures (nursing products or services). For example, continuing education courses can be packaged, marketed, and presented within the organization or taken on the road. Hospitals have moved into home health care, durable medical goods, wellness and fitness programs, and many other ventures. The basic rule for undertaking new ventures is to do sound planning.

EXHIBIT 9-23
Timetable for Strategic and Operational Planning

1. Organization
   Mondays 7–9 A.M. Conference room. Breakfast.
   Attendees: Chief executive officer (CEO), assistants (including for division of nursing), and understudies.
   Agenda: CEO, with input from all others, relates each item to strategic plan. CEO updates and develops written operational plans at meeting or immediately following, then reviews them for next agenda for progress and for strategic plan development.
   Minutes: Prepared and distributed to attendees.
2. Division of Nursing
   Monday 3–4 P.M. Nursing conference room.
   Attendees: Chief nurse executive (CNE), associates, department heads, chairs of clinical consultants, nursing management, and staff nurse committees.
   Agenda: Chairs, with input from CNE and all others, relate each item to strategic plan of division of nursing. These goals and objectives have already been coordinated with the organizational strategic plan. CNE and others update operational plans of division and departments during meeting or immediately following, then review them for next agenda for progress and nursing strategic plan development.
   Minutes: Prepared and distributed to attendees, to CEO, and to selected others.
3. Service and Unit
   CNE and/or associates meet with their nurse managers and representative clinical nurses at mutually determined times and places. The groups have agendas, keep minutes, update written operational plans, and provide feedback to top nurse managers and clinical nurse staff.

Any new venture should have a separate marketing plan. The nurse manager will consult with marketing department personnel and develop a marketing operation plan that will do the following:[76]

- Define problems and opportunities that may confront the new enterprise and product.
- Define the competitive position of the product and set objectives to meet anticipated problems and opportunities.
- Detail work steps, schedules, assignment of responsibility, budgets, and other elements of implementation.
- Describe the monitoring (control) plan.

The marketing plan should be separate from a primary operational plan and should include gathering and analysis of data related to the product or service as it already exists in the area. For example, if the product is continuing education, who will the customers be? They could be nurse managers, nurse educators, RNs, LPNs, or members of other health care disciplines. What is the competition in the market area? Is it local or imported from educational institutions and for-profit companies? Who will pay for the course—employers and/or individuals?

In addition, the operational plan will gather and analyze data that pinpoint possible strengths, weaknesses, problems, and opportunities. It will identify strategies for taking competitive advantages. Each opportunity, problem, strength, and weakness should be addressed by definitive objectives developed into operational plans for advertising, product development, and even personal selling.

Before any new venture is launched, a control plan is made. This plan will include measures of performance, such as numbers or amounts of products or services to be sold within specific time frames. Managers will be assigned responsibility for comparing expected results with actual results and for making corrections in all elements of the plan and its implementation. This plan can be achieved with marketing and operational plan checklists.[77] Exhibit 9-24 illustrates an operational plan for the development of an intermediate cardiac rehabilitation program.

Nursing service planning supports the mission and objectives of the institution. For this reason, the nurse administrator needs to know the plans and programs of the health facility administrator and of other departments in which personnel contribute to the joint effort of providing health care services. The nurse administrator should be a participatory, voting member of all important committees of the institution including those dealing with budgets, planning, credentialing, auditing, utilization, infection control, patient care improvement, the library, or any other committees concerned in any way with nursing service, nursing activities, and nursing personnel.

The nurse administrator who participates in institutional committee work achieves an overall view of agency problems and activities and is in a position to interpret problems, policies, and plans of the agency to nursing personnel. He or she can also interpret nursing needs and problems to personnel of other departments. This planning integrates the nursing care program into the total program of the health care institution.

Business Plans

Business plans are detailed descriptions of the process for ensuring launching of a new product or product line, project, unit, or service. Business plans meet many of the standards for strategic planning as they are projected over an

EXHIBIT 9-24
Division of Nursing–Cardiac Rehabilitation Program

STRATEGIC OBJECTIVE

The patient is provided with an effective patient and patient–family teaching program, which includes guidance and assistance in the use of medical center resources and community agencies that can contribute support to the patient's total needs.

OPERATIONAL OBJECTIVES	ACTIONS	TARGET DATES AND PERSONS RESPONSIBLE	ACCOMPLISHMENTS
Determine cardiologist's perception of the program: goals, resources to be used, breadth of services to be provided, etc.	1. Prepare an agenda for meeting with cardiologist.	Do by July 1, 200x. Swansburg (S) and Perry (P)	The following agenda was developed: • Need for new services. • What will they be? • What will they cost? • What will be charged? • Who will pay? • Where will they be done? • Who will do them? • How many patients? • What equipment and supplies are needed?
	2. Make appointment with cardiologist.	May 3, 200x, at 11 A.M. in Dr. C's office; S and P	May 3, 200x: Had a meeting with Dr. C, the cardiologist. The purpose of this program is to rehabilitate patients following open-heart surgery, angioplasty, and post-MI. It is the intermediate phase between acute care and when they enter "bounce back." The following decision evolved from the meeting: 1. This program will be limited because no other such services are available. 2. Services will include physical exercises, monitoring, progress report by patient, counseling as indicated. 3. Only patients with insurance or ability to pay will be accepted. 4. It will be done in PT on Mon., Wed., and Fri. from 7 to 9 A.M. 5. Equipment and supplies will be in-house. 6. The CV clinical nurse specialist will be the project director.

EXHIBIT 9-24 *(continued)*

OPERATIONAL OBJECTIVES	ACTIONS	TARGET DATES AND PERSONS RESPONSIBLE	ACCOMPLISHMENTS
Meet with the CV clinical nurse specialist and plan the program.	3. Make appointment with nurse D to plan the program.	May 4, 200x, 8 A.M.; S and P with D.	Plan: 1. D will coordinate with PT director. 2. P will figure cost of program by the hour and set charges with accounting office. 3. D will borrow equipment to run the program until the next capital budget. 4. Accomplish this by May 12, 200x.
Have plan completed by May 31, 200x.	4. Set up a control chart to identify when each phase of project will be completed.	May 12, 200x; P.	May 10, 200x: Done. Posted.
	5. Write policy and procedure for the program. Include admission and discharge procedures and emergency plan.	May 31, 200x; D.	May 29, 200x: Draft presented; minor changes needed. May 31, 200x: Done.
	6. Obtain equipment and supplies.	May 31, 200x; D.	May 17, 200x: Done.
	7. Coordinate with PT director.	May 12, 200x; D.	May 17, 200x: Done.
	8. Meet with cardiologist when all this is done.	June 1, 200x; P, S, and D.	June 2, 200x: Met with cardiologist. Dr. C is happy with plan and will be ready to start on July 1, 200x.
Provide for third-party reimbursement.	9. Discuss with insurance companies.	June 15, 200x; P.	June 15, 200x: Insurance reps will visit the program and make decision.
Develop marketing plan.	10. Prepare detailed marketing plan.		Appointment made. Marketing plan is already in operation with announcements mailed to all area cardiologists.
Develop evaluation plan.	11. Prepare evaluation plan.	June 30, 200x; P and D.	D has a good evaluation plan.
	12. Implement program.	July 1, 200x; D.	July 1, 200x: Had our first patient today. Cardiologist was there as required by insurance companies. All went well.
	13. Evaluate the program weekly until stabilized.	D, beginning July 8, 200x.	

extended time period of months or years. Their purpose is to provide sources of information for investors and decision makers, motivation, and measurement of performance.[78] Business plans are the blueprints for ventures. A clinical nurse specialist who decides to enter private practice as a consultant should write a business plan to solidify ideas and prepare for the unexpected.[79]

The following are key elements of a business plan as described by Johnson and others:[80]

1. Introduction: The nature, goals, objectives and desired outcomes of the proposed business.
2. Description of the business: The goals, nature, and history of the sponsoring institution, nature and history of the product, and industry trends.
3. Market and competition analyses: These include the target audience, pricing, promotion, placement, and positioning; data from solid market research are used.
4. Product development: Product description, resources, time frames for development, and quality control plan.
5. Operational plan: The location, facilities, labor force, and equipment.
6. Marketing plan: To market services or products, the mission, marketing research, measurable goals, strategies, and staffing and financial plans.
7. Organizational plan: To recruit qualified employees, an organizational chart and job descriptions.
8. Developmental schedule: To include planning for growth.
9. Financial plan: To secure capital.
10. Executive summary.

Business plans are often categorized as strategic plans. Many of the key elements are the same, although a business plan is more detailed than a strategic plan. Actually, a business plan would be developed for each new venture emerging from a strategic plan.

Exhibit 9-25 is a modified business plan/operational plan for accomplishing objectives related to management improvement and resource management for an intensive care unit.

Practical Planning Actions

Practical day-to-day planning actions of value to the nurse administrator include the following exercises:

1. At the beginning of each day, make a list of actions to be accomplished for the day. Cross off the actions as they are accomplished or at the end of the day. At the beginning of the next workday, carry over actions not accomplished. Either do them first or decide if they are actions that really need to be done. Do not hold tasks over from one day to the next indefinitely.
2. Plan ahead for meetings. If the meeting is a nursing responsibility, prepare and distribute the agenda in advance. Have a secretary call members for their items to be listed on the agenda. Forward nursing items for the agenda of organizational meetings to the appropriate chair in advance. Prepare for the presentation.
3. Identify developing problems and put them in the appropriate portion of the division's operational or management plans.
4. Review the operational or management plan on a scheduled basis. Do this with key managers so that each knows his or her responsibilities for accomplishment of activities.
5. Review the appropriate portions of the division operational or management plan with other nurse managers when counseling them.
6. Plan for discussion of ideas gleaned from professional publications. This activity can be part of a job standard, with different managers assigned specific topics or journals. Doing so may help to integrate research results into practice.
7. Suggest similar practical planning actions to other nurse managers.

Planning will also be necessary to provide programs for orientation and continuing education for nursing personnel so that all will be current in knowledge and practice methods. Improvement of patient care and of other administrative and hospital services necessitates initiation and utilization of and participation in studies or research projects in the health care field. Two additional important areas for planning are (1) educational programs that include student experience in the division of nursing, and (2) evaluation of clinical and administrative practices to determine whether the objectives of the division are being achieved.

Divisional Planning

There are many good reasons for planning; and avoiding duplicated efforts is one of them. Planning will also improve communication throughout the division and the institution and will reduce fragmentation by helping to keep functional units headed in the same direction. Planning is good management training for all nurse managers. During its initial phases, planning will use an objective analysis of the division to determine its current status. The mission, strengths, weaknesses, and environment will be analyzed, and a survey will be performed of how all employees feel about the division. The analysis also will assess the future of the division and the major threats

EXHIBIT 9-25

Operational Plan—Intensive Care Unit

MANAGEMENT IMPROVEMENT: UNIT OBJECTIVES, FEBRUARY 1, 200X

1. Precipitate imaginative thinking to improve existing procedures, capitalize on time expenditure, and introduce modern concepts and materials that directly enhance unit accomplishment.
2. Promote creativity in improving the existing patient environment.
3. Provide more modern concepts of total patient care by constant review and revision of unit administrative/managerial policies.

PLANS FOR ACHIEVEMENT OF OBJECTIVES	ACTIONS	TARGET DATES	ACCOMPLISHMENTS
Plan and implement a continuing unit improvement program.	1. Conduct a continuous review and analysis of unit improvement efforts through:	February	Reviewed and found current for following reasons: Turnover in personnel is fast. Not all objectives were adequately met; need to establish a better way of accomplishing them.
	a. Monthly unit conferences to review and update philosophy and objectives. Strive to accomplish more in each objective area.	February–July	
	b. Patient suggestions	Review each month	
	c. Suggestions of superiors	Daily	Done.
	d. Revision of unit procedures	April	Done. In addition, all nurses were counseled by the charge nurse. Nursing technicians are presently receiving counseling, and all is being documented. Counseling had not been documented in 6 years, except for remarks such as "Things went well and we did our job, so no counseling was needed."
	e. Briefing of all personnel. Discuss philosophy, objectives, job descriptions, performance standards, hospital and nursing service policies and procedures, and unit procedures.	February	
	2. Review equipment and supplies for improvement by addition or deletion.		Disapproved. Disposable tubing was approved, ordered, and in use by June.
	a. Submit work order to alter a locker as a drying cabinet for respirator parts, since moisture provides a growth medium for *Pseudomonas* bacteria.		
	b. Check on status of new floor, piped-in compressed air system, and cardiac monitors.	February–April	New floor to be done by August 1. Compressed air started by March 15. Cardiac monitors arrived April 3. Patient units 1, 3, and 4 were equipped. Unit 4 was designated the maximum monitoring site and is to be used to monitor patients with Swan-Ganz arterial lines and questionable cardiac conditions.

(*continued*)

EXHIBIT 9-25 *(continued)*

PLANS FOR ACHIEVEMENT OF OBJECTIVES	ACTIONS	TARGET DATES	ACCOMPLISHMENTS
Review standardized policies and procedures for implementation of more current concepts of improved care accomplishments.	3. Evaluate all areas of management for current standardized efficiency.		This was done, and cleaning procedures were looked at and improved when they appeared poor. HEPA filters were replaced in February. Wall suction valves were replaced. Pipelines were found to be clogged with secretions, and system had to be purged. Shelves were mounted on wall by four units to replace bedside stands. Respirators, nebulizers, and blenders were mounted on wall above each patient unit. Suction bottles were relocated and outlets changed in an effort to isolate them from the oxygen nebulization units. Swan-Ganz catheters were standardized, and requisitioning was transferred from the unit to central supply. Ambu bags were equipped with corrugated tubing to serve as an oxygen reservoir and deliver a maximum concentration of 99% to 100%. The disposable Aqua-pack nebulizer was deleted, resulting in a $40 per case saving.
	a. Check all areas of infection sources.		
	i. Air exchange and pressure checked quarterly.	February	
	ii. HEPA filters changed quarterly.	February	
	iii. Check wall suction, since filters do not appear to be doing the job.	February	
	iv. Eliminate messy bedside stands.	February	
	b. Improve safety.		
	i. Secure equipment.	April	
	ii. Isolate oxygen nebulization units from suction.	April	
	iii. Send all equipment to central supply for processing.	April	
	iv. Improve efficiency of Ambu resuscitators.	April	
	4. Projected: An anesthesiologist will be assigned to the intensive care unit. All bronchoscopies will be done here. Open heart surgery is still an open and current topic.		

EXHIBIT 9-25

RESOURCE MANAGEMENT

1. Provide, secure, and maintain the appropriate and economical use of supplies and equipment that will permit unit personnel to devote maximum time and care to patient activities.
2. Provide the unit with adequate tools for safe and effective patient care.
3. Provide the unit with conservative utilization and centralization of unit supplies and equipment, thus promoting peak efficiency in meeting patients' needs.

PLANS FOR ACHIEVEMENT OF OBJECTIVES	ACTIONS	TARGET DATES	ACCOMPLISHMENTS
Plan, evaluate, and project needed supplies and equipment that will enhance effective and safe nursing care.	Identify projected needs with unit manager through review of: 1. Unit inventories of equipment and budgetary estimate. 2. Standards for supplies. 3. Availability of supplies and equipment. 4. Economical use of supplies and equipment.	February	Items ordered (projected replacements for 200x–200x): 1 electronic thermometer 1 IV pump 5 transducers 1 ventilator 1 sphygmomanometer 1 Wright respirometer 4 metal storage cabinets 4 Ambu bags 1 blood gas analyzer New cubicle curtains
Plan and execute appropriate utilization of materials.	1. Economical use of expendable supplies and adequate safeguards to prevent misuse and loss. 2. Knowledge of principles of operation of appropriate mechanical equipment and procedures for effecting prompt servicing and repairs.		Items replaced: ECG and defibrillator portable ECG machine spirometers suction regulators Items deleted: 1 electronic thermometer 1 internal/external defibrillator (to dog lab) 2 compressor units Miscellaneous: file card supply system revamped shelving obtained for lower doors Personnel turnover: Projected losses: Ms. Speich, RN, June Ms. Ullman, RN, August Ms. Urbom, RN, May Ms. Malloy, RN, June Mr. Falco, ward clerk, April Projected gains: Ms. Tishoff, RN, May Mr. Robertshaw, RN, May Mr. Angelus, RN, April Mrs. Figuera, unit secretary, April

Myra C. Breck, RN
Nurse Manager, ICU

and opportunities it will face during the next year and the next 5 to 10 years. Planning will engineer a design for monitoring and evaluating divisional performance. This design will involve as many people as possible in planning and managing their areas of responsibility.

Once managers and employees have agreed on objectives, programs and projects, and schedules, employees can control their own jobs and report only when things turn out better or worse than planned.

Planning is such a primary and essential element of management that managers cannot be effective without it.

All planning requires discipline and organization on the part of managers. Planning should be approached logically and calmly; it may threaten the insecure and may even threaten the nurse administrator, who must provide total support in terms of giving or obtaining the resources to accomplish divisional planning. Strategies are developed to address these problems and to ensure that representative nurse managers participate on all planning teams.

Provision of nursing care to patients is the purpose of a division of nursing. Nursing standards require that there will be qualified nursing personnel who will collect data and make nursing diagnoses based on patients' needs and according to patient care standards. Nursing standards further indicate that cooperation among disciplines is expected.

Unit Planning

Planning extends to the operational units of any health care agency; the processes involved are the same. It is in the units that the work for which nursing exists takes place. Planning should be done on a daily, weekly, and long-term basis. Daily planning is related to patient care and includes history taking, assessment, and nursing diagnosis and intervention. It involves matching people to jobs, developing policies and procedures specific to the patient population, identifying educational needs, preparing and conducting educational programs, coordinating patient care activities, supervising personnel, and evaluating the planning process and its results as summarized in Exhibit 9-26. Also included in unit planning are the implementation of theories of nursing care into the management and practice of nursing, an effective and efficient nursing care delivery system, and a system of statistical process control. Unit objectives should be clearly defined and a sound management or operational plan made to achieve them.

Successful Planning

Keeping the responsibility for planning as a line management function is better than creating a separate planning staff of nurses; because nurses who use plans make them effective and productive, they should be the ones to write the plans. Nurse managers ensure the plans are based on data from all sections and not biased by a few. Some people see planning as a management style; planning is a tool as well. Plan for what the health care of the future will be; with inflation and recession, the impact of the local economy on health care needs will always be an issue. Economics is forcing us to teach people to do more for themselves and their families. Nurse managers will certainly have to plan for changes in value systems.

Nurse managers should make decisions about the kind of planning to be undertaken and which management level should perform specific aspects of the planning. Involve personnel in planning activities they will carry out. Teach and combine the elements of planning with other management functions; ensure that all managers are involved. Accept outcomes that are different from those originally planned, as activities may quickly become outdated and require modified plans.

Research studies show that 20% of small businesses that did not perform strategic planning failed, whereas only 8% of small businesses that performed strategic planning failed.[81] Exhibit 9-26 outlines standards for the planning process.

Summary

The basic tools of planning are statements of mission or purpose, vision and values, philosophy or beliefs, and objectives and an active operational or management plan. All managers use such documents to accomplish the work of nursing.

Statements of mission, philosophy, and objectives support each other at different agency levels, from the unit to the service or department and then to the division and finally to the organization.

The statement of mission or purpose gives the reasons an entity exists, whether it is an organization, division, department, or unit. The nursing mission statement pertains to the clinical practice of nursing supported by research, education, and management.

EXHIBIT 9-26
Standards for Planning Process

	YES	NO
1. The plan is written.		
2. It defines the nursing business.		
3. It contains objectives (general and specific goals).		
4. It defines strategies.		
5. It supports the mission.		
6. It details forecasted activities for one year.		
7. It details forecasted activities for longer than one year.		
8. It has been developed with input from clinical nurses and line managers.		
9. It addresses resources (personnel and facilities).		
10. Changes are evident.		
11. Financial plans are included.		
12. Needs are identified and supported.		
13. Priorities are listed.		
14. Timetables are listed.		
15. It is based on current data analysis.		
16. It assesses both strengths and weaknesses.		
17. It derives from a good nursing management information plan.		
18. It is used and modified consistently.		

The statement of philosophy reflects the values and beliefs of the organizational entity. It is translated into action by nursing personnel.

Objectives are concrete statements describing the major accomplishments nurses desire to achieve. Major categorical areas for objectives include the following:

- Organization and use of all resources: human, financial and physical
- Social responsibility
- Staffing
- Requisition of supplies and equipment
- Planning of educational programs
- Innovation
- Marketing
- Evaluation of patient care
- Evaluation of personnel performance

Major strategies of an organization are the planning process; the formulation and use of statements of mission, philosophy, and objectives; and the formulation of organizational plans developed with the broadest possible input.

Planning is the mental process by which nurse managers use valid and reliable data to develop objectives, determine the resources needed, and create a blueprint for achieving the objectives. The major purpose of planning is to make the best possible use of personnel, supplies, and equipment.

Strategic planning sets objectives for long-term nursing activities of one to five years or longer. Although traditionally done by top managers, strategic planning is an important skill for all nurse managers to develop. It ensures survival. Human resource planning will ensure effective use of a scarce commodity, the professional nurse. Strategic planning has a mission, collects and analyzes data, assesses strengths and weaknesses, sets goals and objectives, uses strategies, operates on a timetable, gives operational and functional guidance to nurse managers, and includes evaluation.

Tactical planning is short-term planning. Operational or management plans convert objectives into action and include activities, assignments, deadlines, and provision for accountability. They include goals, objectives, strategies, actions, a timetable, identification of responsible persons, and note of accomplishments. Operational planning is daily, weekly, and monthly planning and can provide data for further strategic and tactical planning.

Planning within the nursing organization is intended to assist in fulfilling the mission of the health care facility. Planning supports the organization's objectives, meshes with the plans of all other departments contributing to provision of total health care needs, and will ultimately provide for optimum support of the nursing agency.

APPLICATION EXERCISES

EXERCISE 9-1 Use Exhibit 9-5, Standards for the Evaluation of Mission Statements of the Nursing Division and Its Departments, Services, and Units, to:

1. Evaluate a mission statement.
2. Develop a mission statement.

EXERCISE 9-2 Use Exhibit 9-9, Standards for Evaluation of Philosophy Statements of the Nursing Division, Department, Service, or Unit, to:

1. Evaluate a philosophy statement.
2. Develop a philosophy statement.

EXERCISE 9-3 Use Exhibit 9-16, Standards for Evaluation of Statements of Objectives for a Nursing Division, Department, Service, or Unit, to:

1. Evaluate objectives.
2. Develop objectives.

EXERCISE 9-4 Use Exhibit 9-22, Standards for Evaluation of Management Plan of Nursing Division, Department, Service, or Unit, to:

1. Evaluate management plans.
2. Develop a management plan.

EXERCISE 9-5 Identify and develop a statement of the planning strategy for a nursing organization or unit.

EXERCISE 9-6 Explore the idea of creating a nursing research council; write its mission, vision, philosophy, and objectives. Create a strategic plan for the present, two years and five years in future projections.

EXERCISE 9-7 Write a summary of a nursing unit, service, department, or division that describes its work, the volume of products and services, marketing activities, trends, financial summary, and impact on employees.

EXERCISE 9-8 Interview a chief executive officer and a chief nurse executive officer of an organization. Determine their orientation to strategic planning. Compare the results. Prepare a list of questions to ask from exhibits in this chapter before doing the interview.

EXERCISE 9-9 Make a management plan for your work for a day; include planning data pertinent to that manager's area(s) of responsibility.

EXERCISE 9-10 List opportunities and threats to nursing, their severity, and the probability that they will occur. Consider technological, economic, demographic, politicolegal, and sociocultural forecasting.

NOTES

1. For a classic article on purpose, philosophy, and objectives, refer to Moore, M. A. (1971). Philosophy, purpose, and objectives: Why do we have them? *Journal of Nursing Administration*, 9–14.
2. Calfee, D. L. (1993). Get your mission statement working! *Management Review*, *1*, 54–57.
3. Crosby, P. (1989). *Running things: The art of making things happen*. New York: NAL-Dutton.
4. Ireland, R. D. & Hitt, M. A. (1992). Mission statements: Importance, challenge, and recommendations for development. *Business Horizons*, *1*, 34–42.
5. Truskie, S. D. (1984). The driving force of successful organizations. *Business Horizons*, *1*, 43–48.
6. Beyers, M. (1984). Getting on top of organizational change: Part 1, process and development. *Journal of Nursing Administration*, 32–39; Gillen, D. J. (1986). Harvesting the energy from change anxiety. *Supervisory Management*, 40–43.
7. Reyes, J. R. & Kleiner, B. H. (1990). How to establish an organizational purpose. *Management Decision: Quarterly Review of Management Technology*, *28*(7), 51–54.
8. Ibid.
9. Spragins, E. E. (1992). Resource-Constructing a vision statement. *Inc.*, 33.
10. Campbell, A. (1992). The power of mission: Aligning strategy and culture. *Planning Review*, *1*, 10–12, 63.
11. Farnham, A. (1993, April 19). State your values, hold the hot air. *Fortune*, 117–124.
12. Henderson, V. (1966). *The nature of nursing*. New York: Macmillan, 15.
13. Yura, H. & Walsh, M. B. (1988). *The nursing process* (5th ed.). New York: Appleton-Century-Crofts, 1.
14. King, I. M. (1968). A conceptual frame of reference in nursing. *Nursing Research*, 27–31.
15. Orem, D. E. (1995). *Nursing: Concepts of practice* (5th ed.). New York: McGraw-Hill, 7.
16. Kinlein, M. L. (1977). *Independent nursing practice with clients*. Philadelphia: J. B. Lippincott, 23.
17. Sussman, G. E. (1985). CEO perspectives on mission, healthcare systems, and the environment. *Hospital & Health Services Administration*, 21–34.
18. Farnham, 1993; Reyes & Kleiner, 1990.
19. Hodgetts, R. M. (1990). *Management: Theory, process, and practice* (5th ed.). Orlando, FL: Harcourt, Brace, Jovanovich, 73–74.
20. Coile, R. C. (2001). Magnet hospitals use culture, not wages, to solve nursing shortage. *Journal of Healthcare Management*, 224–227.
21. Poteet, G. W. & Hill, A. S. (1988). Identifying the components of a nursing service philosophy. *Journal of Nursing Administration*, 29–33.
22. Corporate philosophies. (1988). *Compressed Air Magazine*, 31–34.
23. Ibid.
24. Moore, 1971; 13; Calfee, 1993.
25. Drucker, P. F. (1978). *Management: Tasks, responsibilities, practice*. New York: Harper & Row, 99–102.
26. *Report on the Project for the Evaluation of the Quality of Nursing Service*. (1966). Ottawa, Ontario: The Canadian Nurses Association, 47–48.
27. Drucker, P. F. (1999). *Management challenges for the 21st century*. New York: HarperCollins, 43–44.
28. Drenkard, K. N. (2001). Creating a future worth experiencing: Nursing strategic planning in an integrated healthcare delivery system. *Journal of Nursing Administration*, 362–376.
29. Beckham, J. D. (2004). Strategy: What it is, how it works, why it fails. *Health Forum Journal*, *2*(11), 55–59.
30. Morris, D. E. & Rau, S. E. (1985). Strategic competition: The application of business planning techniques to the hospital marketplace. *Health Care Strategic Management*, 17–20.
31. Cushman, R. (1979). Norton's top-down, bottom-up planning process. *Planning Review*, 3–8, 48.
32. Meier, A. P. (1974). The planning process. *Managerial Planning*, 1–5, 9.
33. Cavanaugh, D. E. (1985). Gamesmanship: The art of strategizing. *Journal of Nursing Administration*, 38–41.
34. Ehrat, K. S. (1983). A model for politically astute planning and decision making. *Journal of Nursing Administration*, 29–35.
35. Ibid.
36. Trexler, B. J. (1987). Nursing department purpose, philosophy, and objectives: Their use and effectiveness. *Journal of Nursing Administration*, 8–12.
37. Fayol, H. (1949). *General and industrial management* (C. Storrs, Trans.). London: Isaac Pitman & Sons, 43–50.
38. Urwick, L. (1944). *The elements of administration*. New York: Harper & Row, 26–34.
39. Rowland, H. S. & Rowland, B. L. (1997). *Nursing administration handbook* (4th ed.). Gaithersburg, MD: Aspen, 13, 32–36.
40. Beyers, M. & Phillips, C. (1979). *Nursing management for patient care* (2nd ed.). Boston: Little, Brown, 41–48.
41. Ackoff, R. L. (1986). Our changing concept of planning. *Journal of Nursing Administration*, 35–40.
42. Schmeling, W. H., Futch, J. R., Moore, D., & MacDonald, J. W. (1991). The interactive planning/management model. *Nursing Administration Quarterly*, 14, 31.
43. Ibid.
44. Curtin, L. (1994). Learning for the future. *Nursing Management*, *25* (1), 7–9.
45. Donovan, H. M. (1975). *Nursing service administration: Managing the enterprise*. St. Louis: Mosby, 50–64.
46. Drucker, P. F. (1978). *Management: Tasks, responsibilities, practices*. New York: Harper & Row, 121–129.

47. Koontz, H. & Weihrich, H. (1988). *Management* (9th ed.). New York: McGraw-Hill, 16.
48. Donovan, 1975, 63–64.
49. Hodgetts, 1990, 123-124.
50. Rowland & Rowland, 1997.
51. Reif, W. E. & Webster, J. L. (1976). The strategic planning process. *Arizona Business*, 14–20.
52. Meier, A. P. (1974). The planning process. *Managerial Planning*, 1–5, 9.
53. Beyers, M. (1984). Getting on top of organizational change: Part 2. Trends in nursing service. *Journal of Nursing Administration*, 31–37.
54. Ibid.
55. Drucker, 1999, 81–85.
56. Ibid., p. 125.
57. Sherman, V. C. (1982). Taking over: Notes to the new executive. *Journal of Nursing Administration*, 21–23.
58. Fox, D. H. & Fox, R. T. (1983). Strategic planning for nursing. *Journal of Nursing Administration*, 11–16; Paul, R. N. & Taylor, J. W. (1986). The state of strategic planning. *Business*, 37–43.
59. Osborne, D. & Gaebler, T. (1992). *Reinventing government.* New York: Plume, 233–234.
60. Odiorne, G. S. (1987). The art of crafting strategic plans. *Training*, 94–96, 98.
61. Ibid.
62. Baldwin, S. R. & McConnell, M. (1988). Strategic planning: Process and plan go hand in hand. *Management Solutions*, 29–36.
63. Peters, T. (1987). *Thriving on chaos.* New York: Harper & Row, 477; Sull, D. N. (1999). Why good companies go bad. *Harvard Business Review*, 42–48, 50–52, 183; Campbell, A. (1999). Tailored, not benchmarked: A fresh look at corporate planning. *Harvard Business Review*, 41–48, 50, 189.
64. Peters, 1987, 615–617.
65. Baldwin & McConnell, 1988.
66. Mercer, Z. C. (1980). Personal planning: An overlooked application of the corporate planning process. *Managerial Planning*, 32–35; Van Mullem, C. et al. (1999). Strategic planning for research use in nursing practice. *Journal of Nursing Administration*, 38–45.
67. Ibid.; Mercy Health Services Nurses Council. (1991). Mercy Health Services: Systemwide redesign of patient care services. *Nursing Administration Quarterly*, 38–45.
68. Fox & Fox, 1983.
69. Jones, D. & Crane, V. (1990). Development of an organizational strategic planning process for a hospital department. *Health Care Supervisor*, *9*(1), 1–20.
70. Begun, J. & Heatwole, K. B. (1999). Strategic cycling: Shaking complacency in healthcare strategic planning. *Journal of Healthcare Management*, 339–352.
71. Amudson, B. A. & Rosenblatt, R. A. (1991). The WAMI Rural Hospital Project. Part 6: Overview and Conclusions. *Journal of Rural Health*, 560–574.
72. Drucker, 1999.
73. Johnson, L. J. (1990). Strategic management: A new dimension of the nurse executive's role. *Journal of Nursing Administration*, 7–10.
74. Cushman, 1979.
75. When the terms *goals* and *objectives* are used, their meaning should be defined. Some references cite goals as being strategic and objectives as being tactical or operational; others do the opposite.
76. Nylen, D. W. (1985). Making your business plan an action plan. *Business*, 12–16.
77. Singleton, E. K. & Nail, F. C. (1985). Guidelines for establishing a new service. *Journal of Nursing Administration*, 22–26.
78. Vestal, K. W. (1988). Writing a business plan. *Nursing Economics*, 121–124.
79. Schulmeister, L. (1999). Starting a nursing consultation practice. *Clinical Nurse Specialist*, *2*, 94–100.
80. Johnson, J. E. (1990). Developing an effective business plan. *Nursing Economics*, *4*, 152–154; Johnson, J. E., Sparks, D. G., & Humphreys, C. (1988). Writing a winning business plan. *Journal of Nursing Administration*, 15–19; Reiboldt, J. M. (1999). Writing a group practice business plan. *Healthcare Financial Management*, *1*, 58–61.
81. Ireland & Hitt, 1992.

REFERENCES

Anderson, M., Cosby, J., Swan, B., Moore, H., & Broekhoven, M. (1999). The use of research in local health service agencies. *Social Science Medicine*, 1007–1019.

"Balanced scorecard" helps fix Overlake strategic plan. (1999). *Healthcare Benchmarks*, 103–105.

Brendtro, M. & Hegge, M. (2000). Nursing faculty: One generation away from extinction. *Journal of Professional Nursing*, 97–103.

Bryan, E. L. & Welton, R. E. (1986). Let your business plan be a road map to credit. *Business*, 44–47.

Chrispin, P. (1996). Decisions, decisions. *Journal of Managerial Medicine*, *10*(6), 42–49, 3.

Cohen, M. (2000). Tools for the practice manager. *New England Journal of Medicine*, 49–50.

Development of an organizational strategic planning process for a hospital department. *Health Care Supervisor*, 1–20.

Edsel, W. M. (1999). How to develop a business plan for your medical group. *Medical Group Management Journal*, 36–39.

Forman, L. (1979). Which comes first, the planning process or the planning model? *Business Economics*, 42–47.

Glen, S. (1999). Educating for interprofessional collaboration: Teaching about values. *Nursing Ethics*, 202–213.

Gray, D. H. (1986). Uses and misuses of strategic planning. *Harvard Business Review*, 89–97.

Hansen, R. D. (1999). Strategic planning: The basics and benefits. *Medical Group Management Journal*, 28–35.

Kelly, K. J. (1992). Administrators' forum. *Journal of Nursing Staff Development*, 90–91.

Kotler, P. & Murphy, P. E. (1981). Strategic planning for higher education. *Journal of Higher Education*, 470–489.

Matthews, P. (2000). Planning for successful outcomes in the new millennium. *Topics in Health Information Management*, 55–64.

McNeese-Smith, D. K. (2000). Job stages of entry, mastery, and disengagement among nurses. *Journal of Nursing Administration*, 140–147.

Mendes, I. A., Trevizan, M. A., Nogueira, M. S., & Sawada, N. O. (1999). Humanizing nurse–patient communication: A challenge and a commitment. *Medical Law*, *18*(4), 639–644.

Moller-Tiger, D. (1999). Long-Range strategic planning: A case study. *Healthcare Financial Management*, 33–35.

Molloy, J. & Cribb, A. (1999). Changing values for nursing and health promotion: Exploring the policy context of professional ethics. *Nursing Ethics*, 411–422.

Nadler, D. A. & Tushman, M. L. (1980). A model for diagnosing organizational behavior. *Organizational Dynamics*, *9*(2), 35–51.

Norris, J. E. S. (1992). Eight steps to strategic planning. *Nursing Management*, 78–79.

Palesy, S. R. (1980). Motivating line management using the planning process. *Planning Review*, 3–8, 44–48.

Paul, R. N. & Taylor, J. W. (1986). The state of strategic planning. *Business*, 37–43.

Pearce, W. H. (1986). I thought I knew what good management was. *Harvard Business Review*, 59–65.

Pender, N. J. (1992). The NIH Strategic Plan. How will it affect the future of nursing science and practice? *Nursing Outlook*, 55–56.

Redman, L. N. (1983). The planning process. *Managerial Planning*, 24–30, 40.

Sabatino, C. J. (1999). Reflections on the meaning of care. *Nursing Ethics*, 374–382.

Schmieding, N. J. (1999). Reflective inquiry framework for nurse administrators. *Journal of Advanced Nursing*, 631–639.

Sechrist, K. R., Lewis, E. M., & Rutledge, D. N. (1999). Data collection for nursing work force strategic planning in California. *Journal of Nursing Administration*, 9–11, 29.

Senge, P. M., Smigh, B., Ross, R. B., & Roberts, C. (1994). *The fifth discipline fieldbook: Strategies & tools for building a learning organization.* New York: Doubleday & Co., Inc.

Siwicki, B. (1999). What's the CEO's role? Why more chief executives are playing pivotal roles in I.T. strategic planning. *Health Data Management*, 76–78, 80–82, 84–85.

Sorrells-Jones, J. & Weaver, D. (1999). Knowledge workers and knowledge-intense organizations, part 3. Implications for preparing healthcare professionals. *Journal of Nursing Administration*, 14–21.

Taft, S. H., Jones, P. K., & Minch, E. L. (1992). Strengthening hospital nursing, part 2: Characteristics of effective planning processes. *Journal of Nursing Administration*, 36–46.

Taft, S. & Stearns, J. (1991). Organizational change with a nursing agenda: Lessons from the strengthening hospital nursing program. *Journal of Nursing Administration*, *21*(2), 12–21.

Thunhurst, C. & Barker, C. (1999). Using problem structuring methods in strategic planning. *Health Policy Planning*, 127–134.

Weaver, H. N. (1999). Transcultural nursing with Native Americans: Critical knowledge, skills, and attitudes. *Journal of Transcultural Nursing*, 197–202.

CHAPTER 10

Staffing and Scheduling

Elizabeth Simms, RN, MSN

> When gathering people together, the first thing is to clarify the rules of engagement. Although this can be tiresome, people must be reminded of the expectations regarding interactions and communication. Deliberations break down most often because the parameters for dialogue were not reinforced and adhered to.
>
> Tim Porter O'Grady and Kathy Malloch

LEARNING OBJECTIVES AND ACTIVITIES

- Describe the components of the staffing process.
- Do a work-sampling study covering a specific period of time.
- Recognize factors influencing planning for staffing.
- Prepare a staffing plan for a nursing unit.
- Determine the modified approaches to nurse staffing and scheduling used by a health care organization.
- Describe the components of a patient classification system (PCS).
- Use a PCS to classify patients on a nursing unit.
- Define and recognize elements of a nursing management information system.
- Identify methods for improving productivity in a health care agency.
- Measure the productivity of the nursing staff on a nursing unit.

CONCEPTS: Staffing philosophy, staffing process, staffing activities, work contract, staffing modules, cyclic staffing, self-scheduling, patient classification systems, productivity.

NURSE MANAGER BEHAVIORS: Uses input from employees to develop and implement a staffing philosophy and staffing policies that inspire personnel to work to their maximum level of productivity; is responsible for staffing and scheduling staff with assignments that illustrate appropriate staffing mix based on scope of practice, competencies, client/resident needs, and acuity of care.

NURSE EXECUTIVE BEHAVIORS: Oversees staffing activities through human resource management that includes use of a patient classification system and provision of qualified nursing personnel in adequate numbers to meet patient care needs; evaluates and revises staffing systems and processes of nursing services to facilitate nurse-sensitive patient/client/family-centered outcomes; oversees measurement of patient/client/resident need for nursing care.

Introduction

Staffing is one of the most important issues in the delivery of health care. It is widely recognized that there is a crisis in nursing. In a survey performed by the American Nurses Association (ANA) in 2001, 7000 nurses reported compromise in the care of patients because of a lack of qualified staff. Up to 20% of nurses are expected to leave the field within 5 years.[1] There is no correlation in increased nursing school enrollments to fill the need created by these exits.[2]

The nursing shortage of this decade is rooted in the following factors:

- The average age of nurses currently employed is 46.
- After age 50, many nurses will work part-time or retire.
- Young professionals choosing health care careers enter medicine more frequently than they do nursing.
- Nursing salaries "plateau" unless nurses make the transition to upper management.
- The plateau offers little financial compensation for nurses wishing to remain at the bedside.[3]

There is strong evidence that an adequate number of nursing staff available to care for and coordinate care among the disciplines has an impact on patient outcomes.[4] In a study conducted in 589 hospitals encompassing 10 states, inverse relationships were recognized between nursing staff levels and negative outcomes for postsurgical patients.[5] In a separate study, the proportion of hours of care provided by nursing staff was inversely related to such adverse events as medication errors, decubitii, and patient complaints.[6]

It is well documented throughout nursing literature that staffing levels can and do affect the clinical outcomes of patients. Job dissatisfaction within the profession, a nursing shortage, and financial pressures contribute to the complexities of these issues.[7]

Staffing Philosophy

Staffing is one of the major problems of any nursing organization, whether that organization is a hospital, nursing home, home health care agency, ambulatory care agency, or another type of facility. Aydelotte has stated that

> Nurse staffing methodology should be an orderly, systematic process, based upon sound rationale, applied to determine the number and kind of nursing personnel required to provide nursing care of a predetermined standard to a group of patients in a particular setting. The end result is prediction of the kind and number of staff required to give care to patients.[8]

Components of the staffing process as a control system include a staffing study, a master staffing plan, a scheduling plan, and a nursing management information system (NMIS). West adds a position control plan and a budgeting plan that integrates all aspects of staffing needs.[9]

Nurse staffing must meet certain regulatory requirements, among which are legal requirements of the Centers for Medicare & Medicaid Services (CMS). This legal standard is further supported by the standards of the Joint Commission on Accreditation of Healthcare Organizations (JCAHO). Other standards include the American Nurses Association (ANA) *Scope and Standards for Nurse Administrators*, the ANA *Standards of Clinical Nursing Practice*, state legislation and state licensing requirements, and boards of nursing.

From all of these standards and from the expectations of the community, of nurses, and of physicians, the nurse administrator will develop a staffing philosophy as a basis for a staffing methodology. Community expectations will be related to economic status, local value and belief systems, and local standards of culture. Nurses' expectations will be related to the same community standards, their own perceptions of the practice of nursing and its components, desired results, and tolerated workload.

Nurse managers can discern various values related to staffing from the nursing division's existing statements of purpose, philosophy, and objectives. A staffing philosophy may encompass beliefs about using a patient classification system (PCS) for identifying patient care needs.[10] A successful nursing leader's personal philosophy should include allowing nursing staff some degree of control within their work environment. Nurses who believe their work environment offers them a higher level of control are more likely to work for improvements rather than leave the organization.[11]

Objectives of nurse staffing are excellent care and high productivity. Professional nurses can develop a statement of purpose that is comprehensive in stating the quality and quantity of performance it is intended to motivate. Purpose statements should be quantified.[12]

Staffing Study

A staffing study should gather data about internal and external environmental factors affecting the staffing requirements of an organization. Aydelotte listed four techniques drawn from engineering to measure the work of nurses, all of which involve the concept of time required for performance:[13]

1. *Time study and task frequency.*
   a. Tasks and task elements (procedures).
   b. Point and time started and ended.
   c. Sample size.
   d. The measurement of *standard time*, which is the sum of average time, plus allowance for fatigue, personal variations, and unavoidable standby.
   e. The measurement of *nursing activity*, which is the frequency of task × standard time.
   f. The *volume of nursing work*, which is the total of all *tasks × standard time.*
2. *Work sampling* (variation of task frequency and time).
   a. Identify major and minor categories of nursing activities.
   b. Determine number of observations to be made.
   c. Observe random sample of nursing personnel performing activities.
   d. Analyze observations. Frequency occurring in a specific category = percentage of total time spent in that activity. Most work sampling studies direct care and indirect care to determine *ratio*.
3. *Continuous sampling* (variation of task frequency and time). The technique is the same as for work sampling, except that:
   a. The observer follows one individual in the performance of a task.
   b. The observer may observe work performed for one or more patients if these tasks can be observed concurrently.
4. *Self-reporting* (variation of task frequency and time).
   a. The individual records the work sampling or continuous sampling on himself or herself.

b. Tasks are logged using time intervals or time tasks start and end.
c. Logs are analyzed.

Many work-sampling studies focus on procedures, ignore standards, and are lacking in objectivity, reliability, and accuracy. The techniques themselves, however, are sound.[14]

According to West, three "cardinal rules" exist for forecasting staffing requirements.[15] The first is to base staffing projections on past staffing history. A data sheet that includes types of task and procedure, average time to complete, measurement of nursing activity, and volume of nursing work is one aspect of such a model. The data can be collected from the PCS reports and census reports. Such data are readily available in most hospitals. Some NMISs, such as Medicus, provide numbers of personnel required, including the mix of RNs, LPNs and NAs. Other data needed are sick time, overtime, holidays, and vacation time; the attrition rate is also important. In some PCSs, these data are built into the staffing formula.

A second rule for staffing is to review current staffing levels. Review of future plans for the institution is the third cardinal rule.[16] Clinical nurses who are involved in staffing plans will have confidence in the plans.

Staffing requires much planning on the part of the nurse administrator. Data must be collected and analyzed. These data include facts about the following:

- The product, that is, the needs of patient care.
- Diagnostic and therapeutic procedures performed by physicians and nurses.
- The knowledge elements of professional nursing translated into the skills of taking a medical history, performing an assessment, providing a nursing diagnosis and prescription, applying care, evaluating, keeping records, communicating, and taking all other actions related to primary health care of patients.

Basic to planning for staffing of a division of nursing is the fact that qualified nursing personnel must be provided in sufficient numbers to ensure adequate, safe nursing care for all patients 24 hours a day, 7 days a week, 52 weeks a year. Each staffing plan must be tailored to the needs of the agency and cannot be determined with a simple worker–patient ratio or formula.

Changing, expanding knowledge and technology in the physical and social sciences, medicine, and economics influence planning for staffing. Health care institutions are treating more clients on an outpatient basis than ever before. New drugs, improved diagnostic and therapeutic procedures, and reimbursement changes have decreased the lengths of hospitalization. The result of decreased length of stay is often an increased inpatient acuity. Standards of the JCAHO, ANA, and other professional and governmental organizations have required the upgrade of health care.

Planning for staffing requires judgment, experience, and thorough knowledge of the requirements of the organization in which the individual nurse administrator is employed. It requires the support of hospital administration, physicians in charge of clinical services, and nursing staff. The basic requirement for staffing is unchanging, regardless of the type or size of the institution: plan for the kinds and numbers of nursing personnel that will give safe, adequate care to all patients and that will ensure that the work of nursing is productive and satisfying.

The following influence planning for staffing:[17]

1. Changing concepts of nursing roles for clinical nursing practitioners and specialists.
2. Patient populations that are changing as birth rates decline and longevity increases.
3. Institutional missions and objectives related to research, training, and many specialties.
4. Personnel policies and practices.
5. Policies and practices related to admission and discharge times of patients, assignment of patients to units, and intensive and progressive care practices.
6. The degree to which other departments carry out their supporting services. Plans should be made to furnish staffing requirements for nursing personnel to perform nonnursing duties such as dietary functions, clerical work, messenger and escort activities, and housekeeping. Whether these services should or should not be carried out by nursing personnel is not the point; the relevance is that the degree to which the situation exists must be considered in any planning. Nurse managers should avoid assuming responsibility for nonnursing services and should encourage the appropriate departments to perform such services. When departments do not do so, nurse managers should have a system of charging the provided services to the appropriate cost center other than the nursing cost center. The services will then become revenue of the nursing cost center.
7. The number and composition of the medical staff and the medical services offered. Nursing requirements will be affected by characteristics of patient populations determined by the size and capability of the medical staff. Several factors affect the quality and quantity of nursing personnel required and influence their placement: special requirements of individual physicians; the time and length of physicians' rounds; the time, complexity, and number of tests, medications, and treatments; and the kind and amount of surgical procedures.
8. Arrangement of the physical plant has a large impact on staffing requirements. Fewer personnel are needed

for a modern, compact facility equipped with labor-saving devices and efficient working arrangements than for one that is spread out and has few or no labor-saving devices. Different staffing is required for a facility that is arranged functionally than for one that is not. If, for example, the surgical suite is not next to the birthing rooms, recovery room, and intensive care units, more staff will be needed to meet acceptable standards of quality and safety. Many other architectural features must be considered, such as the location of specialized units; the location of patient rooms in relation to nursing stations, work rooms, and storage space; and the time required to transport patients to other sections of the hospital for diagnostic or therapeutic services, such as radiography and nuclear medicine.

9. The organization of the division of nursing. Plans should be reviewed and revised to organize the department to operate efficiently and economically with written statements of mission, philosophy, and objectives; sound organizational structure; clearly defined functions and responsibilities; written policies and procedures; effective staff development programs; and planned periodic systems evaluation. Staffing plans for such a department will be different from those that are loosely organized, with overlapping functions and responsibilities, vague or conflicting policies, and poorly defined standards of nursing practice.
10. Data to be analyzed will include number of admissions, discharges, and transfers; patient acuity; amount of supervision needed for ancillary personnel; patient teaching; emergency responses; mode of care delivery; and staff mix.

Staffing Activities

Numerous staffing activities have been identified by Price; he suggests that the nurse administrator assign and identify by name the persons responsible for each activity. Among his suggestions are the following:[18]

1. One person ultimately responsible for each activity should be identified.
2. The category and position of the person who should be responsible for each activity should be identified.
3. The activity should be specified as requiring nursing or nonnursing personnel.
4. The review should be performed for the day, evening, night, weekend, and holiday shifts.

A modified format by Price for gathering data and analyzing responsibility for staffing activities covers the following:

- Recruiting, interviewing, screening, and hiring RNs, LPNs, and NAs.
- Assigning personnel to clinical units and shifts.
- Preparing work schedules in advance.
- Maintaining daily schedules, adjusting for staff absences and patients' needs.
- Calculating turnover and hours of care.
- Checking time cards and payroll.
- Developing policy.
- Handling telephone communication.
- Ensuring contract compliance.

Orientation Plan

The orientation plan offered to new employees can impact both recruitment and retention; orientation is a time when a sense of belonging can be instilled. A main purpose of orientation is to help the nursing worker adjust; it should be a planned program overseen by the education department or a unit based clinical coordinator, with a one-on-one preceptor. Experienced nurses can ease the discomfort of a new work situation by doing the following:[19]

- Encouraging new nurses in the work unit as well as throughout the organization.
- Readily sharing information, and being willing to learn from both new graduates and experienced nurses accustomed to different systems.
- Modeling positive and professional behaviors and attitudes.
- Allowing new employees to establish their own practice patterns.
- Encouraging continuing education in the field.
- Practicing patience!

Exhibit 10-1 gives an example of a nursing orientation.

Policies and procedures should be introduced to the new employee in this phase. As there are too many policies and procedures to be absorbed at once, empower the new employees by enabling them to refer to appropriate sources for reference.

Staffing Policies

Staffing policies are best derived through consultation with clinical nurses. Written staffing policies should be readily available for at least the following areas:

- Vacations, holidays, and sick leave
- Emergency leave
- Weekend shifts: number worked, days considered as "weekend"
- Shift rotation
- Overtime
- Part-time and temporary personnel
- Use of float personnel
- Schedule changes
- Use of educational time

EXHIBIT 10-1
Nursing Orientation—Week 1

MONDAY	TUESDAY	WEDNESDAY	THURSDAY	FRIDAY
8:00–4:30 Personnel Orientation Benefits Performance improvement Employee health Infection control Fire & safety	8:00–10:00 Introduction Philosophy Dress code Staffing Time/attendance Skills Assessment 10:00–10:15 Break 10:15–12:15 Documentation 12:15–1:15 Lunch 1:15–4:30 MAR Medical Policies Medical Exam	8:00–8:15 Computer Class Assignment 8:15–12:00 Code 1 CPR 12:00–1:00 Lunch 1:00–4:30 Clinical Skills RN/LPN BGM Emergency trach R. TPN dressing C. CNA Vital signs Body mechanisms Infection control Legal	8:00–4:30 RN IV Therapy	8:00–8:45 XYZ Eye Center 8:45–9:30 XYZ Organ Center 9:30–9:45 Break 9:45–10:00 Nutrition Service 10:00–11:00 Telephone System 11:00–12:00 Lunch 12:00–4:30 Team Building

- Requests of personnel and management
- The work week

A work contract should be set up between each employee and the organization. The contract should state the date employment is to commence, job classification, job description, work hours, pay rate, full-time or part-time designation, and all other specific points agreed on between the employee and organizational representative.

Staffing the Units

According to JCAHO, staffing effectiveness is defined as "the number, competency, and skill mix of staff as related to the provision of needed services."[20]

Each patient care unit should have a master staffing plan that includes the basic staff needed to cover the unit for each shift. *Basic staff* is the minimum or lowest number of personnel needed to staff a unit and includes fully oriented full- and part-time employees. The number may be based on examination of previous staff records and expert opinion of nurse managers. Basic staff includes all categories: RNs, LPNs, and ancillary personnel for each shift. Exhibit 10-2 shows a formula for determining a core staff per shift. Exhibits 10-3 and 10-4 provide other tools that can be used to assist with staffing. For example, a staffing board showing the number of personnel needed for a period of time, along with a self-scheduling form, can be useful in meeting staffing challenges.

The number of *complementary personnel* is determined next. Complementary personnel are scheduled as additions to the basic group. Financial resources and the availability of personnel will control the total number in both groups. Not ensured a permanent pattern of staffing, complementary personnel provide the flexibility needed to meet short-term and unexpected changes.

Float personnel are not permanently assigned to a station. Managed by a centralized staffing office, they provide flexibility to meet increased patient loads and unexpected personnel absences. They may be cross-trained to a number of different medical milieus, or may specialize in one field. The number and kinds of float personnel can be accurately determined from general monthly records that show absence rates, personnel turnover, and fluctuations in patient care workloads.

Some nurse administrators do not hire *part-time nursing personnel*, who may be an economic or cost-control factor in staffing, because they usually do not receive the same benefits as full-time personnel. Part-time

EXHIBIT 10-2
Formula for Estimating a Core Staff per Shift

The average daily census for a 25-bed medical–surgical unit over a 6-month period is 19 patients. The basic average daily hours of care to be provided are 5 hours per patient per 24 hours. How many total hours of care will be needed on the average day to meet these standards? 19 × 5 = 95 hours. If the workday is 8 hours, this means 95 ÷ 8 = 11.9 or 12 full-time-equivalent (FTE) staff are needed to staff the unit for 24 hours. An FTE is one person working full time (40 hours a week) or several persons who together work a total of 40 hours a week. A total of 12 FTE × 7 days per week = 84 shifts per week, if the staffing is to be the same each day. If each employee works five 8-hour shifts per week, 84 ÷ 5 = 16.8 is the number of FTEs needed as basic staff for this unit.

The number of nursing personnel to cover sick leave, vacations, and holidays or other absences can also be determined and added to the basic staff. This information is determined from a study of personnel policies and use. It is frequently included in patient classification system formulas. Such additional staff may be provided from a float pool.

The next determination to be made is the ratio of RNs to other nursing personnel. If the ratio is determined to be 1:1, how much of the basic staff of 16.8 should be RNs? One half of the total, which would be 8.4 RNs and 8.4 others (LPNs, nurses' aides, orderlies, or nursing assistants). A study of staffing patterns in 80 medical–surgical, pediatrics, and postpartum units in 12 Salt Lake City community hospitals recommends a mix of 58% RNs, 26% LPNs, and 16% aides.[21]

The final determination is how many personnel are needed for each shift. Warstler recommends the following proportions: day, 47%; evening, 35%; and night, 17%.[22] This means that for a total staff of 16.8 personnel, 8 would be assigned to days, 6 to evenings, and 2.8 to nights. Obviously, this is an approximation; other patterns could also be chosen by the nurse administrator.

The number of complementary nursing personnel would be added to this basic staff. They could be a group of one RN, one LPN, and one other, assigned accordingly. The staff is entered into the following table as numbers in parenthesis added to the figure for basic staff.

In an environment that emphasizes reimbursement, complementary personnel may be budgeted as a pool, and may exist as only a portion of basic personnel assigned to a pool.

Basic Staffing Plan for a 25-Bed Medical–Surgical Unit

CATEGORY	DAY	EVENING	NIGHT	TOTAL
RNs	4 + (1)	3	1.4	8.4 + (1)
LPNs	2	2+ (1)	1.4	5.4 + (1)
Others	2	1	0 + (1)	3+ (1)
Totals	8 + (1)	6 + (1)	2.8 + (1)	16.8 + (3)

personnel will be better motivated if they receive some benefits, such as a number of paid holidays and vacation days proportionate to days worked and pay increases when they complete the aggregate days worked by full-time personnel. Their total hours worked can be controlled to fill actual shortfalls.

Staffing Modules

Many different approaches to nurse staffing and scheduling are being explored in an effort to satisfy the needs of employees and meet workload demands for patient care. These include modified work weeks (10- or 12-hour shifts), team rotation, "premium day" weekend nurse staffing, and "premium vacation" night staffing. Such approaches should support the underlying purpose, mission, philosophy, and objectives of the organization and the division of nursing and should be well defined in a staffing philosophy statement and policies. Nurses are like other workers in one respect: they would like to live as normal a home life as possible. In addition, shifts must be staffed and patient care needs met. The successful nurse executive will try to accommodate both by using the best available administrative staffing methodology, which must be considered from the economic or cost–benefit viewpoint, as well as in conjunction with and out of concern for the nursing staff.

Staffing and scheduling are reasons for both turnover and job retention. Understaffing has a negative effect on staff morale, delivery of quality care, and the nursing practice modality. It can close beds. It causes absenteeism resulting from staff fatigue, burnout, and professional dissatisfaction. Conversely, nurse managers must receive value for their money. Economic constraints exist that are further limited by the costs of recruiting, hiring, and orienting new nurses and for overtime and temporary

EXHIBIT 10-3
Staffing Board Showing the Number of Personnel Needed for 6 Weeks

The left row of pegs is coded by category of personnel: RN, LPN, NA (nursing assistant). There are peg holes on the board for 29 persons for 7 weeks. Larger boards can be used. Pegs for scheduling would be color-coded for shifts: day, evening, night, weekend, off, etc.

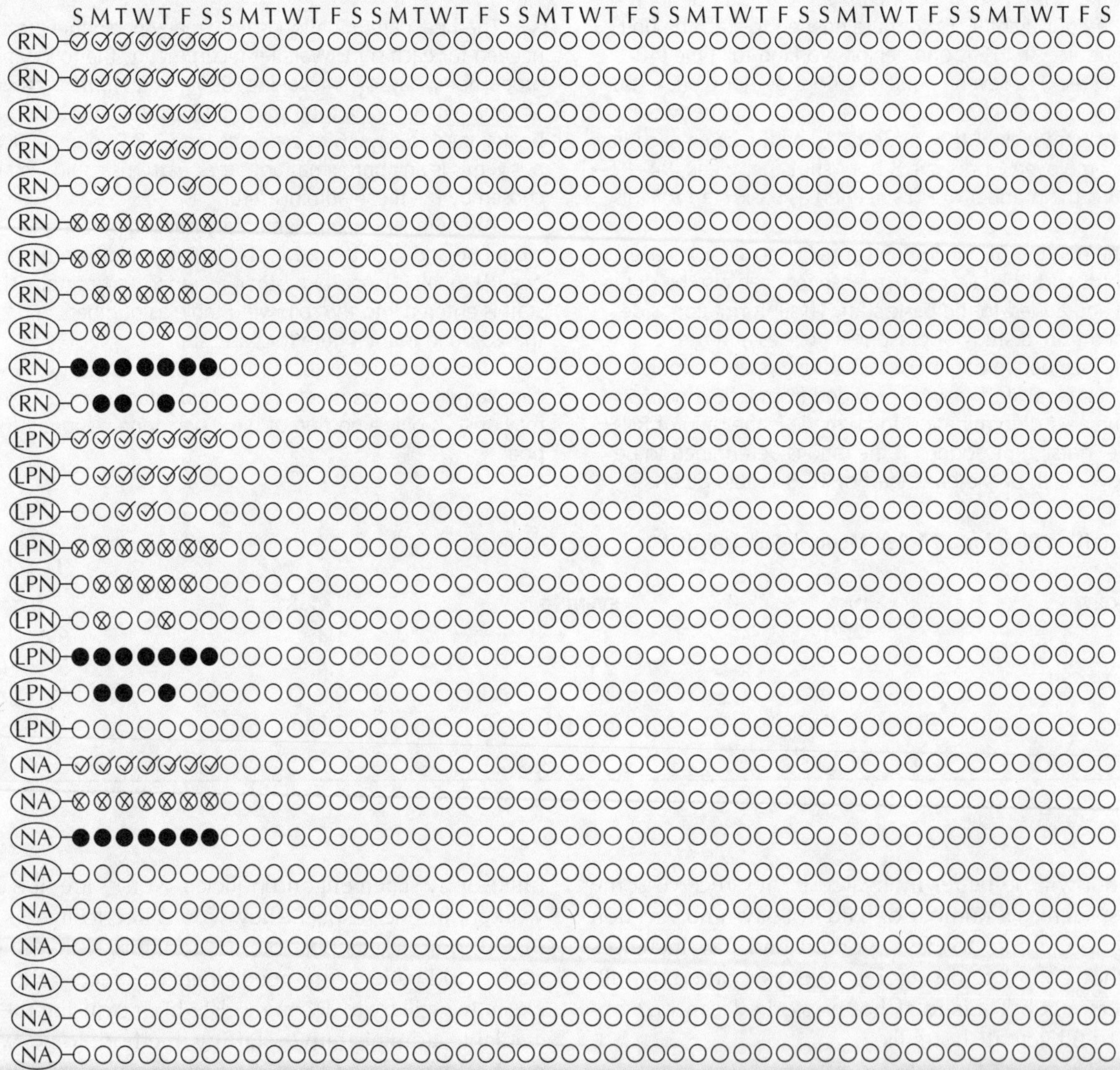

personnel when the environment creates turnover and absenteeism. Overstaffing is expensive and has a negative effect on staff morale and productivity. Staffing and scheduling must balance the personal needs of nurses with the economic and productivity needs of the organization.[23]

Patterns of staffing should be reviewed periodically to determine whether they are meeting the purpose, philosophy, and objectives of the organization and the division of nursing and whether they are practical regarding the numbers and qualifications of personnel. They must be satisfactory to nursing personnel and use available personnel effectively. The ultimate objective of staffing patterns is to ensure that patients' needs are being met.

Cyclic Scheduling

Team rotation is a method of cyclic staffing in which a nursing team is scheduled as a unit. It is used in the team nursing modality.[24]

EXHIBIT 10-4
Self-Scheduling Format

	S	INITIALS	M	INITIALS	T	INITIALS	W	INITIALS	TH	INITIALS	F	INITIALS	S	INITIALS
Week *Jan 15* 11 A.M.	3RNs 1LPN 1NA	JH	5RNs 2LPNs 1NA		4RNs 3LPNs 1NA		4RNs 3LPNs 1NA		4RNs 2LPNs 1NA		5RNs 2LPNs 1NA		3RNs 1LPN 1NA	
3 P.M.	3RNs 1LPN 1NA	JH	5RNs 2LPNs 1NA		4RNs 3LPNs 1NA		4RNs 3LPNs 1NA		4RNs 2LPNs 1NA		5RNs 2LPNs 1NA		3RNs 1LPN 1NA	
7 P.M.	2RNs 1LPN 1NA		4RNs 3LPNs 1NA		3RNs 2LPNs 1NA		3RNs 2LPNs 1NA		4RNs 3LPNs 1NA		3RNs 2LPNs 1NA		2RNs 1LPN 1NA	
11 P.M.	2RNs 1LPN 1NA		4RNs 3LPNs 1NA		3RNs 2LPNs 1NA		3RNs 2LPNs 1NA		4RNs 3LPNs 1NA		3RNs 2LPNs 1NA		2RNs 1LPN 1NA	
3 A.M.	1RN 1LPN 1NA		2RNs 2LPNs 1NA	JH	2RN 2LPN 1NA	JH	1RN 1LPN 1NA	JH	2RNs 2LPNs 1NA	JH	1RN 1LPN 1NA		1RN 1LPN 1NA	
7 A.M.	1RN 1LPN 1NA		2RNs 2LPNs 1NA	JH	2RN 2LPN 1NA	JH	1RN 1LPN 1NA	JH	2RNs 2LPNs 1NA	JH	1RN 1LPN 1NA		1RN 1LPN 1NA	
Week 11 A.M.														
3 P.M.														
7 P.M.														
11 P.M.														
3 A.M.														
7 A.M.														

Each block represents 4 hours of staffing.
Names and Initials:

RN Jane Hatfield JH

Cyclic scheduling is one way of staffing to meet the requirements of equitable distribution of hours of work and time off. A basic time pattern for a certain number of weeks is established and then repeated in cycles. Advantages of cyclic scheduling include the following:

- Once developed, it is a relatively permanent schedule, requiring only temporary adjustments.
- Nurses no longer have to live in anticipation of their time off-duty, because it may be scheduled for as long as six months in advance.
- Personal plans may be made in advance with a reasonable degree of reliability.
- Requests for special time off are kept to a minimum.
- It can be used with rotating, permanent, or mixed shifts and can be modified to allow fixed days off and uneven work periods, based on personnel needs and work period preferences.
- It can be modified to fit known or anticipated periods of heavy workloads and can be temporarily adjusted to meet emergencies or unexpected shortages of personnel.

Because cyclic scheduling is relatively inflexible, it works only with a staff that rotates by policy and personal choice. Personnel who need flexible staffing to meet their personal needs, such as those related to family and educational pursuits, do not generally accept it.

An infinite number of basic cyclic patterns can be developed and tailored to suit the needs of each unit. Patterns should reflect policy, workload factors, and staff preferences. Nursing personnel may use a staffing board (Exhibit 10-3) to develop a pattern and cycle satisfactory to them. A staffing board may be used to show the number of nursing personnel required for each day of the week for 6 weeks.

Self-Scheduling

Self-scheduling is an activity that may make a staff happier, more cohesive, and more committed. It should be planned carefully on a unit (cost center) basis with a written policy in place as a guideline. Planning may use either a self-directed work team or a quality circle technique approach. Personnel are scheduled to work their preferred shift as much as possible, as long as their preferred shifts meet the needs of the unit and balance with the needs of their coworkers. Self-scheduling has been found to shorten scheduling time; increase retention and satisfaction; and reduce conflicts, illness time, voluntary absenteeism, and turnover.

A nurse manager who had 12 RNs with absentee problems asked a nurse administrator how she could reduce these absences. A discussion followed about self-scheduling and the procedures to implement it. Several months later, the nurse manager reported to the nurse administrator that she had implemented self-scheduling and found that only one of the 12 employees still posed an absentee problem. The problems were solved with self-scheduling. The nurse manager then successfully proceeded to use self-scheduling with all other employees who requested it.

Self-scheduling leads to more responsible employees. It meets personal goals such as family, social life, education, child care, and commuting. It is an example of participatory management with decentralized decision making. The planning must include the givens, or rules, to be followed. These rules should be minimal to meet legal and professional standards.[25] Exhibit 10-4 gives an example that can be used to assist with self-scheduling.

Modified Work Week

Modified work week schedules using 10- and 12-hour shifts and other methods are commonplace. A nurse administrator should be sure work schedules are fulfilling the staffing philosophy and policies, particularly with regard to efficiency; such schedules should not be imposed on the nursing staff but should show a mutual benefit to employer, employees, and clients.

The 10-Hour Shift

One modification of the work week is the creation of four 10-hour shifts per week in organized time increments. One potential problem with this model is time overlaps of 6 hours per 24-hour day. The overlaps can be used for patient-centered conferences, nursing care assessment and planning, and staff development. The overlap can also be scheduled to cover peak workload demands, which can be identified by observation, consensus, or self-recording by professional nurses. It can be done by hour or by a block of 3 to 4 hours. Starting and ending times for the 10-hour shifts can be modified to provide minimal overlaps, with the 4-hour gap staffed by part-time or temporary workers.

The 4-day, 10-hour work schedule for night nurses was studied in a hospital that had difficulty recruiting qualified nurses for the night shift. It was found that 10-hour shifts had stabilized staffing in intensive care, with increased productivity and decreased turnover. Turnover on the night shift had been 70% for an 8-month period. Positions stayed vacant longer than for other shifts, and sick time was higher, which increased recruitment and orientation time. Nurses were involved in planning the 4-day, 10-hour night shift schedule. Night nurses agreed to use overlapping hours to assist with day shift care, and the day shift agreed to reduce staff by one FTE. Plans were discussed with and accepted by the union. Personnel assignments and meeting schedules were addressed and resolved through participatory management. The results of these changes included reduced sick time on the 10-hour shift, reduced turnover, increased incentive, increased requests for night shift, and decreased labor hours.[26]

The 12-Hour Shift

A second scheduling modification is the 12-hour shift; in this system, nurses work seven shifts in 2 weeks. They work a total of 84 hours and are paid 4 hours of overtime. Twelve-hour shifts and flexible staffing have been reported to have improved care and saved money because nurses can better manage their home and personal lives.[27] Another commonly used pattern is that of six 12-hour shifts with one 8-hour shift for a total of 80 hours, with no "forced" overtime.

Vik and MacKay report a study of the quality of care by nurses who worked 12-hour shifts versus those who worked 8-hour shifts. It was a matched study of three units each. The Quality Patient-Care Scale was the measuring instrument. Results indicated that patients perceived a significantly higher quality of care from nurses working 8-hour versus 12-hour shifts. Shift patterns worked by nurses do affect the care received by patients. Recruitment and retention of nurses, however, can balance out reduced quality of care when vacancies are high. This study was limited and needs to be replicated.[28]

A research study was done to measure the effect of fatigue from 12-hour shifts on critical thinking. The findings are that there were "no significant differences between levels of fatigue and critical thinking ability in nurses working 8 and 12 hours."[29]

The break-even point for costs is the point at which recruiting, absenteeism, retention, and overtime cost savings equal the shift losses from 12-hour scheduling.[30]

Negative Aspects

The following are some of the disadvantages of 10- and 12-hour shifts:[31]

- Minimum weekend staffing (or excess staff on weekends).
- Unsafe travel times.
- Shift overlaps that decrease total number of personnel on duty.
- Costs for overtime.
- Sleep deficit and fatigue.
- Strain on family life.
- Increased staffing if the schedule is not carefully planned to avoid loss of shifts.
- Possible requirement by state law to pay overtime wages for hours worked in excess of 8 in a day and 40 in a week.
- Less continuity of care, although continuity of care may improve when there are only two shifts per day.
- Less communication among staff.
- Need to develop, maintain, and explain the master schedule.
- More problems managing longer shifts for older nurses.
- Absent days result in greater loss of pay or paid days off.

Working night shifts, split shifts, or extended shifts may create problems such as sleeping on the job, conflicts with family members on other shifts, muddy thinking, and poor memory. Research suggests the following ways to better handle late or rotating shifts:[32]

- Use consistency in working shifts. If possible, work one shift all the time.
- Rotate shifts clockwise, one shift for a week, 48 hours between changing shifts.
- Use caffeine drinks judiciously at work.
- Get enough sleep. Avoid caffeine, alcohol, nicotine, and other sleep-disturbing chemicals for several hours before bedtime.
- Follow the workday routine on days off as much as possible. Change the workday routine if you find yourself feeling as if you are on autopilot.
- Prepare for a new shift by splitting time between sleep and wakefulness.
- Eat healthy snacks such as carrots or apples, rather than heavy foods.
- Drink liquids such as water or juice to stay hydrated.
- Take exercise breaks.
- Talk to coworkers.

The Weekend Alternative

"Weekend specials" have long been an attractive alternative form of scheduling. Not only do they afford the nurse weekdays with which to pursue educational opportunities or to spend time with family, they free "regular" staff from the perceived burden of working every other weekend to balance staffing. At one time, those nurses working two 12-hour shifts on the weekend were paid for a full 40 hour work week with benefits; that pay mode is rarely an option with today's budgetary constraints. There are, however, part-time packages modeled after this weekend schedule that afford greater pay than hours worked, with benefits attached.

"Premium day weekend" nurse staffing is a scheduling pattern that gives a nurse an extra day off duty, called a premium day, when he or she volunteers to work one additional weekend within a four-week scheduling block. This staffing technique could be modified to give the nurse a premium day off for every additional weekend worked beyond those required by nurse staffing policy. This technique does not add directly to hospital costs.[33]

"Premium vacation night" staffing follows the same principle as does premium day weekend staffing. An example is the policy of giving five extra working days of vacation to every nurse who works a permanent night shift for a specific period of time.

Flextime

Nurses often want flexible scheduling to better accommodate their personal lives. Such scheduling options have, in fact, become an essential component of job satisfaction.[34] Flexible time (frequently called *flextime*) schedules have become an increasingly important aspect of employment practices since 1980, when 11.9% of all nonfarm wage and salary workers were reported to be on flextime schedules. They have resulted in improved attitudes and increased productivity as employees have gained more control over their work environment. Employees have been able to adjust to their own bioclocks. Transportation has become more efficient and flexible. Employees have better control of work activities.[35]

To control for weaknesses of previous studies, the New York State government conducted a study of staggered work hours compared with fixed work hours. The study showed the following results:[36]

1. The greatest level of satisfaction and the lowest level of dissatisfaction with the workday was expressed by

employees in agencies with the greatest flexibility in scheduling.

2. Those in agencies with fixed schedules expressed the strongest dissatisfaction and lowest level of satisfaction.
3. Decreased commuting time may improve satisfaction with flextime.

Flexible scheduling improves recruiting, reduces absenteeism, and increases retention by boosting morale.

A study by Imig, Powell, and Thorman indicates that flexible staffing filled vacant positions but did not increase payroll costs, hours per patient day, or overtime. It also decreased absenteeism by 60%. The hospital in this study returned to 8-hour shifts because primary nursing was threatened. In this particular study, there was no change in incidence of medication errors, patient and staff injuries, quality of care plans, complaints, recruitment, or staff attitudes from before to 6 months after flexible staffing. Also, the use of agency nurses was not reduced.[37]

There are multiple scheduling options open for nurse managers to explore. In the case of a staff working 80 hours in a unit (six 12-hour shifts and one 8-hour shift), a need was found between the 7 A.M.–3 P.M. shift and the 11 P.M.–7 A.M. shift. One RN volunteered to work a straight shift five days a week from 3 P.M. to 11 P.M.; her "bonus" was working straight weekdays, with no weekends and holidays off! It is up to the nurse manager and the staff involved to find innovative solutions suitable to their own workplace.

A Flexible Role: Resource Acuity Nurse

At West Virginia University Hospital, top nurse executives established a resource acuity nurse position to provide greater flexibility and ensure adequate staffing during peak workload periods. The executives envisioned having nurses in the position available to provide immediate relief to units when the greatest care needs arose. The resource acuity nurse would stay at the agency for as long as needed.

The nurse managers developed guidelines for undertaking the resource acuity nurse responsibilities:

- Assisting with special procedures, such as central line placement and extensive dressing changes.
- Supporting nursing staff whenever an increased number of patients is returning from the operating room.
- Assisting in cardiac arrests or other emergencies.
- Transferring unstable patients to the intensive care units.

This program has enabled the hospital to better meet the staffing needs of units when workload increases. Since the establishment of the resource acuity nurse position in this organization, nurses' morale has improved, because they know short-term help is more readily available and will be more equitably distributed among units.[38]

Cross-Training

Cross-training of nursing personnel can improve flexible scheduling (as in the example of the resource nurse role). Nurses can be prepared through cross-training to function effectively in more than one area of expertise. They can be kept in similar clinical specialties (such as an ICU cluster) or in families of clinical specialties. To prevent errors and increase job satisfaction during cross-training, nurses assigned to units and in pools require complete orientation and ongoing staff development. Nurses should be provided with policies, job descriptions, and performance evaluations.

Temporary Workers

Nurses have been doing work as temporary agency employees for several decades. They have turned to staffing agencies because they wanted control over their lives, personal and professional. Agency work was the only way they could gain such control until nurse managers and hospital administrators realized the need to apply the science of behavioral technology, including HR management, to nursing. Many organizations are downsizing to make themselves more productive by decreasing overhead, and one result of downsizing is the use of agency or external workers.

The number of temporary jobs, professional and nonprofessional, has increased annually and is now in the millions. In many instances temporary employment has caused workers to experience downward mobility. The lesson for nursing personnel is to gain a reputation for competence in more than one clinical area or in more than one of the areas of clinical practice, teaching, research, and management.

Work forces in today's organizations are leaner and meaner. Temporary employees prevent hiring mistakes by employers and employees. Nearly half of hospitals use temporary workers.

Potential temporary employees should become informed about the temporary agency they will use. They can ask other nurses who have used it about it, screen the agency by telephone to determine customer treatment, visit the agency on a busy Monday morning, and then interview with the agency.[39]

Strategic Staffing

Accounting firms have developed strategic staffing as an approach to downsizing. Strategic staffing analyzes a unit's staffing needs, based on long-term objectives for the unit and organization, to find a combination of permanent and temporary employees with the best skills to meet these needs. Temporary staffing may protect the jobs of permanent or core employees when the temporary employee is used to cover a vacancy while the position or job is analyzed.

Temporary employees may want to sample the work. A variety of professional occupations are represented in the temporary work force. Temporary workers provide relief for overworked permanent employees; many do one-time projects, including internal audits and forensic accounting. They work as trainers of permanent employees. Using temporary employees controls personnel expenses related to benefits, rehiring, and training.

To make strategic staffing work, managers should study staffing once annually, analyzing workload peaks and valleys, looking at the financial blueprint, and communicating with providers and staff.

The warning signs that strategic staffing is required include excessive overtime, high turnover, excessive absenteeism, employees whose skills do not match job requirements, absence of regular staffing planning, missed deadlines, last-minute staffing using temporary employees, lack of a budget line for temporary employees, absence of communication with the HR department, and low employee morale. Obtaining the best temporary workers may require consultation with specialized temporary employment firms.[40]

Temporary workers are cost-effective for small businesses, because they eliminate the expense of an HR department. For large businesses, temporary workers are cost-effective for the flexibility needed for seasonal and short-term work. Using temporary employees also enables employers to evaluate those employees for permanent jobs.[41]

Travel Nursing

A step beyond the nurses who work for local agencies, travel nursing is an increasingly popular career choice. The mobility of society at large has increased the willingness of nursing workers to relocate for weeks- or months-long assignments. Nurses engaged in travel nursing run the gamut from young single professionals with a taste for adventure to older "empty-nesters," free from family ties and ready to experience more than their local health care systems can offer.

"The rapidly growing nursing shortage was the impetus for the development of the travel nursing industry years ago and, as it continues, the shortage will likely fuel the demand for travel nurses in the future."[42] The offer of benefits (401(k)s, health and dental insurance) and a high rate of pay, attracts many applicants; it has become difficult for organizations to match the travel packages available, and many organizations have lost nurses to such enticing offers.

Travel nurses will give organizations the benefit of a fresh outlook, a variety of experiences and a willingness to work within a new system. To their new coworkers, they will give a glimpse of another culture and perhaps share their willingness to learn.

Transfer Fair

In an effort to minimize the negative repercussions of downsizing, one hospital used a "transfer fair" to place staff quickly and fairly. The key participants were as follows:

- Managers with vacancies
- Recruitment staff with a list of vacancies
- Employee relations staff to answer personnel policy questions
- Staff affected by downsizing

Each affected staff member made three choices. Seniority then determined placement, and decisions were made within 48 to 72 hours.

The atmosphere and tone of a transfer fair is gracious, welcoming, professional, relaxed, and supportive. Planners prepare well and make the fair convenient for all shifts. Refreshments are served and top nursing administrators attend.[43]

Magnet Hospitals

In 1982, a groundbreaking study by the American Academy of Nursing identified 41 facilities as "magnet" hospitals, which consistently attracted and retained good nurses and provided excellent nursing care. In response, the Magnet Recognition Program was developed 9 years later by the American Nurses Credentialing Center.[44] In a study of staff nurses working in 14 magnet hospitals, those attributes identified as essential to delivering quality care were as follows:

- Organizational support for education.
- A work force of clinically competent nurses.
- Positive relationships between nurses and physicians.
- Autonomy in nursing practice.
- A client-centered culture.
- Control of nursing practice.
- Perception of adequate staffing.
- The support of nursing administration.

In the face of chronic understaffing, many hospitals use competitive wages and benefits to attract nurses. Competitive wages are important, but they are not the ultimate tool for attraction and retention of nurses. "Current health care concerns mandate innovative, culture-based approaches to recruiting and retaining staff."[45]

Patient Classification Systems

The component of a traditional system of nurse staffing that is essential to all facets of the total system is patient classification. A patient classification system (PCS), which quantifies the quality of nursing care, is essential to staffing nursing units of hospitals and nursing homes. In selecting or implementing a PCS, a representative committee of hospital administration, nurse managers, and clinical nurses should be used.

The primary aim of patient classification is to be able to respond to the constant variation in the care needs of patients.[46]

Classification systems originated in the 1960s, when R. J. Connor's doctoral research work resulted in the development of a classification tool for hospitals to better use nursing staff. Three categories of patient acuity, with guidelines describing typical characteristics, were identified:

- Category I: Self-care
- Category II: Intermediate care
- Category III: Total care

Connor's guidelines described the time necessary for the care of a patient in each category. He created a staffing algorithm using a patient index:

$$I = 0.5N_1 + 1.0N_2 + 2.5N_3$$

in which I represents the patient care index, and N the number of patients in each category. The constant (0.5, 1.0, 2.5) represents the amount of direct care in hours and the subscripts (1, 2, 3,) represent the specific classification level.[47]

Purposes

The committee will identify the purposes of the PCS to be purchased or developed. Among such purposes are the following:[48]

- *Staffing*. The system will establish a unit of measure for nursing, that is, time, which will be used to determine numbers and kinds of staff needed. Perceived patient needs can be matched with available nursing resources.
- *Program costing and formulation of the nursing budget*. A prescribed unit of time will be used to determine the actual costs of nursing services. Profits and losses of nursing can then be determined.
- *Tracking changes in patient care needs*. A PCS gives nurse managers the ability to moderate and control delivery of care services, adjusting intensity and cost.
- *Determining values for the productivity equation: output divided by input*. Reducing input costs reduces the cost of each output (time unit). In the prospective payment system (PPS), this output measure has been the discharged patient. Outputs become the criteria for measuring nursing productivity, regardless of quality. PCSs provide workload indices as productivity measures.
- *Determining quality*. Once a standard time element has been established, staffing is adjusted to meet the aggregate times. A nurse manager can elect to staff below the standard time to reduce costs, making a decision to reduce quality by reducing times and costs. It is best to do this in collaboration with clinical nurses. These nurses can assist with developing and applying more efficient procedures and protocols, which can involve rearrangement of the physical setting and the assembling of equipment and supplies. Involvement by clinical nurses will increase their trust and respect, improve their attendance and work habits, improve work force stability, and reduce errors.

Desired Characteristics

A PCS should do the following:[49]

1. Differentiate intensity of care among definitive classes.
2. Measure and quantify care to develop a management engineering standard.
3. Match nursing resources to patient care requirements.
4. Relate to time and effort spent on the associated activity.
5. Be economical and convenient to report and use.
6. Be mutually exclusive, counting no item under more than one work unit.
7. Be open to audit.
8. Be understood by those who plan, schedule, and control the work.
9. Be individually standardized as to the procedures needed for accomplishment.
10. Separate requirements for registered nurses from those of other staff.

Components

The first component of a PCS is a method for grouping patients or patient categories. Johnson describes two methods of categorizing patients. Through factor evaluation, each patient is rated on independent elements of care, each element is scored (weighted), scores are summarized, and the patient is placed in a category based on the total numerical value obtained. In prototype evaluation, each patient is categorized to a broad description of care requirements.[50]

Johnson describes a prototype evaluation with four basic categories (self-care, minimal, moderate care, extensive care) and one category for a typical patient requiring one-on-one care. Each category addresses activities of daily living, general health, teaching and emotional support, and treatments and medications. Data are collected on average time spent on direct and indirect care. For example, under activities of daily living aspects of eating, grooming, excretion, and comfort are identified. At a minimal care level, the patient requires help in preparing food and positioning or encouragement to eat, but can feed his or her self.

A second component of a PCS is a set of guidelines describing the way in which patients will be classified, the frequency of classification, and the method of reporting the data. The third component of a PCS is the average amount of time required for care of a patient in each category.

A method for calculating required staffing and required nursing care hours is the fourth and final component of a PCS. The sum of the standard times for each category multiplied by the number of patients in that category plus the indirect care time equals required hours of patient care. Dividing this value by the number of hours staff actually works each shift results in the number of staff required to work each shift.[51]

The Commission for Administration Services in Hospitals (CASH) system of patient classification is an example of the prototype evaluation type. CASH rates patients by intensity of care and establishes a category relating to nursing hours required based on patients' ability to feed and bathe themselves with supervision; mobility status; special procedures and treatments; and observational, institutional, and emotional needs. The CASH design is quantified by determining the nursing care time associated with the critical indicators.

The GRASP® PCS uses a workload measurement design to evaluate the categories of tasks that nurses perform in providing patient care and identifies how much nursing time is required for each task. The time is then totaled.[52] GRASP® is a factor evaluation design, as is Medicus.

General agreement exists that three to five categories of patient acuity are sufficient for a PCS. Alward argues that four categories are best to reduce variance and statistical probability of error. She also states that the factor evaluation instrument is better than the prototype system because the former prevents ambiguity and overlap among the categories.[53] Research has indicated that different PCSs can generate different hours of workload and related nursing workload.[54]

Examples

Nursing Models

PCSs based on a model of nursing are rare. Auger and Dee describe one based on the Johnson Behavioral System Model, which has eight behavioral subsystems: ingestive, eliminative, affiliative, dependency, sexual, aggressive-protective, achievement, and restorative. Patient behaviors and nursing interventions were rank-ordered for four categories of patient acuity, with category 1 identified as reinforcing independent behaviors in adaptive areas and providing supervision. Category 4 denotes care provided on a one-to-one basis for eight hours per shift, as, for example, in suicide observations. In this model, specifically in the eliminative subsystem, patients' behaviors that might be noted include absence of bowel and bladder control, and excessive diaphoresis. Nursing interventions would include implementing a behavioral program for toilet training, bedwetting, and encopresis. Other systems would be assessed with nursing interventions identified to address the behaviors.

Auger and Dee list four advantages to relating nursing models to PCSs:[55]

1. Providing a frame of reference for the systematic assessment of patient behaviors and the development of nursing intervention.
2. Providing a frame of reference for all practitioners in the clinical setting.
3. Providing a theoretical framework of knowledge and behavior.
4. Providing for consistency and continuity of care.

Dee and Auger emphasize orientation and teaching of all new personnel so the system will be used effectively. This is true of all PCSs, and of their use to make decisions about admissions.

In-House Versus Purchased

Purchased PCSs are very expensive and must be modified for specific hospitals. An in-house PCS can be developed using work analysis techniques. Methods for developing such systems are described in several references; most use observation or self-reporting techniques. In the self-reporting techniques, personnel are trained to list activities they perform at timed intervals. Observation on a continuous or internal basis can be costly in time and money. Self-reporting is cheaper, but employees must be trained.[56]

Alward states that it is more realistic to use the budget to determine staffing. She suggests selecting a prototype or factor-evaluation classification instrument and revising it to conform to the division's nursing practice.[57]

Nyberg and Wolff describe a PCS that calculates the total time, direct and indirect, needed to care for each patient by unit, shift, and job classification. The required time is compared with actual and budgeted nursing time per patient. This system has been found to identify patient care trends, improve efficiency of staffing, and justify budgeting changes. It has been used for utilization review, using access to admitting and working diagnoses, surgical procedures, physician–consultants, patient classification categories, and a list of all daily nursing care activities. When hospitalization is not justified, a chart review is done. This computerized system determines nursing costs per patient by unit, Medicare patients and non-Medicare patients by diagnosis, and average and total costs of Medicare and non-Medicare patients. In one 2-week period, Medicare patients required 10% more nursing resources per day and 40% more nursing time for their entire hospitalization.[58]

Computer Models

There are also personal computer models of PCSs. One of these, described by Grazman, has modules for planning nursing care and dealing with the budget. This system projects the number of hours of care, for each of four patient levels, that will meet budgetary and program delivery constraints of the staffing parameters. It is a staffing system that addresses the "demand" function based on planning and the "management" function based on a blending of planning and actual situations. Thus, the input variables can be changed and the budget renegotiated. This model plans nursing time and resource allocation daily, based on patient case mix and census. It gives the nurse manager control over resource use.[59]

Adams and Duchene describe a PCS that includes nursing diagnosis with related cause, nursing care goals, and potential patient outcomes. It is an in-house system, the advantages of which include the following:[60]

- Knowledge of the data tool.
- Ability to alter the system to accommodate changes in procedural time standards.
- Ability to make changes in staffing levels.
- Ability to make percentage alterations of time given to indirect care activities.

This PCS produces a plan of care, with acuity used as the basis of determining staffing needs.

Problems

One of the major problems of PCSs is maintaining reliability and validity. This can be addressed through continuing education and quality checks. A calendar can be established to have external personnel from staff development or another nursing department or unit perform a classification after one is done by unit personnel (interacter reliability). This classification can be done monthly or more or less often, depending on the results. Patients can be monitored on different days and different shifts, with a stratified random sample of 15% or 20% of the patient census. Simple percentage agreement of 90% or higher indicates satisfactory reliability. If agreement is below 80%, the system should be reviewed and adjusted.

A calendar can also be established to take a unit rotation work sample to determine whether procedures or tasks change with time and technology. The calendar can be used as an annual spot-check. Validation of PCSs varies. A questionnaire can be used to evaluate nursing staff's satisfaction with hours of care. Validity can also be tested by an expert panel of nurses. Patient category descriptions or critical indicators of nursing intervention and patient requirement lists should be reviewed annually according to standards. The PCSs must be altered when results of quality checks or work samples so indicate.

Orientation and continuing education are the best methods of ensuring reliability and validity. The nursing staff must find the PCS credible. If nurses believe that the classifications are accurate and useful, they will try to rate patients accurately. They need periodic classes to be updated, and they must be kept well informed. Managers must support the use of a valid and reliable PCS, because it indicates the institution's commitment to quality patient care.

Nursing should orient other department heads and physicians to the use of PCSs. Admission and placement of patients are related to PCS outcomes.[61]

Practicing nurses want the PCS to provide more staff. Managing nurses want to use it to validate staffing and scheduling and to permit variable staffing. These objectives must be kept in harmony.

Fixed Ratio Staffing

A second method of determining the level of staffing necessary to deliver patient care is a fixed-ratio pattern, predetermined by nursing administrators and frequently based on historical data from PCSs, productivity reports, and admit/discharge data. Its major negative aspects include its disregard for the type of patient and for the education and experience level of the nursing staff.

The American Nurses Association California (ANA/C) lobbied for and facilitated the creation of the nation's first law mandating nurse-staffing ratios for acute care hospitals. AB 394, authored by Assemblywoman Sheila Kuehl, was signed into law by Governor Gray Davis (CA) on October 10, 1999. Despite a tentative agreement for implementation by January 2002, it was not until January 2004 that the regulations stipulated within the law were implemented. Among those regulations are the following:[62]

- Nurse staffing is determined based on the severity of illness and the need for specialized equipment.
- Registered nurses must receive an orientation to the area assigned; orientation and competency validation is required for temporary personnel.
- Nursing positions are mandated; ancillary positions are not.
- Both the education and experience levels of the nurse are to be factored in with acuity levels when determining staffing patterns.

Nursing Management Information Systems

Hanson defines a management information system (MIS) as "an array of components designed to transform a collective set of data into knowledge that is directly useful and applicable in the process of directing and controlling resources and their application to the achievement of specific objectives."[63]

The nursing management information system (NMIS) includes these five elements:[64]

1. Quality of patient care to be delivered and its measurement.
2. Characteristics and care requirements of patients.
3. Prediction of the supply of nurse power required for components 1 and 2.
4. Logistics of the staffing program pattern and its control.
5. Evaluation of the quality of care desired, thereby measuring the success of the staffing itself.

A management information system is basic to a sound system of staffing, of scheduling, and of classification of patients. It provides shift reports of personnel by type needed and assigned, staffing and productivity data by unit and area, average data on the intensity of care needed by class of patient and the cost per time unit of patient care.[65]

Staffing is a major reason to have an NMIS. A personal computer can be used to show, via menus and printouts, the number of nurses required by time slot, restrictions, off-duty policy, continuous or other than intermittent days off, cyclical schedules, and single rotations.[66]

Information stimulates action through management decision making. Data do not; they must be processed to be useful. Information must be timely to be useful. The following is the process for establishing any MIS:[67]

1. State the management objective clearly.
2. Identify the actions required to meet the objective.
3. Identify the responsible position in the organization.
4. Identify the information required to meet the objective.
5. Determine the data required to produce the needed information.
6. Determine the system's requirement for processing the data.
7. Develop a flowchart.

Productivity

"The most valuable asset of the twenty-first century institution, whether business or non-business, will be its knowledge workers and their productivity." Frederick Winslow Taylor set the stage for scientific management in developing a method for job analysis and eliminating unneeded motions. Scientific management makes the worker productive.[68]

Definition

Productivity is commonly defined as output divided by input. Hanson translates this definition into the following:

$$\frac{\text{Required staff hours}}{\text{Provided staff hours}} \times 100 = \text{Percent productivity}$$

For example:

$$\frac{\text{380.50 Required staff hours}}{\text{402.00 Provided staff hours}} \times 100 = 94.7\% \text{ productivity}$$

Productivity can be increased by decreasing the provided staff hours while keeping the required staff hours constant or increasing them. These data become information when they are related to an objective that indicates variances.[69] Because health care resources are limited, the nurse manager is faced with the task of motivating clinical nurses to increase productivity.

Productivity in nursing is related to both efficiency of use of clinical nursing in delivering nursing care and the effectiveness of that care relative to its quality and appropriateness. Brown suggests that US productivity can decline with increased labor costs without corresponding increases in performance. This decline can be due to factors such as inexperienced workers, technological slowdown from outdated equipment and decreased research and development, government regulations, a diminished work ethic, increased size and bureaucracy in business and industry, and erosion of the managerial ethic.[70]

Measurement

In developing a model for an MIS, Hanson details several formulas for translating data into information. He indicates that in addition to the productivity formula, *hours per patient day (HPPD)* are a data element that can provide meaningful information when provided for an extended period of time. HPPD is determined by the formula:

$$\frac{\text{Staff hours}}{\text{Patient days}} = \text{HPPD}$$

For example:

$$\frac{\text{52,000 Staff hours}}{\text{2883.5 Patient days}} = 18.03 \text{ HPPD}$$

Staff hours are calculated as:

52,000 Staff hours = 25 FTEs × 2080 work hours per year

2883.5 Patient days = 7.9 Average daily census (ADC) × 365 days per year.

No allowance is made for personal time such as coffee breaks, meals, vacations, holidays, sick time, and decreased census time. The figure of 18.03 HPPD may be a high provision of HPPD even for intensive care.

Another useful formula is for budget utilization:

$$\frac{\text{Provided HPPD}}{\text{Budgeted HPPD}} \times 100 = \text{Budget Utilization}$$

$$\frac{\text{18.03 Provided HPPD}}{\text{16.0 Budgeted HPPD}} \times 100 = \text{112.7\% Budget utilization}$$

The result would have been over budget if the provided hours had been the net of personal time. Because they were not, the HPPD provided may be highly productive. The adequacy of the budget is determined as:

$$\frac{\text{Budgeted HPPD}}{\text{Required HPPD}} \times 100 = \text{Budget adequacy}$$

or,

$$\frac{\text{16.0 Budgeted HPPD}}{\text{18.03 Required HPPD}} \times 100 = \text{88.74\% Budget adequacy}$$

Obviously, if the required HPPD are equal to the provided HPPD and exceed the budgeted HPPD, productivity is high because of budget inadequacy. According to Hanson, all data become information when related to the objective.[71] Staffing should be defined in terms of the goal of HPPD to be provided. This goal will relate to productivity, budget utilization, and budget adequacy. Whether it will be effective or not depends on measurement of quality of outcomes.

Davis writes that productivity in nursing is the volume and quality of products divided by the cost of producing and delivering them. It is directly related to what nurses do and how they do it. Systems have been developed to determine nursing cost per patient per shift. For example, at University Hospital of Cleveland, the following formula is used:

Nurse competence rank × Hourly salary rate
× Required nursing hours
× Care acuity
= Nursing cost per patient

For example:[72]

Clinician III × $25.00
× 3 hr
× 5
= $1,125.00 per shift

One could conclude that the more acutely ill patients are, the more licensed nurse contacts they require.

Smith, Mackey, and Markham developed a productivity monitoring system for the recovery room. The performance ratio was the required FTEs divided by worked FTEs. The data were used to decide whether to fill vacant positions and to develop a budget.[73]

Mailhot reported an analysis of problems in an operating room: poor physical environment, inadequate financial support, poor systems, and low morale. The department was overstaffed by 10 FTEs. Task forces used brainstorming and open forums to solve the problems. They used Lewin's force field analysis, putting complex decision alternatives through an outcome matrix, developing needed evaluation tools, and using pilot projects to test all changes. The task forces made 87 changes in one year. In addition, the task forces marketed services to patients and surgeons, provided management training for operating room managers, analyzed operating room procedures, and held an open day between director and staff once every 6 weeks during which each person could see the director. They reduced the staffing by 38 FTE positions and the budget by $1.5 million in 3 years. Job satisfaction surveys indicated improvement.[74]

High input for low output produces low productivity and high output for low input produces high productivity. Thus, the objective of a nursing productivity model is low input for high output.

Productivity Model Differences

Producers of services do not fit the same productivity models as do producers of material goods. Marked discretion exists in determining both expected and actual role performances of nurses who do not produce physical outputs. For this reason, nursing prescriptions such as "emotional support" are difficult to measure. Patient outputs or outcomes can be measured by client satisfaction and client condition on discharge.

Greater emphasis has been placed on the nursing process than on nursing outcome. Haas defines efficiency as the relationship of personnel assigned and time spent to materials expended, as well as capital and management employed, for the greatest economy in use. Productive nurses must balance their personal energies and their institution's resources with their own effectiveness.[75]

Curtin proposes that productivity in nursing is related to the application of knowledge. Professional productivity must be measured by means of efficacy, effectiveness, and efficiency in applying knowledge. Curtin indicates that these processes can be objectively measured by using the following guidelines:[76]

1. Objective measures of efficacy: years of formal education, levels of academic achievement, evidence of continuing education and skill development, and years of experience.
2. Objective measures of effectiveness: demonstrated ability to execute job-related procedures, prioritize activities correctly, perform according to professional

and legal standards, record appropriate information clearly and concisely, and cooperate with others.

3. Objective measures of efficiency: Promptitude, attendance, reliability, precision, adaptability, and economical disposition of resources.

Curtin and Zurlage acknowledge that human services such as nursing are difficult to test, to return, or to exchange if they are unsatisfactory. These authors propose a system for measuring nursing productivity that includes a nursing productivity equation, an equation relating nursing productivity ratio to hospital revenue, and a nursing productivity index.[77]

Improving Nursing Productivity

The first step toward improving productivity is to study or measure it as it exists. For example, the personnel of an education department decided to improve their productivity. They considered using a time-based method versus a value-based method in developing the productivity system.

A time-based method of productivity considers the length of time required to do each task. The first steps of a time-based method are to review the literature, do a time study, and then compare the results with those in the literature. This is done for activities unique to the unit. Units are then assigned to activities according to the estimated time for completing each. The time-based method does not give priority to activities.

A value-based system considers the value of activities to the institution. Steps for developing a value-based system of productivity include listing activities, grouping them by their value to the institution, and assigning units of productivity. The HR department should be involved in developing a productivity system.

The McKay-Dee education department at McKay-Dee Hospital Center (Ogden, Utah) uses data-collection tools that provide useful methods to better understand productivity from a qualitative and quantitative perspective.[78]

The reported knowledge and skills from improved nursing productivity add to the theory of nursing management. Rabin writes that professionals can impose productivity values on themselves. Managers should develop managerial goals and values. They need a standard of performance for themselves. Professionals must commit themselves to fostering innovative attitudes and technologies, stimulating performance by commitment to constructive action and followup, living up to standards of practice, keeping up-to-date, and being receptive to public review. Most professions can develop measurable standards of performance and productivity using online spreadsheets and software programs such as Lotus or Excel.[79]

Employers should measure nursing output objectively and pay for it accordingly in salary, benefits, and promotions. Some progress has been made in nursing in the form of standards of practice, clinical ladders, and models of peer review. These tools, along with respect for the individual dignity of nurses, support for their personal commitment to professional goals, and support for the integrity of their professional judgments, need to be enacted in the workplace.[80]

Productivity can be managed and improved through the following:[81]

- Planning that increases the variations between inputs and outputs by:
  - Outputs increasing, inputs decreasing.
  - Outputs increasing, inputs remaining constant.
  - Outputs increasing faster than inputs.
  - Outputs remaining constant, inputs decreasing.
  - Outputs decreasing more slowly than inputs.
- Involving staff; soliciting staff's ideas and recommendations.
- Creating challenges.
- Showing interest in the staff's achievement and concerns.
- Praising and rewarding good performance; using incentives such as staff development, books and tuition reimbursement, paid meals, bonuses, and vacation days.
- Setting the climate for productivity by asking nurses what makes them productive, acting on their suggestions, and measuring the results.
- Having a meaningful set or family of easily understood outcome measures for which data are available or easy to gather and over which workers have some control.
- Monitoring workload changes in staffing requirements with established standards.
- Combining support with employees' understanding, motivation, and recognition.
- Increasing the ratio of professional to nonprofessional staff.
- Placing admitted patients based on resource availability.
- Using approaches such as work simplification and workflow analysis.
- Making an organizational diagnosis of problems, resources, and realities.
- Stimulating nurse managers and clinical nurses to want to achieve excellence.
- Setting targets for increasing output annually without additional capital or employees.
- Having personnel keep and analyze time diaries to determine personal improvement actions. Setting personal objectives, and measuring performance against them.
- Making a commitment to improved productivity, effectiveness (doing the right things), and efficiency (doing things right).

- Seeking new products and services and new methods and ways of producing them. Seeking new and useful approaches to old problems.
- Maintaining concern about the process and methods of producing nursing care.
- Reducing the costs of what nurses do by returning unused budgeted funds.
- Improving aesthetics: the quality of work life and the pleasantness and beauty of the environment.
- Applying the ethical policy statements of professional nursing organizations.
- Improving use of time.
- Gaining the confidence of peers.
- Recognizing the need to do better.

Personnel working in service areas can improve productivity by doing the following:[82]

- Focusing on organizational strategy, customer service, mission, and results rather than on methodology.
- Using self-directed work teams to break jobs into observable tasks and responsibilities.
- Observing and then making changes or providing training to correct deficiencies.
- Watching for problems such as repetition, duplication, recurring delays, and waste of resources.
- Observing the outcome of the person's work by splitting the job into four main areas: managing self, resources, and activities and working with others. Suggestions for the key skills required are analytical thinking, ability to learn, adaptability, positive self-image, emphasis on results, good time management, concern for standards, ability to influence others, and independence.
- Providing feedback that is specific, constructive, and frequent.

Case Study

At the Presbyterian Hospital of Dallas, a study revealed that more time was spent on clerical functions, telephone calls, and reporting patient conditions to other caregivers than on direct patient care. Several actions were taken that greatly improved productivity:[83]

- A fax machine network was instituted between nursing units and the pharmacy, reducing the number of telephone calls and medication errors.
- A keyless narcotics system was installed that included personnel pass codes. The main control system was in pharmacy, but nurses could enter their personal pass code at the narcotics cabinet. This reduced time wasted to search for keys and produced an audit trail.
- A unit beeper system with eight beepers was purchased at a local store for $375. Beepers given to every staff member at the beginning of each shift made nursing assistants feel valued.

Summary

Staffing and scheduling are major components of nursing management. A nursing division needs a practical and written philosophy that guides all staffing and scheduling activities and that is acceptable to the staff.

Staffing studies can be used to determine staffing needs related to personnel skills, numbers of personnel, and time and workload requirements. There are as many possible approaches to staffing as there are nursing managers and staff to create them. Staffing innovations are key to the satisfaction, and therefore retention, of nurses.

Staffing can be planned with models that calculate workload requirements from patient classification data, or at the discretion of nursing administration with fixed-ratio staffing.

Productivity, the unit of output of nursing, is a focus of increasing interest to nurse managers. It must include quality care indicators that can be observed and measured.

> Productivity, quality of care, and a safe and healthy workplace are all enhanced when concern for the individual seeking health care services is the top priority and when nursing administrators assure:
>
> - adequate numbers of clinically competent staff,
> - positive working relationships among the health care team,
> - autonomy and accountability for nursing practice, adequate compensation, commensurate with responsibilities, education, and experience,
> - access to education and research,
> - access to appropriate technologies, and promotion of evidence-based practice.[84]

APPLICATION EXERCISES

EXERCISE 10-1 Based on the information listed below, use Exhibit 10-2, Formula for Estimating a Core Staff per Shift, to do the following exercise.

1. The average daily census (ADC) of a unit is 29 patients.

EXERCISE 10-1 (continued)

2. The basic average daily hours of care to be provided are 6 hours per patient per 24 hours.
3. The workday is 8 hours.
4. Determine the following:
   a. The total hours of care needed on the average day to meet these standards.
   b. The total number of FTEs needed to staff the unit for 24 hours.
   c. The number of 8-hour shifts needed per week.
   d. The number of FTEs needed as basic staff for this unit.
5. Using the Salt Lake City Community Hospital recommendation of staff mix, determine the mix of RNs, LPNs, and aides.
6. Using Warsler's proportion for staffing shifts, determine the number of FTEs for days, evenings, and nights.
7. Create a table for basic staffing for this unit. Do not add complementary staff without a specific reason for doing so.

EXERCISE 10-2

Use cyclic scheduling, and then self-scheduling to schedule a staff of six RNs and one NA for a period of one month. In the self-scheduling section, you may use any combination of schedules effective for unit coverage and satisfactory to the staff.

EXERCISE 10-3

Use Hanson's formula to determine productivity of each nursing unit for a division or department of nursing:

$$\frac{\text{Required staff hours}}{\text{Provided staff hours}} \times 100 = \text{Percent productivity}$$

EXERCISE 10-4

Identify at least 12 activities that can be done to improve productivity in a division or department of nursing in which you work.

NOTES

1. Rewick, D. & Gaffey, E. (2001). Nursing system makes a difference. *Health Management Technology*, *1*, 24–26.
2. Materra, M. D. (2001). Nurses' problems are yours. *Medical Economics*, 4.
3. Coile, R. C., Jr. (2001). Magnet hospitals use culture, not wages, to solve nursing shortage. *Journal of Healthcare Management*, 224–227.
4. Page, A. (Ed.). (2004). *Keeping patients safe: Transforming the work environment of nurses.* Washington, DC: The National Academies Press.
5. Kovner, C. & Gergen, P. J. (1998). Nurse staffing levels and adverse events following surgery in US hospitals. *Image: Journal of Nursing Scholarship*, 315.
6. Blegen, M. A., Goode, C. J., & Reed, L. (1998). Nurse staffing and patient outcomes. *Nursing Research*, 43–49.
7. White, K. (2003). Effective staffing as a guardian. *Nursing Management*, 20–24.
8. Aydelotte, M. K. (1973). *Nurse staffing methodology: A review and critique of selected literature*. Washington, DC: US Government Printing Office, 3.
9. West, M. E. (1980). Implementing effective nurse staffing systems in the managed hospital. *Topics in Health Care Financing*, 11–25.
10. Althaus, J. N., Hardyck, N. M., Pierce, P. B., & Rodgers, M. S. (1982). Nurse staffing in a decentralized organization: Part I. *Journal of Nursing Administration*, 34–39.
11. Parker, L. (1993). When to fix it and when to leave: Relationships among perceived control, self-efficacy, dissent, and exit. *Journal of Applied Psychology*, *78*(6), 949–959.
12. Minetti, R. C. (1983). Computerized nurse staffing. *Hospitals*, 90, 92; Shaheen, P. P. (1985). Staffing and scheduling: Reconcile practical means with the real goal. *Nursing Management*, 64–69.
13. Aydelotte, 1973, 26–31.
14. Bell, H. M., McElnay, J. C., & Hughes, C. M. (1999). A self-reported work sampling study in community pharmacy practice. *Pharmacy World Science*, 210–216; Upenieks, V. V. (1998). Work sampling: Assessing nursing efficiency. *Nursing Management*, 27–29; Urden, L. D. & Roode, J. I. (1997). Work sampling: A decision-making tool for determining resources and work redesign. *Journal of Nursing Administration*, 34–41; Cardona, P., Tappen, R. M., Terrill, M., Acosta, M., & Eusebe, M. I. (1997).

Nursing staff time allocation in long-term care: A work sampling study. *Journal of Nursing Administration*, 28–36; Miller, M. E., James, M. K., Langefeld, C. D., Espeland, M. A., Freedman, J. A., Martin, D. M., et al. (1996). Some techniques for the analysis of work sampling data. *Statistical Medicine*, 607–618.

15. West, 1980, 16.
16. Ibid., 17.
17. Schroder, P. J. & McKeon, K. L. (1990). What is a safe staffing pattern for locked long-term and acute care units for adults? *Journal of Psychosocial Nursing*, *28*(12), 36–37.
18. Price, E. M. (1970). *Staffing for patient care*. New York: Springer, 12.
19. Steed, C. K. (2004). Eating our young isn't practiced here. *Nursing 2004*, 43.
20. JCAHO. (2001). Accreditation process improvement: Introduction to staffing effectiveness presentation. Retrieved September 3, 2004 from http://www.amda.com/caring/april2002/staffing.htm.
21. Study questions all-RN staffing. (1983). *RN*, 15–16.
22. Warstler, M. E. (1972). Some management techniques for nursing service administrators. *Journal of Nursing Administration*, 25–34.
23. American Hospital Association (AHA). (1985). *Strategies: Flexible scheduling*. Washington, DC: Author.
24. Froebe, D. (1975). Scheduling: By team or individually. In *Staffing: A Journal of Nursing Administration Reader*. Wakefield, MA: Contemporary Publishing.
25. Rondeau, K. V. (1990). Self-Scheduling can increase job satisfaction. *Medical Laboratory Observer*, 22–24; Teahan, B. (1998). Implementation of a self-scheduling system: A solution to more than just schedules. *Journal of Nursing Management*, 361–368; Irvin, S. A. & Brown, H. N. (1999). Self-scheduling with Microsoft Excel. *Nursing Economics*, 201–206.
26. Ricci, J. A. (1984). 10 Hour Night Shift: Cost vs. Savings. *Nursing Management*, 34–35, 38–42.
27. Fagin, C. M. (1982). The economic value of nursing research. *American Journal of Nursing*, 1844–1849.
28. Vik, A. G. & MacKay, R. C. (1982). How does the 12-hour shift affect patient care? *Journal of Nursing Administration*, 12.
29. Washburn, M. S. (1991). Fatigue and critical thinking on eight- and twelve-hour shifts. *Nursing Management*, 80A–CC, 80D–CC, 80 F–H–CC.
30. Lant, T. W. & Gregory, D. (1984). The impact of 12-hour shift: An analysis. *Nursing Management*, 38A–38B, 38D–38F, 38H.
31. AHA, 1985; Arnold, B. & Mills, E. (1983). Care-12: Implementation of flexible scheduling. *Journal of Nursing Administration*, 9–14; Mech, A., Mills, M. E., & Arnold, B. (1984). Wage and hour laws: Their impact on 12-hour scheduling. *Journal of Nursing Administration*, 24–25; Metcalf, M. L.; Mitchell, R. J. & Williamson, A. M. (2000). Evaluation of an 8-hour versus a 12-hour shift roster on employees at a power station. *Applied Ergonomics*, 83–93; Bourdouxhe, M. A., Queinnec, Y., Granger, D., Baril, R. H., Guertin, S. C., Massicotte, P. R., et al. (1999). Aging and shift work: The effects of 20 years of rotating 12-hour shifts among petroleum refinery operators. *Exp Aging Research*, 323–329; Federwisch, A. (1998, November 23). Shift priorities. *HealthWeek*, 28–32; Erwin, J. (1998, November 9). Staying alert. *HealthWeek*, 20.
32. Ancona, P. (1994, February 19). Working shifts can be dangerous to your health, experts say. *San Antonio Express-News*, pp. 1F–2F.
33. Fisher, D. W. & Thomas, E. (1975). A "premium day" approach to weekend nurse staffing. In *Staffing: A Journal of Nursing Administration Reader*. Wakefield, MA: Contemporary Publishing.
34. Robb, E. A., Determan, A. C., Lampat, L. R., Scherbring, M. J., Slifka, R. M., & Smith, N. A. (2003). Self scheduling: Satisfaction guaranteed? *Nursing Management*, 16–18.
35. McGuire, J. B. & Liro, J. R. (1986). Flexible work schedules, work attitudes, and perceptions of productivity. *Public Personnel Management*, 65–73.
36. Ibid.
37. Imig, S. I., Powell, J. A., & Thorman, K. (1984). Primary nursing and flexi-staffing: Do they mix? *Nursing Management*, 39–42.
38. O'Donnell, K. (1992). A flexible role: Resource acuity nurse. *Nursing Management*, 75–76.
39. Bruzzese, A. (1994, April 19). Companies turning to temps to fill voids in workplace. *San Antonio Express-News*, pp. 1C, 7C.
40. Messmer, M. (1992). Strategic staffing. *Management Accounting*, 28–30.
41. Hicks, L. (1993, December 12). The rise in temps. *San Antonio Express-News*, pp. 1-H, 6-H.
42. Randolph, L. (2003). Tracking travel trends. *Nursing Management Supplement 4*, 9–11.
43. Tuttle, D. M. (1992). A "transfer fair" approach to staffing. *Nursing Management*, 72–74.
44. Kramer, M. & Schmalenberg, C. (2004). Essentials of a magnetic work environment: Part 1. *Nursing 2004*, 50–54.
45. Kramer, M. & Schmalenberg, C. (2002). Essentials of magnetism. In M. McClure & A. Hinshaw (Eds.) *Magnet hospitals revisited: Attraction and retention of professional nurses*. Kansas City, MO: American Nurses Publishing.
46. Fagerstrom, L. & Rainio, A. K. (1999). Professional assessment of optimal nursing care intensity level: A new method of assessing personnel resources for nursing care. *Journal of Clinical Nursing*, 369–379.
47. Connor, R. J. (1961). A work sampling study of variations in nursing workload. *Hospitals*, *35*(9), 40–41.
48. Herzog, T. P. (1985). Productivity: Fighting the battle of the budget. *Nursing Management*, 30–34; Porter-O'Grady, T. (1985). Strategic planning: Nursing practice in the PPS. *Nursing Management*, 53–56; Johnson, K. (1984). A practical approach to patient classification. *Nursing Management*, 39–41, 44, 46; Schroeder, R. E., Rhodes, A. M., & Shields, R. E. (1984). Nurse acuity systems: CASH vs. GRASP. *Nursing Forum*, 72–77; Alward, R. R. (1983). Patient classification systems: The ideal vs. reality. *Journal of Nursing Administration*, 14–18; Nyberg, J. & Wolff, N. (1984). DRG panic. *Journal of Nursing Administration*, 17–21.
49. Schroeder, Rhodes, & Shields, 1984.
50. Johnson, 1984.
51. Ibid., 41.
52. Schroeder, Rhodes, & Shields, 1984.
53. Alward, 1983.
54. O'Brien-Pallas, L., Leatt, P., Deber, R., & Till, J. (1989). A comparison of workload estimates using three methods of patient classification. *Canadian Journal of Nursing Administration*, 16–23.
55. Dee, V. & Auger, J. A. (1983). A patient classification system based on the behavioral system model of nursing: Part 2. *Journal of Nursing Administration*, 18–23.
56. Alward,1983.
57. Ibid.
58. Nyberg & Wolff, 1984.
59. Grazman, T. E. (1983). Managing unit human resources: A microcomputer model. *Nursing Management*, 18–22.
60. Adams, R. & Duchene, P. (1985). Computerization of patient acuity and nursing care planning. *Journal of Nursing Administration*, 11–17.
61. Giovannetti, P. & Mayer, G. G. (1984). Building confidence in patient classification systems. *Nursing Management*, 31–34; Alward, 1983.

62. American Nurses Association (ANA). (1999, October 13). Press Release. Retrieved September 1, 2004 from http://www.nursingworld.org/pressrel/1999/pr1013.htm.
63. Hanson, R. L. (1982a). Applying management information systems to staffing. *Journal of Nursing Administration*, 5–9.
64. Aydelotte, 1973, 26.
65. Halloran, E. J. & Kiley, M. (1984). Case mix management. *Nursing Management*, 39–41, 44–45.
66. Moores, B. & Murphy, A. (1984, July 4). Planning the duty rota, one, computerized duty rotas. *Nursing Times*, 47–48; Canter, D. (1984, July 4). Planning the duty rota, two, back to basics. *Nursing Times*, 49–50.
67. Hanson, 1982a.
68. Drucker, P. F. (1999). *Management challenges for the 21st century*. New York: HarperCollins, 135–140.
69. Hanson, R. L. (1982b). Staffing statistics: Their use and usefulness. *Journal of Nursing Administration*, 29–35.
70. Brown, D. S. (1983). The managerial ethic and productivity improvement. *Public Productivity Review*, 223–250.
71. Hanson, 1982b. The formulas are Hanson's; applications are the author's.
72. Davis, D. L. (1984). Assessing and improving productivity in the operating room. *AORN Journal*, 630, 632, 634.
73. Smith, J. L., Mackey, M. K. V., & Markham, J. (1985). Productivity monitoring: A recovery room system for economizing operations. *Nursing Management*, 34A–D, K–M.
74. Mailhot, C. B. (1985). Setting OR's course toward greater productivity. *Nursing Management*, 42I, J, L, M, P.
75. Haas, S. A. W. (1984). Sorting out nursing productivity. *Nursing Management*, 37–40.
76. Curtin, L. (1984). Reconciling pay with productivity. *Nursing Management*, 7–8.
77. Curtin, L. L. & Zurlage, C. L. (1986). Nursing productivity: From data to definition. *Nursing Management*, 32–34, 38–41.
78. Waterstradt, C. R. & Phillips, T. L. (1990). A productivity system for a hospital education department. *Journal of Nursing Staff Development*, 139–144.
79. Rabin, J. (1983). Professionalism and productivity. *Public Productivity Review*, 217–222; DiJerome, L., Dunham-Taylor, J., Ash, D., & Brown, R. (1999). Evaluating cost center productivity. *Nursing Economics*, 334–340.
80. Curtin, 1984.
81. Fralic, M. F. (1982). The modern professional and productivity. Annual Meeting of the Alabama Society for Nursing Service Administrators, Huntsville, AL; Hanson, R. L. (1982c). Managing human resources. *Journal of Nursing Administration*, 17-23; Kaye, G. H. & Utenner, J. (1985). Productivity: Managing for the long term. *Nursing Management*, *1*, 12–13, 15; Haas, 1984; Davis, 1984; Brown, 1983.
82. Ancona, P. (1993, July 24). How to measure productivity and improve effectiveness among workers. *San Antonio Express-News*, p. 1B.
83. Gilliland, M., Crane, V. S., & Jones, D. G. (1991). Productivity: Electronics saves steps-and builds networks. *Nursing Management*, *1*, 56–59.
84. American Nurses Association (ANA). (2004). *Scope and standards for nurse administrators* (2nd ed.), 4.

REFERENCES

Althaus, J. N., Hardyck, N. M., Pierce, P. B., & Rodgers, M. S. (1982). Nurse staffing in a decentralized organization: Part II. *The Journal of Nursing Administration*, 18–22.

Bermas, N. F. & Van Slyck, A. (1984). Patient classification systems and the nursing department. *Hospitals*, 99–100.

Domrose, C. (2000, January 10). A good day's sleep. *HealthWeek*, 22.

Evans, C. L. S. (1984). A practical staffing calculator. *Nursing Management*, 68–69.

Flynn, E., Heinzer, M. M., & Radwanski, M. (1999). A collaborative assessment of workload and patient care needs. *Rehabilitation Nursing*, 103–108.

Gebhardt, A. N. (1982). Computers and staff allocation made easy. *Nursing Times*, 1471–1473.

Harrington, C., Kovner, C., Mezey, M., Kayser-Jones, J., Burger, S., Mohler, M., et al. (2000). Experts recommend minimum nurse staffing standards for nursing facilities in the United States. *Gerontologist*, 5–16.

Henney, C. R. & Bosworth, R. N. (1980). A computer-based system for the automatic production of nursing workload data. *Nursing Times*, 1212–1217.

Jecmen, C. & Stuerke, N. M. (1983). Computerization helps solve staff scheduling problems. *Nursing Economics*, 209–211.

Jelinek, R. C., Zinn, T. K., & Brya, J. R. (1973). Tell the computer how sick the patients are and it will tell how many nurses they need. *Modern Health*, 81–85.

Joint Commission on Accreditation of Healthcare Organizations (JCAHO). (2004). *2004 comprehensive accreditation manual for hospitals*. Chicago: Author.

Linna, M. (2000). Health care financing reform and the productivity change in Finnish hospitals. *Journal of Health Care Finance*, 83–100.

Lloyd, R. & Goulding, J. (1999). Nursing ratios shift up. *Health Service Journal*, 28.

Mcue, M, Mark, B. A., & Harless, D. (2003). Nurse staffing, quality, and financial performance. *Journal of Health Care Finance*, *29*(4), 64–76.

Nurse staffing law may herald benchmarks. *Healthcare Benchmarks*, 137–138.

Purdum, T. S. (1999, October 13). New California law sets fixed nurse-to-patient ratios. *San Antonio Express-News*, p. 6A.

Ritter-Teitel, J. (2002). The impact of restructuring on professional nursing practice. *Journal of Nursing Administration*, *32*(1), 31–38.

Ritter-Teitel, J. (2004). Registered nurse hours worked per patient day. *Journal of Nursing Administration*, *34*(4), 167–169.

Robertson, R. H. and M. Hassan. (November 1999). Staffing intensity, skill mix and mortality outcomes: The case of chronic obstructive lung disease. *Health Service Management Research*, 258–268.

Seago, J. A., Spetz, J., & Mitchell, S. (2004). Nurse staffing and hospital ownership in California. *Journal of Nursing Administration*, *34*(5), 228–237.

Snyder, J. & Nethersole-Chong, D. (1999). Is cross-training medical/surgical RNs to ICU the answer? *Nursing Management*, 58–60.

Sochalski, J., Estabrooks, C. A., & Humphrey, C. K. (1999). Nurse staffing outcomes: Evolution of an international study. *Canadian Journal of Nursing Research*, 69–88.

Spetz, J. (1999). The effects of managed care and prospective payment on the demand for hospital nurses: Evidence from California. *Health Service Research*, 993–1010.

Stuerke, N. (1984). Computers can advance nursing practice. *Nursing Management*, 27–28.

Van Slyck, A. (1999). Improving productivity: A payer/provider debate. *Journal of Nursing Administration*, *29*(1), 51–56.

CHAPTER 11

Principles of Budgeting

Denise Danna, RN, DNS, CNAA, CHE

LEARNING OBJECTIVES AND ACTIVITIES

- Discuss concepts of budgeting.
- Identify budget-planning steps.
- Identify stages of the budget.
- Examine elements of cost accounting in a health care organization.
- Define selected terms related to budgeting.
- Differentiate between direct and indirect costs.
- Differentiate among fixed, variable, and sunk costs.
- Describe various budgets: operating or cash budget, personnel budget, supplies and equipment budget, capital budget.
- Discuss the budget as a controlling process.
- Discuss monitoring of the budget.
- Discuss motivational aspects of the budget.
- Discuss cutting the budget.
- Observe preparation of the budget for an agency or a cost center.
- Describe the elements of managed care and their impact on patients.
- Explain the effects of managed care relative to managers, nurses, physicians, health care organizations, and other providers.

CONCEPTS: Budget, budgeting, cost center, budget stages (calendar), cost accounting, fixed costs, variable costs, sunk costs, direct costs, indirect costs, activity-based costing, revenue budgeting, expense budgeting, operating budget, cost-to-charge ratio, zero-base budgeting, cost-benefit analysis, negative cash flow, service units, chart of accounts, inventory, financial standards, performance budgeting, personnel budget, supplies and equipment budget, capital budget, managed care, fee-for-service reimbursement, indemnity insurance plans, health maintenance organization (HMO), capitation, preferred provider organization (PPO), contracting.

NURSE MANAGER BEHAVIORS: Is involved in the development of personnel, supplies, equipment, and capital budgets, with expenditures projected. Solves problems resulting from managed care, and promotes interests of patients and personnel.

NURSE EXECUTIVE BEHAVIORS: Decentralizes budget development for personnel, supplies, equipment, and capital expenditures and for projected revenues to cost-center managers. Provides budget guidance through budget stages and provides cost-center managers with current reports of expenditures and revenues while they manage all aspects of their budgets. Assists personnel in maximum understanding of their health care benefits. Empowers professional nurses to produce quality outcomes for patients, personnel, and insurers within an environment heavily influenced by managed care.

Introduction

Because the amount and quality of nursing services depend on budgetary plans, nurses should become proficient in budgeting procedures. This proficiency will provide the resources necessary for safe and effective nursing care. With limited resources and in a competitive market, health care organizations must use personnel and material resources wisely and efficiently. The enlightened nurse knows that the person who controls the budget is the person who controls nursing services. The costs of nursing services have been identified for many years, but the income earned from nursing services has been included in "bed and board" on the budget sheets. Achieving reimbursement for nursing services means that many government regulations and third-party payer policies must change to allow for direct payment to nursing providers, based on the amount of care given and the skills of the persons giving it.

Budgeting is an ongoing activity in which revenues and expenses are managed to maintain fiscal responsibility and fiscal health. The nurse manager has financial responsibility; is accountable for managing the nursing budget; and makes all of the decisions about how to adjust the nursing budget to manage programs and costs, including those related to adding and dropping programs, expanding and contracting programs, and modifying revenues and expenses within the nursing unit.

Basic Planning

Planning yields forecasts for one year and for several years. The budget is an annual plan, intended to guide effective use of human and material resources, products, or services and to manage the environment to improve productivity. Budgetary planning ensures that the best methods are used to achieve financial objectives. It should be based on valid objectives to provide a product or service that the community needs and for which it will pay. In nursing, budgetary planning helps ensure that clients or patients receive the nursing services they want and need from satisfied nursing workers. A good budget is based on objectives; is simple, flexible, and balanced; has standards; and uses available resources first to avoid increasing costs.

There is no formula for the form, detail, or periods covered by budgets. Each budget system is designed for the situation at hand and must take into consideration the character of the company, the company's position, and the nature of the plans involved. Ordinarily, the budget system is most detailed in aspects of operations most important to the firm's success. Furthermore, the period covered by the budget varies with the nature of the plans and with the degree of accuracy possible in the preparation of estimates.[1]

A nursing budget is a systematic plan that is an informed best estimate by nurse administrators of revenues and nursing expenses. It projects how revenues will meet expenses, and it projects a return on equity, that is, profit. The budget should be stated in terms of attainable objectives to maintain the motivation of nurses at the unit or cost-center level. The nursing budget serves three purposes:

1. To plan the objectives, programs, and activities of nursing services and the fiscal resources needed to accomplish them.
2. To motivate nursing workers through analysis of actual experiences.
3. To serve as a standard to evaluate the performance of nurse administrators and managers and to increase awareness of costs.

These purposes should include the group's mission, strategic plans, new programs or projects, and goals.

Managing the financial end of nursing through an operational budget obviously can create a new sense of involvement for nurses. The budget can be a strong support for developing written objectives for the nursing division and for each of its units. It can provide motivation for effective planning and standards by which to evaluate the performance of nurse managers.[2] Effective planning provides for contingencies by indicating which programs or activities can be reduced or eliminated if budget goals are not met.

Procedures

Decentralized budgeting involves the nursing unit managers and their staff in the process. Nursing service is labor-intensive, which is reflected in the fact that the first six budget-planning steps pertain to labor. Note that only steps 7 and 8 are concerned with nonlabor expenses. The steps are as follows:[3]

1. Determine the productivity goal. The director of nursing services and the nurse manager determine the unit's productivity goal for the coming fiscal year.
2. Forecast the workload. The number of patient days expected on each nursing unit for the coming fiscal year is calculated.
3. Budget patient care hours. The expected number of hours devoted to patient care for the forecasted patient days is calculated.
4. Budget patient care hours and staffing schedules. The budgeted patient care hours are reflected in recommended staffing schedules by shift and by day of the week.
5. Plan nonproductive hours. Vacation, holiday, education leave, sick leave, and similar hours are budgeted for the coming year.
6. Chart productive and nonproductive time. To aid in the planning process, a graph is used to show nurses how the level of forecasted patient days, and therefore the staffing requirements, are expected to increase and decrease during the year. Productive time

is the time spent on the job in patient care, administration of the unit, conferences, educational activities, and orientation.

7. Estimate costs of supplies and services. The supplies and services to be purchased for the year are budgeted.
8. Anticipate capital expenses. The expected capital investments for the coming year are included in the budget.

These eight steps result in a proposed budget that goes to the nursing administrator for review. After preliminary acceptance, this budget is sent to the accounting department, where the forecasted patient days are translated into expected revenue. The budgeted productive and nonproductive times are converted into dollars, as are the costs for supplies, services, and other operating expenses that will be allocated to a given nursing unit for the coming year. A pro forma operating statement is then returned to the director of nursing for review with the nurse manager. Once the director of nursing and the nurse manager accept the budget, it is returned to the accounting department and forwarded with the rest of the agency manager's budgets to administration and the board of directors.[4]

People who pay high prices for health care want accountability of both costs and quality of service. The nursing budget can be a shared responsibility, with unit budgets being prepared with staff involvement at the clinical level. The planning and controlling processes are ongoing. Through their participation, clinical nurses enhance their professional stature. A budget prepared and executed as a shared experience becomes an object of ownership to a staff that will put forth effort to work within its framework.

Managing Cost Centers

A *cost center* is a given area of assigned accountability for both direct and indirect expenditures. A department of nursing is a cost center, as are each of its units, each clinic, in-service education, surgical suites, long-term care, home health care, and any other section with a nursing mission in which nurses provide services to clients. Each cost center is assigned a code. A reference (Seawell, 1994) is available for a uniform accounting and reporting system for hospitals. An organization may use this coding system, usually referred to as the patient care system. Work load measurements, sometimes referred to as performance classifications or units of measure, are necessary. The unit of measure for each cost center is identified as a specific, quantitative statistic, such as inpatient days or number of tests. Each cost center has a manager, called the cost-center manager, who is responsible for identifying needs for equipment and programs to maintain progress at the current level of technology in the unit.

Each cost center is an internal department dealing with distribution of services and products. The cost-center manager is responsible for determining the cost of such services or products and how they are distributed within the organization. Two types of cost centers are mission, or revenue-producing, and service cost centers. Examples of mission centers are radiology and laboratory departments. These centers have monetary income related to the purpose of the organization. A service center is a support center that provides a service to other units and charges for that service; no exchange of revenue takes place. The unit served adds the costs of these support services to its costs of output.[5] Examples of support centers are food service, purchasing, and laundry.

Budgeted costs within the cost center are broken down into subcodes. This promotes better budgetary planning and control because items are specifically identified during the budget planning process. Also, each item purchased is charged to (deleted from) the balance shown for that specific subcode.

Relationship of Budget and Objectives

One of the chief planning activities is to identify the objectives of the nursing division and each of its units, including developing a management plan with a budget for each objective. One of the first sources of budgetary information is the nursing objectives. By using these objectives, nurse managers see the benefit of developing pertinent, specific, and practical budgeting objectives.

Budget Stages

For practical purposes, the nursing budget follows three stages of development: formulation, review and enactment, and execution. The entire budgeting process is given a specific time frame, and a target date is assigned for each step. (See Exhibit 11-1.) During the fiscal year of the execution stage of budgeting, the formulation and review and enactment stages for the next fiscal year are carried out. The budget stages are sometimes labeled forecasting, preparation, and control, respectively.[6]

Formulation Stage

The formulation stage is usually a set number of months (six or seven) before the start of the fiscal year for the budget. During this period, procedures are used to obtain an estimate of the funds needed, funds available, expenses, and revenues. Financial reports of expenses and revenues of the previous fiscal year and the year to date will be analyzed by the chief nurse executive, department heads, and cost-center managers.

EXHIBIT 11-1
The Budget Calendar

FORMULATION STAGE

1. Develop objectives and management plans.
2. Gather all financial, historical, and statistical data and distribute to cost-center managers.
3. Analyze data.

REVIEW AND ENACTMENT STAGE

4. Prepare unit budgets.
5. Present unit budgets for approval.
6. Revise and combine into organizational budget.
7. Present to budget council.
8. Revise and present to governing board.
9. Revise and distribute to cost-center managers.

EXECUTION STAGE

10. Direct and evaluate expenses and receipts.
11. Revise budget if indicated.

One of the first steps in writing a budget is gathering data for accurate prediction of expenses (costs) and revenues (income). This task can be developed into a system. Primary sources of data are the objectives for the division of nursing and for each cost center. Each program and activity needs to have an estimated cost placed on it. If in-service educators want new audiovisual equipment, they should not walk into the nurse administrator's office and expect to have it next week or next month. Purchasing this equipment should be planned for six to seven months before the next fiscal year begins, and it may be budgeted for any quarter or month within that fiscal year. In surveying the objectives, nurse administrators and managers evaluate the previous year, review the philosophy, and rewrite the objectives for the future.

Other data include programs from other departments that will require use or expansion of nursing resources, expansion of nursing clinics and client teaching programs, travel costs for attendance at professional and educational meetings, incentive awards, library requirements, clinical and office supplies and equipment, investment equipment and facilities modification on a five-year plan, and contracts for items such as intravenous pumps and oxygen equipment. Data can be obtained from historical financial records of the organization.

Among the cost-center reports that will assist the nurse manager are the following:

- Daily staffing reports
- Monthly staffing reports
- Payroll summaries
- Daily lists of financial categories of patients
- Biometric reports of occupancy
- Biometric reports of workload
- Monthly financial summaries of revenues and expenses

Review and Enactment Stage

Review and enactment are budget development processes that put all the pieces together for approval of a final budget. Once the cost-center managers present their budgets to the budget council, the chief nurse executive will consolidate the nursing budget. The budget officer will then further consolidate the budget into an organizational budget. The chief executive officer of the organization and the governing board will then give their approval. Throughout this process, conferences will be held at which budget adjustments are made. Nurses can sell a budget by using a marketing strategy, anticipating challenges, being persuasive without being emotional, and working toward a win–win situation.[7]

Execution Stage

The formulation stage and the review and enactment stage of the budget are planning activities. Execution of the budget involves directing and evaluating activities. The nurse administrators and managers who planned the budget execute it. Revisions in execution of the budget are scheduled at stated intervals, usually once or twice during the fiscal year. Certain procedures are followed for evaluating the budget at cost-center levels. Budgets are prepared for either fiscal years that coincide with government budgets or calendar (fiscal) years, depending on the policy of the organization.

Cost Factors

Cost is money expended for all resources used, including personnel, supplies, and equipment. The volume of service provided is the greatest factor affecting costs. Others factors include length of patient stays, salaries, prices of material, case mix, seasonal factors, and efficiencies (such as simplification of procedures and quality management to prevent errors that increase patient complications and increase costs). Still other factors that have an impact on costs are regulation and competition for market share; third-party payers; the age and size of the agency; type and amount of services provided; the agency's mission; and relationships among nurses, physicians, and other personnel.

Expenses

Expenses are the costs of providing services to patients. They are frequently called *overhead*, and include wages and salaries, fringe benefits, supplies, food service, utilities, and office and medical supplies. As part of the budget, expenses are a collection or summary of forecasts for each cost center's account.

Full costs include both direct and indirect expenses. Although direct costs such as nursing can be traced to the source, indirect costs such as utilities, telephones, or purchasing services are allocated to the source department by a standard formula.

Expense Budgeting

Expense budgeting is the "process of forecasting, recording, and monitoring the manpower, materials and supplies, and monetary needs of an organization in such a manner that the operation of the various components of the organization can be controlled."[8] The components of expense budgeting are cost centers. Purposes of expense budgeting include the following:

- To predict labor hours, material, supplies, and cash flow needs for future time periods.
- To establish procedures for making comparative studies.
- To provide a mechanism for determining when changes in procedures need to be made, provide gross information on the kinds of changes needed, and provide evidence that control has been established or reestablished.

Historical trends are the single best inexpensive indicator available to the institution. They are valid for prediction of present and future trends.

Types of Expenses/Costs

Fixed, Variable, and Sunk Costs

Fixed costs are not related to volume. They remain constant as volume increases and decreases over a period of time. Among fixed costs are depreciation of equipment and buildings, salaries, benefits, utilities, interest on loans or bonds, and taxes.

Variable costs do relate to volume and census (patient days). They include items such as meals and linen. Supplies are usually volume-responsive, meaning that total costs increase or decrease according to use. The cost of supplies varies by patient census, physician orders, and diagnosis. For example, the cost of surgical dressings increases when a patient's wound has drainage and dressings must be changed frequently. Also, the cost of supplies increases or decreases with the census. For this reason, every cost center should have an established unit of measure for productivity. This unit may be numbers of tests, procedures, patients of a specific acuity type, hours or minutes of service, or discharges. Most activities include elements of both fixed and variable costs. For example, personnel costs and utility costs can be both fixed and variable because a minimum is required for each.

Sunk costs are fixed expenses that cannot be recovered even if a program is canceled. Advertising is a good example.[9]

Direct and Indirect Costs

Direct costs are the costs of providing the product or service and are often considered to be those directly related to patient care, such as personnel costs and the variable cost of supplies. The definition of direct costs varies by department. In areas not involved in direct patient care, each department incurs its own category of direct costs.

Indirect costs are those incurred in supporting the provision of the product or service, are not directly related to patient care, and include utilities, administration, housekeeping, and building maintenance. As previously mentioned, however, they are direct costs for the source department. Some indirect costs are fixed, such as depreciation and administration. Others, such as laundry and accounting, are variable. All indirect costs are allocated or transferred by a specific method to the departments that use the service.

Every hospital has a method to establish costs, including the Hospital and Hospital Health Care Complex Cost Report Certification and Settlement Summary, commonly known as the Centers for Medicare & Medicaid Services (CMS) Cost Report. In a few agencies the method is more refined. Nurse administrators should become informed about the methods favored by their organizations.

Cost Accounting

A *cost-accounting* system assigns all costs to cost centers. Periodically, usually monthly, reports of costs are provided to cost-center managers, but they do not reflect all costs. Many indirect costs are allocated only once a year in the CMS Cost Report. Included are costs of items such as utilities, accounting, administration, data processing, and admitting. Informed and influential nurse managers use these cost allocations when preparing budgets. Such allocations are usually hidden in the operational budget under the category of "room costs."

Cost assignments to cost centers are made on the basis of direct costing if they are direct costs of patient care. Otherwise, they are made by transfer costing from a patient care support department or by cost allocation if they are not related to direct patient care or support. Job order sheets are used to account for all services to patients. Direct overhead costs that cannot be identified with specific services rendered are allocated based on some other measurement, such as square feet of floor space.

Service Units

Service units are measurable units of productivity or volume for identifying and counting costs. They must be measurable, known to managers, and affected by volume. The number of service units produced measures productivity.

Unit of Service

The *unit of service* is a measurement of the output of agency services consumed by the patient. In the surgical suite and recovery room, it is measured in minutes or hours; in the emergency room, it is the number of visits or time and procedures; and in the nursing units, it is based on the acuity category of patients and hours per day expressed as a targeted number. Types of measurement include procedures, patient days, patient visits, and cases.

With the increased sophistication of information systems, it is easier for nurse managers to become involved in identifying and costing service units, which can be quantified by hours of nursing care per category of acuity of illness.

Chart of Accounts

A chart of accounts that includes a number and table for each cost center is subdivided into major classifications and subcodes (see Seawell, 1994). Examples are salaries and wages, employee benefits, medical and surgical supplies, professional fees, purchased services, utilities, other direct expenses, depreciation, and rent. These classifications are divided into further subcategories.

To assign items to the correct cost center, one must record all movement of labor and materials between cost centers. All benefits must be charged to the appropriate cost center by some established method, and so must all purchases, including shared ones. This is usually done using allocated shares of service units.

Amortized expenses are deferred charges allocated to units over a specified period of time. They include depreciation charges for aging plant and equipment in addition to prepaid items. Prepaid items usually are charged monthly as service units. Other deferred expenses include unamortized borrowing costs and costs incurred for capital expansion or renovation programs.

Inventory and Cost Transfer

Identifying actual costs of any service unit is improved through an accurate system of inventory control. Based on the number of orders or requisitions for any item, the appropriate proportion of its costs can be transferred to the cost center that ordered the items.

Financial Accountability

In accepting financial accountability, nurses' first duty is to their patients, who have given them their trust. Nurses should be accountable to themselves for their work, to their professional peers, to their employers, and to taxpayers in publicly funded institutions.

In one way or another, patients pay the costs of health care. They may do so through insurance premiums, taxes, or benefits or from their own pockets. Financial accountability means that nurses and others can account for the efficient spending of the money paid for health care.

Nurse managers need information on the costs of all services provided by their own and competing institutions. This information, in turn, can be provided to clinical nurses, who should know what it costs to do their work. Cost consciousness leads to waste reduction and effective cost management.

Some managers mistakenly believe that controlling nursing labor power and expenditures can control overspending. Holding nurses accountable for their budgets, including both revenues and expenses, can rectify this misconception.

The Cost of Nursing Care

To determine the cost of nursing care, one must consider several factors. Nursing charges should be quantifiable. A patient acuity system serves this purpose. The patient acuity system usually separates patients into four or five levels of nursing care and enumerates nursing requirements for each level. Charges could be set by level and negotiated with third-party payers. These costs could be separated from the cost of nonnursing requirements. Nonnursing tasks could then be reassigned to ensure that the charges for nursing care reflect the actual cost of providing such care.

A second method of costing nursing services is determining what share of total agency cost is attributable to nursing. This will vary by diagnosis-related group (DRG) or by patient acuity. An industry-wide effort for each region could produce standards for nursing costs and charges. Otherwise, a majority of the health care institutions in the United States would need to undertake research to determine nursing costs and charges on an agency-specific basis. Multinational corporations, of course, can apply research studies across member institutions.

Activity-Based Costing

Drucker recommends activity-based costing that accounts for the total process of doing business from personnel, supplies, material, and parts to installation and service of products. Health care organizations will know and manage the costs of the entire economic chain, tying the costs to all sources of payment. To do this requires foundation, productivity, competence, and resource allocation information. Personnel perform to meet specific expectations, and they are evaluated accordingly. Old organizational structures are replaced with new cost centers that support activity-based costing, in which managers turn data into information through analysis and interpretation that lead to action.[10]

Definitions

Budget

According to *Webster's New Twentieth Century Dictionary, Unabridged (2nd ed.)* a budget is "a plan or schedule adjusting expenses during a certain period to the estimated or fixed income for that period." Herkimer states, "An effective budget is the systematic documentation of one or more carefully developed plans for all individually supervised activities, programs, or sections. The budget is a tool which can aid decision makers in evaluating operating performance and projecting what future operations might produce."[11]

A budget is an operational management plan, stated in terms of income and expenses, covering all phases of activity for a future division of time. It is a financial document that expresses an operation's plan of action. In the division of nursing, it sets the limits of financial support, thereby controlling the extent and quality of nursing programs. The budget determines the number of kinds of personnel, materials, and financial resources available for patient care and for achievement of the stated nursing objectives. It is a financial policy statement. Budgeting is the process whereby objectives and plans are translated into financial terms and evaluated using financial and statistical criteria.

Revenue

Revenue is the income from sales of products and services. Nursing revenue traditionally has been included with room charges. Increasingly, it is being unbundled from the room rate as a separate charge per patient acuity category and per visit, day, or procedure.

Revenue can include assets, such as accounts receivable and income-producing endowments. The latter can be restricted to specific purposes. Buildings, land, and other items can be assets if they produce income or are capable of producing income. Total income is frequently termed *gross income*; the excess of revenues over expenses is known as *net income* or *profit*.

Revenues also come from research grants, gift shops, donations, gifts, rentals of cots and televisions, parking fees, telephone charges, and vending machines. Revenues may be elements of product lines such as orthopedic services that include orthopedic nursing, traction equipment, and prostheses. In hospitals, revenue may refer to sources such as Medicare, Medicaid, third-party payers (insurance companies), and patients.[12]

Revenue Budgeting

Revenue budgeting, or *rate setting*, is the process by which an agency determines revenues required to cover anticipated costs and to establish prices sufficient to generate these revenues. Not all patients (purchasers) pay an equal share of an agency's costs, which complicates the process.

To remain viable, any business must generate sufficient revenues to cover operating costs and make a profit. These revenues include increases in working capital, capital replacements, and inflation adjustments.

Nonprofits use profits to improve plants and services; profits do not go to stockholders or owners. Profit appears as a positive balance on account ledgers. Fundamental to the rate-setting process are adequate statistical data, historical and projected, for implementing the rate-setting method to be employed. On a departmental basis, these data include volume of services, current rate, allocated costs, and rate increase constraints. The goal is to obtain the greatest impact from a minimum cumulative rate increase in a cost-management environment. This can be accomplished by increasing rates in high-profit departments while instituting rate reductions in low-profit departments so that they offset each other. Revenues are often budgeted before expenses. This is necessary to determine how much revenue will be available.

Patient Days

Patient days are used to project revenues. They are commonly used as units of service to compute staffing. Patient day statistics are usually derived from census reports that are done daily at midnight and summarized monthly for the year to date and annually. A patient admitted on May 2 and discharged May 10 is charged for nine patient days. Exhibit 11-2 illustrates the number of patient days per unit for one month.

Fiscal Year

The *fiscal year* (FY) is the budgetary or financial year. It may be the calendar year in some organizations, beginning on January 1 and ending on December 31. Many organizations use October 1 to September 30 as the fiscal year. Some use July 1 to June 30 to coincide with budget decisions of state legislatures and the US Congress. In the latter examples, the fiscal year overlaps two calendar years.

Year to Date

The term *year to date* (YTD) describes the accumulated units of service at a particular point in the fiscal year. If the fiscal year begins October 1, the year-to-date patient days for December 31 would be the summary for 92 days.

Average Daily Census

The census is summarized for a specific number of days and divided by that number of days. For example, the *average daily census* (ADC) for the month of May would be the total patient days for May divided by 31. In Exhibit 11-2, the number of patient days for May is 7975. When this is divided by 31, the average daily census is 257.

Hours of Care

Hours of care have traditionally been the number of hours of care allocated per patient per day (24 hours) on a unit. With the use of patient acuity rating systems, hours of care can be determined to the hour or even to the fraction of an hour. Patients usually fall into one of

EXHIBIT 11-2
Sample of Patient Day Census

	CURRENT YEAR			YEAR TO DATE		
	MAY	OCC (%)	APRIL	CURRENT YEAR	OCC (%)	PREVIOUS YEAR
NURSING STATION						
3rd Floor	1,014	79.8	833	9,792	78.6	8,650
4th Floor	811	76.9	718	7,834	75.8	7,255
5th Floor North	526	65.3	524	5,300	67.1	4,838
5th Floor South	622	77.2	592	5,587	70.7	5,603
6th Floor	792	71.0	866	8,730	79.8	8,176
7th Floor	850	68.5	895	9,086	74.7	8,885
8th Floor North	376	60.6	383	4,624	76.1	2,393
8th Floor South	303	69.8	274	3,253	76.4	1,729
9th Floor North	526	84.8	501	5,332	87.7	2,690
9th Floor South	481	77.6	506	5,118	84.2	2,617
MINU	104	83.9	89	1,041	85.6	432
SINU	73	58.9	84	964	79.3	471
Burn Unit	173	79.7	188	1,723	81.0	1,912
Labor and Delivery	138	37.1	99	1,228	33.7	1,258
CCU	206	83.1	148	1,848	76.0	1,937
Clinical Research Unit	137	73.7	132	1,342	73.6	1,361
EAU	23	0.0	7	390	0.0	634
MICU	213	85.9	191	2,099	86.3	2,291
PICU	169	54.5	112	1,612	53.0	1,834
SICU	229	92.3	207	2,175	89.4	2,302
NTICU	209	84.3	87	1,891	77.8	2,277
Total	7,975	73.2	7,436	80,969	75.3	79,086

four or five patient acuity categories, each of which is assigned a specific number of hours of care per patient day.

Caregiver

Each nurse who works with patients is called a *caregiver*. In nursing, the three common types of caregivers are registered nurses (RNs), licensed practical nurses (LPNs), and nurse aides (NAs) or extenders. Most personnel budgets have a ratio of RNs to other caregivers. Considerable research supports an all-RN caregiver staff. The current cost-management environment often alters this goal.

Case-mix

The patient's acuity of services is known as a *case-mix*. Case-mix refers to the type of patients cared for by the institution. Some of the variables included in the case-mix are diagnosis, comorbidities, and treatment patterns.

Budgeting Approaches

Zero-Base Budgeting

Zero-base budgeting is a method of budgeting used to control costs. In a zero-base budget, the budgeting process starts from zero, and everything must be justified by each new budget cycle. A previous activity can be included in the budget, but its relation to the current organizational objectives must justify funding for it. In theory, each function in a zero-base budget must stand on its own merits, and the merits of each function are reviewed annually. All labor power and costs are recalculated, and decisions are made about whether to continue the function and at what levels.

Program Budgeting

Program budgeting is a part of budget planning. Items such as continuing education programs, employee benefits fairs, and health promotion programs should be incorporated into the annual budget. The budget for each program should enumerate fixed expenses, such as rent, advertising, fixed speaker fees, and department overhead, and variable expenses, such as for food, handouts, and per-person honorarium speaker fees. Some costs, such as those for advertising, are unrecoverable even if the program is canceled. They are sunk costs and should be in the cost center budget as well as in the individual program's budget.

EXHIBIT 11-3
Break-Even Analysis

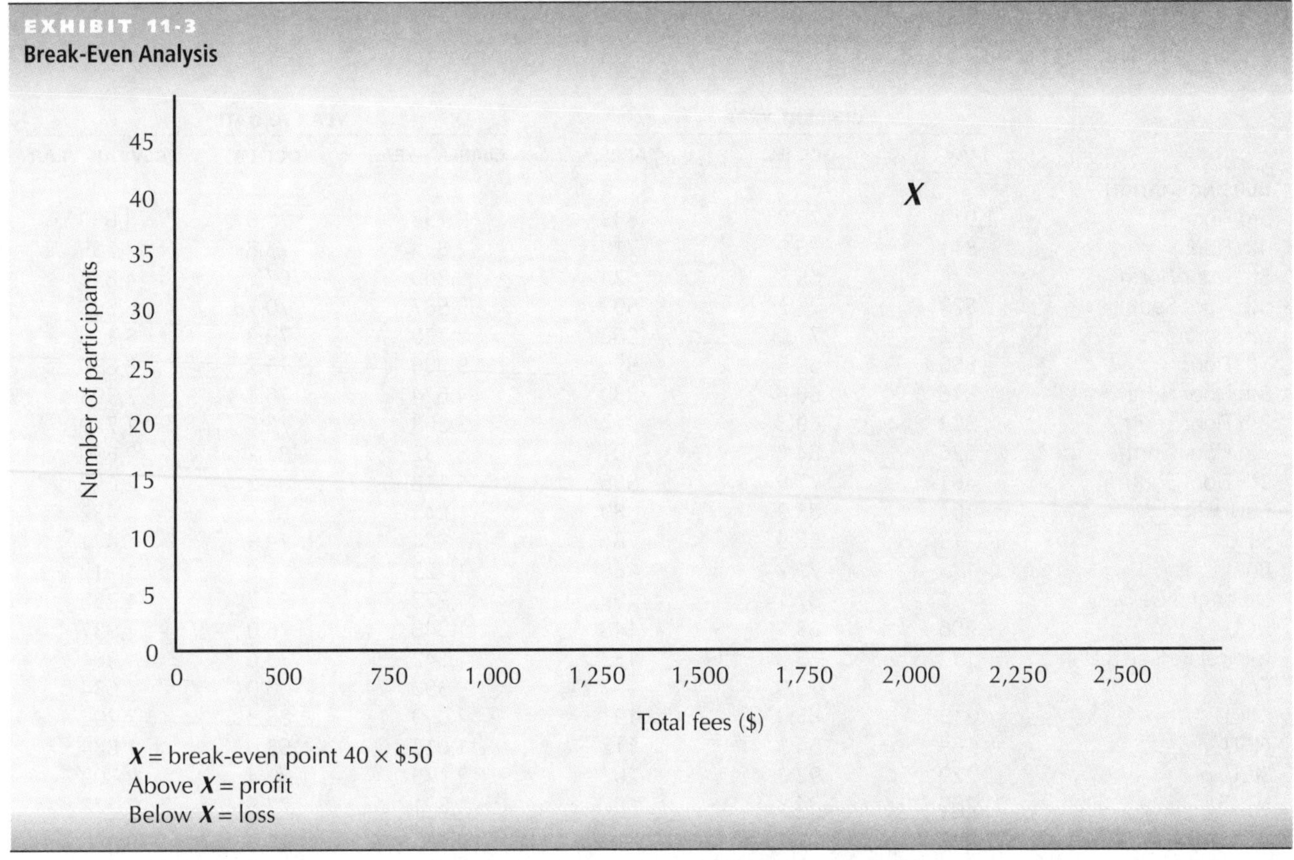

X = break-even point 40 × $50
Above ***X*** = profit
Below ***X*** = loss

Program budgets should include a break-even analysis. If the cost of the program is $2000 and the reasonable charge is $50 per participant, the break-even point is 40 participants. A break-even chart can be made for each program (see Exhibit 11-3). Income above the break-even point is profit; below it is loss.

The point at which the cost to carry out a program is equal to the cost to cancel it is called the *least-loss point*. If enough people have registered to pay the sunk costs, the net loss will be the same whether the program is canceled or held. It may be good public relations to carry out a program at the least-loss point.[13]

Flexible Budgeting

Flexible budgeting takes into account variations or ranges from low to high points.[14] This approach requires a well-prepared and educated nurse manager. It determines a range of volume instead of an actual volume, which is much more difficult to plan and manage.[15]

Fixed Budgeting

A *fixed budget* is based on a fixed annual level of volume. For example, the annual number of x-rays performed is divided by 12, giving a monthly average of x-rays. This approach to budgeting does not take seasonal or monthly variations into consideration.[16]

Types of Budgets

Operating Budget

The *operating budget* is the overall plan identifying expected revenues and expenses, both fixed and variable, for the forthcoming fiscal year. It is an annual budget that includes the cash budget and the capital budget. In addition, the operating budget identifies the source and nature of expected revenues and expenses. The operating budget determines the per diem and other charges to be made to the patient.

Cost-to-Charge Ratios

Cost-to-charge ratios are convenient tools for computing the cost of providing a service. For example, if the charge to a patient for fiber optic laboratory services is $1000, and the cost-to-charge ratio is 0.815626, then the cost to the hospital for these services is approximately $815.63. This cost includes the expense of running the fiber optic laboratory and a portion of the hospital's overhead cost. In some instances, the cost-to-charge ratio is greater than one, which means the cost of operating these cost centers is greater than the charges.

The hospital has two types of cost centers. The first is the revenue-producing cost center, such as the fiber optic laboratory, which bills patients for services provided.

The second type is the overhead cost center, such as the accounting department, which exists to support the revenue-producing centers. The cost of the overhead cost centers is allocated to the revenue-producing centers by various statistical methods. For example, utility costs are allocated to revenue-producing departments based on the square footage of space they occupy. Accounting department costs, however, are allocated based on the size of the operating budget of each revenue-producing cost center. The cost-to-charge ratio is computed by dividing the total cost of the cost center, both direct and overhead, by the total charges for the same department.

Cost-Benefit Analysis

Cost-benefit analysis is a planning technique that answers the following questions:[17] What are the costs of pursuing a goal, an objective, a program, or a specific nursing intervention? How do costs compare with the benefits? Is the project worthwhile? Comparison of different nursing interventions for the same nursing diagnosis or problem results in using the least costly interaction to achieve similar or better results. The intervention used is then cost-effective.

Operating or Cash Budget

The *cash budget* is the actual operating budget in detail, usually excluding the capital budget. A cash budget indicates whether cash flow will be adequate to meet anticipated payments, such as debt obligations, including replacement and expansion of facilities, unanticipated requirements, payroll, payment for supplies and services, and a prudent investment program. Cash receipts come from third-party payers, tuition, endowment fund earnings, and sales of food, gifts, and services.

The cash budget is the day-to-day budget and represents money coming in and going out. It is advisable to have cash reserves so that cash flow and the money coming in will pay the bills. Otherwise, revenues must be sped up or payment of bills slowed down. Cash reserves should not be excessive; they may represent money that should be working for the organization. Cash budgets show revenues and expenses, whereas operating budgets show plans. They are usually considered integrated entities.[18]

Negative Cash Flow

The four major factors that influence negative cash flow are as follows:

1. Time lag between delivery of services and collection of payments.
2. The difference in cycles between the timing of net income and flow of cash.
3. Lag created by the large up and down cycles of volume during different seasons (cash deficit during a busy census cycle or surplus during a low census cycle).
4. Labor expense (60% to 70% of operating expense) paid out in salary and wages does not cycle concurrently with collections.

To maintain solvency, cash flow must be managed carefully and cycles of cash shortage planned for appropriately. The cash budget should plan for the ability to borrow cash during shortfalls, the investment of excess cash, and the strict monitoring and reporting of lost charges and of the billing and collecting process. The cash budget is a part of the total budget and is apportioned to departments based on individual cost-center activity.

Developing the Operating Budget

Operating budget information supplied to the chief nurse executive, department heads, and cost-center managers includes a budget worksheet and a worksheet that explains budget adjustments (see Exhibits 11-4 and 11-5). The budget worksheet depicts information by the account number and subcode of each cost center and lists prior-year expense, original budget, and annualized expense. This form usually is provided during the new budget formulation stage, and the annualized expense is the projected total expense if current rates continue to the end of the fiscal year. The column headed Budget Adjustment is empty so that the cost-center manager can fill in the budget expenses for the projected fiscal year. The column Approved Budget is the budget that has been approved by the Finance Department along with Administration after reviewing the requested adjustments. Note in Exhibit 11-4 that the cost-center manager had projected an increased budget of $1000 for subcode 6000, supplies. This amount was reduced to an annualized projection of $650 (subcodes 6100 and 6200), at the annual budget meeting.

Also in Exhibit 11-4, note that subcode 8200, maintenance and repairs, was increased by $100 (from $800 to $900). This increase was justified on the adjustment explanation (Exhibit 11-5). Overall, increases were approved for subcodes 8200 (maintenance and repair), 9200 (travel), and 9300 (airfare). A total budget for supplies and minor equipment for this cost center was approved for $2,925. Exhibit 11-5 shows the adjustment explanation for subcodes 8200 and 9200.

Osborne and Gaebler refer to the operational budget as the *expenditure control budget*. It sets up accounts for various major expenditures. These authors recommend shifting among accounts as needed, and allowing departments to carry over into the new budget what they do not spend. A recommended formula for establishing

EXHIBIT 11-4
Budget Worksheet

Operating Expenses

SUBCODE	DESCRIPTION	PRIOR-YEAR EXPENSE	ORIGINAL BUDGET	ANNUALIZED EXPENSE	BUDGET ADJUSTMENTS	APPROVED BUDGET
6000	Total–Supplies	.00	1,000	$915		$650
6100	Forms	860	.00	200		$200
6200	Books	450	.00	450		$450
6434	Brochures	398	.00	.00		
6660	Film rental	100	.00	.00		
Total Supplies		**1,808**	**1,000**	**650**		
8000	Total–Repairs & Maintenance	.00	1,360			
8200	Main. & Repair	100	.00	800	$900	$1,190
8310	Minor Equip.	675	.00	100		$100
8524	Telephone	185	.00	190		$190
Total Repairs & Main.		**960**	**1,360**	**1,090**		
9000	Total–OCE		.00	1,370		
9200	Travel	1,345	.00		$685	$1,085
9300	Airfare	800	.00		200	$400
9600	Entertainment	275	.00		220	
Total Other Controllable		**2,420**	**1,370**	**420**		
Account Total		**5,188**	**3,730**	**2,160**		

Total $2,925

EXHIBIT 11-5
Adjustment Explanation for Fiscal Year 2004

Emergency Department Budget Unit: Supplies and Minor Equipment, Fiscal Year 2004.

SUBCODE	DESCRIPTION	BUDGET ADJUSTMENT	JUSTIFICATION
8200	Maintenance & Repairs	100	Ice machine is breaking more frequently
9200	Travel	685	Two extra conferences for JCAHO
9300	Airfare	200	As above

an expenditure control budget is: same as previous year plus account for inflation and growth or decline plus any carryover funds. Management should apply additional money for the new initiatives. The strengths of such a mission-driven budget include the following:[19]

- Every employee has an incentive to save money.
- Resources are freed up to test new ideas.
- Managers have the autonomy they need to respond to changing circumstances.
- A predictable environment is created.
- The budget process is enormously simplified.
- Money can be saved on auditors and a budget office.
- Management can focus on other important issues.

Personnel Budget

Most budgets for nursing personnel are based on quantitative workload measurements, such as a patient acuity system. A computer software program usually produces staffing requirements by shift and day. It produces an acuity index for each patient, and the formula indicates needed staff by skill mix (RN, LPN, CNA) and by shift. It also compares actual staffing with that required, and a summary can be provided by month and year. Each day either the unit secretary or nurse enters the acuity rating for each patient into a computer.

Exhibit 11-6 is a nursing personnel budget based on a patient-acuity rating system. The ADC is obtained from

EXHIBIT 11-6
Nursing Personnel Budget

NURSING BUDGET

1. The personnel budget is based on total number of hours of care needed which is determined by the acuity levels (1–4).

PATIENT ACUITY LEVEL	HHPD (HOURS PER CARE PER PATIENT DAY)
1	4.0 hours
2	6.4 hours
3	10.5 hours
4	16.0 hours

2. The staffing formula is:

$$\frac{\text{Average census} \times \text{nursing hours} \times 1.4 \times 1.14}{7.5}$$

3. The total nursing personnel needed for an ADC and specific patient acuity is presented below. The total nursing personnel also includes unit secretaries.

UNIT	ADC	ACUITY	HHPD	RN	LPN	CNA	OTHER	TOTAL
				MEDICAL				
Oncology	17.1	3.0	10.5	24	2	12	4	42
BMT	8.2	4.0	16.0	22	0	6	2	30
Telemetry	22.3	2.0	6.4	18	3	9	6	36
4S	19.4	1.0	4.0	9	2	6	3	20
MICU	8.0	4.0	16.0	27	0	0	3	30
Total				**100**	**7**	**33**	**18**	**158**
				SURGICAL				
Orthopedics	30.0	2.0	6.4	26	5	10	6	47
SICU	8.0	4.0	16.0	27	0	0	4	31
4CW	20.3	2.0	6.4	22	0	6	3	31
5CW	26.7	2.0	6.4	28	1	7	3.5	39.5
Total				**103**	**6**	**23**	**16.5**	**148.5**
				WOMEN'S & INFANTS				
NBN	18.4	2.0	6.4	21	0	4	4.0	29
NICU	19.3	4.0	16.0	65	0	0	4.5	69.5
L & D***	28	0	7	3.5	38.5			
Women's	24.1	2.0	6.4	25	2	6	2	35
Total				**139**	**2**	**17**	**14**	**172.0**
				INPATIENT REHABILITATION				
3 East	11.7	2.0	6.4	9	1	6	4	20

*** No acuity system

records produced in the admissions office. It is the result of dividing the total patient days for a unit for 1 year by 365 days. Census reports are generated daily, monthly, and annually by a computer.

Acuity is the sum of all acuities for 1 year divided by 365 days. This figure is also generated daily, monthly, and annually. The nursing hours are generated from the acuity standard listed in item 1 of Exhibit 11-6. Application of a staffing formula for preparing the personnel budget for a specific unit is illustrated in Exhibit 11-7.

In planning the personnel budget, the nurse has quantitative information related to staffing and can accurately predict the number of full-time equivalents (FTEs) needed for patient care. Other considerations must be weighed at the same time: Will there be a pay increase next year? If so, it must be calculated and budgeted. Will benefits increase or decrease? They must also be budgeted. If new programs are being implemented, do they require additional labor power? Will this labor power come from cutbacks in other programs, or from

EXHIBIT 11-7
Calculating the Nursing Personnel Budget

The staffing formula is

$$\frac{\text{Average census} \times \text{nursing hours} \times 1.4 \times 1.14}{7.5}$$

Example: Oncology Unit

- Average daily census = 17.1
- HHPD = 10.5
- 1.4 is a constant representing 7 days in a week with a full-time employee working 5 days a week: 7 ÷ 5 = 1.4
- 1.14 is a constant which allows for 0.14 FTE for vacation, sickness, etc. for each 1.0 FTE
- 7.5 is one workday

$$\frac{17.1 \times 10.5 \times 1.4 \times 1.14}{7.5} = 38 \text{ FTEs}$$

The budgeted staffing for the Oncology Unit consists of 24 RNs, 2 LPNs, and 12 CNAs. In addition, the unit has 4 unit secretaries.

added FTEs? See Exhibit 11-8 for adding new positions to the budget.

Personnel account for the largest portion of the nursing budget. When one is preparing budgets for clinics, emergency departments, recovery rooms, operating rooms, delivery rooms, and home care, one must have quantitative data, such as numbers of visits, procedures, and deliveries. Records of length of time required for each activity can be obtained by using management–engineering techniques in which visits, procedures, or other activities are charted over a period of time.

Data should be collected over a representative period to show the actual hours worked by shift and by day. These data will indicate fluctuations in the workload by shift and by day of the week. Use a second data sheet to determine the total number of patients in the emergency department area at any one time, including patients in a holding status. Conversion of these data into graphs provides information to compare staffing with workload. These data will provide the following information:[20]

- Current nursing hours available per patient visit.
- Fluctuations in available hours by shift and by day.
- Fluctuations in workload by time of day.
- Fluctuations in ratio of staffing levels to patient load.

Piper writes that the basic staffing of an emergency room should be calculated to handle a *critical mass*, the staffing level required to handle an unexpected emergency. In addition to quantitative data, the nurse administrator should collect qualitative data from the staff to assist in containing stress, determining mix of staff, and improving support services. Data can be compared with those from other institutions. The result will then be translated into personnel dollars.[21]

In the process of budgeting, the nurse manager knows how much each decision will cost and whether it involves numbers and kinds of personnel or amounts and kinds of supplies and equipment. Few nurse managers have the luxury of a budget that provides all of the resources that can be used. Hard decisions must be made. These decisions are easier to substantiate when work loads are quantified. If the patient dependency or acuity system is reliable and valid and has quality checks on the raters, it will provide data that justify the personnel budget. When the number of adult patients of the highest acuity level increases from 24 to 32 per shift and day, the budget must be adjusted. Comparisons must be made to determine whether other levels have decreased. Estimates must be made as to whether the increases and decreases are permanent or temporary. Then the budget decisions are made.

Nurse managers study fluctuation trends in patient census and use these data for minimum staffing requirements to determine the percentage of time to staff one nurse less and the percentage of time to staff one nurse more per shift. The salary expense for the one time that one nurse less per shift is needed should be subtracted from the budget. The salary expense for the one time that one nurse more per shift is needed should be added to the budget. The result is an improved salary expense budget result.

Strategies to reduce budget overages include the following:[22]

- Maintain good staff retention.
- Use nurse extenders to perform non-RN functions.
- Monitor and control unscheduled absenteeism.
- Implement an effective on-call system.
- Institute a "flex-team" in related clinical areas to avoid overtime and agency nurse expenses.
- Create a large pool of part-time nurses.
- Budget according to trends.
- Negotiate for a reasonable budget that considers turnover and orientation.

EXHIBIT 11-8
New Position Requisition

1. Job Title: ______
2. Department: ______
3. FTE Status:
   - Full time
   - Part time
   - Permanent
   - Temporary: If temporary, provide finishing date ______
   - Exempt
   - Non-Exempt
4. Expected Starting Date: ______
5. Hours/Shift: ______
6. Description of Essential Job Duties: ______
7. Justification for New Position (i.e., new program/increased volume): ______
8. Requirements essential for position (i.e., licensure, education): ______
9. Advertising:
   - Yes
   - No
10. Preferred publication: ______
11. Approvals:
    Supervisor: ______ Date: ______
    Human Resources: ______ Date: ______

Nonproductive Full-Time Equivalents

Nonproductive FTEs are hours for which an employee is paid but does not work. Nonproductive FTEs include vacation days, holidays, sick days, education and training time, jury duty, leave for funerals, and military leave. These nonproductive hours must be determined and added to personnel expenditures as replacement FTEs. An FTE is based on 2080 hours per year. If the nonproductive FTE average is to be used for personnel budgeting, the human resource (HR) department payroll section will provide it. For example:

Average vacation FTE	12.5 days
Average holiday FTE	7.0 days
Average sick days FTE	3.5 days
Average training and education FTE	3.0 days
Average other leave FTE	1.5 days
Total	27.5 days, or 220.0 hours

The total work time is 2080 hours less 220 hours; the actual work time is 1860 hours. The percentage of nonworked to total hours paid is 10.6%. The percentage of nonworked to worked hours is 11.8%.

A cost-center manager prepares the budget according to management rules. The budget should include a line item for replacement FTEs to cover nonproductive FTEs by assigning a fixed amount to each person's paid time off. An option is to determine percentage of nonproductive FTEs and add this total to the budget. This information is then used for staffing determination, as are seasonal fluctuations for vacations, census, and other pertinent factors.[23]

Supplies and Equipment Budget

The supplies and equipment budget is part of the operating or cash budget. It includes all supplies and equipment used in provision of services, except capital equipment and supplies charged directly to patients.

Minor equipment includes items such as sphygmomanometers, otoscopes, and ophthalmoscopes. Minor equipment costs less than the base amount set for capital equipment. If the base amount is $500, all equipment under $500 appears as minor equipment in the supplies and equipment budget.

Generally, the director of materials management furnishes the total cost of supplies and equipment per cost center to the accounting office, which generates a cost per patient day. This cost is used for budgeting purposes, and increases for inflation are a decision of top management. Based on projected patient days and revenues, decisions can be made to increase or decrease the supplies and equipment budget.

Controlling the amounts of supplies can decrease costs and equipment kept in inventory. Nurse managers should look at the inventories they control and reduce them according to usage.

Factors that might influence the supply and equipment aspects of the budget include new program development in the institution, new physicians, and product upgrades. A product evaluation committee may be very cost-effective.

Product Evaluation

Product Evaluation Committee

A product evaluation committee usually has as its members representatives of nursing, central supply, infection control, finance, purchasing, administration, and education. The committee is usually chaired by the materials manager. This committee is responsible for evaluation and purchase of supplies and equipment. The following are among its goals:

- Standardization, with all units using the same products
- Lower prices through higher volumes
- Providing a clinical perspective in focusing on the quality of the product for improved patient care
- Minimizing inventory levels wherever possible
- Decreasing the cost of education and training by standardization

Thus systematic control of the introduction of patient care products into the institution is achieved. Exhibit 11-9 presents a product evaluation checklist used to justify the product under consideration.

The following is a suggested process for product evaluation by a committee:[24]

1. Determine objectives of product evaluation.
2. Define use of the product with input from potential users.
3. Define objectives for each evaluation project.
4. Do initial review of various products: features, techniques for use, and prices.
5. Select products for evaluation and evaluate techniques for use, staff acceptance, and problems.
6. Conduct in-service tests to use products.
7. Use simple closed-ended questions, open-ended questions, and rating scales to evaluate the product.
8. Compile and analyze data, including costs, cost savings, conversion cost, and reimbursement potential. The Deming theory of working with one supplier to improve products is noted in Chapter 17.
9. Make a decision for purchase.

EXHIBIT 11-9
Product Evaluation Checklist

The purpose of product evaluation is to provide a mechanism to ensure that the evaluation of products emphasize quality of care and cost containment. A checklist will be completed for products that have been selected for evaluation. The checklist will be submitted to the Director of Material Management for consideration by the Product Evaluation Committee. The checklist must be reviewed by your Department Director before submitting it to the Director of Material Management. An example of the questions needed for the committee are provided below:

1. Name and purpose of the product.
2. Is this product new, a replacement, or an upgrade?
3. What is the price and costs of this product? (purchase price, installation, training, staff, facility, service agreement)
4. How dependable is this product?
5. What type of service and vendor support will be provided?
6. What is the patient benefit from this product?
7. What resources are required to support this product? (staff, education, plant/environmental requirements)
8. How do the financials look? Where will the funds to pay for this product come from?
9. Are revenues generated by this product?
10. How and what is the reimbursement potential?
11. What is the anticipated utilization of this product? If it is a replacement or upgrade, what is the utilization of the current product?
12. Can the facility potentially hold or increase market share with this product?

Capital Budget

A capital budget is usually separate from the operating budget (see Exhibit 11-10). A capital budget projects the planned costs of major purchases. Each capital budget item is defined in terms of dollar value and is an item of equipment that is used over a period of time. The budget provides for depreciation of each item in the capital budget, sets aside the amount of depreciation in an escrow

EXHIBIT 11-10

Capital Budget Requested Fiscal Year 200x–200x: Metropolitan Memorial Hospital

DEPT.	ITEM	QUANTITY	AMOUNT
66h & 7th	Beds & misc. pat. furn.	85	$200,000.00
Admin	Pneumatic tube system	1	75,000.00
Anest	Capnograph-portable	1	4,200.00
Anest	Trans. Mon.- inc NIPB & O2 Sat	1	9,200.00
Anest	Ventilators	2	5,050.00
ER Med	Pro Pac 106	1	13,790.00
Bio Med	Safety tester	1	1,695.00
Blood Bk	Table top centrifuge	1	2,000.00
Blood Bk	Automated cell washer	1	6,250.00
Cath Lab	Pulse oximetry	1	2,600.00
Cath Lab	Dynamap	1	3,800.00
Clin. Lab	Miscellaneous equipment	1	250,000.00
Dialysis	Dialysis machine	1	25,000.00
Dietary	Refrigerator-bakery	1	3,500.00
Dietary	Refrigerator-bakery	1	6,950.00
Dietary	Refrigerator-cook area	1	3,500.00
Dietary	Refrigerator-PFS	1	3,100.00
Dietary	Meat slicer	1	3,500.00
ER	New monitoring system	1	160,000.00
ER	Propak monitor	1	3,500.00
Envir	High-speed burnisher	4	8,000.00
Envir	Slow-speed buffers	2	1,600.00
GI Lab	Video processor CV-100	1	20,000.00
CVStation	Blood pressure monitor	1	4,500.00
CVStation	Stress test system	1	20,000.00
CVtation	ECG management system	1	70,000.00
MICU/CCU	Faceplates-central monitors	12	4,920.00
Nursing	Medication carts	17	25,000.00
Nutri	Computer & printer	1	2,011.00
OR	Laparoscopic video system	1	30,165.00
OR	Electrosurgical cautery	2	17,200.00
PACU	RR stretchers	10	20,000.00
Plant Op	4000-watt portable generator	1	1,495.00
Plant Op	8 ch. OPS card for telephone switch	1	1,337.00
Radio	Rebuilt film processor	1	12,000.00
Res. Th	Sterile pass-through drier	1	12,567.00
SPD	Washer decontaminator	1	75,000.00
Staff Dev	Overhead projector	1	700.00
Staff Dev	CPR manikin	1	5,641.00
Total requested Metropolitan Memorial Center			$1,114,771.00

account, and uses this account to finance new capital budgets. Depreciation records the declining value of a physical asset. In addition, department heads are required to justify and set priorities on capital budget items (see Exhibit 11-11). The exact definition of what constitutes a capital budget item with regard to dollar amount and life expectancy varies among hospitals.

Capital budgets also deal with maintenance, renovations, remodeling, improvements, expansion, land acquisition, and new buildings. The financial manager for nursing is the nurse manager, who should evaluate past decisions and advise the nurse administrator whether they were good or bad.

All proposals for capital equipment must be fully evaluated for amount of use, method of payment, safety, replacement, duplication of service, and every other conceivable factor, including the need for space, personnel, and facility renovation. The needs and desires of the medical staff should be considered. Staff involvement in planning helps ensure wise purchases of capital equipment.

A strategic capital-budgeting method based on principles of decision analysis can help health care organizations allocate capital effectively when meeting requests for capital expenditures. The eight steps of the strategic capital-budgeting method are establishing evaluation criteria, classifying proposals by area of investment, ensuring that proposals are complete and easy to understand, determining costs of proposals, rating proposals with respect to individual criteria, setting priority weights for criteria, calculating weighted value scores for each proposal, and ranking proposals by cost-benefit ratios. The results provide a reliable basis for optimal capital allocation.[25]

The capital budget must address increased forms of competition, dwindling financial resources, and regulatory constraints. Management should enhance conditions under which effective planning and capital budgeting increase the agency's chance of long-term survival. Capital budgeting is a part of the overall budget planning process for the organization and not an entity unto itself. When each entry or item in the capital budget list has been analyzed and reduced to the amount available, the budget is again tabulated. It is now ready to present to the board of directors. With the board's approval, the list is distributed to cost-center managers, who prepare requisitions for purchase. The purchasing department prepares bid specifications, with input from cost-center managers. Purchases are finalized based on results of bids submitted by vendors who meet the required specifications. Finally, purchases are entered into the depreciation budget schedule. The latter is published by American Hospital Publishing and is considered the standard for the industry. The following are a few examples of the composite estimated useful lives of depreciable hospital assets: boiler house (30 years); masonry building, wood/metal frame (25 years); bed, electric (12 years); and otoscope (7 years). For budgetary purposes, the nurse manager should have access to the entire publication.[26]

When evaluating capital equipment, one should evaluate similar products one at a time. When purchasing capital equipment, one should determine whether it can be upgraded or must be replaced when the technology improves. One should consider construction, durability, modularity, warranty, availability of parts, and service agreements as part of the total cost of equipment. One should also consider leasing rather than buying.[27]

Part of the capital equipment budgeting process includes estimating the use of each item. For revenue budgeting purposes, a price or charge should be assigned to the use of each item. The cost-center manager can then determine the break-even point at which the item will be paid for.

Performance Budgeting

Performance budgeting focuses on the activities of a cost center such as indirect care, direct care, and quality monitoring. Each activity has objectives with specific financial resources, and the focus is on what is expected to be accomplished. Performance is evaluated based on a variety of outputs. Flexible budgeting that evaluates actual costs based on actual workload is an improvement over traditional budgeting but is a limited evaluation of nursing performance. Performance budgeting is an improvement over flexible budgeting because it ties performance to financial resource consumption. The steps involved are as follows:[28]

1. Define the performance activities or area of accomplishment for the cost center, which may include direct care, improved quality of care, nursing staff satisfaction, patient satisfaction, productivity, and innovation.
2. Identify the line-item operating-budget costs for the cost center being evaluated. These costs will be manager and clinical salaries, education costs, supplies, and overhead.
3. Define how much of the resources represented by each line item are to be devoted to each of the performance areas.
4. Choose measures of performance for each performance area, budget an amount of work for each area, and determine the budgeted cost per unit of work based on these measures.

The performance budget evolves or is converted from the operating budget. Potential output measures are

EXHIBIT 11-11
Capital Equipment Requisition Form

1. Project description: ______________________ 2. Date: ______________________
3. Submitted by: ______________________ 4. Department: ______________________
5. Equipment requested: ______________________ 6. Useful life: ______________________
7. Justification for equipment: 8. How often will equipment be requested/utilized?
   - Regulatory
   - New service
   - Replacement
   - Upgrade
9. Equipment description: ______________________
10. Impact to other departments: ______________________
    - Plant operations (renovation, installation)
    - Bio-Med
    - ISD
    - Education department
    - Other
11. Costs:
    - Equipment Costs: ______________
    - Renovation/installation: ______________
    - Service agreement:: ______________
    - Personnel: ______________
    - Education/Training: ______________
    - Shipping: ______________
    - Storage: ______________
12. For any equipment $5,000 or over, an equipment evaluation must be completed.
    _____ Yes _____ No (attach evaluation form)
13. For any equipment $25,000 or over, a financial pro forma must be completed.
    _____ Yes _____ No (attach pro forma)
14. Approvals:
    Department Director: ______________________ Date: ______________________
    Administrator: ______________________ Date: ______________________

proxies and consist of both process and outcome measures. These output measures may include the following:[29]

- Compliance with patient care plan procedures, with the goal of a percentage reduction in errors.
- Improved compliance costs (the fix, which is usually additional resources of some kind).
- Staffing decisions using reduced management time.
- Cost reduction.
- Increased productivity.
- Increased patient and staff satisfaction.
- Innovation and planning.
- Direct care.
- Indirect care.

Multiple measures can be developed for each performance area.

Revenues

The sources of nursing revenue or for securing a financial base for nursing include grants, continuing education, private practice, community visibility, health care for students and staff, health maintenance organizations, city health departments, professional corporations, and nurse-managed centers.

Operating room nursing is an example of a cost that can be billed as a source of revenue. Determining the level of care needed for different procedures and the room charges, based on use of supplies and equipment, and billing the services separately may be considered revenue. In computing the nursing charges, the cost of nursing personnel per case can be determined from the records. To this can be added the cost of preparation time for assembling supplies and equipment and setting up the room, preoperative and postoperative patient visits, nursing administration, and staff development. Room costs include environmental services and maintenance.[30] Using product-line strategy, nursing divisions can sell a number of product lines, such as staff development programs, consultation services, home health services, wellness programs, and computer software.

The Controlling Process

Now that we have seen the nursing budget from its planning and directing aspects, we can turn to its controlling or evaluating aspects. The budget establishes financial standards for the division of nursing and through the division's cost center for each nursing unit. Daily, weekly, monthly, and quarterly feedback provides information to compare managerial performance with the established standards. The results are used to make adjustments. What kind of feedback do nurses need relative to their budgets and cost control? Nurses need information to determine whether their goals are being met. Are they exceeding the budget? Is the excess both for costs and for revenues? Are the supplies and expenses of the quantity and quality planned? Is the equipment being purchased and installed as scheduled? Are employees being recruited and used effectively to produce the expected quality and quantity of nursing services? Is employee morale good? What adjustments need to be made? Where are the problems, and who is responsible for them?

Budget processes should be flexible to allow for increased and decreased volume of business. The hospital's finance department provides cost-center managers with needed biometric information to make adjustments in staffing and in use of supplies. The colossal mistakes of budgeting are made in the control area. Variations in budget should be used as a tool for decision making, and not as an instance or reactionary intervention to make arbitrary cuts that result in unrealistic operating budgets for line managers.[31]

Monitoring the Budget

Various techniques have been described for monitoring the budget; however, all budget objectives should contain procedures for quality review, including identification of a team to perform such a review. If a program is not successful—that is, if it is not meeting objectives or is running above predicted costs and below predicted revenues—then a decision should be made about whether to rework or cancel it. Although very difficult, making this decision is essential to good control. The technique of canceling budgeted programs is sometimes referred to as sun setting. A nurse manager should accept the responsibility for "sun setting" programs that are costly and unprofitable.

In developing the nursing budget, it is necessary that the unit structures for nursing administration are comparable in type and quantity of workload. Developing and providing financial policies and guidelines is most successful when the top administrative team works with the budget monitor. The nurse administrator is part of this team and brings to its meetings standards of service that are defensible (such as data on workload, including numbers and types of procedures, patients, surgical operations, and visits). These policies should reflect the long-term plans of the governing board.

Part of the information furnished to nurse administrators and managers is in the form of reports, which include statistical reports of revenues and expenditures for the current year. Exhibit 11-12 illustrates financial information that is needed by the cost-center manager and the nursing administrator.

Note that the account number at the head of the table in Exhibit 11-12 is 2-7010. The prefix 2 denotes that the account balance does not turn over at the end of the fiscal year. The cost center or department is 7010. Financial

EXHIBIT 11-12
Accounting System Report

Account: 2-7010
Department: 7010

Fiscal Year Ending 200x
January–October (83% fiscal year elapsed)
Medical/Surgical Unit—Expense

SUBCODE	DESCRIPTION	BUDGET APPROVED	ACTUAL CURRENT MONTH	ACTUAL YTD	OPEN ENCUMBRANCES	REMAINING BUDGET	PERCENT USED
1000	Pool–Salary & Wages	901,053				901,053	0
1100	Professional Salary		72,533	775,790		775,790-	$
1200	Nursing Asst Salary		4,085	50,947		50,947-	$
1300	Secretary Salary		4,347	53,168		53,168-	$
1400	Orderly Salary		3,936	52,195		52,195-	$
1500	Students		14,898	1,518		14,898	100
1600	Accurred Salaries	32,791	11,462	32,791			100
	Salaries	$948,742	97,881	979,789		31,047-	103
2000	Pool–Empl Benefits	55,722				55,722	0
2100	FICA	112		112			100
2200	Health Insurance	59,973	5,887	59,973			100
2300	Retirement	62,158	5,591	62,158			100
2400	Disability	4,869	526	4,869			100
2500	Life Insurance	2,569	264	2,569			100
	Employee Benefits	**185,403**	12,268	129,681		55,722	70
3000	Pool–Med/Surg	10,000				10,000	0
3100	Med & Surg Supplies	185,000	22,000	185,000			100
3110	Drugs	2,317	1,100	2,317			100
3114	Solutions	44,000	10,000	44,000			100
	Med/Surg Supplies	241,317	33,100	231,317		10,000	96
4000	Pool–General Supply						0
4010	Office Supplies	1,010	220	1,009			100
4120	Forms	1,490	1,090	400			100
4134	Copying	35	30	36			100
4260	Dietary	620	50	620			100
4330	Linen Bedding	215		215			100
4440	Housekeeping Supply	2,880	350	2,880			100
	General Supplies	6,250	650	5,850			100

(continued)

EXHIBIT 11-12 *(continued)*

Account: 2-7010
Department: 7010

Fiscal Year Ending 200x
January–October (83% fiscal year elapsed)
Medical/Surgical Unit—Expense

			ACTUAL				
SUBCODE	DESCRIPTION	BUDGET APPROVED	CURRENT MONTH	YTD	OPEN ENCUMBRANCES	REMAINING BUDGET	PERCENT USED
5000	Minor Equipment	450				450	0
	Total Expenses	1,382,212	143,899	1,346,637	400	35,725	97
	Account Total	**1,382,212**	**143,899**	**1,346,637**	**400**	**35,725**	**97**

OPEN ENCUMBRANCE STATUS

P.O. ACCOUNT	P.O. NUMBER	DATE	ORIGINAL DESCRIPTION	LIQUIDATING ENCUM.	CURRENT EXPENDITURES	LAST ACT ADJUSTS. ENCUM.	DATE
2-7010-4120	D3333	4/10/04	Print-All	400.00		400.00	10/4/04

transactions, including purchase orders for supplies and minor equipment, as well as the payroll, are identified with this cost center number and are charged by the purchasing and accounting departments to this number and to the appropriate subcodes 1000 through 5000. Table columns indicate the operational budget, the actual expenditures for the current month and for the fiscal or budget year, open encumbrances, and the balance available. Because 83% of the fiscal year (which begins January 1) has elapsed, these figures have some relationship to the Percent Used column. Although 103% of the budgeted salary has been used, only 70% of employee benefits have been used, which indicates a use of overtime plus part-time employees working less than the 20 hours per week required to qualify for benefits. Zero percent of the budgeted money for minor equipment has been spent to date. Total budget expenses were 97%, indicating a variance of 10% overspending. This report serves as a control for nurse managers, but the expenditure of budgeted money for any one subcode could cause the total expenses to date to be greater than the percentage of fiscal year elapsed without creating an alarm. In this instance, overspending should be related to increased census and revenue.

Exhibit 11-13 informs the nurse managers of the specific financial transactions that took place during the month of October. These transactions can be checked against Exhibit 11-12.

Information on revenues is reported in a similar manner. Exhibit 11-14 illustrates the inpatient revenue for the Medical–Surgical Unit, which includes nursing and hotel services. All the revenue is credited to nursing. The revenue account is 2-40815, and the cost center is the same as for expenses, 7010. The budgeted revenues for the year are listed, as are the revenues for the month and for the fiscal year. Note that although 83% of the fiscal year has elapsed, only 76% of the budgeted revenues have been charged, a variance of 7%. Also, Exhibit 11-15 indicates that 76% of budgeted equipment revenues have been billed.

Because the amount billed (that is, the unit's revenues), 76%, is less than the 83% of fiscal year elapsed, the nurse managers can note that revenues are currently lower than expenses, which is a negative financial report. The manager's goal is to improve this financial status by the end of the fiscal year.

Additional financial information can be furnished to each nurse manager, including summary reports in whole dollars and for all cost centers supervised. This can be done by subcode, by subcode and cost center, or by any unit or department.

Rollover funds are also included in the financial reports that can be provided to the chief nurse executive and nurse managers. Balances in these funds are carried over into the next fiscal year to be spent at any future date. The chief nurse executive, a department head, or a cost-center manager can manage rollover funds.

Motivational Aspects of Budgeting

Budgeting can be a motivating force for personnel if current programs must increase in effectiveness and efficiency to remain; if decentralization and staff involvement provide an increased sense of responsibility and satisfaction; and if merit increases, promotions, and bonuses are tied or linked to budgetary performance.

EXHIBIT 11-13
Accounting System Report

Report of transactions for FY ending 200x

Distribution code = 600
Medical–Surgical Unit—Expense

Acct: 2-7010
Dept: 7010

SUBCODE	DESCRIPTION	DATE	REF.	J.E. OFFSET ACCOUNT	CURRENT REV/EXP	ENCUMBRANCES	BATCH REF.	BATCH DATE
1100	Payroll Expense	10/07	60001	0-11181-128CR	35,017.03		TTS584	10/7
1100	Payroll Expense	10/21	60001	0-11181-128CR	37,516.33		TTS588	10/21
1100	Total Profess. Salary				72,533.36			
1200	Payroll Expense	10/07	60001	0-11181-128CR	2,115.98		TTS584	10/07
1200	Payroll Expense	10/21	60001	0-11181-128CR	1,969.04		TTS588	10/21
1200	Total Asst. Salary				4,085.00			
1300	Payroll Expense	10/07	60001	0-11181-128CR	2,012.56		TTS584	10/07
1300	Payroll Expense	10/21	60001	0-11181-128CR	2,334.44		TTS588	10/21
1300	Total Secretary Salary				4,347.00			
1400	Payroll Expense	10/07	60001	0-11181-128CR	1,936.22		TTS584	10/07
1400	Payroll Expense	10/21	60001	0-11181-128CR	1,999.78		TTS588	10/21
1400	Total Orderly Salary				3,936.00			
1500	Payroll Expense	10/07	60001	0-11181-128CR	751.56		TTS584	10/07
1500	Payroll Expense	10/21	60001	0-11181-128CR	766.44		TTS588	10/21
1500	Total Student Salary				1,518.00			
	Susp Corr/Accr Sal	9/30	R3490	0-12000-140CR	35.00		JJV002	10/10
	Susp Corr/Accr Sal	9/30	R3490	0-12000-140CR	55.00		JJV002	10/10
	RVS Acc Sal & Wage	10/01	06510	0-14300-110DP	21,462.00–		JJV001	10/10
	RVS Acc Sal & Wage	10/01	06510	0-14300-110DP	35.00–		JJV001	10/10
	RVS Acc Sal & Wage	10/01	06510	0-14300-110DP	65.00–		JJV001	10/10
	Accrued Sal & Wgs	10/31	06500	0-14300-128CR	32,924.00		JJV019	10/31
1600	Total Accrued Salaries				11,462.00			

(continued)

EXHIBIT 11-13 *(continued)*

SUBCODE	DESCRIPTION	DATE	REF.	J.E. OFFSET ACCOUNT	CURRENT REV/EXP	ENCUMBRANCES	BATCH REF.	BATCH DATE
2200	Payroll Expense	10/07	60001	2-66000-170CR	65.81		TTS588	10/07
2200	Payroll Expense	10/21	60001	2-66000-170CR	5,821.12		TTS588	10/21
2200	Total Health Ins.			5,886.93				
2300	Payroll Expense	10/07	60001	2-66000-170CR	2,659.96		TTS588	10/07
2300	Payroll Expense	10/21	60001	2-66000-170CR	2,930.66		TTS588	10/21
2300	Total Retirement				5,590.62			
2400	Payroll Expense	10/21	60001	2-66000-170CR	526.48		TTS588	10/21
2400	Total Disability				526.48			
2500	Payroll Expense	10/21	60001	2-66000-170CR	264.04		TTS588	10/21
2500	Total Life Insurance				264.04			
3100	Inventory Exp Alloc	10/31	06526	0-14100-130CR	22,000.00		JJV027	10/31
3100	Total Med/Surg Supplies				22,000.00			
3110	Pharmacy Distrib–Oct	10/31	07500	4-50730-214CR	1,100.00		JJV033	10/31
3110	Total Drugs				1,100.00			
3114	Inventory Exp Alloc	10/31	07524	0-121000-120CR	10,000.00		JJV027	10/31
3114	Total Solutions				10,000.00			
4010	Inventory Exp Alloc	10/31	07526	0-12100-T40CR	220.00		JJVO27	10/31
4010	Total Office Supplies				220.00			
4120	Inventory Exp Alloc	10/31	07508	4-69669-965CR	400.00		JJVO26	10/31
4120	Total Forms				400.00			
4134	Xerox Expense	10/31	07501	4-60960-960CR	30.00		JJVO28	10/31
4134	Total Copying				30.00			
4260	Inventory Exp Alloc	10/31	07506	0-12100-144CR	50.00		JJVO27	10/31
4260	Total Food Expense				50.00			
4440	Inventory Exp Alloc	10/31	07564	0-12100-140CR	350.00		JJV028	10/31
4440	Total Housekeeping Sup.				350.00			
	Account total				143,899.00	400.00		

EXHIBIT 11-14
Accounting System Report

Fiscal Year Ending 200x
January–October (83% of fiscal year elapsed)
Distribution Code = 600
Medical–Surgical Unit—Revenue

Acct: 2-40815
Dept: 7010

			ACTUAL				
CODE	**DESCRIPTION**	**APPROVED BUDGET**	**CURRENT MONTH**	**FISCAL YEAR**	**OPEN ENCUMBRANCES**	**REMAINING BUDGET**	**PERCENT USED**
030							
0/0	Inpatient Revenue	2,345,200–	225,800–	1,782,352–		562,848–	76
	Total Revenues	2,345,200–	225,800–	1,782,352–		562,848–	76
	Account Total	2,345,200–	225,800–	1,782,352–		562,848–	76

EXHIBIT 11-15
Accounting System Report

Fiscal Year Ending 200x
January–October (83% of fiscal year elapsed)
Distribution Code = 600
Medical–Surgical Unit—SP & D—Revenue

Acct: 2-40818
Dept: 7010

			ACTUAL				
SUBCODE	**DESCRIPTION**	**APPROVED BUDGET**	**CURRENT MONTH**	**FISCAL YEAR**	**OPEN ENCUMBRANCES**	**REMAINING BUDGET**	**PERCENT USED**
030	Inpatient Revenue	1,895,000–	201,647–	1,440,200–		454,800–	76
	Total Revenues	1,895,000–	201,647–	1,440,220–		454,800–	76
	Account Total	1,895,000–	201,647–	1,440,220–		454,800	76

Cutting the Budget

When the budget must be cut, planning is a vital aspect of the process. Budget cuts happen as hospital admissions and stays decrease and reimbursement changes. The form and the process of nursing management can determine the course of events when the budget has to be cut.

A nursing administration that delegates decision making to the lowest level and encourages participative management is an effective administration. When clinical nurses are informed at the unit level and invited to give their input, they can help with suggestions for cutting costs. They will gladly implement and support the activities they recognize as resulting partly from their input. A nursing organization that promotes self-direction at the levels of clinical nurse, nurse manager, clinical consultant, and executive nurse will support direction to reduce costs and to increase productivity and profits. For example, when a hospital CEO discovered that self-pay patient care was the only category not reviewed for use of resources, a clinical nurse established a review process. Physicians and other health care professionals supported this process.

Nursing budgets are enormous, and budgets for a single unit can run into hundreds of thousands of dollars per year. Pay awards or increases must be met by budget cuts (personnel cutbacks), use of less expensive supplies and techniques, or increased productivity. The latter requires more paying patients, shorter stays, and increased sales of all paying services. When personnel cuts are to be made, nursing is vulnerable. Some cuts can come from all services, but nursing has greater numbers. The nurse manager who controls these numbers daily, weekly, and yearly has greater credibility. Many sources indicate that turnover is costly. The cost of turnover of personnel low on the salary scale is sometimes weighed against the higher cost of employees who are at the top of the salary scale. An assumption is made that long-time employees are better satisfied with their jobs and do better work. This assumption needs to be validated through research.

As workload data indicate shifts from one unit to another, resources also must be shifted. Asking for volunteers, moving vacated positions, and using PRN pools can do this. Inpatient procedures in hospitals have shifted to outpatient procedures either in hospitals or at ambulatory surgery centers. New reimbursement rates, which are part of a system of ambulatory patient classifications, have been issued by CMS and will affect revenues from ambulatory services. Many more diagnostic procedures are now being done on an outpatient basis; as a result, inpatients are often a sicker group, requiring more nursing care.

Because nurse administrators control multi-million-dollar budgets, they are powerful people. They are also vulnerable to personnel cuts. Much of this vulnerability stems from external controls imposed by state and federal governments and health insurance companies. Power comes from the ability of nurse administrators to use knowledge and skills in defending, directing, and controlling their budgets. They learn to hold the line on staffing and overtime and monitor for the appropriate use of supplies and equipment.

Legitimate Budget Activities

Health care organizations should be managed like other businesses. Charges should be determined from costs and should include allowance for profits or return on equity and for bad debts. The practice of cost shifting to make certain services revenue producers should be stopped.

Oszustowicz suggests the following seven-step system by which total financial requirements eventually determine the gross patient revenue equal to meet the financial needs of a department:[32]

1. Detail demand for nursing services and equipment needs.
2. Detail direct expenses.
3. Detail indirect expenses.
4. Detail working capital requirements.
5. Detail capital requirements.
6. Detail earnings (profit) requirements.
7. Detail deductions from patient revenues.

Reimbursement

Introduction

With the continued escalation of health care costs, the health care system has evolved to emphasize managed care. Basically, there are four major sources of revenue for health care providers: charges, retrospective reimbursement, prospective reimbursement/DRGs, and managed care.[33] The following sections will concentrate on managed care.

The US Health Care System

The US health care system has many components: patients, insurers, and employers; providers such as hospitals, ambulatory care services, home health services, long-term care facilities, physicians, nurses, allied health personnel, pharmacists and pharmacies, and providers of durable medical equipment; and federal, state, and local public health services. As costs have increased, physicians who have been reimbursed based on fees for services are increasingly being reimbursed by capitation through contracts with managed care insurers, or they have themselves become employees of the managed care insurers. Employees have switched from indemnity insurance plans to managed care plans. Exhibit 11-16 outlines the sequential development of health care insurance in the United States.

EXHIBIT 11-16
Historical Development of Health Care Insurance

1929 Blue Cross
1935 Social Security Act
1946 Hospital Survey and Construction Act (Hill–Burton)
1964 Hill–Harris Hospital and Medical Facilities Amendments
1965 Public Law 89-97, Medicare and Medicaid
1982 Public Law 97-248, Tax Equity and Fiscal Responsibility Act (TEFRA)
1983 Public Law, 98-21, Social Security Amendments Prospective Payment System
1985 Consolidated Omnibus Budget Reconciliation Act (COBRA)
1986 Gramm–Rudman Deficit Reduction Amendment and Omnibus Budget Reconciliation Act
1987,
1988 Omnibus Budget Reconciliation Act (OBRA)
1989 Physician Payment Review Commission
1994 Medicare Choice Act
1996 Health Insurance and Accountability Act
1997 Balanced Budget Act

Indemnity insurance plans cover bills from most providers and pay most health care bills by charges or costs, with some deductibles or copayments. Indemnity plans are fast disappearing as employers and governments switch to managed care plans. As health care costs have soared, employers have increased employees' share of indemnity insurance premiums. Indemnity insurance plans do not keep costs down. Indemnity insurers are changing to become organizers and administrators of managed care networks and subsequently deliverers of health care. This transformation is reducing the number of insurers.[34]

In the new managed care environment, many providers are integrated into insurance plan services through individual contracts and subcontracts. Clients accept the providers of these contract services, thus limiting their choices regarding most health care provider services. Clients receive a total package of health care dictated by the contracts between employers and insurers.

Managed Care

Managed care is a patient care system that includes insurance companies, employers, providers, and clients. Most enrollees of managed care plans are employees of businesses that contract for health insurance as a benefit. Many plans accept individual enrollees, particularly plans that enroll Medicare beneficiaries. Managed care is also the process by which health care benefits are monitored for purposes of cost management, resulting in limitation of benefit coverage and access to health care benefits. Managed care organizations manage the distribution of health care dollars, use of services, and access to benefits.

Organizations and Alternative Delivery Systems

Patients now accept health care plans that limit their freedom of choice. The following sections discuss some of these plans.

Health Maintenance Organizations

Financing of health maintenance organizations (HMOs) is done by capitation, in which there is a predetermined payment per patient or per service. Managed care is designed to cut costs.

The HMO is defined as

> a prepaid health plan delivering comprehensive care to members through designated providers, having a fixed periodic payment for health care services, and requiring members to be in a plan for a specified period of time (usually 1 year). A group HMO delivers health services through a physician group that is controlled by the HMO unit or contracts with one or more independent group practices to provide health services. An individual practice association (IPA) HMO contracts directly with physicians in independent practice, and/or contracts with one or more associations of physicians in independent practice, and/or contracts with one or more multispecialty group practices. Data are based on a consensus of HMOs.[35]

HMOs have the following characteristics:

- Utilization risks are shifted from payer to provider.
- Competition draws consumers to less costly services when they have a choice of plans.
- Use of preventive care and ambulatory facilities decreases hospital admission rates, lowering insurance costs by 10% to 40%.
- Use of primary care physicians and nurse practitioners at fixed salaries decreases the use of expensive surgeons and specialists.
- HMOs eliminate unneeded facilities such as hospitals, operating rooms, and radiation therapy units.
- Paperwork and overhead are reduced.
- HMOs provide organized, cooperative care for individuals and families.
- Enrollees make appointments with gatekeeper physicians or nurses, mostly family practice physicians, internists, and pediatricians.
- Gatekeepers control all referrals to specialists.
- Enrollees pay a small fee per visit and for medications.
- Gatekeepers control unneeded procedures, both diagnostic and therapeutic.

- HMO plans contract for discounted prices with various providers, such as hospitals, laboratories, radiologists, physician specialists and pharmacists.
- HMO plans emphasize complete patient care, management of chronic illnesses, education, disease prevention, and wellness. Oxford Health Plans hired 20 nurse practitioners because they are trained to provide services for disease prevention and health promotion. These registered nurse practitioners perform more preventive care and are reimbursed at the same rate as physicians.
- HMOs make physicians business-oriented practitioners.
- HMO plans do mass customization to give each of a mass of customers what the customer desires.
- HMOs offer capitated payments, one price per enrollee.
- HMOs reduce the risks of unneeded procedures, such as caesarean sections and hysterectomies.
- Half of HMO physicians are paid flat fees that are incentives to reduce care.

Although HMOs are the most common type of managed care organization, many more millions of people belong to other types, which are discussed in the following sections.

Preferred Provider Organizations

In a PPO, a group of providers acts as health care brokers providing services to a group of patients at reduced fees. PPOs have the following characteristics:

- PPOs contract with consumers through employers and insurers and with providers, including physicians, hospitals, and allied services.
- PPO services are discounted, and patients have no out-of-pocket expenses.
- In PPOs, patients are limited to using the listed providers or paying larger fees for out-of-network providers.
- PPOs are intermediaries between payer and subscriber groups, furnishing marketing and administrative services.
- PPOs set their own size, number of staff specialists, geographic availability, time limits for claims and payments, and other features.
- PPOs place hospitals but not physicians at risk. Physicians are paid discounted rates for a steady flow of patients.

Arguments that the traditional physician–patient relationship will be destroyed are inconsequential because these relationships will soon disappear. Working people want efficiency; they do not want to sit in a physician's office waiting for hours past their appointed time. Given adequate information, they will make choices about their care, and they should. The old concept of withholding information is outmoded and dangerous and in some cases illegal (i.e., informed consent). The objective of all competitive health care plans is to provide quality care less expensively. There are approximately 1036 PPOs in the United States and more than 50.2 million enrollees.[36]

Health Care Cost Coalitions

Health care cost coalitions (HCCCs) are organizations of employers, and sometimes unions, that effectively bargain for better rates and parity with Medicare, Medicaid, and other insurers. They work to develop PPOs and utilization review programs.

Prudent Buyer Systems

Prudent buyer systems are characterized by joint purchasing arrangements, purchasing consortia composed of multiple providers, and competitive bidding for exclusive contracts.

Health Promotion and Wellness Programs

Increased education and awareness enable these programs to emphasize illness prevention.

Hospital Physician Organizations

The hospital physician organization (HPO) is a relatively new entity. Its objective is to combine and reduce overhead, which can be done by sharing services such as billing.

Provider-Sponsored Organizations (PSOs)

Provider-sponsored organizations (PSOs) are networks of physicians and hospitals that are their owners. Approximately 84 PSOs exist in the United States. Supporters of PSOs say they are health providers engaged in treating patients, whereas HMOs are insurance companies that invest in stocks, bonds, and other liquid assets. PSOs offer less risk to providers than do HMOs because providers receive only part of their income from the PSO.[37]

Enrollment

More than 78.8 million people were enrolled in 647 HMOs in 1998, which means that one out of every four Americans was enrolled in an HMO. The 647 HMOs are divided in one of the following managed care plans: 322 (50%) enrolled in IPAs, 21 (32%) in mixed-model plans, and the remaining 115 (17%) enrolled in either a network model, group, or staff model.[38] HMO enrollments are shown in Exhibit 11-17.

Advantages

Managed care has reined in skyrocketing medical costs. Medical care inflation, the lowest since 1973, has increased since 1997 to pay for rollbacks and decreasing profits.

EXHIBIT 11-17
HMO Enrollments for 1980 to1998

YEAR	NUMBER OF PLANS	ENROLLMENTS (IN THOUSANDS)
1980	236	9,100
1985	393	18,894
1989	590	32,493
1990	556	33,622
1991	559	35,052
1992	559	27,199
1993	540	39,783
1994	547	43,443
1995	550	46,182
1998	651	64,800

Managed care has a number of advantages, including the following:

- Managed care puts patients first by making clinical decisions before economic ones.
- Managed care limits patients' time to get appointments.
- Managed care offers fast-track treatment for life-threatening conditions.
- The US Department of Health and Human Services is responsible for ensuring due process for Medicare HMO enrollees. It can require a written notice describing the reason for denial of a service, provide clear information on how to appeal an HMO decision, and require expedited consideration in time-sensitive medical situations.
- Managed care holds the interests of third parties at bay.
- Medicare rules limit financial penalties against physicians in managed care plans for referrals or expensive procedures.
- By law, new mothers in managed care plans cannot be forced out of hospitals in less than 48 hours.
- Laws can limit gag rules.
- Most HMO enrollees receive the care they need. Sixty percent are highly satisfied (this number ranged from 45% to 77% depending on the HMO). Of enrollees, 10% would not recommend HMOs.[39]
- Profit motives may be checked.
- Managed care plans receive better quality report cards than indemnity insurance plans.

If improvements are made, managed care will lead to better-informed consumers. Treatment guidelines for managed care plans will be developed that people can trust. Conservative treatment may cost less and have better outcomes. For example, $1000 worth of physical therapy may be better for a herniated disk than would a $15,000 operation. In a study of Californians under 65 years of age who had appendicitis, 25.8% of HMO members had ruptured appendices versus 29.3% of patients in fee-for-service plans. Patients in managed care plans have a place to voice complaints. Of female HMO members at Scripps Clinic (La Jolla, California), 95% receive mammograms, whereas the national average is about 75%. Mammograms can detect breast cancer and result in earlier treatment.[40]

Problems

The following are among the problems associated with managed care:

- Gag clauses in contracts between the plan and physician forbid disclosures that advise patients on medically necessary but expensive treatment options. Gag clauses limit care, undermine trust, and are negative to clinical independence. Presidential orders prohibit gag rules for Medicare patients (5.7 million or 8.8% of beneficiaries) and the 7.8 million recipients of Medicaid. The managed care industry has promised not to restrict patient–doctor communications.
- Managed care limits choices by denial of referral to specialists.
- Managed care promotes less research.
- Managed care plans have conflicting formularies and incompatible information systems.
- Physicians must pursue approvals and correct inappropriate denials.
- Physicians are rewarded for providing less care.
- Money goes to corporate salaries and profits (20% of total expenses).
- High-risk patients are screened out. Services to sick and disabled persons are limited. Patients are dumped into public facilities. The poor, the sick, and the elderly have limited access, low satisfaction, and poor outcomes.
- Because more people are now in the managed care system, they have a harder time accessing needed care and therefore visit doctors more frequently because they become sicker.
- Members with rare medical conditions sometimes encounter problems in obtaining appropriate treatment. This problem can be solved with a point-of-service option that permits clients to go to any physician by paying an additional fee.
- Plans have a tendency to look only at statistical averages and fail to understand the individuality of patients. As a result, plans fail to recognize that complex medical problems cannot always be standardized into predetermined treatment paths.

Contracts

Under managed care, contracts are a way of life for insurers, employers, health care providers, and consumers.

Consumers usually obtain their contracts through employers and should carefully study the provisions of their contract coverage. Insurers have contracts with both employers and health care providers. To avoid legal pitfalls and maximize profits, health care providers must have a thorough knowledge of the terms of their contracts with insurers. Contract terms include coverage limits, criteria for authorization of services, identification of all the provider parties to the contract, automatic renewal, criteria for termination of contracts, credentialing processes, criteria for accepting or rejecting patients, liability insurance requirements, grievance procedures, provision for contract changes, utilization review requirements, provision for timely payment of claims, provision for continuity of care and payment when contracts are terminated, avoidance of unnecessary record keeping, and provision for assignments when insurers are bought and sold. Providers of health care need to know all state laws regulating managed care insurers.[41]

Nurses frequently provide services, and particularly home care services, under managed care contracts. Other nurses are case managers for insurers and employers. Nurses involved in negotiating managed care contracts need access to good cost data, including fixed and variable costs. Other needed data include the benefits package, and patient and physician demographics, including practice patterns. Legal counsel is a necessity in contract negotiations under managed care. All nurse managers need knowledge of managed care contracts affecting their patients.

In an HMO, the client may have the option of choosing a primary care provider who is a nurse. This nurse may receive a monthly fee (capitation) to provide appropriate primary care services, including prior approval for specialty care, hospitalization, surgery, and simple emergencies. The nurse provider has a contract negotiated with the HMO. When nurse providers reduce the costs of health care, they benefit from bonuses paid by the HMO for reducing costs, provided the nurse providers have such clauses in their contracts. Nurse providers may consider negotiating contracts that provide an exclusive relationship with the HMO whereby they contract only with that HMO. Other contract negotiations include sign-on bonuses and additive fee-for-service payments for particular services such as transportation, intensive outreach, and health education.[42] See Exhibit 11-18 for a managed care contract checklist.

EXHIBIT 11-18

Questions to Ask When Choosing a Managed Care Plan

1. Are your physicians on salary or capitiation?
2. Do your physicians get bonuses for keeping costs down?
3. How does your plan address the need for basic medical research?
4. How does your plan address the need for education of health professionals?
5. How does your plan measure quality?
6. What have been the results of measuring quality?
7. How does your plan credential physicians? Are all specialists board certified?
8. What other health professionals does your plan credential?
9. What is the average time for a person to get an appointment with a physician?
10. What is covered by the plan? Prescription drugs? Preventive care? Hearing and eye care? Dental care? Podiatry? Mental health care? Chiropractic care? Medical supplies and equipment? Home health care? Nursing home care? Rehabilitation?
11. What is not covered by the plan? What are the specific exclusions?
12. What copayments are required by the plan? Deductions? Specify.
13. What are the costs of the plan? How much is my employer paying?
14. Is there a point-of-service option allowing care by certain providers outside the plan? How does it work?
15. Are there maximum amounts the plan will pay for particular services?
16. Who are the physicians in the plan? Is there access to specific specialists and hospitals, or is such access restricted?
17. Are physicians' offices conveniently located?
18. Do the hospitals affiliated with the plan meet my needs?
19. Do enrollees like the plan? Check with consumer groups, the media, and other employees.
20. How many members disenrolled during the past 3 years? Why?
21. How many primary care physicians left the plan during the past 3 years? Why?
22. How does the plan handle emergency or urgent care?
23. How does the plan handle emergency or urgent care outside the service area?
24. Is the plan accredited? (http://www.ncqa.org.)
25. How does the plan handle complaints?

Economic Implications

Managed care, whether by for-profit or not-for-profit organizations, has a number of economic implications. Profits of mental health managed care plans are enormous. Administrative and profit-loading costs are seldom below 40%.[43] Unnecessary mastectomies, heart bypass procedures, and prostate surgeries are reduced under managed care plans. Health care premiums rose only 2% in 1995. Some companies encourage workers to choose the best HMOs by discounting monthly premiums.[44] Overuse of medical services and administrative inefficiencies result in $200 million in unnecessary costs each year.[45]

Whether the organization is designated as not for profit or for profit, profit is the ultimate goal of managed care. The not-for-profit organization needs to make a profit to stay in business. By law, any profits must be reinvested in the business or used to reduce premiums. For-profit organizations want to make profits for their shareholders. Business is about providing employment, providing value for customers, developing skills of employees, developing capabilities of suppliers, and earning money for shareholders.

Having reached maximum savings through managed care, health care costs are expected to rise. This increase will be partly a result of higher costs for technology and drugs, which have risen three times faster than the costs of other components of health care. Also, legislators and employers tell the insurers they must cover a certain minimum level of service and a minimum number of persons who have preexisting or serious conditions. Physicians are demanding higher compensation.[46]

Ethical Implications

Successful managed care organizations will recognize all players as stakeholders in a community. These organizations will conduct business in an ethical manner. They will make long-term commitments to employees, customers, suppliers, and other stakeholders. Doing so will give these organizations a competitive advantage.

Whether the results of myth or fear, the following are some of the ethical questions raised by managed care:

- Will the poor, the elderly, and the uninsured continue to be forced to accept fewer costly procedures and face early death?
- Will patients' rights force physicians to inform patients of the right to physician-assisted suicide?
- Should people, including those in need, receive uncompensated care?

Implications for Consumers

Most consumers are not in managed care plans voluntarily but because of choices made by their employers. Consumers need to be informed and vigilant so they can use the services effectively and efficiently. Many physicians belong to several plans, and several plans have many physicians from whom to choose. Thus, physician choice for consumers can be broad.

Practice Implications

Nurse–midwife numbers are increasing. Physicians and hospitals are hiring nurse practitioners. Because nurse practitioners are less expensive than are physicians, and because they score high in patient satisfaction, managed care organizations are interested in hiring them. Nurse practitioners provide quality time and personal attention and apply their expert skills to patient care.

HMOs also determine practitioners' credentials and set practice guidelines that result in less qualified providers and less stringent rules.

Research Implications

Research is unprofitable in the managed care environment. Because research expands the frontiers of medical knowledge, less funding for research has serious implications for health care.

Quality Implications

A system for rating HMO quality allows consumers to differentiate between an HMO that may be great at answering the phone from one that does an excellent job of detecting breast cancer.[47]

Criteria for rating HMOs may include the following:

- Meets industry standards of accreditation by the National Committee for Quality Assurance (NCQA). The Health Plan Employer Data and Information Set (HEDIS) measures aspects of plans such as physicians' credentials, affiliation with the Joint Commission on Accreditation of Healthcare Organizations accredited hospitals, and board certification.
- Measures satisfaction of physicians and members.
- Tracks members' health, measuring and addressing risk-taking behavior.
- Uses hard-nosed outcome measures, including morbidity and mortality.
- Develops prevention and screening tools to keep people healthy through early detection.
- Encourages perinatal care during first trimester of pregnancy, resulting in low caesarean section rates and high rates of normal delivery.
- Allows employers to perform independent surveys of contract plans using outcome measures.[48]

The three major contenders in the movement for health care quality are:[49]

1. The National Committee for Quality Assurance, which judges 50 different characteristics.
2. John Ward's Medical Outcomes Survey. The survey evaluates the general health of persons. It may be effective over time.
3. The Foundation for Accountability (FACCT). FACCT develops standards for judging how well HMOs handle specific illnesses.

It is difficult for persons to agree on and thus to standardize quality measurements. Insurers and providers often select treatment based on the least expensive outcome rather than on morbidity and mortality rates. If they are to access quality care, consumers need knowledge of ways in which providers deliver care without increasing costs; of how consumers can be assertive about obtaining needed services; about data linked to expected care and treatment outcomes; about best practices that are benchmarks, including critical paths for specific diagnoses and procedures; and about data on morbidity and mortality related to all health care providers.[50]

Health maintenance organizations with thick rosters of physicians may be laggards in providing quality care. These contracted physicians practice medicine the way in which the HMO dictates. The best HMOs may have fewer physicians and a central office. Aetna has large numbers of physicians and offers financial incentives to keep costs down. In 1996, the average physician worked for 13 HMOs, with 13 sets of criteria. Physicians who are on salary use treatments that work best and thus maintain quality. This fact can be proven; for example, Kaiser Permanente HMO scores higher on quality measures than does Aetna.[51]

Hospitals are beginning to use a program developed by General Motors for measuring quality, called Purchased Input Concept Optimization with Suppliers (PICOS). PICOS purports to eliminate waste, streamline operations, and improve customer satisfaction. A hospital using PICOS guides a small team of 8 to 10 key employees to examine a process, identify waste, and redesign the process to reduce or eliminate the waste. Health care providers look at waiting times, billing procedures, and duplication of work.[52]

Patients may be satisfied with physicians and access to them, although physicians may not know the latest treatment for a patient's condition. It is easy to find satisfied customers who are healthy.

Self-surveys may inflate customer satisfaction. Independent surveys are best, although the results may comply with the wishes of those who pay for them.

Among good independent surveyors are the Sachs Group, Evanston, Illinois; Care Data; Center for the Study of Services Annual Guide, which rates 400 HMOs; and the NCQA HEDIS 3.0 Report.

Management Implications

As managed care plans and enrollments increase, managers of all health care provider organizations face the need to maintain financial stability. To do this, they become experts in negotiating contracts, planning new ventures, and reorganizing their organizations to make maximum use of human resources. Successful managers provide leadership that empowers employees to provide maximum quality outcomes for their patients. As managers pursue these functions, they oversee evaluation techniques that are simple to administer and lead to quality improvement.

Summary

It is important for nurses to have a working knowledge of the objectives of budgeting and of component costs. Every activity that takes place in a health care agency costs money. A standard must exist for assigning costs to user departments. The nursing department should pay its user share, and no more. Knowledge of the cost-accounting system will provide accurate information for budgeting and for cost management.

Efficient nurse managers use a budget calendar that covers formulation, review and enactment, and execution stages of the total budget process.

The major elements of nursing budgets are personnel, supplies and equipment (minor), and capital equipment. Generally, equipment that costs less than a fixed dollar amount is included in the supplies and equipment budget. A product evaluation committee is useful for ensuring that supplies and equipment will promote effective and efficient patient care. The capital equipment budget includes equipment that costs more than a fixed dollar amount; it is prepared separately from the supplies and equipment budget.

Evaluation is an administrative aspect of budgeting that in itself serves as a controlling process. Decentralization vests control at the lowest competent level of decision making. Good budget feedback is essential if the budget is to be an effective controlling process. Good feedback includes information about revenues and expenses as well as internal comparisons of projected and actual budgets. The budget can motivate professional nurses to facilitate their development of innovations.

The belief that budgets are beyond comprehension can sabotage a nurse's effectiveness. Spiraling health care costs, cost-management efforts, and increasing accountability from individual cost centers should serve as an impetus for nurses to learn at least the fundamentals of budgets and the budgeting process. Assuming the responsibility for budget work increases the nurse's potential realm of planning, predicting, and reviewing programs within the nurse's jurisdiction.

Like a nursing care plan, the budget is an activity guidance tool. It is a plan expressed in monetary terms and carried out within a time frame. To be an effective caregiver, the nurse must know how to develop and use a nursing care plan. Similarly, to be most effective as a manager, the nurse manager must know how to develop and use a budget.

One main competency the nurse manager must possess is understanding information and managed care. Managed care is replacing fee-for-service and indemnity insurance plans. The objectives of this transformation are reduced costs and increased profits. Although problems still exist with managed care, they are gradually being solved—some with federal and state legislation.

APPLICATION EXERCISES

EXERCISE 11-1 Develop a performance budget for a cost center to be used as a model for a health care organization.

EXERCISE 11-2 Every hospital prepares the Hospital and Hospital Health Care Complex Cost Report Certification and Settlement Summary, commonly known as the Medicare Cost Report. Obtain the latest one for your employing or clinical experience hospital. Select a nursing cost center and complete Exhibit 11-19, Preparing a Budget for a Unit or Project.

This exercise has acquainted you with the Medicare Cost Report. You can use projected medical inflation rates to prepare a budget for the following year. For instance, if the inflation rates are projected to be 8%, multiply all costs by 1.08 to project and budget costs. Note that intensive care units are budgeted separately. All other inpatient units are grouped as Adults and Pediatrics (General and Routine Care). To separate these units for revenue and expenditures, make the following calculations:

1. Select a patient care unit of a hospital: ______________________
2. Determine the number of patient days of occupancy for this unit (from the biometric records): ______________________
3. From the Medicare Cost Report determine:
   - 3.1. Total direct and indirect costs: $__________
   - 3.2. Total patient days: __________
   - 3.3. Divide the total direct and indirect costs $__________ by total patient days __________ = $__________ cost per patient day.
   - 3.4. Patient days for unit (from 3.2) __________ × cost per patient day (from 3.3) __________ = $__________, or approximate expenses for the nursing unit for this year.

For help, refer to Swansburg, R.C. & Sowell, R. L. (1992). A model for costing and pricing nursing service. *Nursing Management*, 33–36; Swansburg, R. C. (1997). *Budgeting and financial management for nurse managers*. Sudbury, MA: Jones and Bartlett.

EXHIBIT 11-19

Preparing a Budget for a Unit or Project

Unit _______ Revenue Center Number _______

Direct Expenses (Directly Assigned)	
Salaries (attach position questionnaire for new ones)	$______.___
Employee benefits	$______.___
Personnel services	$______.___
Supplies	$______.___
Other	$______.___
Total Direct	$______.___
Indirect Expenses	
Depreciation of capital buildings and fixtures	$______.___
Capital equipment (movable)	$______.___
(attach requests for new items)	$______.___
Worker's compensation	$______.___
Life insurance	$______.___
Communications	$______.___
Data processing	$______.___
Purchasing	$______.___
Admitting	$______.___
Patient accounts	$______.___
General administration	$______.___
Plant operations	$______.___
Biomedical	$______.___
Laundry	$______.___
Housekeeping	$______.___
Nursing administration	$______.___
Patient transport	$______.___
Preparation	$______.___
Central supply	$______.___
Pharmacy	$______.___
College of nursing (or other college)	$______.___
Interns and residents	$______.___
Other	$______.___
Total Indirect	$______.___
Total Costs (Direct + Indirect)	$______.___
Total Charges or Revenues	$______.___
Cost-to-Charge Ratio (Divide total costs by total charges or revenues.)	$______.___
divided by	$______.___
minus	$______.___
or	______%

EXERCISE 11-3 Choose several managed care products. Identify the costs to the patient enrolled in a managed care plan and compare them with the costs to a patient for the same products in an indemnity health insurance plan.

EXERCISE 11-4 Attend a marketing session given by a managed care company. Analyze the presentation. What are the advantages and disadvantages for the patient?

EXERCISE 11-5 From information in this chapter, prepare a short questionnaire (10 to 15 questions) pertaining to the services provided for managed care enrollees. Identify and interview two persons: one who is a managed care plan enrollee and one who is an indemnity insurance plan enrollee. Compare the problems and advantages of the two plans.

EXERCISE 11-6 John Kay, director designate of Oxford University's new School of Management Studies, asks the question: "What is a company's purpose if it is not to maximize shareholder value?"[53] With a group of your peers, discuss how the values evident in a world of managed care can be integrated to meet the goals of this statement with the goals of quality health care for clients.

EXERCISE 11-7 Locate and read five recent articles on managed care published in nursing journals. Summarize the implications for the nursing profession.

NOTES

1. Johnson, R. W. & Melicher, R. W. (1982). *Financial planning*. Boston: Allyn & Bacon.
2. Baker, J. D. (1991). The operating expense budget, one part of a manager's arsenal. *AORN Journal*, *54*(4), 837–841; Klann, S. (1989). Mastering the OR budgeting process is key to success. *OR Manager*, 10–11.
3. Althaus, J. N., Hardyck, N. M., Pierce, P. B., & Rodgers, M. S. (1981). *Nursing decentralization: The El Camino experience*. Gaithersburg, MD: Aspen.
4. Whitman, G. R. (1991). Analyzing and forecasting budgets. In C. Birdsall (Ed.), *Management issues in critical care* (pp. 287–307). St. Louis: Mosby.
5. Ibid.
6. Anthony, R. N. & Young, D. W. (1988). *Management control in nonprofit organizations* (4th ed.). Chicago: Irwin.
7. Klann, 1989.
8. Huttman, B. (1964). Taking charge: Selling your budget. *RN*, *1*, 25–26.
9. Covert, R. P. (1982). Expense budgeting. In W. O. Cleverly (Ed.), *Handbook of health care accounting and finance* (pp. 261–278). Rockville, MD: Aspen.
10. Talbot, G. J. (1983). Key for successful program budgeting. *The Journal of Continuing Education in Nursing, 14*(3), 8–10.
11. Drucker, P. F. (1999). *Management challenges for the 21st century*. New York: HarperCollins, 111–129.
12. Herkimer, A. G., Jr. (1978). *Understanding hospital financial management*. Rockville, MD: Aspen, 132.
13. Hoffman, F. M. (1984). *Financial management for nurse managers*. East Norwalk, CT: Appleton-Century-Crofts, 9.
14. Talbot, 1983.
15. Rowland, H. S. & Rowland, B. L. (1992). *Nursing administration handbook* (3rd ed.) Gaithersburg, MD: Aspen, 174.
16. Ibid., 175.
17. Ibid., 174.
18. Buchan, J. (1992). Cost-Effective caring. *International Nursing Review, 39*(4), 117–120.
19. Campbell, R. K. (1989). Understanding the management process and financial and managerial accounting, part IV: Cash flow analysis and budgeting. *Diabetes Education*, 126–127, 129.
20. Osborne, D. & Gaebler, T. (1992). *Reinventing government*. New York: Plume, 119–124.
21. Piper, L. R. (1982). Basic budgeting for ED nursing personnel. *Journal of Emergency Nursing*, 285–287.
22. Ibid.
23. Tzividies, E., Waterstraat, V., & Chamberlin, W. (1991). Managing the budget with a fluctuating census. *Nursing Management*, 80B, 80F, 80H.

24. Planning your replacement budget. (1990). *Journal of Nursing Administration*, 3, 17, 24.
25. Dickerson, M. (1988). Product evaluation: A strategy for controlling a supply and equipment budget. In H. C. Scherubel (Ed.), *Patients and purse strings* (pp. 2, 465–468). New York: National League for Nursing.
26. Kleinmuntz, C. E. & Kleinmuntz, D. N. (1999). A strategic approach to allocating capital in healthcare organizations. *Healthcare Financial Management*, 52–58.
27. Arges, G. S. (1998). *Estimated useful lives of depreciable hospital assets*. Chicago, IL: American Hospital Publishing.
28. Aronsohn, B. & Deal, N. (1992). Navigating the maze of capital equipment acquisition. *Nursing Management*, 46–48.
29. Finkler, S. A. (1991). Performance budgeting. *Nursing Economics*, 404–408.
30. Ibid.
31. Palmer, P. N. (1984). Why hide the revenue produced by perioperative nursing care? *AORN Journal*, 1122–1123.
32. McGrail, G. R. (1988). Budgets: An underused resource. *Journal of Nursing Administration*, 25–31.
33. Oszustowicz, R. J. (1979). *Financial management of department of nursing services*. New York: National League for Nursing, 1–10.
34. Westmoreland, D. (1995). Managing costs and budgets. In P. Yoder-Wise, *Leading and managing in nursing*. St. Louis, MO: Mosby, 256.
35. Loomis, C. J. (1994, July 11). The real action in health care. *Fortune*, 149–153, 155–157.
36. US Census Bureau. (1999). *Statistical abstract of the United States 1999* (118th ed.). Washington, DC: Author, 149.
37. http://www.thirteen.org/archieve/mch.
38. Gonzales, P. Health care battle pits doctors against insurance firms. (1997, March 30). *San Antonio Express-News*, p. 13A.
39. InterStudy. (1999). *The competitive edge, 9:1: HMO Industry Report*.
40. Study says health care costs, access troubling to many. (1996, October 23). *San Antonio Express-News*, p. 6A.
41. Faltermayer, E. (1994, October 31). Will the cost cutting in health care kill you? *Fortune*, *24*, 221–222, 226, 228, 230, 232.
42. Hogue, E. E. (1994). Contracting with managed care providers. *Journal of Home Health Care Practice, 6*(2), 17–23.
43. Jenkins, M. & Torrisi, D. L. (1995). Nurse practitioners, community nurse centers, and contracting for managed care. *Journal of the American Academy of Nurse Practitioners*, 119–123.
44. Olian, C. (1997). HMO: Managed or mangled? *Public Citizen Health Research Group Health Letter*, 3–5.
45. HMO backlash spurs wave of restrictive legislation. (1996, March 15). *San Antonio Express-News*, p. 10B.
46. Loomis, 1994.
47. Lamiell, P. (1997, April 12). With savings peaked, health-care costs may rise. *Austin American-Statesman*, p. D2.
48. Spragins, E. (1996, June 24). Does your HMO stack up? *Newsweek*, 56–61, 63.
49. Quinn, J. B. (1997, February 10). Is your HMO OK—or not? *Newsweek*, 52.
50. Ibid.
51. How HMOs are destroying medical trust [Review of the book *Health against wealth: HMOs and the breakdown of medical trust*]. (1997). *Public Citizen Health Research Group Health Letter*, *1*, 1–4.
52. Spragins, E. E. (1997, April 7). Take my freedom, please! *Newsweek*, 81.
53. Driscoll, K. (1997, April 13). Hospitals take lesson in quality improvements from GM. *San Antonio Express-News*, p. 3H.

REFERENCES

Allen, E. (2000, January 12). Baptist Health Systems lays off about 100 staffers. *San Antonio Express-News*, p. 2E.

American Hospital Association (AHA). (1980). *Managerial cost accounting for hospitals*. Chicago: Author.

Applegeet, C. J. (1989). AORN's budget: Planning and forecasting uncover future needs. *AORN Journal*, 212, 214.

Bauerhaus, P. I. (1996). Creating a new place in the competitive market. *Nursing Policy Forum*, 18–20.

Benchmark data, improved productivity help team save $6.9 million in labor costs. (1998). *Data Strategic Benchmarks*, *18*,170, 161.

Borgelt, B. B. & Stone, C. (1999). Ambulatory patient classifications and the regressive nature of Medicare reform: Is the reduction in outpatient health care reimbursement worth the price? *International Journal of Radiation Oncology and Biological Physics*, 729–734.

Brown, B. (1999). How to develop a unit personnel budget. *Nursing Management*, 34–35.

Bunch, D. (1995). The next frontier in managed care. *AARC Times*, 48–49.

Butler, K. (1996). Managed care: Emerging issues in clinical ethics. *ASHA*, 7.

Cericola, S. A. (1995). Facing challenges of managed care. *Plastic Surgical Nursing*, 219.

Cochran, J., Sr. (1979). Refining a patient-acuity system over four years. *Hospital Progress*, 56–60.

Coile, R. C., Jr. (1995). Integration, capitation, and managed care: Transformation of nursing for 21st century health care. *Advanced Practice Nursing Quarterly*, 77–84.

Cokins, G. (1998). Why is traditional accounting failing managers. *Hospital Materials Management Quarterly*, 72–80.

Conway-Welch, C. (1996). Trends in health care impact on nursing education. *NSNA Imprint*, 37–38.

Corder, K. T., Phoon, J., & Barter, M. (1996). Managed care: Employers' influence on the health care system. *Nursing Economics*, 213–217. D'Andrea, G. (1996). Introduction to managed care. *Journal of AHIMA*, 42–46.

Davidson, J. R. & Davidson, T. (1996). Confidentiality and managed care: Ethical and legal concerns. *Health and Social Work*, 208–215.

Davis, G. S. (1996). Learning the ropes of contracting. *Provider*, 32–34.

Day, B. (2000, April 14). BHS lays off 290 workers. *San Antonio Express-News*, pp. 1D, 8D.

Department of Health and Human Services (DHHS), Health Care Financing Administration (HCFA). (1999, July 30). Medicare program; changes to the hospital inpatient prospective payment systems and fiscal year 2000 rates. Final rule. *Federal Register*, 41489–41641.

Drucker, P. F. (1990). The emerging theory of manufacturing. *Harvard Business Review*, 94–100.

Emery, D. W. (1999). Global theory and the nature of risk, part 2. Towards a choice-based model of managed care. *Physician Executive*, 62–66.

Esmond, T. H., Jr. (1982). *Budgeting procedures for hospitals*. Chicago: American Hospital Publishing.

Esterhuysen, P. (1993). Budgeting: A serious matter. *Nursing News*, 8.

Finkler, S. A. (1992). *Budgeting concepts for nurse managers* (2nd ed.). Philadelphia: W. B. Saunders.

Flaherty, M. (1998, August 17). Fight over rights. *HealthWeek*, 1, 30.

Geyman, J. P. (2003). The corporate transformation of medicine and its impact on costs and access to care. *JABFP*, *16*(5), 443–454.

Goetz, J. F. & Smith, H. L. (1980). Zero base budgeting for nursing services: An opportunity for cost containment. *Nursing Forum*, 122–137.

Goodroe, J. H. & Murphy, D. A. (1994). The algebra of managed care. *Hospital Topics*, 14–18.

Gray, B. (1995). Managed health care plans pose employment risk for NPs. *NP News*, *3*(3), 1, 8.

Grimaldi, P. L. (1985). HMOs and Medicare. *Nursing Management*, 16, 18, 20.

Hahn, A. D. (1998). Payment reform will shift home care agency valuation parameters. *Healthcare Financial Management*, 31–34.

Hallows, D. A. (1982, August 4). Budget processes and budgeting in the new authorities. *Nursing Times*, 1309–1311.

Hancock, C. (1982). The nursing budget. *Nursing Mirror*, 47–48.

Hauser, R. C., Edwards, D. E., & Edwards, J. T. (1991). Cash budgeting: An underutilized resource management tool in not-for-profit health care entities. *Hospital Health Services Administration*, 439–446.

Hicks, L. L. & Boles, K. E. (1984). Why health economics? *Nursing Economics*, 175–180.

HMOs win physician support but quality questions remain. (1985). *Medical Staff News*, 3.

Hutchins, B. (1996). Managing cost and quality. *REHAB Management*, 25–26.

Hutton, J. & Moss, D. (1982, August 11). Budgetary control: The role of the director of nursing services and treasurers. *Nursing Times*, 1364–1365.

Johnson, K. P. (1982). Revenue budgeting/rate setting. In W. O. Cleverly (Ed.), *Handbook of health care accounting and finance* (pp. 279–311). Rockville, MD: Aspen.

Kaden, R. J. (1998). Ensuring adequate payment for the use of new technology. *Healthcare Financial Management*, 46–52.

Kilty, G. L. (1999). Baseline budgeting for continuous improvement. *Hospitals Materials Management Quarterly*, 29–32.

Kin, C. S. (1995). Managed care: Is it moral? *Advanced Practice Nursing Quarterly*, 7–11.

La Violette, S. (1979). Classification systems remedy billing inequity. *Modern Healthcare*, 32–33.

Liebler, J. G. & McConnell, C. R. (2004). Management principles for health professionals (4th ed.). Sudbury, MA: Jones and Bartlett.

Lin, H. C., Xirasagar, S., & Tang, C. H. (2004). Costs per discharge and hospital ownership under prospective payment and cost-based reimbursement systems in Taiwan. *Health Policy and Planning*, *19*(3), 166–176.

Lyne, M. (1983, November 23). Grasping the challenge. *Nursing Times*, 11–12.

Mackelprang, R. & Johnson, P. B. (1995). Managed care: Balancing costs, quality and access. *SCI Psychosocial Process*, 175–178.

Marriner, A. (1980). Budgetary management. *The Journal of Continuing Education in Nursing*, 11–14.

Matson, T. & Georgoulakis, J. (1999). Outpatient PPS will create hospitals' greatest challenge. *Health Care Strategic Management*, 10–13.

Maturen, V. & Van Dyke, L. (1996). Using outcome-based critical pathways to improve documentation. *Home Health Care Management Practice*, 48–58.

McCarty, P. (1979). Nursing administrators control millions. *The American Nurse*, 1, 8, 19.

Mendlen, J., Goss, S., & Heist, K. (1996). Managing data for managed care. *Provider*, 66–68.

Moore, K. F. (1996). Cost or quality when selecting a health plan? *Nursing Policy Forum*, 24.

Narayanasamy, A. (1990). Evaluation of the budgeting process in nurse education. *Nurse Education Today*, 245–252.

Negotiating managed care contracts. (1996). *Laboratory Medicine*, 587–596.

Netzel, L. (1995). A primer on capitation: Another step in managed care. *The Surgical Technologist*, 16–18.

Orem, D. E. (1995). Nursing concepts of practice (5th ed.). New York: McGraw-Hill.

Osley, M. (1995). Legislative update. *Journal of Legal Nurse Consulting*, 12–13.

Petersen, B. A. (1996). Nurse-midwifery in a managed care environment. *Journal of Nurse Midwifery*, 267–268.

Phoon, J., Corder, K., & Barter, M. (1996). Managed care and total quality management: A necessary integration. *Journal of Nursing Care Quality*, 25–32.

Potter, L. (1999). The managed care contract: Survival or closure. *Nursing Administration Quarterly*, 58–62.

Rowsell, G. (1981). Economics of health care. *AARN Newsletter*, *37*(7), 6–8.

Roybal, H., Baxendale, S. J., & Gupta, M. (199). Using activity-based costing and theory of constraints to guide continuous improvement in managed care. *Managed Care Quarterly*, 1–10.

Rulon, V. (1996). Measurement systems beyond HEDIS: The evolution of healthcare data analysis in managed care. *J AHIMA*, 48, 50–52.

Ruskowski, U. (1980). A budget orientation tool for nurse managers. *Dimensions in Health Service*, 30–31.

Sandler, R. H. (2000). Managed costs, mismanaged care. *Health Letter*, 1–2.

Schirm, V., Albanese, T., & Garland, T. N. (1999). Understanding nursing home quality of care: Incorporating caregivers' perceptions through structure, process, and outcome. *Quality Management Health Care*, 55–63.

Seawell, V. L. (1994.) *Chart of accounts for hospitals: An accounting and reporting reference guide*. Burr Ridge, IL: Probus.

Shmueli, A. & Glazer, J. (1999). Addressing the inequity of capitation by variable soft contracts. *Health Economics*, 335–343.

Sonberg, V. & Vestal, K. E. (1983). Nursing as a business. *Nursing Clinics of North America*, *18*(3), 491–498.

Sparer, M. S. (1996). Medicaid managed care and the health reform debate: Lessons from New York and California. *Journal of Health Politics, Policy and Law*, 433–460.

Spitzer-Lehman, R. (1995). Managed care: What's ahead. *Surgical Services Management*, 18–21.

Starck, P. L. & Bailes, B. (1996). The budget process in schools of nursing: A primer for the novice administrator. *Journal of Professional Nursing*, 69–75.

Suver, J. D. (1982). Zero base budgeting. In W. O. Cleverly (Ed.), *Handbook of health care accounting and finance* (pp. 353–391). Rockville, MD: Aspen.

Swansburg, R. C. & Swansburg, P. W. (1988). *The nurse manager's guide to financial management*. Rockville, MD: Aspen.

Talone, P. (1996). Ethics and managed care: Beyond helplessness. *MEDSURG Nursing*, 212–214.

Thurgood, J. (1993). Definitions and explanations of the new financial vocabulary. *British Journal of Nursing*, 295–296.

Towers, J. (1996). What do you lnow about NCQA? *Nursing Policy Forum*, 30.

Trofino, J. (1984). Managing the budget crunch. *Nursing Management*, 42–47.

Vracin, R. A. (1982). Capital budgeting. In W. O. Cleverly (Ed.), *Handbook of health care accounting and finance* (pp. 323–351). Gaithersburg, MD: Aspen.

Ward, D. L. (1993). Operational finance and budgeting. In P. R. Kongstvedt (Ed.), *The managed care handbook* (2nd ed., pp. 281–298). Gaithersburg, MD: Aspen.

Wild, J. & Imbrogno, L. (1996). Market changes create need for practice budgets. *Healthcare Financial Management*, 77–78.

Willock, M. & Motley, C. (1998). Financial and material management. *International Anesthesiology Clinic*, 41–57.

Zachry, B. R. & Gilbert, R. L. (1992). Director of nursing planning and finance: A new role. *Nursing Management*, 24–28.

CHAPTER 12

The Directing Process

Linda Roussel, RN, DSN
Russell C. Swansburg, Ph.D, RN

The leader lives in the space between action and potential, anticipating the next step and translating the process for others.

Tim Porter O'Grady
Kathy Malloch

LEARNING OBJECTIVES AND ACTIVITIES

- Describe benchmarking as a means of directing improved patient care delivery services.
- Define *directing*.
- Describe the nature of the directing function of nursing management with relation to the physical acts of directing.
- Make a plan for delegating duties, tasks, and responsibilities.
- Make a plan for using management by objectives (MBO).
- Use a set of standards to evaluate the directing function.
- Differentiate between content (exogenous) theories of motivation and process (endogenous) theories of motivation.
- Describe Maslow's hierarchy of needs.
- Describe nurse dissatisfaction as it relates to productivity and the nurse's role as a knowledge worker.
- Describe nurse satisfaction as it relates to applications of behavioral science.
- List examples that indicate the value of career planning, communication, self-esteem, and self-actualization as management strategies.

CONCEPTS: Directing (leading), delegating, management by objectives, organizational development, benchmarking, Six Sigma, motivation, content theories of motivation, process theories of motivation, self-esteem, self-actualization, self-concept.

NURSE MANAGER BEHAVIORS: Implements management plans through the process of supervision; provides extrinsic conditions of work in quality and quantity that maintain minimal job satisfaction.

NURSE EXECUTIVE BEHAVIORS: Develops and implements management plans through the process of delegating decision making to the lowest organizational entity. Encourages management by objectives and other directing activities that develop the conditions for individual and organizational effectiveness. Directs human resource personnel to develop working conditions to satisfy and retain the best workers at high levels of productivity.

Introduction

The nurse administrator faces growing challenges in directing and leading health care organizations. Evidence-based management practices underscore the need to refine the directing and leading processes. "The patient care delivery models and staffing of the future will be very different as integration of technology and availability of people will change how things are done today."[1] Change and innovation models are essential to the directing processes, as they provide an infrastructure through which to redesign the work and environment of nursing. As Watson writes, "[m]uch work still needs to be done to determine the critical elements of care that must be performed by the nurse, what can be delegated, and what constitutes appropriate oversight of delegated tasks."[2]

The American Organization of Nurse Executives (AONE), the professional association for nurse executives and nurse leaders, states that leadership is necessary to create work environments that will attract and retain nurses. AONE delineated three education and research priorities for nurse leaders in 2004:[3]

1. Stewards of leadership. "In this role, AONE wants to promote evidence-based leadership, mentor aspiring leaders, and engage in effective succession planning."[4]

2. Implement and evaluate future care delivery models. "The goal is to design and develop patient care delivery models that leverage new technologies, improve provider and patient safety, honor diverse work, and support quality care and satisfying work for nurses."[5]
3. Create positive and healthy work environments in nursing and health care. The nurse administrator is responsible for directing and leading organizations that promote professional growth and continuous learning.[6]

Directing the health care organization and motivating its work force are pivotal to creating positive staff and patient care outcomes.

Directing

Fayol states that a manager must know how to handle people and must be able to defend his or her point of view with confidence and enthusiasm. The manager learns continuously and educates people at all levels for success in their assigned tasks.[7]

Fayol stated that command occurs when the manager gets "the optimum return from all employees of his unit in the interest of the whole concern."[8] To do this, the manager must know the personnel; eliminate the incompetent; understand binding agreements with employees; set a good example; conduct periodic audits; confer with chief assistants to focus on unity of direction; not become mired in detail; and have as a goal unity, energy, initiative, and loyalty among employees.[9] Fayol defines coordination as creating harmony among all activities to facilitate the work and success of the unit.[10] In modern management, command and coordination are often labeled *directing* or *leading*.

According to Urwick, it is the purpose of command and the function of directing to see that individual interests do not interfere with the general interest.[11] Directing protects the general interest and ensures that each unit has a competent and energetic head. Command functions to promote *esprit de corps* and to carefully select a staff that can be of most service.[12] It is Urwick's premise that bringing in new blood rather than promoting from within may incite resentment. Urwick describes the need for a grievance procedure, for common rules to be observed by all, and for regulations that allow for self-discipline. Managers should explain regulations and cut red tape. They should "decarbonize," that is, clean out rules and regulations as needed.[13]

Rowland and Rowland state that directing "initiates and maintains action toward desired objectives" and is "closely interrelated with leadership."[14] These authors suggest that a manager's choice of leadership style will be the major factor in directing. Among the activities of directing are delegation, communication, training, and motivation.[15]

Leading is another acceptable term for the directing function. All of the effective principles of nursing management are to be applied by nurse leaders. They begin with accomplishing the mission, goals, and objectives of a division, department, or unit. Because statements of mission, goals, objectives, philosophy, and vision direct the work of all nursing personnel, it is important that these statements be functional. All leading or directing activities will be guided by these statements. The actions of nurse leaders should inspire nursing personnel to produce services and products that please customers and maintain the vitality of the organization. The following are activities related to the leading or directing function:[16]

1. Implementing the theory (knowledge) base of nursing.
2. Making and using strategic and tactical plans with input from nursing personnel. Facilitating operational planning.
3. Facilitating the achievement of the organizational mission, vision, goals, and objectives.
4. Providing and maintaining resources: people, supplies, and equipment.
5. Maintaining morale.
6. Providing education and training programs to maintain competence.
7. Providing, interpreting, and maintaining standards in the form of policies, procedures, rules, and regulations.
8. Facilitating maximum communication.
9. Coordinating among disciplines.
10. Providing leadership.
11. Facilitating and maintaining intrapersonal relationships.
12. Counseling and coaching.
13. Acting to inspire trust, teamwork, and cooperation.
14. Resolving conflict.
15. Using controlling (evaluating) processes that increase and maintain quality and productivity.
16. Facilitating group dynamics.
17. Organizing human resources.
18. Maintaining the physical plant.
19. Assisting personnel with directing their own careers.
20. Promoting the implementation of new nursing roles involving nurse practitioners and case managers, who direct all activities related to process and outcomes.
21. Facilitating nursing research and implementing its results in practice.

Nurse managers oversee the work of nursing personnel. It is incumbent on nurse managers to have up-to-date knowledge and skills so they can develop satisfied nursing workers. This requires that nurse managers facilitate and coach nursing workers in becoming self-managers who produce quality outcomes, work cooperatively within nursing and among other disciplines, do peer review, maintain their knowledge and abilities, and hold themselves accountable for their performances.

In the 9,9 Grid style developed by Blake and Mouton, the directing function of management is described by the following statement: "I keep informed of progress and influence subordinates by identifying problems and revising goals or action steps with them. I assist when needed by helping to remove barriers."[17]

What separates good leaders from great leaders is the understanding and development of facilitation skills.[18]

Directing and Nursing Administration

Directing is a physical act of nursing management, the interpersonal process by which nursing personnel accomplish the objectives of nursing. To understand fully what directing entails, the nurse manager examines the conceptual functions of nursing management, that is, planning and organizing.[19] From the statement of mission or purpose, the statement of beliefs or philosophy, the vision statement, and the written objectives of the organization, the nurse manager develops management plans, the process by which methods and techniques are selected and used to accomplish the work of the nursing unit. Directing is the process of applying the management plans to accomplish nursing objectives. It is the process by which nursing personnel are inspired or motivated to accomplish work. Three of the major elements of directing are embodied in supervision of nursing personnel: motivation, leadership, and communication.[20]

Nurse administrators know something of human nature. Associates are hired and must be managed as total human beings who respond to many institutions within society: church, school, government, family, service organizations, professional societies, and so forth. Similarities and differences exist between supervisors and subordinates, who are complex human beings with needs for physiological well-being, safety, achievement, and human associations. People react to the stresses and strains of a fast-paced society and may need some time for solitude if they are to function effectively and survive. Most individuals place their own concerns before those of others. They enjoy work when the benefits exceed the costs, and they take a job that meets their established priorities for income and, perhaps, for social life.

People can be led and will accept leadership for various reasons, among them admiration, power, income, and safety. The zest with which they pursue achievement of the objectives of the nursing division, department, service, or unit will correspond with the leader's ability to create an internal environment that inspires them to work at the levels of their capabilities. A person who accepts an administrative position must develop and use leadership abilities. These include the following:

- Identification of training and education needs of individuals and establishment of programs to meet such needs.
- Establishment of a system of performance appraisal to identify personal competencies; assignments and promotions based on competency, including performance.
- Development of trust and subsequent delegation of responsibility and authority for decision making.

A good leader will contribute to creating a work environment that has the following properties:

- Jobs that offer a living wage as well as adequate work.
- Group identity and group purpose, that is, the opportunity to work with others.
- Pleasant surroundings and coworkers.
- Interesting work.
- Recognition that employees' work is valued and well done.
- Opportunity for accomplishment and challenge.
- Harmony between organizational and individual goals: equality of opportunity to be safe and secure, to achieve differently, to have choices about shifts, to have job enlargement, and to be recognized as an individual.

A nurse leader who is also a nurse manager is in many ways different from subordinates. He or she is the one who persuades the group to work to achieve organizational objectives. The nurse leader knows more about organizational policies, goals, new programs, and plans for change. He or she is believed to have good judgment based on breadth of experience. He or she controls the careers of subordinates. The nurse leader is expected to behave in a socially acceptable manner, to exhibit personal qualities acceptable to subordinates, and to demonstrate skill in leadership, communication, and motivation techniques.

Nurse managers encourage and inspire their workers every step of the way.

Effective directing increases subordinates' contributions to the achievement of nursing management goals and creates harmony between nursing management goals and nursing workers' goals. Effective directing is the management function wherein the nurse manager acts as facilitator and coach. The effective facilitator and coach provides the education needed for primary nurses and case managers to become leaders and managers. Nurse managers teach nursing personnel to work in self-managed teams. Personnel learn to do planning, self-scheduling, personnel management, and budgeting; to effect change; to make decisions and solve problems; and to build teams for doing research.[21]

Delegating

Delegating, a technique of time management, is a major element of the directing function of nursing administration.[22] It is an effective management competency by which nurse managers get the work done through their employees. One of the criticisms of new nurse managers is that they emerge from clinical nurse roles and fail to identify with their management roles. These nurses have been rewarded for their nursing, not for their skill in leading other nurses. Delegation is a part of management; it requires professional management training and development to accept the hierarchical responsibilities of delegation.

Nurse managers need to be able to delegate some of their own duties, tasks, and responsibilities as a solution to overwork, which leads to stress, anger, and aggression.

As nurse managers learn to accept the principle of delegation, they become more productive and come to enjoy relationships with the staff. They learn to delegate by purposefully thinking about the delegation process, carefully planning for it, gaining knowledge of clinical nurses' capabilities, planning and implementing effective interpersonal communications, and being willing to take risks. As they learn to delegate, they are freed of daily pressures and time-consuming chores and have time to manage. Concepts from clinical delegation can also be applied as an overall model for delegation. Hansten and Jackson outline the following priorities for delegation:

- Know your world (practice, organization)
- Know your organization (communication channels, collaboration, resolution)
- Know your practice (professional, technical, amenity, based on outcomes)
- Know yourself (barriers, benefits)
- Know your delegate (competency, motivation)

While essentially a clinical delegation model, the concepts described require critical thinking skills, knowledge, and careful planning.[23]

The following list suggests ways for nurse managers to successfully delegate:[24]

1. Train and develop subordinates. They are an investment. Give them reasons for the task, authority, details, opportunity for growth, and written instructions, if needed.
2. Plan ahead. It prevents problems.
3. Control and coordinate the work of subordinates but do not peer over their shoulders. To prevent errors, develop ways of measuring the accomplishment of objectives with communication, standards, measurements, feedback, and credit. Nursing employees want to know the nurse manager's expectations of them. They understand expectations when clear, consistent messages and behaviors exist. They understand expectations from clearly defined jobs, work relationships, and expected results.
4. Followup by visiting subordinates frequently. Spot potential problems of morale, disagreement, and grievance. Expect employees to make suggestions to improve work, and use the feasible ones.
5. Coordinate to prevent duplication of effort.
6. Solve problems, and think about new ideas. Encourage employees to solve their own problems, and then give them the autonomy and freedom to do so.
7. Accept delegation as desirable.
8. Specify goals and objectives.
9. Know subordinates' capabilities, and match the task or duty to the employee. Be sure the employee considers the task or duty important.
10. Agree on performance standards. Relate managerial references to employee performance.
11. Take an interest in employees.
12. Assess results. Expect what is clearly and directly asked for as the deadline for completing and reporting arrives. The nurse manager should accept the fact that employees will perform delegated tasks in their own style.
13. Give appropriate rewards.
14. Do not take back delegated tasks.

Build professional nurses' self-esteem by delegating as much of the authority for nursing practice as possible. Professional nurses want authority over their practice and can be educated to perform management tasks related to it. Nurse managers will determine what authority to delegate through communication with clinical nurses. Authority should be commensurate with assigned responsibility. As professional nurses gain individual self-esteem, organizational self-esteem follows. Employees respond to participation in decision making and gain satisfaction with their jobs and the organization.

Organizational self-esteem will be enhanced by the following qualities:[25]

- Managerial interest in employees' well-being, status, and contributions, and concern and support for their personal problems, personal development, and comfort.

- Job variety from delegation that provides job enlargement, autonomy, significant work, and use of skills and abilities the employees value. Delegation that enlarges an employee's job develops his or her sense of responsibility, general understanding, and job satisfaction. As part of a successful knowledge base, professional nurses learn effective strategies for managing tasks, including increasing workloads, establishing priorities, and delegating responsibility.
- A climate or work environment that bolsters cohesiveness and trust.
- Management's faith in and recognition of the rewards of self-direction.

Reasons for Delegating

The following are five reasons for delegating:[26]

1. Assigning routine tasks.
2. Assigning tasks for which the nurse manager does not have time.
3. Problem solving.
4. Changes in the nurse manager's own job emphasis.
5. Capability building.

The nurse manager should be careful not to misuse the clinical nurse by delegating tasks that can be done by nonnurses or nonlicensed personnel. This error can be avoided by consulting with clinical nurses to determine what authority they want.

Techniques for Delegating

Nurse managers at all levels, from nurse executive to department or unit head and from unit head to clinical nurse, can prepare lists of duties that can be delegated. Delegation includes authority to approve, recommend, or implement. The list of duties should be ranked by time required to perform them and their importance to the institution. One duty should be delegated at a time.

What Not to Delegate

Do not delegate the power to discipline, responsibility for maintaining morale, overall control, a "hot potato," jobs that are too technical, or duties involving a trust or confidence.[27] These complicated areas of nursing management require specialized knowledge and skills. Nurse managers who handle these responsibilities should be well educated in the sciences of management and behavioral technology. Delegating these duties and responsibilities will cause clinical nurses to assume that managers are incompetent to handle these areas of nursing leadership and management.

Barriers to Delegating

Barriers to delegating can exist in the delegator, delegatee, or situation. For example, barriers in the delegator relate to preference for operating by oneself, insecurity, fear of being disliked, lack of confidence in associates, and refusal to allow mistakes. From the delegatee's perspective, barriers include lack of experience, lack of competence, avoidance of responsibility, disorganization, overload of work, and immersion in trivia. The situation may also provide barriers such as no tolerance for mistakes, understaffing, criticism of decisions, and confusion in responsibilities and authority.

Management by Objectives

Management by objectives (MBO) was first advocated by Peter Drucker and made famous by George Odiorne, who defined it as "a process whereby the superior and subordinate managers of an organization jointly identify its common goals, define each individual's major areas of responsibility in terms of the results expected of him [sic], and use these measures as guides for operating the unit and assessing the contribution of each of its members."[28]

Odiorne further defines MBO as a system for making organizational structures work, of bringing about vitality and personal involvement in the hierarchy by means of statements of what is expected from everyone involved and measurement of what is actually achieved. It stresses ability and achievement rather than personality.[29]

Management by objectives allows the individual nurse to contribute to the common goal of the enterprise while nurse managers focus on the business goals. MBO promotes high standards, focusing on the job and not on the manager or the worker. Applying Drucker's MBO theory accomplishes this; nurse managers know what to expect of employees. Just like their nurse managers, nursing staff should know for what they will be held accountable.[30]

Management by objectives spells out the results expected of the clinical nursing unit itself and in relation to other units. It emphasizes teamwork and team results and includes short- and long-term objectives, as well as tangible and intangible objectives. Intangible objectives include development of the individual, performance and attitude of workers, and public responsibilities. Objectives should include those that indicate the contributions to higher levels of the enterprise.

Management by objectives allows people to control their own performance and measure themselves. Through MBO, clinical nurses make demands of themselves. Nurse managers will assume that clinical nurses want to be responsible, want to contribute, want to achieve, and have the strength and desire to do so. According to Drucker,

> What the business enterprise needs is a principle of management that will give full scope to individual strength and responsibility, as well as common direction to vision and ef-

fort, establish team work, and harmonize the goals of the individual with the commonwealth. Management by objectives and self-control make[s] the commonwealth the aim of every manager. It substitutes for control from outside the stricter, more exacting, and more effective control from inside. It motivates the manager to action, not because somebody tells him [sic] to do something or talks him into doing it, but because the objective task demands it. He acts not because somebody wants him to but because he himself decides that he has to—he acts, in other words, as a free man.

I do not use the word "philosophy" lightly; indeed I prefer not to use it at all; it's much too big a word. But management by objectives and self-control may properly be called a philosophy of management. It rests on a concept of the job of management. It rests on an analysis of the specific needs of the management group and the obstacles it faces. It rests on a concept of human action, behavior, and motivation. Finally it applies to every manager, whatever his level and function, and to any organization whether large or small. It ensures performance by converting objective needs into personal goals. And this is genuine freedom."[31]

Procedure and Process

Educating the Process

The education of the MBO process should begin with the nurse managers of the enterprise. Managers will learn the characteristics of the process, the objectives of initiating an MBO program, the procedures to be used, and the methods for evaluating the program's effectiveness. During this educational program, nurse managers can simulate the procedures to be used.

Once nurse managers are educated, all nursing employees are given similar educational opportunities. Employees will be made aware of the necessity for writing and working toward their personal objectives as they seek to achieve those of the organization. They will be taught the value of synergy of personal and organizational objectives, and they will be asked to bring their written lists of objectives to the first meeting with their superior.

First Meeting

The first MBO meeting should be held in quiet surroundings, with sufficient time for discussion. The nurse manager should put the employee at ease. Most survival and safety needs of nurses are reasonably satisfied. Nurses' social, ego, and self-fulfillment needs are predominant at this time. As the nurse presents each personal objective, the nurse manager relates it to an objective of the enterprise. Thus, the manager creates the conditions for fulfilling the nurse's needs, including the removal of obstacles, encouragement of growth, and provision of guidance.

During this first meeting, the nurse manager and clinical nurse set goals that are specific, promote teamwork, are measurable (in the sense that they can be quantified or described qualitatively), and are attainable. Goals should involve enough risk to challenge but not defeat. They should include objectives that are routine, solve problems, are creative or innovative, and result in personal development.[32]

At the end of the first meeting, both the nurse manager and clinical nurse should be satisfied with the written objectives. Each will have a copy of these objectives. The nurse manager and the clinical nurse will part with an understanding of mutual expectations on how future meetings will progress, and they will have set a time for the next meeting.

Actions

Between meetings, employees perform work that meets their mutual objectives. They should periodically review these objectives and summarize their accomplishments.

Second Meeting

Conditions for the second MBO meeting will be the same as for the first meeting. The meeting will provide a time for evaluation of results, review, appraisal, and the setting of further goals.

The employee should be encouraged to spell out gratifying and exhilarating experiences, do self-examination, and relate his or her thoughts about work. The nurse manager should listen and make the employee feel safe while helping him or her to have a person-to-organization fit.

The manager examines his or her own reactions without criticizing the employee, which helps build trust and confidence as well as an ethical relationship. In doing so, the manager and employee establish an organizational climate for personal and organizational achievement.[33]

Management by objectives should include appraisal of managers by subordinates. Subordinates will appraise how well the manager helps employees do their jobs, supports them, assists with problems, and demonstrates proficiency and visibility.[34]

Both nurse manager and employee should exit the second meeting with a sense of accomplishment. This does not mean the employee will not be made aware of deficiencies or shortcomings. Deficiencies and shortcomings will be recognized in the form of needed additions or changes, increased progress, and even deletions. All will be tied to patient care and organizational development. The feedback process tells the employee what is expected and when an error has been made.

The process will be repeated at intervals, with dates and times agreed on at each meeting. At the end of an appraisal period, a performance results contract will be signed by both the employee and the supervisor and sent to the personnel department to be included in the employee's record. The performance appraisal can be used to identify promotion potential and to determine merit pay increases.

Problems with Management by Objectives

Management by objectives must be viewed as genuine and fair by all employees. It must allow for errors and for adjustments that result from work constraints and individual capabilities. The following are some specific problems of MBO:

1. Top management is not supportive. To be effective MBO must be supported and carried out at all levels, and it must be monitored closely.
2. Inconsistency exists among managers. This can be fixed or avoided by increased awareness of both parties. Periodic summative evaluation conferences can help uncover these inconsistencies.
3. Goals are too easy or are unattainable. Employees sometimes fear that they will be subjected to goals of increasing difficulty. Frank discussion will help resolve this problem. Employees have to be able to meet increasing personal needs as they climb the career ladder. These can be recognized and satisfied through MBO.
4. Conflicts between goals and policies exist. When this occurs, policies should give way to goals unless they would violate a safety or legal standard.
5. Accountability is beyond the control of employees. When this occurs, the nurse manager helps modify the goal and makes allowance for the difference, which can be done by decreasing accountability or increasing authority. Factors beyond the employee's control should not be evaluated.
6. Employees have a lack of commitment. Determine the cause, if possible, and produce interactions that will increase commitment. Discuss the problem frankly, and encourage the employee to be specific in a plan to cope with it. Do not threaten.

Management by objectives is a superb tool if the objectives are (1) simple, (2) focused on what's important, (3) genuinely created from the bottom up (the objectives are drafted by the person who must live up to them, with no constraining guides), and (4) a "living" contract, not a form driven exercise. MBO should promote flexibility.[35]

Some management writers recommend management by results (MBR) rather than MBO. When using MBR, managers should be sure the key results include quantity, quality, and cost of outcomes. Subjectivity and favoritism should be avoided because they sow resentment and distrust. Objectives should be set high and pushed even higher using the new level as the expected base, with quality as the fundamental objective. Workers should be rewarded with bonuses or in any other way possible. It is best to reward groups so that people share information and work together.[36]

When using MBR, follow these principles:[37]

1. Employees are capable of crafting solutions to problems because they know the system and its problems.
2. Use budget systems that fund outcomes rather than inputs.
3. Outcomes are measures of the volume of something produced and of quality.
4. Two thirds of workers today work more with their minds than with their bodies.
5. The work force comes from a society with great cultural diversity.

MBO is a total management process that includes planning, organizing, directing (leading), and controlling (evaluating). Exhibit 12-1 lists the standards for evaluating the directing function of nursing management.

Organizational Development

Management by objectives is needed for organizational development (OD) and vice versa. Organizational development allows the organization to be managed against goals and for results. OD occurs as management skills and organizational processes are applied to shape and develop the conditions for human effectiveness. These conditions include the following:[38]

- Interpersonal competence. The individual has high expectations, respect for others, honest relationships, freedom to act, and a team orientation.
- Meaningful goals. The goals are understandable, desirable, attainable, and synergistic. The individual influences the goals.
- Helpful systems. Users understand and control systems because systems are goal-oriented and provide feedback. Users adapt to and adopt systems.
- Achievement and self-actualization. As the organization grows, the individual grows. People are committed to goals, are highly motivated, and have high trust and minimal dissatisfaction.

The management philosophy should permit these conditions for human effectiveness to occur. In addition, it should emphasize meaningful work in which the doers are involved in all aspects of the job. Managers should delegate decisions and ensure that the decisions are made, limits are known, support is provided, and accountability is met by evaluating results.

Benchmarking and Six Sigma Strategies

Management by objectives provides a mechanism in which an organization can compare goal setting to goal attainment. Another method of comparison used by organizations is benchmarking. "Benchmarking is simply comparison of one's own activity or results with the

EXHIBIT 12-1
Standards for Evaluating the Directing Function

1. Managers have established a medium by which nursing workers feel free to ask for advice, counsel, and consultation.
2. Necessary written directions are available in the form of policies, procedures, standards of care, job analyses, job descriptions, job standards, and nursing care plans. They are clearly stated and current and are kept to a minimal number.
3. A training program is in effect that meets nursing employees' needs as they perceive them. They participate.
4. Supervisors are competent in needed knowledge and skills of administration and clinical specialization.
5. Nurse managers periodically work evening, night, weekend, and holiday shifts to keep abreast of clinical and administrative behaviors peculiar to these shifts.
6. The nurse administrator has operationalized the American Nurses Association (ANA) *Scope and Standards for Nurse Administrators*.
7. The nurse managers have operationalized the ANA *Standards of Clinical Nursing Practice*.
8. Nurse managers are knowledgeable about and apply the appropriate standards of the Joint Commission on Accreditation of Healthcare Organizations, National League for Nursing, Medicare, and Medicaid.
9. The nurse administrator uses techniques of operations analysis. (This service is available at no charge to member hospitals of the American Hospital Association and its state affiliates.)
10. Nurse managers use a system of management by objectives or results.
11. The nurse administrator works with the consent and knowledge of patients and solicits input from consumers regarding nursing services desired.
12. Nursing unit personnel are organized into and working as direct care personnel and clerical personnel.
13. Nurse managers use the physical plant to the best advantage for patients and personnel.

level of activity or results of another department or organization."[39] External benchmarking sources include Joint Commission on Accreditation of Healthcare Organizations (JCAHO), the American Society for Testing and Materials (ASTM), and American Health Information Management Association (AHIMA), which provide best practice models within their respective industries.[40] Such benchmarks provide measures to direct a quality organization and work force. Six Sigma is also an approach to quality management and continuous improvement. This strategy is based on measurement and statistical analysis and incorporates process improvement teams to minimize variation from the desired norms. Teams work together through a process described as DMAIC:[41]

Define (project goals and customers/clients, both internal and external)

Measure (processes to determine performance)

Analyze (determine root cause(s) of defect)

Improve (eliminate defect)

Control (future process performance)

A theory of nursing management explores the cause–effect relationship between clinical nurses and their performances. It has as its objectives the removal of controls that create distrust, fear, and resentment and the promotion of conditions that provide opportunities for clinical nurses to achieve their goals. Motivating the work force is important to the overall function of directing. Understanding motivation theory and developing strategies to advance positive work force development serve to increase productivity and quality outcomes.

Theories of Motivation

Motivation is a concept used to describe both the extrinsic conditions that stimulate certain behavior and the intrinsic responses that demonstrate that behavior. The intrinsic response is sustained by sources of energy, termed motives—often described as needs, wants, or drives. All people have motives. Motivation is measured by observable and recorded behaviors. Deficiencies in needs stimulate people to seek and achieve goals to satisfy these needs. Consider the following questions.

- Why do some registered nurses pursue an area of nursing specialization to the extent of continuously acquiring new knowledge and skills that enable them to make rapid and accurate nursing diagnoses and prescriptions?
- Why does a pediatric nurse pursue development of a role that extends professional practice into areas such as teaching parents to enjoy their children, providing followup health observations of high-risk newborns, and teaching health practices to the parents of newborns after they have been discharged to their homes?
- Why does that nurse go a step further and teach others to extend themselves and then write articles to provide the information for everyone?
- Why does a mental health nurse pursue a role in off-duty time as a cotherapist of a group in addition to rotating shifts as a staff nurse?
- Why does another nurse work to conduct a psychodrama therapy program and ask for the privilege of answering mental health consultations for medical and surgical patients?

- Why does a professional nurse work many hours as a committee member for a district nurses' association?
- Why do some nurses perform positively and others negatively?
- Why do some people always act with truthfulness, integrity, and candor to support principles they believe in, whereas others remain silent and passive?
- Why are some nurses goal-oriented and others not? Why are some nurses actively dedicated to improving the quality of people's lives, whereas others merely exert minimal effort to maintain it?
- What makes some nurses come to work on time, work hard and without error, maintain a pleasant demeanor, and meet all standards of performance, appearance, and behavior, whereas others do just the opposite? Some persons do not do well in an organization. This does not mean that these persons are not useful; the organization may be lacking the means of making them productive, useful, satisfied employees.

The answer to all the preceding questions is motivation. Some nurses are motivated to excel and be creative; others put forth just enough effort to do the job. To get goods and services to the customer, managers must care about people and their motivations. Managers' beliefs about motivation are reflected in their personal management styles.

Theories of motivation have been classified into content theories and process theories.[42] Work motivation theories have also been classified as dealing either with exogenous causes or with endogenous causes.[43] Exogenous theories focus on motivationally relevant independent variables that can be changed by external agents (such as organizational incentives and rewards) and social factors (such as leader and group behavior). There are seven exogenous theories: motive–need theory, incentive–reward theory, reinforcement theory, goal theory, personal and material resource theory, group and norm theory, and sociotechnical system theory. Exogenous theories are content theories, four of which are presented here.[44]

Content Theories

Content theories of motivation focus on factors or needs within a person that energize, direct, sustain, and stop behavior. The most widely recognized work in motivation theory is that of Maslow. Although not universally accepted because of its lack of scientific evidence or research base, Maslow's work is universally known.

Many managers attempt to use Maslow's work as they turn to a human behavior approach to management.

Like every science, nursing is a human creation stemming from human motives; having human goals; and being created, renewed, and maintained by human beings. As are other scientists, nurses are motivated by physiological needs, including the need for food; needs for safety, protection, and care; social needs for gregariousness, affection, and love; ego needs for respect, standing, and status, leading to self-respect or self-esteem; and a need for self-fulfillment or self-actualization, characterized by integrity, responsibility, magnanimity, simplicity, and naturalness. Many nurses, but not all, are also motivated by cognitive needs for knowledge and understanding. They voraciously question others; read textbooks, journals, and patients' charts; and regularly pursue courses in their specialties and in the liberal arts (particularly the humanities). Other nurses are motivated by aesthetic needs for beauty, symmetry, simplicity, completion, and order and by their need to express themselves. How many of these needs are related to a nurse's desire to keep learning and applying new knowledge and skills? What can the nurse manager do to spark in a nurse the motive of curiosity that sets in motion a desire to understand, explain, and systematize? These and many other human needs may serve as the primary motivations for a person pursuing a career in nursing who wants to update and expand knowledge and skills. The motivation may be a feeling of identification and belonging with people in general, love for human beings, a desire to help people, the need to earn a living or express oneself, or a combination of all these needs working together. An individual's needs are diverse and unique.[45]

Alderfer, who reduced Maslow's hierarchy of needs from five to three, developed a second content theory of motivation: existence (E), relatedness (R), and growth (G) (the term ERG theory). To compare Alderfer's scheme with Maslow's, existence needs correspond to physiological and safety needs; relatedness needs to belongingness, social, and love needs; and growth needs to self-esteem and self-actualization.

Whereas Maslow's theory proposes that the next level of needs emerges when the predominant (satisfaction–progression) ones have been fulfilled, Alderfer's theory adds a frustration–regression process. When higher-level needs are frustrated, people will regress to the satisfaction of lower-level needs.[46]

Limited research is available to support or sustain the ERG theory. As with other theories of motivation, nurse leaders should become familiar with it and use its implications as appropriately as possible.

Herzberg did research on a third content theory, which he labeled a two-factor theory of motivation. One set of factors—dissatisfiers—is extrinsic conditions or hygiene factors. This set includes salary, job security, working conditions, status, company policy, quality of technical supervision, and quality of interpersonal relations among peers, with supervisors, and with subordinates.

These factors must be maintained in quantity and quality to prevent dissatisfaction. These conditions become dissatisfiers when not equitably administered, causing low performance and negative attitudes. The other set of factors—satisfiers—are intrinsic conditions or motivators, which include achievement, recognition, responsibility, advancement, the work itself, and the possibility of growth. They create opportunities for high satisfaction, high motivation, and high performance. The individual must be free to attain intrinsic conditions. Both factors, hygiene and motivation, must be done simultaneously. Herzberg's research has been criticized for its limited sample of 200 accountants and engineers and for being simplistic.[47]

McClelland proposed and researched a fourth content theory of motivation closely associated with learning concepts, the learned needs theory. The three primary groups of learned needs acquired from the culture are the need for achievement, the need for affiliation, and the need for power. McClelland used the Thematic Apperception Test (TAT) to measure the need for achievement. He contended that needs can be learned through organizational and nonorganizational meetings. Persons high in the need for achievement want to set their own performance goals, which they prefer to be moderate and achievable. They want immediate feedback, and they like responsibility for solving problems.[48]

Many nursing personnel enjoy working together and are motivated by these affiliations. In some situations, such as in nursing homes, nurses do not get the recognition they need from clients, so they look for it from colleagues. Many nursing personnel want to talk and socialize with each other on the job. They enjoy and prefer group–centered work activities, teamwork, interdependence, dependability, and predictability. The nurse educator works with these nurses to maintain this affiliation need at a mutually acceptable level.[49]

Process Theories

Endogenous theories deal with process or mediating variables such as expectancies and attitudes "that are amenable to modification only indirectly in response to variation in one or more exogenous variables." Four endogenous theories are:[50]

1. Arousal–activation theory, which focuses on internal processes that mediate the effects of conditions of work on performance.
2. Expectancy–valence theory, which focuses on people's expectations that their efforts will result in good performance and on valued outcomes.
3. Equity theory, which focuses on fair treatment; inputs from the employee will result in equal inputs from the employer.
4. Intention–goal theory, which focuses on performance as determined by commitment to goals.

Most behavior within organizations is learned behavior: perceptions, attitudes, goals, emotional reactions, and skills. Practice that occurs during the learning process results in a relatively enduring change in behavior.

Skinner advanced a process theory of motivation called operant conditioning, also called behavior modification. Learning occurs as a consequence of behavior. Behaviors are the operants; they are controlled by altering the consequences with reinforcers or punishments.

Positive or desired behaviors should be rewarded or reinforced. Reinforcement motivates, increasing the strength of a response or inducing its repetition. Continuous reinforcement speeds up early performance. Intermittent reinforcement at fixed or variable ratios sustains performance. Research indicates higher rates of response with ratio rather than with interval schedules. Reinforcers tend to weaken over time, and new ones have to be developed.

Undesirable organizational behavior should not be rewarded. Negative reinforcement is a situation which occurs when desired behavior occurs to avoid negative consequences of punishment. Although frequently used, punishment creates negative attitudes and can increase costs. Behaviorists believe that people will repeat behavior when consequences are positive.

Behavior modification research uses a scientific approach. Application of behavior modification is occurring in large companies, and benefits or results claimed include improved attendance, productivity, and efficiency and cost savings. Reinforcers center on praise, recognition, and feedback. The problem-solving method is used to apply behavior modification:[51]

1. Identify and define (observe and measure) the specific behavior.
2. Measure or count the occurrences.
3. Analyze the antecedents, behaviors, and consequences (ABCs) of the behavior.
4. Perform positive reinforcement, negative reinforcement, or punishment, or extinguish the behavior. Positive reinforcement is best because people repeat behavior that is rewarded and avoid behavior that is punished.
5. Evaluate changes. Provide feedback for reinforcement or correction. Give positive reinforcement while discussing areas that need improvement. Give feedback at all steps of performance, not just at outcomes. Followup reinforcement motivates people to put plans into effect because of the attention generated: somebody cares and is paying attention. Structured followup can include review sessions between clinical nurse and nurse leader, interdisciplinary or intradisciplinary team review of outcomes, review of collected data, or direct consultation.

Critics of the behavior modification theory consider rewards to be bribes.

A second process theory of motivation is Vroom's expectancy theory, which postulates that a person voluntarily controls most behaviors and therefore is motivated. There is an effort-performance expectancy, or a person's belief that a chance exists for a certain effort to lead to a particular level of performance. The performance–outcome expectancy or belief of this person will have certain outcomes. Given choices, the individual selects the one with the best expected outcome. Research on expectancy theory is increasing although not systematic or refined. This process is a complicated one in which unconscious motivation is avoided.[52]

Equity theory is a third process theory. Persons believe they are being treated with equity when the ratio of their efforts to rewards equals those of others. Equity can be achieved or restored by changing outputs, attitudes, the reference person, inputs or outputs of the reference person, or the situation. Research on equity theory has focused on pay.[53]

A fourth process theory of motivation is the goal-setting theory of Locke. This theory is based on goals as determinants of behavior. The more specific the goals, the better the results produced. Research indicates that goals are a powerful force. Goals must be achievable; their difficulty level should be increased only to the ceiling to which the person will commit. Goal clarity and accurate feedback increase security.[54]

Maslow

Maslow's theory of motivation is a positive one and is based on a holistic–dynamic theory. At the base of a needs system are the physiologic needs, based on homeostasis, a condition of constancy of body fluids, functions, and states. The constancy is maintained automatically by uniform interaction of counteracting processes. Human beings do not just eat; they eat selectively to maintain homeostasis. The same is probably true of other physiological needs, although not all physiological needs are homeostatic. Some are relatively independent of each other while at the same time interdependent. For example, smoking may satisfy the hunger need in some persons. Some needs are in opposition to each other, such as the tendency to be lazy and the desire to be industrious.

Maslow proposed that human needs are organized in a hierarchy of prepotency: higher needs emerge as lower ones are satisfied. When the physiological needs are satisfied, they no longer motivate the human being. However, a person tolerates deprivation of a long-satisfied need better than one that has been long or previously deprived.

When unsatisfied, physiological needs are the most prepotent, the strongest, of human needs. A starving person will steal food and perform other acts that threaten his or her safety. The dominance of a physiological need changes the individual's philosophy for the future.

Safety needs are the second group in the hierarchy. Among these are security, protection, dependency, and stability; freedom from anxiety, chaos, and fear; need for order, limits, structure, and law; and strength in the protector. Satisfaction of these needs influences a person's values and philosophy of life. What threatens the safety of nursing? Are nurses threatened by increased consumer interest in their shortcomings, which may lead to consumer control of practice? What motivates people? Is it a fear of the high cost of extended illnesses and results of poor care? The average person likes law, order, predictability, and organization, which may be one reason that people resist change. Insurance programs, job tenure, and savings accounts are expressions of safety needs. People prefer familiar to unknown things. Today's managers are often threatened by the new generation of personnel who question regulations and use the law to achieve their goals.

Once the physiological and safety needs have been satisfied, the needs for love, affection, and belonging emerge. Most nurses in practice today have had their physiological and safety needs satisfied. Now they want to be part of a group or family with love, acceptance, friendliness, and a feeling of belonging. Are these needs thwarted by frequent moves? How are the needs of the individual, as well as those of the organization, satisfied? A society that wants to survive and be healthy will work to satisfy these needs. Otherwise, people will be maladjusted and exhibit severe emotional and behavioral pathology.

Human beings want to gain new knowledge, to solve problems, to bring order, and to explore, and they will voluntarily face dangers to do so.

Two categories emerge under the fourth set of needs, the esteem needs. All people share these needs. First, they desire strength, achievement, adequacy, mastery and competence, confidence before the world, independence, and freedom. Second, they desire reputation or prestige, status, fame and glory, dominance, recognition, attention, importance, dignity, or appreciation. A person whose self-esteem is satisfied has feelings of self-confidence, worth, strength, capability, adequacy, usefulness, and being needed in society. For self-esteem to be stable and healthy, it must be based on known or deserved respect. The reason for self-esteem must be known and recognized by its recipient.

Finally, at the pinnacle of the hierarchy of needs is the emotional gold—the need for self-actualization, the effort of people to be what they can be. Nurses want to become everything that they are capable of becoming, to achieve their potential, to be effective nurses, to be creative, and to meet personal standards of performance.

Certain conditions are prerequisites to satisfying basic needs. When basic needs are thwarted, the individual feels threatened. These necessary conditions include the following:

- Freedom to speak—communication
- Freedom to do what one wishes to do without harming others—choice of jobs, friends, and entertainment
- Freedom to express oneself—creativity
- Freedom to investigate and seek information
- Freedom to defend oneself—justice, fairness, honesty, and orderliness in the group

The hierarchy of needs is not a simple classification. Individuals order their needs differently. Some place self-esteem before love; others place creativity before all else. Certain people have low levels of aspiration. Permanent loss of love needs results in a psychopathic personality.

A long-satisfied need may become undervalued. A person who has never been deprived of a particular need does not regard the need as important. If two needs emerge, a person will probably want the more basic one satisfied first. People who have loved and been well loved and who have had many deep friendships can hold out against hatred, rejection, or persecution.

Most normal persons in our society have partially satisfied and partially dissatisfied basic needs at the same time. They may have more satisfied physiological needs and correspondingly fewer satisfied self-actualization needs. New needs emerge gradually and are more often unconscious than conscious. Basic needs are common throughout different cultures. Most behavior is multidetermined: all of the basic needs are involved. A single act of an individual could be analyzed to show how it addresses physiological needs, safety needs, love needs, esteem needs, and self-actualization needs. Not all behavior is internally motivated; some is stimulated externally. Some is highly motivated, some weakly, and some not at all. Some is expressive and some rote. A gratified or satisfied need is not a motivator of behavior. Healthy persons are primarily motivated by the need to develop and actualize their fullest potential and capabilities.

Usefulness to Nurse Managers

Motivational theory has been used in a number of studies of behavior modification for smoking cessation, weight control, exercise, and general reduction of cardiovascular risk factors. To date, modifying risk-taking behavior has had limited positive results. For example, because nicotine is known as a highly addictive substance, motivational theory may have to be combined with other treatment regimens to sustain cessation of smoking. The same may be true of other risk-taking behaviors. This area presents an opportunity for nurses to expand motivational research to include identifying factors that contribute to sustaining risk-taking behavior, including psychological profiles.[55] Results of such research are important in managing patients and personnel.

Knowledge of motivation theories is essential to improving the job performance of employees. Individual employees have different needs and goals. Nurse managers will learn and use motivation theories selectively.

Although many theories exist and much has been written about motivation, there is no easy way to motivate employees. Human motivation is diverse, subtle, and complex. To use the available information on motivation effectively, the nurse manager will study it and select and use those elements that appear to be practical and workable.

Some theories of motivation are contradictory. They provide useful knowledge when used selectively and carefully. Theories of motivation are constructs, because they cannot be directly observed and measured.[56]

Dissatisfactions

Nurse managers who apply learned approaches to change within nursing organizations can alleviate dissatisfactions of nurses.

Productivity

Nurses respond negatively and become dissatisfied when managers use force, control, threats, and repeated applications of institutional power. Productivity decreases or stagnates. The new breed of nurses questions authority and gives loyalty to those who earn it. An attitude of mutual respect between clinical nurses and managers is essential to productivity.

To promote mutual respect, free interaction and communication must take place in which expectations are clarified and feedback on performance is given through role modeling of expected and desired performance. In addition, promises that cannot be fulfilled must be avoided. In more than 7 of 10 working relationships, the employee does not know what is expected of him or her. Expectations must be clear. In a productivity attitude test developed and administered to production workers by Pryor and Mondy over a 2-year period, 75% of respondents said that their supervisors did not keep promises they made. Broken promises anger employees and decrease productivity.[57]

Nurse managers are powerful models for staff. They are emulated, whether their example is good or bad. The obvious implication is that nurse managers must do self-assessment and modify their behavior to assume roles beneficial to both staff and organization.

Like other workers, nurses work to survive and meet their needs and aspirations. The complexity of the technological environment of patient care can lead to specialization and the depersonalization of jobs and work. This alienates nursing employees, and the quality of their work declines.

Nurse as Knowledge Worker

Nurses are knowledge workers. Their basic economic needs are related to other human needs or human values. Drucker suggests that knowledge workers are productive only with self-motivation, self-direction, and achievement. People are motivated to work based on Maslow's hierarchy of needs. Even when satisfied, a need remains important. Economic rewards that are not properly dispensed create dissatisfaction with work and become deterrents to job satisfaction and productivity.[58] Pay is part of the social or psychological need of nurses. Nurses perform work of equal difficulty and want economic rewards of equal value to those of other knowledge workers. They also want rank, power, and status commensurate with those of other knowledge workers.

More formal education and skills translate into higher real incomes and increased living standards. Boosts in investments in education, research and development, and updated equipment result in increased productivity. Ideas rather than physical resources result in added economic value. Highly skilled workers can switch jobs more easily, and therefore spend less time unemployed, than can unskilled workers. Money invested in education is an investment in the economic health and future of the United States.[59] Educated people are mobile. Nurses can move laterally to jobs in other organizations.

The nurse as knowledge worker is self-directed and takes responsibility. Rewarding and reaffirming self-direction and responsibility produce learning; fear produces resistance. Education makes fear a demotivator. Psychological manipulation is only a replacement for the carrot-and-stick approach to management. It does not work.

The role of discipline is to eliminate marginal friction. If used to drive nurses, discipline causes resentment and resistance; it demotivates. Direction and control are useless in meeting ego needs. Needs thwarted or otherwise not satisfied lead to sick or negative behavior. To focus on needs already satisfied is ineffective; however, employees will demand more of what they already have unless attention is given to self-esteem and self-actualization. In such a situation money becomes the only means available to satisfy needs. Inflation increases the demand because it takes more money to satisfy other desires. This increased demand, however, destroys the usefulness of money and material rewards as incentives and managerial tools.

Nurses are independent adults who want to be treated with dignity and respect—as adults and as partners. The organizational perspective should be that it is practicing clinical nurses who achieve health care productivity gains, and not capital spending and automation.

Nursing personnel retreat from association and identification with organizations in which they cannot meet their perceived care requirements. Nurses may believe they are competent and able to do good work; however, they are dissatisfied because organizational resources are not allowing them to live up to the standard of care they consider appropriate. Nurses care, and because they care, they are dissatisfied.

Satisfactions

Science of Human Behavior

How do we apply the knowledge of the social sciences so that our human organizations will be truly effective? We have the knowledge just as surely as we have the knowledge of physical sciences to develop alternative sources of energy. Application of knowledge in both physical and social sciences, however, is expensive and time-consuming.

Theory X and Theory Y

Douglas McGregor's theories of leadership and motivation remain influential. Unfortunately, his Theory X has not been replaced by his Theory Y. Theory X, as he described it for the world of business, is summarized in the following points:[60]

1. Management is responsible for organizing the elements of productive enterprise—money, materials, equipment, people—in the interest of economic ends.
2. With respect to people, this is a process of directing their efforts, motivating them, controlling their actions, and modifying their behavior to fit the needs of the organization.
3. Without this active intervention by management, people would be passive—even resistant—to organizational needs. They must therefore be persuaded, rewarded, punished, and controlled; their activities must be directed. This is management's task—in managing subordinate managers or workers. We often sum it up by saying that management consists of getting things done through other people.

Behind this conventional theory there are several additional beliefs—less explicit, but widespread:

4. The average person is by nature indolent—he or she works as little as possible.
5. He or she lacks ambition, dislikes responsibility, and prefers to be led.
6. He or she is inherently self-centered, indifferent to organizational needs.
7. He or she is by nature resistant to change.
8. He or she is gullible, not very bright, the ready dupe of the charlatan and the demagogue.

How many nurse managers demotivate practicing nurses by falling into the trap of voicing the very statements embodied in Theory X? How may nurse managers motivate practicing nurses by applying the following precepts of Theory Y?[61]

1. Management is responsible for organizing the elements of productive enterprise—money, materials, equipment, people—in the interest of economic ends.
2. People are not by nature passive or resistant to organizational needs. They have become so as a result of experience in organizations.
3. The motivation, the potential for development, the capacity for assuming responsibility, and the readiness to direct behavior toward organizational goals are all present in people. Management does not put them there. It is the responsibility of management to make it possible for people to recognize and develop these characteristics for themselves.
4. The essential task of management is to arrange organizational conditions and methods of operation so that people can achieve their own goals best by directing their own efforts toward organizational objectives.

McGregor's Theory Y was used to change personnel behavior in a skilled nursing facility. An "audit process created unit expectations which provided a sense of accomplishment, personal growth and motivation to seek more responsibility." The staff was provided with extensive in-service education. "Noting," the leaving of notes for the responsible staff person to correct noncompliance, was accepted as peer review to foster responsibility and accountability. The goal was to manage personnel to meet their needs for self-respect and improvement.[62]

Nurse Managers and Motivation

The first manager known to tackle the problem of productivity was Robert Owen (1771–1858) in his textile mill in Lanark, Scotland, in the 1820s. Owen is known as a manager who related to the work, the worker, the enterprise, and the manager.[63] His knowledge of technical skills and their applications, along with his use of underlying motivational theory, made him a forerunner in participatorial organizations.

Nurse managers should apply techniques, skills, and knowledge, including knowledge of motivational theory, to help people obtain what they want out of nursing work. At the same time these efforts should be directed so as to achieve the objectives of the institution and the division of nursing.

To persuade people to apply their skills to achieve nursing and organizational goals requires many things on the part of the nurse manager: brilliance and sensitivity to people; energy and negotiating skills; gaining people's attention so that their aspirations and emotions are melded with those of a leader, the profession, and the organization for which they work; and integrity so that people will be controlled only to the extent necessary. To successfully lead today's nurses toward accomplishing the goals of nursing, nurse leaders should do motivational research or at least be aware of the findings of motivational research and apply them to personnel management. Through intuition, observation, and knowledge, the nurse's objectives are mixed with those of leaders (and consequently those of nursing management and the nursing profession). The objectives will be restated so that when approved by the group they are seen as desirable ones to attain. This process requires intellectual skills that open nurses' hearts and minds, analysis of their perceptions, and synthesis of their perceptions with those of leadership. To achieve results will require mental agility, emotional intensity, and communication and negotiation skills.

Motivational research is a prime subject for continuing education for nurse leaders.

Several authors make a good case for saying that one person cannot motivate another and that motivation lies within the individual. The choice of action lies with the individual. Incentives should be meaningful to the individual, and motivation should be stimulating on an individual basis. The organization has a set of standards it wants met in providing care that is satisfactory to patients. Nurses want remuneration for providing that care, which they provide best as part of an organized group. Interaction between employee and employer is essential to a contract. For interaction to be successful, rapport and involvement must exist. A successful contract depends on the employer's authority to give or withhold rewards and the employee's level of aspiration. Does the nurse want to advance if risks increase? To find out nurses' needs and aspirations, ask them. Note their individual responses to a variety of work assignments and incentives. A person will seldom respond to being seen as just a number. Personnel policies must provide support to supervisors. Communication that identifies needs is not an invasion of privacy but rather a realistic approach that leads to mutual trust and frankness among people.[64]

Motivation is an emotional process; it is psychological rather than logical. The nurse leader should first learn how a nurse wants to feel and then help that nurse use the tools that will encourage attainment of those feelings. These tools may derive from associations with people on the job that make the nurse feel accepted, performance of those acts for which he or she is highly skilled, and recognition for a satisfactory performance.

Motivation is basically an unconscious process. When asked why he or she did a certain thing, a nurse may not be able to give an answer. Even though a person's basic motives are hidden and intangible, his or her actions make sense to him- or herself.

Motivational patterns are learned early and followed for years. There is no conscious selection, judgment, or decision making involved in 95% of what people do.

Each person is unique, with the key to behavior lying within the self. A leader uses judgment to figure out why each person reacts in a given way to a certain situation. Within each individual, motivating needs differ from time to time. The key is to figure out which need is currently predominant.

Human beings, including nurses, motivate themselves. The nurse leader will provide or deprive practicing nurses of the opportunity to satisfy their needs.[65]

The motivational theory under discussion asserts that a person—if freed to some extent, by his or her presence in an affluent society, from the necessity to use most of his or her energy to obtain the necessities of life and a degree of security—will by nature begin to pursue goals associated with higher-level needs. These include needs for a degree of control over his or her fate, for self-respect, for using and increasing his or her talents, for responsibility, and for achievement (both in the sense of status and recognition and in the sense of personal development and effective problem solving). Thus freed, he or she will also seek in many ways to satisfy more fully his or her physical needs for recreation, relaxation, and play. Management has been well aware of the latter tendency; it has not often recognized the former, or at least it has not taken into account its implication for managerial strategy.

Hard Approach Versus Soft Approach to Nursing Management

What are the effects of a hard approach to personnel management (i.e., coercion and disguised threats, close supervision, and tight controls over behavior)? Experience has shown that such an approach causes resistance, including the restriction of output, militant unionism, and subtle but effective sabotage of the objectives of management.

Nurses turn to labor organizations when they fail to achieve results from their supervisors and when authoritarian managers manage from the top down. These managers use job descriptions, performance standards and evaluations, rules, pay incentives, promotions, management objectives, and dismissal threats. Nurses are not consulted on any of these management tools and activities.

The soft approach to personnel management, such as permissiveness, satisfying people's demands, and achievement of harmony, has been proven to cause indifferent performance, with expectations of receiving more and giving less. As a consequence, many managers try to take a middle-of-the-road approach.

Observation and the evidence of the social sciences indicate that employees' behavior shapes itself to management perceptions. This behavior does not result from individual nature but from the nature of organizations, management philosophy, policy, and practice. The nurse leader looks for simple, practical, immediate ideas to solve personnel problems. There are no magic wands, but that does not mean there are no solutions.

Solutions

Career Planning

Career planning is a continuous process of self-assessment and goal setting. It is a cooperative venture between the organization and the employee, the career counselor (who could be a mentor or sponsor) and the individual nurse. Career planning is an organized system with short- and long-term career goals fitted to those of the organization.

To build a career development program requires major effort. An advisory committee can be formed. Staff development personnel can be career counselors. The real goal is the self-development of a career plan for every nurse, a plan fostered by the nursing organization. For this reason the individual nurse is best involved in the entire career development program from its inception. Most nurses will benefit from participation in a career development program, even if it improves only the quality of their working lives. The following outline details the major activities of a career development program:[66]

1. Assess the future goals and labor power needs of the nursing organization with relation to recruitment, promotion, hiring, placement, retention, and turnover.
2. Develop job structures with career paths and qualifications, including career opportunities within the nursing organization.
3. Recruit qualified applicants, including those already employed within the nursing organization.

4. Assess applicants on an individual basis for personal expectations. Why are they making this career choice? What are their needs, motivators, and job satisfiers? What stresses make them frustrated and dissatisfied? What stresses excite them? What are their career goals? How does their present performance relate to their career goals? What are their competencies and interests? What potential performance will be needed to achieve their career goals?
5. Develop an individual career development plan for the individual nurse.
6. Provide developmental opportunities for the individual nurse to achieve career goals.

Communication

Producing quality nursing products and services requires highly motivated practicing nurses. Nurse leaders can motivate nurses by sharing information about the organization. Consultative leaders consult with nurses on problems, solutions, and decisions, and they share information about results.

Teamwork

Nurse leaders can motivate practicing nurses by encouraging teamwork. Teams can be built from work groups to discuss and resolve work-related issues. Teams should have identifiable output; inclusive membership; leaders with carefully circumscribed authority; agreement on purpose; rules of procedure; and measurable goals, resources, and feedback. Teams are successful because they pool interpersonal skills, knowledge, and the expertise needed to accomplish goals effectively and efficiently.

By using teams, Hewlett-Packard has cut labor costs, reduced defects, solved vendor problems, eliminated jobs, decreased inspections, cut scrap production, and reached targets ahead of schedule. Teamwork helps workers achieve personal recognition, raise self-esteem, and increase motivation and commitment. It is stimulated by trust, support, completion, acknowledgment, communication, and agreement.[67]

Teamwork raises the spirits of nurses during a time of economic recession, cutbacks, and curtailment of capital expenditures.

Teamwork is used to clarify the purpose or mission of a department or unit, to define a vision of the process and product of team effort, to identify blocks and barriers to team members' vision, to look at ways the work group members support each other, to make requests and agreements about how each can work better with others on the team, and to plan the team's work goals and activities and commit each member to accomplishing them. The result is an effective team in which each member feels personally satisfied.[68]

Team processes are developmental. A summary of the developmental stages of teams as described by Farley includes four stages: orientation, adaptation, emergence, and production. Farley describes the characteristics, team leader tasks, member tasks, and ideal outcomes for each of these four stages.[69]

Self-Esteem

Having self-esteem means having a stable, firmly based, usually high evaluation of oneself. Self-esteem involves having self-respect and self-confidence. Being held in esteem by others because of one's personal accomplishments and reputation provides status and recognition, makes one feel appreciated and respected, and increases one's self-esteem. It satisfies one's desire to have strength among family, friends, colleagues, supervisors, patients, visitors, and others.[70]

Self-esteem is gained through strength, achievement of goals, adequacy, mastery, confidence, and independence. Exhibit 12-2 shows examples of self-esteem based on strength. Self-esteem entails satisfying the desire for achievement of personal, professional, and organizational goals, as illustrated in Exhibit 12-3. Self-esteem

EXHIBIT 12-2

Examples of Self-Esteem Through Strength

1. Educators have strength when they know that other employees want to hire them because of their demonstrated influence with nurses, physicians, and others. They have self-esteem when this gives them satisfaction.
2. Nurse administrators have strength when chosen by top management to expand their spheres of responsibility to direct other departments and when recognized by other administrators for skills and knowledge—being consulted by legislators or leaders in nursing and health care. They have self-esteem when this gives them satisfaction.

EXHIBIT 12-3

Examples of Self-Esteem Through Achievement of Goals

1. A professional nurse satisfies the desire for self-esteem by running for and winning a government office or an office in some service or professional organization.
2. A professional nurse satisfies the desire for self-esteem by achieving credentials such as certification, an advanced degree, or computer skills.
3. A professional nurse manager satisfies a desire for self-esteem by lowering the absenteeism and turnover rates of personnel in the nursing division.

comes from satisfaction of the desire for adequacy, that is, feeling worthwhile as a person in society and as a worker. (See Exhibit 12-4.) Self-esteem involves satisfying the desire for mastery of and competence in the knowledge and skills needed to perform a role as a member of a family, and as a citizen and in clinical practice, management, education, or research. (See Exhibit 12-5.) Self-esteem comes from acquiring a feeling of confidence in the face of the world. (See Exhibit 12-6.) Self-esteem involves satisfying the desire for independence and freedom. A person must be free to speak, to act without hurting others, to express himself or herself, to investigate and seek information, and to defend himself or herself. Each person must be treated with justice, fairness, honesty, and orderliness in the group (see Exhibit 12-7).

Other terms can be used to describe self-esteem. These include valuing oneself or estimating one's worth. Our goal is to value ourselves highly, to consider ourselves favorably, to appreciate and think well of ourselves. We also want others to have a high regard for us, to honor and admire us.

In terms of Maslow's hierarchy of needs, self-esteem is a higher-level need in the ego category. It emerges after physiological, safety, belonging, and love needs are fairly well gratified. Although self-actualization needs are higher in the hierarchy, this hierarchy does not follow the same order in everyone. Rarely are self-esteem needs fully satisfied.

EXHIBIT 12-4
Examples of Self-Esteem Through Adequacy

1. A professional nurse feels that she is a good wife and mother because she can work a schedule compatible with her husband's, be involved in the activities of her family, and save money for her children's college education.
2. A staff nurse in the recovery room feels she has the time to assess, plan, and give good care and attend to good documentation of care. She even has an opportunity to obtain reading references needed to keep professional knowledge and skills updated.

EXHIBIT 12-5
Examples of Self-Esteem Through Mastery

1. A nurse educator involves clinical nurses in preparing strategic objectives for a unit. The plan is approved by the organization's administrators.
2. A clinical nurse is selected to implement a theory of nursing about which the nurse is considered an authority.

EXHIBIT 12-6
Examples of Self-Esteem Through Confidence

1. A professional nurse goes to work confident of his or her ability to perform as well as any other nurse, and better than some; of his or her ability to learn whatever is needed to do a job well; that his or her abilities will be recognized and that credit will be given; that full merit pay will be earned; and that the employer's standards as well as those of the ANA, the JCAHO, and other internal and external agencies can be met.
2. A professional nurse decides to win support and run as a candidate for president of the district nurses' association and wages a successful campaign.

EXHIBIT 12-7
Examples of Self-Esteem Through Independence

1. A supervisor decides to learn something about joint practice as a modality of nursing and obtains information and writes a position paper on it. The administrator suggests making a plan to practice it. The supervisor sets a specific schedule to orient and gain approval of the clinical nurses and then the physicians who use the unit.
2. Clinical nurses are given complete freedom to manage the care of their patients, including coordination with personnel of x-ray, medical laboratory, nutrition and food service, and with physicians and others.

People meet their esteem needs in different ways. They are influenced by culture, including the culture of the organization in which they work. The ends or results of achieving self-esteem are more important than the roads taken to achieve those ends or results. All human beings want to be esteemed, unless they are pathological. Persons lacking self-esteem feel inferior, weak, helpless, and discouraged. They become indolent, passive, resistant to change, irresponsible, and unwilling to follow a dialogue. In the workplace, persons lacking self-esteem focus on salary and benefits, making unreasonable demands for economic benefits. They can become neurotic or emotionally ill when they lack self-esteem.[71]

People want a good reputation and to have prestige; they want respect or esteem from others. They want to be recognized, to have attention, to be important, and to be appreciated.

Meeting the self-esteem needs of employees is of great significance to managers in nursing. Most nurses work in bureaucratic organizations such as hospitals, home health care agencies, nursing homes, and clinics.

In such places, work is organized to meet many concerns such as those of the organization, physicians, and the routines and personnel of other departments. The lower levels of the hierarchy have few opportunities to meet nurses' ego needs. Nurses schedule care of their patients around everyone else. They are the servants of the organization.

Direction and control are useless in motivating professional nurses whose social, ego, and self-fulfillment needs are predominant. Intellectual creativity is a characteristic of professional nurses who do not get ego satisfaction from wages, pensions, vacations, or other benefits of work. The job itself must be satisfying and fun if professional nurses are to satisfy their self-esteem needs. Professional nurses get their ego needs met by having a voice in decision making. They will commit to organizational objectives when they are allowed to determine the steps to take to achieve them. Nurses want to collaborate with other professionals, both internal and external to the environment in which they work.

Full use of their talents and training is another desire of professional nurses. They want critical attention paid to the nature of nursing as a clinical practice discipline, to the organization of nursing functions, and to job challenges. They do not want close and detailed supervision. One reason for the success of primary nursing has been the control professional nurses have over the nursing of patients who are their primary responsibility. This success will continue if management gives attention to a career development plan. Such a plan's logical evolution is a joint practice in which physicians and nurses collaborate to give total care to patients. Professional nurses want opportunities to develop within their professional careers as clinical nurses. Career ladder progression must relate to clinical practice.[72]

What can management do to meet nurses' needs for self-esteem? Management can set the conditions under which professional nurses become committed to organizational goals and exercise self-control and self-direction, which leads to creativity.

What do managers get from their jobs? Freedom? Social satisfaction? Opportunities for achievement? Knowledge? The ability to create? Who gets the reward and for what? Who must provide the opportunities for increased dignity, achievement, prestige, and social satisfaction?

Strategic planning by top management can involve professional clinical nurse participation. The strategic plan can then be submitted to the department level for input by clinical nurses and other professionals. They will critique the plan, strengthen it, and make it one to which nurses can commit. This management process will be a difficult task, the accomplishment of which gives professional nurses new knowledge and skills, opportunity for creativity, and recognition and prestige in the eyes of others, thus meeting nurses' ego needs for self-esteem.

In the area of performance evaluation, nurse managers can again set the stage for meeting the self-esteem needs of professional nurses who want to be evaluated, promoted, rotated, and transferred in terms of their clinical or other personal career motivations. Self-evaluation in which individuals plan and appraise their contributions to organizational objectives promotes self-esteem. Conventional performance appraisal attacks it.[73]

It is obvious that management can create the conditions under which professional nurses can meet their esteem needs. Management can make nurses feel good about themselves by providing adequate staffing to give good nursing care; by correct placement and orientation to achieve mastery, independence, and freedom; by respecting them for a job well done; and by encouraging deserved respect from coworkers and employees.[74]

Self-esteem involves the personhood of all professional nurses, be they managers, clinical nurses, researchers, or teachers. Each person should enrich the esteem of another person and should be the peer pal, mentor, sponsor, and guardian of the person within the profession. Esteem results in leading and influencing. One can listen to other people, treat them as individuals, show earnest exhilaration in responding to their creativity, offer ideas for improvement, and share the excitement of their successes and victories. Success provides a good positive self-image and builds self-esteem. It avoids the pain of failure.[75]

Self-Actualization

Self-actualization is defined by Maslow as an ego need at the top of the needs hierarchy. Self-actualization does not exist in isolation. In some persons, it may be no stronger than is the love and belonging need or the self-esteem need.

Self-actualized persons have the following characteristics:

- Ability to see reality more clearly than do others.
- Comfort with and attraction to the unknown.
- Creativity in whatever they do and perceive.
- Less defensiveness and artifice than others have; acceptance and adjustment to their own shortcomings.
- Discomfort when they are not doing something to improve their shortcomings, prejudices, jealousies, envy, and other faults of humanity.
- Autonomous codes of ethics.
- Ability to conform easily when no great issues are involved.

- Acceptance of their own nature, human nature, the realities of social life, and the constraints of physical reality.
- Problem-centered, not ego-centered.
- Broad and universal values.
- Deeply democratic, as opposed to authoritarian, natures; thus they respect others.
- A strong sense of right and wrong, of good and evil.
- Not interested in hostile humor. Their humor is of a philosophical bent, stated only to produce a laugh.
- Self-movers.
- Detachment and objectivity in conditions of turmoil.

Self-actualized people like solitude and privacy. Although they generally want to help the human race and can sometimes feel like strangers in a strange land, their relationships with others are profound and their circle of friends is small. They love children and humanity but can be briefly hostile when that hostility is justified for the good of others. In social terms, self-actualized people are godly but not religious. They are not conventional, but they conform to social graces with tolerance. They can be radical.

Self-actualized people develop detachment from the culture. They become autonomous and accepting.

Maslow indicates that living at the higher need level is good for growth and health, both physically and psychologically. Self-actualized persons live longer, have less disease, sleep and eat better, and enjoy their sexual lives without unnecessary inhibitions. For them, life continues to be fresh, thrilling, exciting, and ecstatic. They count their blessings.

Self-actualized people have mystic or peak experiences. These are natural experiences. Happiness can cause tears. It comes from appreciation for poetry, music, philosophy, religion, interpersonal relationships, beauty, or politics. The peak experience can come from doing or from sensing.

Self-actualized people merge or unify dichotomies, such as selfishness, considering every act to be both selfish and unselfish. They perceive work as play and duty as pleasure. The purpose of higher needs is a "healthward" trend—when people experience them, they place a higher value on them.

Self-actualized people are "metamotivated." Their motivations are for character growth, character expression, maturation, and development. They place more dependence on self-development and inner growth than they do on the prestige and status of others' honor.

Self-actualizing people are not perfect. They can be (or can be perceived to be) joyless; mundane; silly, wasteful, or thoughtless in habits; boring, stubborn, or irritating; superficially vain or proud; partial to their own productions, family, friends, or children; temperamental; ruthless; strong and independent of others' opinions; shocking in language and behavior; concentrated to the point of absent-mindedness or humorlessness; mistaken; or needing improvement. They can feel guilt, anxiety, sadness, self-castigation, internal strife, and conflict.

The satisfaction of higher needs requires more preconditions, such as more people, larger scenes, longer runs, more means and partial goals, and more subordinate or preliminary steps. To achieve the higher needs requires better environmental conditions.

Pursuit and gratification of higher needs have desirable civic and social consequences: loyalty, friendliness, and civic consciousness. People who are living at this level make better parents, spouses, teachers, and public servants. They also create greater, stronger, and truer individualism. They are synergistic.

One possible conclusion is that the self-actualized person achieves a highly satisfactory quality of life and that this quality of life extends from the gratified self-actualized person into society. The social environment of work, family, community, government, and the like can positively influence gratification or satisfaction of the higher-level needs.

Applying these insights to nursing, the nurse leader would selectively apply knowledge and skills of the social and behavioral sciences to create an environment or climate in which practicing nurses can become self-actualized. In doing so, nurse managers themselves become self-actualized, and the products and services of nursing increase in quantity and quality.

Although critics of Maslow's work say it is based on too narrow a population, the theory is widely accepted and used. Maslow analyzed the profiles of 60 subjects, including Lincoln, Jefferson, Einstein, and Frederick Douglass. He suggested that the self-determined population might be limited to being from 5% to 30% of the total (another prediction criticized by other scientists).[76]

Self-Concept

Self-concept has been analyzed as a nursing diagnosis. Its components are in body image, self-esteem, and personal identity. The nursing diagnoses under "human responses pattern, perceiving," include body image disturbance, personal identity disturbance, and chronic low or situational self-esteem disturbance. Self-concept results from experience and is a determinant of behavior. LeMone adapted Roy's definition of self-concept as follows: "Self-concept is a composite of thoughts, values, and feelings that one has for one's physical and personal self at any given time, formed from interactions with the environment and with other people, and directing one's behavior."[77]

Maslow emphasized self-actualization as the motivating force in developing one's unique self-concept.

Other Activities to Stimulate Motivation

Motivation is stimulated by activities such as job enrichment; praise; empowerment; employee stock ownership plans; lateral promotions; inclusion in organizational actions; and focus on vision, values, and strategy. (Some of these activities or strategies have been discussed in other chapters.)

All employees should be able to describe the values of their employer. These values are identified, defined, prioritized, and communicated through means such as booklets and orientation programs. Values are critical in empowerment. Managers should emphasize the value of people by trusting, respecting, and encouraging them. They should tie rewards to values of teamwork, innovation, safety, growth, and profitability and provide employees with financial and nonfinancial rewards.

Taking the following actions capitalizes on the power of a value-driven management system:[78]

- Identify, define, and prioritize critical values through communication and involvement at all organizational levels, including board support.
- Measure the organization's perceptions of the defined values and possible areas of conflict.
- Assess customer–client perceptions of the degree to which they feel company actions conform to these values.
- Audit current management practices to evaluate the extent to which they direct, support, and reinforce desired outcomes.
- Modify leadership styles, management systems, and action programs to close the gap between desired and perceived behaviors.
- Develop a reward system that reinforces selected values and confronts and acts on the lack of performance.

Managers should motivate employees by including them in the group's mission. Employees are motivated by detailed explanations, praise, tangible rewards, and constructive criticism. They need time to improve unsatisfactory performance, and when they cannot do so, they should be encouraged to seek another post within the organization.[79]

Firms are using flexible work plans to cut costs and keep the best people. These plans, which reduce forced layoffs, include the following (the companies surveyed included DuPont, Philadelphia Newspapers, IBM, and Avon Products):[80]

- Paternity leave or work-at-home policies. Of firms surveyed in 1987 by Hay/Haggins Company, none had such policies. By 1991, nearly half offered paternity leave, and 14% offered telecommuting options. Flexible hours policies increased from 35% in 1987 to 40% in 1991. These numbers have expanded greatly, and there is even a work-at-home online magazine. Web sites have a wealth of information on flexible hours and on paternity leave policies.
- Reduced work week schedules, job sharing, unpaid leaves of absence, and early retirement.
- Rearranged workdays to allow parents to attend children's school functions or meet other personal and family needs.
- Child care assistance.

Setting personal goals is a way of planning ahead. Doing so provides momentum to employees because it means that they have decided to pursue what they want and to obtain the necessary qualifications. Evaluating job satisfaction as a means of developing foal can also be a useful exercise in goal attainment. Exhibit 12-8 through 12-10 provide tools for setting and evaluating goals, as well as assessing job satisfaction. It is important that they recognize their personal limitations and abilities and use that awareness to initiate the changes needed to achieve their goals. Social and leadership goals gained from aspects of living, such as family, community, and church, are often overlooked credentials for achieving self-improvement and self-fulfillment.

Summary

Effective directing will result in greater harmony in the actions of supervisors and employees and in the achievement of the objectives of personnel as well as of the enterprise. Directing will be most effective when employees have leaders who provide direct personal contact. Directing that encourages leadership, motivation, and communication techniques and emphasizes the human aspects of managing individuals is most desirable. Personal and motivational goals are met as the nurse is motivated to be ambitious and responsible, to show initiative, to be proud of fellow nurses and the employing institution, to welcome change, and to demonstrate individual abilities.

The following rule will lead to successful leadership in nursing: find out where nurses want to go and what they want to accomplish, and bring these goals into line with those of the organization. Then nurses will accomplish organizational goals as they achieve their own. Effective leadership can be fostered by nursing administrators who desire to improve their directing or leading activities.

APPLICATION EXERCISES

EXERCISE 12-1 Look at the statements of mission, philosophy, vision, and objectives of a division of nursing in which you work as a student or an employee.

1. What is the work of the unit or division?
2. What is the implication for the directing function of the unit or division?

EXERCISE 12-2 *Scenario:* Jennie Lynd, RN, has been working in the newborn nursery for one year. Her performance in caring for babies, teaching parents, and supporting other unit personnel has been exemplary. She has been told this. Jennie Lynd tells her nurse manager she is interested in transferring to the pediatric intensive care unit. With a group of your peers, decide how the nurse manager should handle this request.

EXERCISE 12-3 *Scenario:* As a nurse manager, Ms. Pressley, RN, has studied career development theory because she believes that clinical nurses do not really have careers. This is particularly true when a clinical ladder is nonexistent. Ms. Pressley plans to counsel her clinical nurses regularly and to push for a clinical promotion ladder that recognizes advanced competence, education, and certification. This activity falls within the directing category of management. Compare Ms. Pressley's actions with those of several other nurse managers you know or have known. Summarize your findings.

EXERCISE 12-4 Select one or more goals you would like to accomplish in the unit in which you work as a student or employee. Make a management plan to accomplish them.

1. Cover your individual objectives.
2. Be discussed and adjusted with your boss.
3. Have a plan for achieving each objective.
4. Set a time to evaluate accomplishments with your boss.

EXERCISE 12-5 Use Exhibit 12-1, Standards for Evaluating the Directing Function, to evaluate one of the entities in the organization where you work as a student or employee. Identify one concrete example for each standard. Summarize your results. If the directing function does not meet the standards, use a problem-solving approach and implement a plan of improvement.

EXERCISE 12-6 Use Exhibit 12-8, Future Goals Worksheet, to develop a list of goals. Once you have them written down, you can evaluate them using Exhibit 12-9, Goal Evaluation Checklist.

EXHIBIT 12-8
Future Goals Worksheet

You should set goals in at least three areas:

1. **Personal Goals.** What would you really like to do with your life? Write down the personal goals you want to accomplish. Examples are "Become a role model for the profession," "Achieve as a writer in the field of staff development," or "Serve people who need but lack the means to buy health care."

   ____

   ____

2. **Family Goals.** Do you want to save money to travel? To put yourself and your family through school? To supplement a primary income? To buy something special? You may want to discuss these goals with your spouse and children, but write down your family goals.

   ____

   ____

3. **Professional Goals.** Do you want to become a professor, a director of nursing, a consultant in nursing care of cancer patients, a clinical researcher, something outside of nursing altogether? Write down your professional goals.

   ____

   ____

EXHIBIT 12-9
Goal Evaluation Checklist

STANDARDS FOR EVALUATING GOALS	YES	NO
1. I have reviewed my short-term goals within the past 3 months.		
2. I have reviewed my long-term goals within the past year.		
3. My goals reflect my personal philosophy or beliefs and the purpose or reason I want to achieve them.		
4. My goals can be measured or verified as being achieved.		
5. I have set my goals in the priority or sequence in which I want to accomplish them.		
6. My goals are clear to me. They are specific and indicate actions to take to achieve them.		
7. My goals are flexible and realistic so that I will have as many opportunities as possible.		
8. I have the resources to accomplish my goals.		
9. My goals are stated for a specific job.		

EXERCISE 12-7 Small Group Session

1. Write a statement that provides a vision of what you want to accomplish in stimulating the motivation of your peers or employees. (20 minutes)
2. Outline a process for accomplishing this vision. (20 minutes)
3. Report.

EXERCISE 12-8 Complete Exhibit 12-10, Checklist for Assessing Job Satisfaction, and use it to develop goals that you can achieve. Don't forget that all responsibility for personal satisfaction in life is ultimately your own. We have to take action to help ourselves, to be informed, to become better educated, to improve our interpersonal relationships, and to make our lives meaningful.

EXHIBIT 12-10

Checklist for Assessing Job Satisfaction

IN MY CURRENT JOB I AM	YES	NO OR INSUFFICIENT
Happy with being able to help others.		
Intellectually stimulated and challenged.		
Given opportunity to progress educationally.		
Learning new skills.		
Sharpening old skills.		
Learning a new discipline.		
Qualifying for more responsibility.		
Qualifying for more respect.		
Given opportunities to attend staff meetings, patient care conferences, and staff-development programs.		
Rewarded for doing my job well.		
Adequately paid.		
Given opportunity for advancement.		
Given opportunity to innovate and be creative.		
Given opportunity to choose shifts and hours of work.		
Given opportunity to be a leader.		
Given opportunity to grow as a bedside nurse.		
Able to trust my supervisors and peers.		
Supported by administration.		
Communicated with by administration.		
Being paid for my total knowledge and experience.		
Confident of job security.		
Working with adequate staffing.		
Feeling satisfied with my accomplishments.		
Supported by nursing management in resolving physician–nurse conflict.		
Able to resolve peer conflict.		
Adequately paid for overtime.		
Given opportunity to schedule extra time off above and beyond holidays and vacation.		
Given opportunity to schedule my working hours.		
Prepared to function as a team leader or charge nurse.		
Supported by competent professional nurses who assist and teach me.		

EXHIBIT 12-10 *(continued)*

My job satisfaction could be increased by:

____

____

Identify specific steps to gather the information or make the changes that will help you reach your goal.

____

____

One of my job satisfaction goals is:

____

____

As a step toward reaching this goal I will talk to: ______________________________

about: ____

and I will undertake the following activities myself:

____

____

EXERCISE 12-9 *Scenario:* Ms. Sanchez has been director of nursing of a 250-bed hospital for 8 years. Although her management operation has followed traditional patterns, she has read extensively on the subject and has been taking business administration courses in the evenings at the state university. Ms. Sanchez has decided to make some management changes in her department.

Although meetings with members of the nursing staff had been held on a scheduled basis, they were never productive and served mainly as a medium for information to flow from management downward. Ms. Sanchez carefully planned an agenda for her next staff development faculty meeting and distributed it a week in advance. An item of new business on the agenda was to write specific objectives for these meetings that would benefit the members and ultimately the nursing employees throughout the institution. At the same time, Ms. Sanchez would present a working draft of an operational plan for accomplishing the objectives of the department of nursing. The staff development nurse group would be asked to discuss the departmental mission, philosophy, objectives, and operational plan to determine whether the statements express a vision that would motivate nursing personnel.

At the meeting, Ms. Sanchez was pleased with the active participation by the members. They had many suggestions for changes and for additional activities that would be helpful in achieving the mission, philosophy, objectives, and operational plan. During the discussion Ms. Sanchez learned about many major dissatisfactions of these personnel. For example, they did not understand the personnel rating system and wanted to know how she arrived at decisions for promotions. One of the suggested activities for accomplishment of objectives was that job standards be written and that they use the ANA standards for nursing practice as a basis for them. The members appointed an ad hoc committee to do this, without the prodding of Ms. Sanchez, and they set a target date for completion. It was their intent to help Ms. Sanchez strengthen the objectivity of the rating system, thereby giving them input into the promotion process. The members also made plans to expand the project through inclusion of representatives of the entire nursing staff.

(continued)

EXERCISE 12-9
(continued)

Next, Ms. Sanchez asked if the statements of the department's mission, philosophy, objectives, and operational plan should be presented to all the nursing staff, and a large majority of members agreed that they should. They also recommended that Ms. Sanchez do this, because the staff would be impressed with being able to discuss these important statements with the boss. A suggestion was made that Ms. Sanchez meet with the staff of each unit; the ad hoc committee members wrote a schedule that was acceptable to her. The committee then decided to assist unit personnel with developing or revising statements of mission, philosophy, and objectives, and operational plans for each of the units and to have them done by a specific date.

Ms. Sanchez discussed means of encouraging the nursing staff to be more productive and better satisfied with their working conditions. Several suggestions were made by the staff development nurse group. These included modifications in policies related to the uniform, staffing, and time schedules. The nurses also stated that many nursing personnel had expressed the desire to become more involved in unit in-service education and other nursing activities but had not been encouraged to do so. Ms. Sanchez said she would welcome all suggestions for change but that she could not guarantee that all would take place immediately, because some would have to be approved by the hospital administrator. If Ms. Sanchez did not agree with any of the recommendations she would tell the people involved the reasons why. They agreed that this was acceptable to them, and the meeting was adjourned. From this scenario:

1. Identify a factor that encourages or discourages freedom to speak, that is, communication.
2. Identify a factor that encourages or discourages freedom to do what one wishes to do without harming others, that is, choice of jobs, friends, or entertainment.
3. Identify a factor that encourages or discourages freedom to express oneself, that is, creativity.
4. Identify a factor that encourages or discourages freedom to defend oneself, justice, fairness, honesty, or orderliness in the group.
5. Identify a factor that encourages or discourages freedom to investigate and seek information.

EXERCISE 12-10

Scenario: Ms. Rather is in charge of pediatric unit in-service education and encourages employees to discuss their families and their off-duty activities. They tell her of their hopes and dreams and even of confidential personal happenings. Mr. Pottinger is in charge of in-service education on an intensive care unit. He gives personnel needed supervision and training and supports them well while on duty. He lets it be known that he does not want to know anything about employees' personal lives unless it relates to their work.

1. Which nurse exhibits the best understanding of motivational theory?
2. What motivational theory has been exhibited by the nurse you selected?

EXERCISE 12-11

Using Herzberg's two-factor theory of motivation and the items in Exhibit 12-10, Checklist for Assessing Job Satisfaction, do the following:

1. Summarize the results of the extrinsic conditions, hygiene factors, or dissatisfiers related to yourself and your job.
2. Summarize the results of the intrinsic conditions, motivators, or satisfiers related to yourself and your job.

EXERCISE 12-12 Self-Esteem Exercises

1. List the strengths or abilities to influence others that you have and that give you self-esteem. How can you improve them?
2. List the personal, professional, and organizational goals of achievement that make you think well of yourself. How can you improve them?
3. List the things that make you feel adequate in your personal life and your job. How can you improve them?
4. List two or more major areas in which you have achieved mastery and competence. List one or more in which you desire to achieve mastery and competence.
5. List those qualities that give you confidence in the face of the world. How can they be enlarged or improved?
6. List those areas in which your desire for independence and freedom are limited. How can your independence and freedom be expanded?
7. List those activities that tell you that you have a good reputation and the respect of others. Indicate whether your reputation and the respect come from patients, visitors, supervisors, physicians, personnel, or others.
8. List those activities that give you feelings of self-confidence, value, strength, or being useful and needed in the world.
9. List those activities that make you feel inferior, weak, helpless, and discouraged.

EXERCISE 12-13 The following is a list of matched pairs of personal characteristics. Complete the list by circling the characteristic in each pair that you think applies to you, and write a statement summarizing your personal characteristics. Make a plan to change any personal characteristics you believe should be changed to improve your self-esteem.

Personal Characteristics

A	B	A	B
Vivacious	Languid	Honest	Dishonest
Intelligent	Stupid	Truthful	False
Bright	Dull	Accurate	Deceptive
Clever	Clumsy	Confident	Pessimistic
Funny	Solemn	Respectful	Rude
Courteous	Rude	Pleasant	Obnoxious
Prompt	Late	Candid	Deceitful
Tolerant	Prejudiced	Courageous	Fearful
Gracious	Surly	Decent	Gross
Unpretentious	Complacent	Unselfish	Egotistic
Sincere	Devious	Having integrity	Fraudulent
Friendly	Antagonistic	Sincere	Sly
Humble	Arrogant		

Source: Swansburg, R. C. & Swansburg, P. W. (1984). *Strategic career planning and development for nurses.* Rockville, MD: Aspen, 76.

EXERCISE 12-14 The following is one approach to developing standards for the motivation aspects of nursing leadership.

Standards for the Evaluation of the Motivational Aspects of Nursing Leadership

STANDARDS

There is evidence to show that the nurse administrator demonstrates knowledge of the following:

1. Maslow's hierarchy of needs: The manager demonstrates ability to identify employees' physiological, safety, social, esteem, and self-actualization needs, and to create work situations that help meet their needs.
2. Modern motivational theory that relates needs to behavior.
   a. Argyris's immaturity–maturity theory: The manager attempts to make jobs challenging and subordinates as independent as they are capable of being.
   b. Herzberg's two-factor theory of motivation: The manager attempts to prevent dissatisfaction through providing hygiene factors and prompt satisfaction through motivators.
   c. Expectancy theory and learned behavior: The manager promotes an environment in which subordinates see a high probability of achieving objectives that are desirable, and the manager reinforces satisfactory performance with recognition.
      i. Vroom's expectancy theory: The manager recognizes the productivity of subordinates and recommends promotions accordingly, causing them to expect such outcomes.
      ii. Porter and Lawler's theory: The manager acts so that subordinates expect rewards based on performance.
   d. Equity or social comparison theory: The manager recognizes that subordinates adapt and weigh what they give to the enterprise against rewards or benefits.

Apply the standards for evaluation of the motivational aspects of directing nursing personnel, and determine whether there is adequate evidence to show that nurse managers are using modern motivational theory at division, department, service, or unit levels. Summarize your findings.

If the nurse managers are not meeting the standards, discuss with them how they can devise and implement programs to identify and meet the needs of personnel. Summarize your results.

NOTES

1. Watson, C. (2004). Evidence-Based management practices: The challenge for nursing. *Journal of Nursing Administration*, *34*(5), 207–209.
2. Ibid., 208.
3. American Organization of Nurse Executives (AONE). (2004). *2004–2006 strategic plan*. Washington, DC: Author.
4. Watson, 2004, 207.
5. Ibid., 207.
6. AONE, 2004.
7. Fayol, H. (1949). *General and industrial management* (C. Storrs, Trans.). London: Sir Isaac Pitman & Sons, 82–96.
8. Ibid., 97.
9. Ibid., 97–98.
10. Ibid., 103.
11. Urwick, L. (1944). *The elements of administration*. New York: Harper & Row, 77.
12. Ibid., 81–82.
13. Ibid., 90–96.
14. Rowland, H. S. & Rowland, B. L. (Eds.). (1992). *Nursing administration handbook* (3rd ed.). Gaithersburg, MD: Aspen, 10.
15. Ibid., 11.
16. Kron, T. & Durbin, E. (1987). *The management of patient care: Putting leadership skills to work* (10th ed.). Philadelphia: W. B. Saunders, 155–176; Douglass, L. M. (1988). *The effective nurse: Leader and manager* (3rd ed.). St. Louis: Mosby, 115; Strickland, D. & O'Connell, O. C. (1998). Saving your career in the 21st century. *Journal of Case Management*, *1*, 47–51; Retsas, A. (2000). Barriers to using research evidence in nursing practice. *Journal of Advanced Nursing*, 599–606; Neal, J., Brown, T., & Rojjanasrirat, W. (1999). Implementation of a case coordinator role: A focused ethnographic study. *Journal of Professional Nursing*, 349–355; Beal, J. A. (2000). A nurse practitioner model of practice in the neonatal intensive care unit. *MCN: American Journal of Maternal/Child Nursing*, 18–24.
17. Blake, R. R. & Mouton, J. S. (1985). *The managerial grid III* (3rd ed.). Houston: Gulf Publishing, 94.
18. Schulte, T. (1999). Facilitating skills: The art of helping teams succeed. *Hospital Materials Management Quarterly*, 13–26.
19. Arndt, C. & Huckabay, L. M. D. (1980). *Nursing administration: Theory for practice with a systems approach* (2nd ed.). St. Louis: Mosby, 92–106.
20. Koontz, H., O'Donnell, C., & Weihrich, H. (1990). *Essentials of management* (5th ed.). New York: McGraw-Hill, 300.
21. Swansburg, R. C. (1977). *The directing function of nursing service administration*. Hattiesburg, MS: The University of Southern Mississippi School of Nursing, 3–5.
22. Schroeder, R. E. (1998). Using time management to achieve balance. *Medical Group Management Journal*, 20–26, 28.
23. Hansten, R. I. & Jackson, M. (2004). Clinical delegation skills: A handbook for professional practice (3rd ed.). Sudbury, MA: Jones and Bartlett Publishers, 3–4.

24. Beegle, B. B. (1970). Don't do it—Delegate it! *Supervisory Management*, 2–6; Matejka, J. K. & Dunsing, R. J. (1987). Great expectations. *Management World*, 16–17.
25. Matejka & Dunsing, 1987.
26. Rowland & Rowland, 1992, 69–70.
27. Ibid.
28. Odiorne, G. S. (1965). *Management by objectives*. New York: Pitman, 55–56.
29. Ibid.
30. Drucker, P. F. (1973). *Management: Tasks, responsibilities, practices*. New York: Harper & Row, 430–442.
31. Ibid., 441–442.
32. Bell, M. L. (1980). Management by objectives. *Journal of Nursing Administration*, 19–26.
33. Levinson, H. (1970). Management by whose objectives? *Harvard Business Review*, 125–134.
34. Ibid.
35. Peters, T. (1987). *Thriving on chaos*. New York: Harper & Row, 603–604.
36. Osborne, D. & Gaebler, T. (1992). *Reinventing government*. New York: Plume, 156–158.
37. Ibid., 160–168.
38. Beck, A. C., Jr. & Hillman, E. D. (1975). OD to MBO or MBO to OD: Does it make a difference? In A. T. Hollingsworth & R. M. Hodgetts (Eds.), *Readings in basic management* (pp. 190–196). Philadelphia: W. B. Saunders.
39. Liebler, J. G. & McConnell, C. R. *Management principles for health professionals* (4th ed.). Sudbury, MA: Jones and Bartlett Publishers, 270.
40. Ibid., 270.
41. Breyfogle, F., Cupello, J., & Meadows, B. (2000). *Managing six sigma: A practical guide to understanding, assessing and implementing the strategy that yields bottom-line success*. Indianapolis: John Wiley and Sons.
42. Hodgetts, R. M. (1990). *Management: Theory, process, and practice* (5th ed.). Orlando, FL: Harcourt, Brace, Jovanovich, 460.
43. Katzell, R. A. & Thompson, D. E. (1990). Work motivation. *American Psychologist*, 144–153.
44. Ibid.
45. Maslow, A. H. (1970). *Motivation and personality* (2nd ed.). New York: Harper & Row; http://www.accel-team.com/motivation/theory.
46. Gibson, J. L., Ivancevich, J. M., & Donnelly, J. M., Jr. (1994). *Organizations: Behavior, structure, processes* (8th ed.). Burr Ridge, IL: Richard D. Irwin, 151–193.
47. Hodgetts, 1990, 478–479; McGregor, D. (1966). *Leadership and motivation*. Cambridge, MA: MIT Press; http://www.accel-team.com/human–relations.
48. Gibson, Ivancevich, & Donnelly, Jr., 1994, 176–177.
49. Murphy, E. C. (1984). What motivates people to work? *Nursing Management*, 61–62; Gordon, G. K. (1982). Developing a motivating environment. *Journal of Nursing Administration*, 11–16; http://www.accel-team.com/human–relations.
50. Katzell & Thompson, 1990.
51. Gibson, Ivancevich, & Donnelly, Jr., 1994, 168–193; Roach, K. L. (1984). Production builds on mutual respect. *Nursing Management*, 54–56; Youker, R. B. (1985). Ten benefits of participant action planning. *Training*, 52, 54–56.
52. Gibson, Ivancevich, & Donnelly, Jr., 1994; www.accel-team.com/motivation/theory.
53. Ibid.
54. Ibid.
55. Fleury, J. (1992). The application of motivational theory to cardiovascular risk reduction. *Image*, 229–239; www.accel-team.com/human–relations.
56. Gordon, 1982.
57. Roach, 1984; Pryor, M. G. & Mondy, W. (1978). Mutual respect key to productivity. *Supervisory Management*, 10–17.
58. Drucker, 1973, 176, 195–196.
59. Konstam, P. (1992, February 12). Greenspan joins cry for better education. San Antonio Express-News, p. G1.
60. McGregor, 1966, 5–6.
61. Ibid., 15.
62. Griffin, M. (1988). Assumptions for success. *Nursing Management*, 32U–32X.
63. Drucker, 1973, 23.
64. Lancaster, J. (1985). Creating a climate for excellence. *Journal of Nursing Administration*, 16–19; Ackerman, L. (1970). Let's put motivation where it belongs: Within the individual. *Personnel Journal*, 559–562.
65. Miller, M. (1968). Understanding human behavior and employee motivation. *Notes & Quotes*; McGregor, 1966, 211–212.
66. Kleinknecht, M. K. & Hefferin, E. A. (1982). Assisting nurses toward professional growth: A career development model. *Journal of Nursing Administration*, 30–36; Crout, J. C. (1984). Care plan for retaining the new nurse. *Nursing Management*, 30–33; Swansburg, R. C. & Swansburg, P. W. (1984). *Strategic career planning and development for nurses*. Rockville, MD: Aspen.
67. Allender, M. C. (1984). Productivity enhancement: A new teamwork approach. *National Productivity Review*, 181–189.
68. Cornett-Cooke, P. & Dias, K. (1984). Teambuilding: Getting it all together. *Nursing Management*, 16–17.
69. Farley, M. J. (1991). Teamwork in perioperative nursing: Understanding team development, effectiveness, evaluation. *AORN Journal*, 732–733.
70. Maslow, 1970.
71. Fuszard, B. (Ed.). (1984). *Self-actualization for nurses: Issues, trends, and strategies for job enrichment*. Rockville, MD: Aspen, 140.
72. McGregor, 1966.
73. Fuszard, 1984.
74. Ibid., 40.
75. Ibid., 207.
76. Maslow, 1970.
77. LeMone, P. (1991). Analysis of a human phenomenon: Self-Concept. *Nursing Diagnosis*, 126–130.
78. Ginsburg, L. & Miller, N. (1992). Value-driven management. *Business Horizons*, *1*, 23–27.
79. Hicks, L. (1994, March 17). Motivation key to successful employment. *San Antonio Express-News*, pp. 1E–2E.
80. Trost, C. (1992, February 18). To cut costs and keep the best people, more concerns offer flexible work plans. *Wall Street Journal*, p. B1.

REFERENCES

Al-Shehri, A. (1992). The market and educational principle in continuing medical education for general practice. *Medical Education*, *26*, 384–387.

Ash, S. (1992). A big job: How to psych yourself up. *Supervisory Management*, 9.

Astra, R. L. & Singg, S. (2000). The role of self-esteem in affiliation. *Journal of Psychology*, 15–22.

Barber, A. E., Dunham, R. B., & Formisano, R. A. (1992). The impact of flexible benefits on employee satisfaction: A field study. *Personal Psychology*, 55–75.

Blanchard, K. & Johnson, S. (1982). *The one minute manager*. New York: William Morrow.

Dearhammer, W. G. (1991). Con: Promotion calls for proper preparation. *Business Credit, 1*, 27–28.

Donadio, P. J. (1992). Capturing the principles of motivation. *Business Credit*, 40.

Dowless, R. (1992). Motivating salespeople: One order of eEmpowerment, hold the carrots. *Training, 16*, 73–74.

Emblen, J. D. & Gray, G. T. (1990). Comparison of nurses' self-directed learning activities. *Journal of Continuing Education in Nursing, 21*(2), 56–61.

Erdman, A. (1992, August 10). What's wrong with workers? *Fortune*, 18.

Farley, M. J. (1991). Teamwork in perioperative nursing: Understanding team development, effectiveness, evaluation. *AORN Journal*, 730–738.

Fong, C. M. (1993). A longitudinal study of the relationship between overload, social support and burnout among nursing educators. *Journal of Nursing Education*, 24–29.

Franklin, A. J. (2000). Invisibility syndrome: A clinical model of the effects of racism on African-American males. *American Journal of Orthopsychiatry*, 33–41.

Ginnodo, W. L. (1985-1986). Consultative management: A fresh look at employee motivation. *National Productivity Review*, 78–80.

Hanks, J. H. (1992). Empowerment in nursing education: Concept analysis and application to philosophy, learning and instruction. *Journal of Advanced Nursing, 17*, 607–618.

Hayes, E. (1993). Managing job satisfaction for the long run. *Nursing Management*, 65–67.

Hotter, A. N. (1992). The clinical nurse specialist and empowerment: Say good-bye to the fairy godmother. *Nursing Administration Quarterly*, 11–15.

Kipnis, D. (1987). Psychology and behavioral technology. *American Psychologist*, 30–36.

Leclerc, G., Lefrancois, R., Dube, M., Hebert, R., & Gaulin, P. (1999). Criterion validity of a new measure of self-actualization. *Psychology Report*, 1167–1176.

Lublin, J. S. (1992, February 13). Trying to increase worker productivity, more employers alter management style. *Wall Street Journal*, pp. B1, B7.

MacDicken, R. A. (1991). Managing the plateaued employee. *Association Management*, 37–39, 57.

Margotta, M. H., Jr. (1991). Pro: Continuing education leads to promotion. *Business Credit*, 26–28.

Maslow, A. H. (1964). *Religion, values and peak experiences*. Columbus, OH: Ohio State University Press.

Maslow, A. H. (1968). *Toward a psychology of being* (2nd ed.). New York: Van Nostrand Reinhold.

Mayo, E. Elton Mayo's Hawthorne experiments, motivation theory, financial motivation. (2000) Retrieved October 3, 2004 from http://www.accel-team.com/motivation/hawthorne.

Meyers, M. E. (1992). Motivating high-tech workers. *Best's Review-Life-Health Insurance Edition*, 86–88.

Nikolajski, P. Y. (1992). Investigating the effectiveness of self-learning packages in staff development. *Journal of Nursing Staff Development*, 179–182.

Pell, A. R. (1992). Motivation: Praise. *Manager's Magazine, 67*(8), 30–31.

Peters, T. (1992, July 21). Gee Whiz: Wow factors significant. *San Antonio Light*, p. B3.

Peters, T. (1992, February 11). "Must do" ideas help keep business afloat. *San Antonio Light*, p. B8.

Rigdon, J. E. (1992, May 26). Using lateral moves to spur employees. *Wall Street Journal*, pp. B1, B5.

Rondeau, K. V. (1992). Morale boosters for off-shift staff. *Medical Laboratory Observer*, 40–41.

Ross, H. T. & Oumsby, M. M. (1990). Teamwork breeds quality at hearing technology. *National Productivity Review*, 321–327.

Sayers, W. K. (1990). ESOPs are no fable. *Small Business Reports*, 57–60.

Slotterback, Carla. (2000). Carla Slotterback's Portfolio.

White, J. A. (1992, February 13). When employees own big stake, it's a buy signal for investors. *Wall Street Journal*, p. C1.

Wing, D. M. & Oertle, J. R. (1999). The process of transforming self in women veterans with post-traumatic stress disorder resulting from sexual abuse. *International Journal of Psychiatric Nursing Research*, 579–588.

CHAPTER 13

eNursing

Richard J. Swansburg, RN, BSN, MSCIS

LEARNING OBJECTIVES AND ACTIVITIES

- Record a synopsis of what your electronic information environment is like today, and try to envision what you believe it will be like in five years.
- Differentiate between the various types of networks.
- Illustrate uses for applications software.
- Identify and discuss the purpose of various information systems.
- Develop a confidentiality and security plan.

CONCEPTS: Confidentiality, data, database, information, Internet, intranet, multimedia, network, security, spreadsheet, technology, word processing.

NURSE MANAGER BEHAVIORS: Advocates and supports computer technology that affects nursing operations.

NURSE EXECUTIVE BEHAVIORS: Plans, develops, and evaluates information technology that improves nursing operations, including management, education, research, and clinical practice. Does so with input from representative nurses.

Introduction

I started working with computers and information technology in 1982. The changes that have occurred in the years since have amazed me. Computers are now a common part of our life. We encounter them in our automobiles, home appliances, and home electronics. We have personal computers in the home with access to the Internet. Automatic teller machines, debit cards, and electronic banking are now the norm for dealing with money. Retail services are driven by electronic inventory and point of sale systems. Computers and information systems in the workplace are a fact of life.

> Today, we are often told, we live not simply in an age of information, but in an age of excessive information. The amount and availability of information seem to be increasing at an exponential rate. We feel that our entire world is moving, changing, mutating, at an accelerated pace. Our interactions with this world of information seem plagued by an increasing sense that we cannot keep up, can't take it all in, that we are being overwhelmed by information, deluged by data: the sense of an "information overload."[1]

The challenge of advocating and using new technology will be critical for the management of health care in constant transition. "As the business world changes at an ever-increasing rate, many of us are finding that our jobs require us to constantly enhance our skills and develop new ones—possibly some we never thought we'd need. Today, staying in place means falling behind, and no one can afford to do that in our technology-driven world."[2] Nurses will have to assimilate the knowledge and expertise required to understand and interact with this constantly changing technology, and then they must be capable of teaching this new knowledge and expertise to others.

The focus of future computer communication will be one of a more simplistic user interface, which will be built around the use of multimedia that interacts with the user through sight, sound and voice and evolves based upon patterns of use. It will seamlessly integrate all the tools, technologies, and information that may be located in geographically distributed and often highly differentiated hardware and software environments. The issue of location has already become somewhat irrelevant with the advent of the global network we call the Internet.

Ethical and legal issues will need to be advanced in scope to address new and changing technology. Concepts of privacy, confidentiality, and security should be instilled in nursing personnel not only in terms of operational guidelines (data and physical security, policies and procedures) but also in terms of professionalism and responsibility. Control of information needs to be taught as a management issue, not a technical one.

Historical Perspective

In 1642, Blaise Pascal created a calculating device that could add or subtract with the turning of little wheels. In 1834 Charles Babbage theorized a new machine that he called the Analytical Engine; this machine was to be programmable with the ability to calculate and store results. Even though this machine was never built, Lady Augusta Ada Loveless created a set of instructions for it in 1842. She is credited with being the first computer programmer.

Herman Hollerith developed the first electronic computing device in the 1880s. This machine was used to calculate the US census in 1890. The results of the census were completed in 6 weeks, much less time than the 7 years it took to count the census of 1880. In 1909, the electronics world was changed with the development of the vacuum tube by Lee deForest. The term computer bug was coined in 1945 when a moth flew into a computer at the Naval Weapons Center. In 1946, the first electronic computer, called the ENIAC (Electronic Numerical Integrator and Computer), was developed at the University of Pennsylvania.

In 1947 John Bardeen, Walter Brattain, and William Shockley achieved an electronic milestone with the discovery of the transistor. The next monumental change in electronics happened in 1959 with the creation of the integrated circuit by Jack Kilby and Robert Noyce. The transistor and the integrated circuit have massively reduced the size of computing hardware. The integrated circuit is the building block of today's computers.

In 1962, John Licklider introduced the idea of a global network. He imagined the ability to access data from anywhere on a set of globally connected computers. In 1968, the precursor to the Internet appeared in the form of ARPANET (Advanced Research Projects Agency Network). In 1971, Ray Tomlinson sent the first electronic message. In 1973, Vinton Cerf and Bob Kahn developed the Transmission Control Protocol (TCP). The first personal computer (PC), the Altair 8800, debuted in 1974. In 1980, Tim Berners-Lee created HyperText Markup Language (HTML). In 1981, Xerox pioneered the use of the mouse and graphical user interface (GUI). In 1983, the Department of Defense coined the term *Internet*, and TCP was adopted as the standard protocol [changing in effect to TCP/IP (Internet Protocol)]. In 1991, the University of Minnesota developed Gopher, the first browser for surfing the Internet. Finally, in 1993, Dave Thompson and Marc Andreesen introduced the graphical Web browser.

Current Information Technology

Today's information technology puts us in a period of major transition. The advancement of new technology can be overwhelming. A critical challenge is to prove that this technology will provide for the efficient delivery of quality health care while reducing the cost of that care. We also have a whole generation of workers that views information technology as a normal part of life. These workers are prepared to acquire, implement, and use newer technology. Health care should not lag behind other industries in the use of emerging technology.

We are caught between the desire to use today's knowledge efficiently and the desire to implement tomorrow's technology. What this means is that there is an incredible amount of new technology in the world that many of us aren't using yet. Instead we are concentrating on finding solutions to some of the older challenges:[3]

- Moving information between multiple locations and entities;
- Sharing this information in real time;
- Developing real, effective automated scheduling systems;
- Building a totally electronic medical record;
- Using Internet-based technologies for professional enhancement and patient care improvement;
- Integrating disparate systems; and
- Working toward a paperless delivery system.

Implementing these solutions is a long-term project. The organization has to develop and put into practice a business plan for integrating the technology. This often requires a reengineering of the organization with huge changes to its infrastructure and workflow processes. Many organizations are looking for a single vendor to deliver and support turnkey enterprise information technology systems; unfortunately, mature solutions aren't widely implemented, and organizations often have to choose a vendor from only a handful of viable candidates.

Workplace technology involves many systems. Legacy systems (text-based information systems that reside on mini and mainframe computers) continue to be integral because of their historical information and because they provide for the most rapid delivery of information to thousands of concurrent users. Often, the legacy system is the corporate or organizational information system that is used by everyone. Secondary information systems are specialized departmental information systems relevant to the area in which we work. Applications software for personal and group productivity includes communications, database management, word processing, spreadsheets, and personal information management systems. Finally, we must also consider access to the Internet.

These dissimilar systems usually reside at different locations on different hardware and software platforms. Local area networks (LANs) and wide area networks (WANs) provide us with the connections to access these systems. The standard for a LAN connection is 10 or 100 megabit Ethernet running over copper wiring, and the standard for a WAN connection is a T1 data line leased from the local telephone provider. Some organizations have implemented mobile computing. In this environment, the health care professionals are issued notebook computers that use wireless radio technology to access the network. This allows the end users to take their computers and move about the facility while staying connected to the systems they need.

As of this writing, the newest technology is moving toward the use of interactive multimedia. In these applications, the user interacts with text, voice, music, images, animation, and video. This technology has potential for education and telemedicine. Multimedia educational material is being developed for patients and health care practitioners alike. Some devices can simulate medical environments, such as an ER, OR, or ICU for training purposes. Telemedicine brings the patient and health care practitioner face to face regardless of their geographical locations.

Future Information Technology Trends

The future of information technology begins with the resolution of two of today's most pressing problems: communications bandwidth and the integration of systems. *Bandwidth* refers to the amount of data or information that can be moved across a particular communications medium over a given period of time.[4] Optical fiber is currently the material of choice to provide increased bandwidth. The seamless integration of systems is coming about with the incorporation of the Internet into all of today's emerging technologies.

One vision of the future is that of a wireless world in which everything and everyone is connected to a network that is "always on, always there." Objects are alive with intelligence, and technologies evolve to change the form of everyday things.[5] Real streaming audio and video will be the norm for the integration of the health care environment. All parties will be connected (patients, doctors, nurses, health care organizations, etc.). Even intelligent equipment will be involved to monitor, make recommendations, and possibly act. Everything will become part of the electronic medical record.

Simulation, virtual reality, and robotics will become common tools. A wearable computer, most likely incorporated into protective eyewear, will be the means for managing all interaction. A video screen will become part of the lens, or a projector will generate holographic images. A microphone will capture speech as well as all other audio input. Speakers will play for us whatever sound it is that we wish to hear. A possible alternative to a wearable computer is the merging of computer technology directly into our biological processes.

Gordon Moore and Ray Kurzweil predict that the next big technological revolution will occur by 2010 to 2020. Moore declared that technological advances will double the capacity of intergrated circuits every 18 to 24 months. This theory predicts that transistors will be so small around 2010 that they will be incapable of functioning reliably. New advances in technologies must be achieved. Kurzweil believes that as technology evolves, the period between advances becomes shorter, and the benefits from prior developments interact, causing the rate of progress to accelerate further.[6] New technologies that could exponentially increase the power of computing are now on the foreseeable horizon.

The progress of information technology will improve the quality of life for most of us. Work will become more enjoyable as machines perform some of the manual labor and assist us in the decision support process. There will be a price, though, as low-skill and middle management positions are lost. Personnel will constantly need to upgrade their skills in what will become a lifelong process. Organizations will compete for the more effective, higher-skilled workers. These workers will also be in a better position to demand higher salaries and better working conditions.

Computer Networking

Networks are the infrastructure of today's world of electronic technology. They are the conduits by which we use computers to transfer information from one location to another. A network can be a mini or mainframe computer with terminals attached to it, two personal computers connected together in your home, or all the computing devices in the world that are attached to the Internet. Networks include a number of components, including client and server computers, client and server network software, network protocols, network adapters, physical transport media, hubs, switches, bridges, routers, and other analog and digital data transmission equipment.

Two standards form the basis of today's networking. They are the establishment of the 802 project by the Institute of Electrical and Electronics Engineers (IEEE) and the adoption of the Open Systems Interconnect (OSI) model by the International Organization for Standardization (ISO). The IEEE 802 project provides us with standards for the implementation of various network topologies, whereas, the OSI model provides us with a common point of reference for describing the communications process across these networks. Exhibit 13-1 presents the IEEE 802 standards, and Exhibit 13-2 presents the OSI model.

EXHIBIT 13-1
The IEEE 802 Standards

STANDARD	DESCRIPTION
802.1	Higher level interface
802.2	Logical link control
802.3	Ethernet
802.4	Token-bus
802.5	Token-ring
802.6	Metropolitan area networks
802.7	Broadband
802.8	Fiber optic
802.9	Integrated services local area network
802.10	Interoperable local area network security
802.11	Wireless local area network
802.12	Demand priority
802.14	Cable-TV-based broadband communication network
802.15	Wireless personal area network
802.16	Broadband wireless access

EXHIBIT 13-2
The OSI Model

NO.	LAYER	USAGE
7	Application	Provide application services
6	Presentation	Adapt the data to suit the receiver
5	Session	Set up and maintain a communication session
4	Transport	Transport data between two programs
3	Network	Transport data across a network
2	Link	Transport data across a link
1	Physical	Convert data to electricity/light/radio

EXHIBIT 13-3
Example of Labor and Delivery and Operating Room LAN Domains

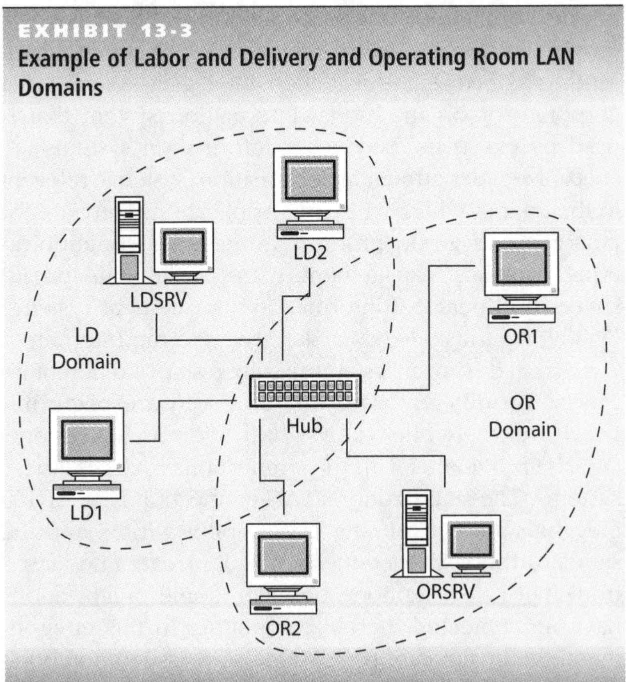

Several issues need to be explored in any discussion of computer networking. One is the physical representation and implementation of the network, and the other is the logical usage of the physical network. Let's develop an example to help us get the gist of this. Let's say that we work in a hospital where the Operating Room and Labor and Delivery reside on the same floor. They have separate client/server information systems with a departmental server for each. All of the computers are attached using copper wiring to a hub in a centralized wiring closet. Exhibit 13-3 illustrates this setup.

Now physically we have one network, and logically we could have one network. But we are going to divide these computers into two workgroups or domains. We can associate the client computers LD1 and LD2, along with the server computer LDSRV, with the domain LD. Similarly, we can associate the client computers OR1 and OR2 and the server computer ORSRV with the domain OR. Clients in either of the domains can be totally unaware that the other domain exists, even though they both pass their information on the same physical network. We'll expand upon these issues as we discuss other topics in this section.

Local Area Networks (LAN) and Wide Area Networks (WAN)

For practical purposes, computer network technology can be broken down into two main types, LANs and WANs. A LAN is a network of computers considered local to each other, meaning that all of the computers are within the same room or building. A WAN is a network of two or more groups of computers or computing devices that are remote from each other and are connected by telecommunications equipment.

Design, implementation, and management are crucial issues in networking. Depending on the size and needs of an organization, these tasks can range from very simple to extremely complex. Another variable that affects these issues is the willingness of an organization to spend money. Quite often an organization will make a conscious choice to use inferior products and a lower speed network, only to find out that the installed network fails in its purpose.

In designing a LAN, we should plan for the future. This means we should consider the possibilities of technological changes and expansion of the network. The most important area to concentrate on in the design process is arguably the cabling strategy. A wireless network would provide for the ultimate in end user convenience and mobility. Unfortunately, at present wireless is limited by bandwidth, though it is likely to improve. If we choose a wired network, we should promote a cabling strategy that provides for maximum bandwidth.

The wiring closet that contains the hubs and switches should be centrally located within the LAN area. We should minimize the cable lengths between the attached computers and the wiring closet. In larger organizations, there should be separate wiring closets for departments with a large number of users or buildings with more than one floor. These wiring closets will all be connected by a "backbone" LAN, which will also support connections for server computers, routers, and telecommunications equipment. The routers and telecommunications equipment provide WAN access to other organizational sites and the Internet. Exhibit 13-4 shows what a university WAN might look like with a campus and two remote hospital sites.

Implementation of our network builds upon our design. Client PCs and servers are attached using network interface cards (NIC). All computers that participate on the network, clients, and servers must have network software installed to manage the communication between them. For the servers, such network operating systems (NOS) include Microsoft Windows NT, Novell Intranetware, and UNIX. This communication process starts with some type

EXHIBIT 13-4
Example of a University WAN

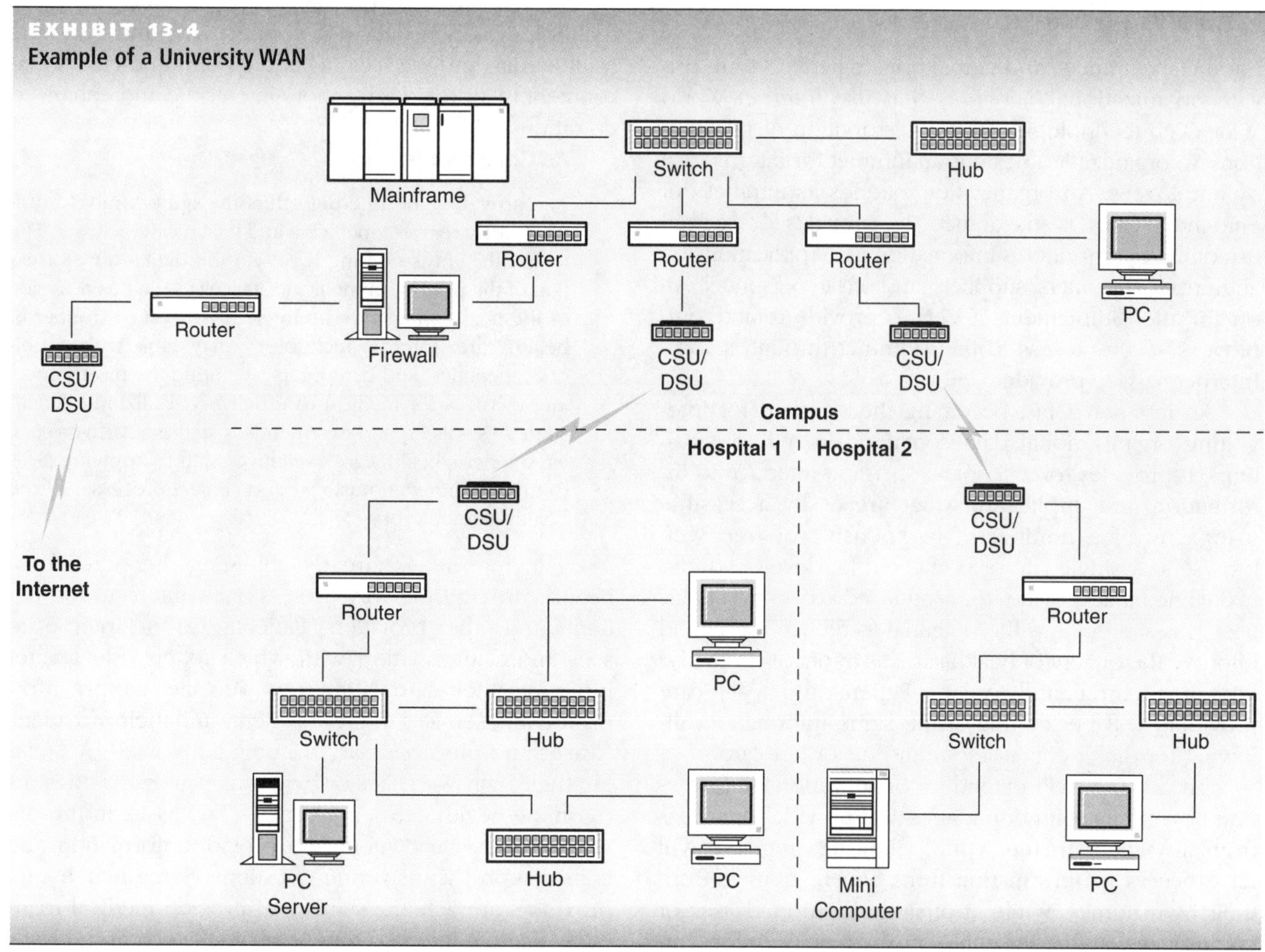

of authentication procedure in which the client is required to login. Once the client has been authenticated, LAN resources are made available based upon security policies. These resources typically include shared disk space, software, and printers.

Network management is an ongoing process that begins before the first client is attached to the network. Numerous personnel are involved in the practice of network management. Network staff are involved in the installation, configuration, and support of computers, cables, hubs, switches, routers, and telecommunications equipment. Troubleshooting a network problem may require expensive equipment and can be tedious and time-consuming. Routine monitoring should be done to evaluate capacity and performance and, if necessary, to tune the network. Finally, we need continuing network administration related to server and user management. Server administration includes the maintenance of shared resources and the daily backup of data. User administration includes the maintenance of client IDs and the security relationships between users and shared resources.

Intranets, Extranets, and Virtual Private Networks (VPNS)

Intranets, extranets, and virtual private networks are private organizational networks that use Internet/World Wide Web technologies for the distribution of information. An organization designs an intranet for internal use by employees. An organization extends its intranet out onto the Internet as an extranet. This provides for external use of the organization's information and applications by authorized customers, suppliers, and offsite personnel. An organization implements a VPN to provide remote employees secure access to their intranet through a local Internet service provider (ISP).

An intranet is fast becoming the standard for integrating organizational data contained in multiple systems. It provides for a simple, consistent interface to information and applications that are easily accessible using any of a number of inexpensive or free Web browsers. A single site or portal can be developed and maintained that provides for centralized access by all parties. This strategy has the potential to reduce errors and improve the quality of health care, as information can be kept more current and accurate. Patients and health care providers will be looking at the same information, allowing for direct patient input into his or her care.

An extranet will extend an organization's information beyond its solid boundaries and provide for access from anywhere in the world. Clinical caregivers will have access to information from patient homes, from their own homes, while at offsite education classes or conferences, and even while on vacation. Vendors, insurers, and regulating agencies will have a common gateway for obtaining information from and providing information to the health care organization.

A VPN provides the organization with economical and flexible remote access with a stronger degree of security. Special software can be required on the client PC to connect to the organization's intranet. This software interacts with software on the organization's intranet to manage authentication and encryption. Questions to ask before buying or creating a VPN include the following: How many people need remote access, and who are they? What hardware, software, and administration costs are involved in a dedicated remote access server? What other long distance and telecommunications costs are in the mix? What additional security does the organization need when using the Internet?[7]

The Internet

The Internet is essentially a globally implemented WAN: a network of tens of millions of computers connected by the same TCP/IP protocol. Using routers and domain name servers (DNS), the Internet provides us with the capability to communicate with any one of these computers. Add to this the integration of Web browsing technology, open database connectivity, and real-time multimedia, and we have a simple point-and-click environment that provides for more interactive and enhanced communications.

As Coile writes,

> The arrival of the Internet offers the opportunity to fundamentally reinvent medicine and health care delivery. The "e-health" era is nothing less than the digital transformation of the practice of medicine, as well as the business side of the health industry. The Internet is the next frontier of health care. Internet technology may rank with antibiotics, genetics, and computers as among the most important changes for medical care delivery. Utilizing e-health strategies will expand exponentially in the next five years, as America's health care executives shift to applying IS/IT to the fundamental business and clinical processes of the health care enterprise.[8]

The Internet is already changing the practice of health care and the way professionals interact with patients and other providers. Patients use the Internet to seek more information with which to provide greater input into their care. Numerous Web sites supply information and services to these patients and their providers. Nurses and physicians are becoming involved by creating their own Web sites or by going to work as advisors to online health care companies. They assist in the design of Web site content and provide information and consultation by answering questions. Some health care providers are actually starting to provide medical treatment over the Internet. New legal, regulatory, and privacy issues arise as medical practice moves to a new setting.

The first step toward this new health care system is the implementation of electronic medical records. Any data or information that can be captured and maintained electronically can be more easily and quickly accessed. The extension of this information onto the Internet via a private extranet has the potential to improve the quality of care as well as patient and provider satisfaction. Patients can access the Internet from home and complete electronic forms for medical and social histories, lists of allergies and medications, and insurance and payment options. This can be done prior to a doctor's visit or admission to the hospital. After an appointment, patients would be able to review information for accuracy and changes. Doctors and nurses would also have the ability to access this information from any place.

The next step in virtual health care proposes to use the Internet to provide all the services of a doctor's visit except the physical exam. This lack of touch bothers some patients' rights advocates and the American Medical Association (AMA).[9] Is this impersonality a step in the right direction? It may be a significant improvement in the delivery of health care to rural or remote populations where providers are just not available. Through the use of computers and multimedia, patients can be evaluated and treated for minor illnesses and injuries. The addition of emergency medical technicians or advanced practice nurses and diagnostic medical equipment makes the treatment of major medical problems more feasible.

Nurses and physicians are already using the Internet for consultation, research, and decision support. Consultation is a normal part of the delivery of health care, and now with the Internet it can be done from anywhere. Today, nurses search online literature to obtain the most current nursing research about rare diseases. They visit chat rooms and newsgroups to ask questions and to seek reassurance and support in their delivery of nursing care. Physicians use evidence-based medicine to access the most recent medical research and practice guidelines. They use video conferencing at the point of care to consult with peers concerning their evaluation of diagnoses and treatments. Health care providers are already using all available resources to improve their decision support process; the Internet may provide for more timely, accurate information that will reduce errors and improve the quality of care.

The Internet is also changing education. It has now become an ideal vehicle for the delivery of full multimedia instruction on demand. This is useful not only for the patient education process, but also for our own continuing or higher education as providers. Today there are Internet sites that deal specifically with AIDS, diabetes, gerontology, hepatitis, nutrition, oncology, renal disease, wellness, and other health-related topics. They provide various degrees of information and education based on ownership and purpose. The primary issue surrounding the use of public sites relates to the quality of information that is provided. Currently there are no standards for the publication of information unless the site is controlled by a governing organization, such as the AMA or the CDC. Private provider extranets can be customized to meet the specific needs of patient populations.

Continuing and higher education for nursing are available over the Internet. Online learning provides up-to-date knowledge in a convenient environment. Thousands of continuing education programs require only a registration fee to use. The higher education process is more complex: the admission process does not guarantee acceptance, and there may be requirements that cannot be met over the Internet. For the latter reason, you should look for a school that is within commuting distance. Distance learning programs are geared toward RNs who want to further their education, often associate's degree nurses seeking baccalaureate degrees or baccalaureate degree nurses seeking master's degrees or doctorates.

Health care businesses must reengineer their information technology to focus on Internet/extranet/intranet development. Many business aspects of the health care industry involve information communication between two or more parties. The electronic transfer of bills and payments between providers and payers, for instance, has been taking place for a number of years. Extranets that allow providers to check on the status of claims and payers to audit patient care records are just becoming widespread.

Marketing is a part of the health care business environment. Organizations market their facilities, products, and services to patients and health care providers; making the organization visible on the Internet makes good sense. Organizations can actively recruit patients who are seeking particular services and an openness of information communication. Organizations can post openings for professional caregivers, and professionals can submit online resumes and communicate with human resources personnel directly. Organizational employees can access their personnel records to obtain information about education and credentialing, vacation and sick time, and even insurance and retirement benefits.

The sale of health care supplies and appliances can also involve the Internet. Providers should be able to connect to vendors online and order their supplies. A dynamic inventory system can track usage and reorder supplies over the Internet. Providers could request bids for products and vendors could submit responses. Patients could connect to the providers or possibly directly to the vendors and purchase needed supplies and appliances. These changes improve cost, convenience, efficiency, and service.

Finally, through all of this we must not forget about privacy and security. These are primary issues that everyone is raising red flags over. Today, loss of personal privacy ranks as one of the top concerns of most people.

The government in 1996 passed the Health Insurance Portability and Accountability Act (HIPAA). This act provided for an initial three-year period to pass legislation that would regulate the healthcare industry's management of patient records. "The goal is not to inappropriately restrict access, but to restrict inappropriate access."[10] What's the best way to deal with these issues? We'll discuss this in greater detail in its own section.

General-Purpose Applications Software

Nurse managers should be prepared to support the increased use of information technology in all areas of nursing. Part of this support includes a fundamental degree of computer literacy and the acceptance of a microcomputer as a professional work tool. Many nurses use computers in the performance of their daily duties in such areas as patient care documentation, budgeting, policy and procedure documentation, personnel records, patient and staff education, scheduling, research, and inventory management. The general-purpose applications available for nurses include communications, database management, spreadsheets, word processing/publication, personal information management, graphic editing and presentation, and Internet browsing software.

A number of office suites exist that integrate these applications into a single bundle. Integrated suites provide the easy ability to share information between applications. For example, spreadsheets, database information, and graphics can be inserted directly into word processing documents such as memos, letters, and reports. When the numbers in a spreadsheet or the information in a database is changed, the corresponding information in the memo or report is automatically updated. In addition, all the applications can provide a shared look and feel with similar menus, toolbars, and keyboard shortcuts. They can also incorporate a common macro, scripting, or programming language that allows for the automation of repetitive and complex tasks.

Communications

Communications software provides the foundation for access among computers. Such access may be dedicated (the link is maintained even when it is not in use) or not dedicated (the link is maintained only while being used). Dedicated links tend to be business related with direct access to the organization's information resources through a LAN connection. Nondedicated links tend to be home- or small-business-related with the need for intermittent access to remote information resources. With advances in digital communications services, such as integrated services digital network (ISDN) and digital subscriber line (DSL), dedicated links are becoming the standard.

We tend to take for granted the communications software to support our LAN attachments (local and remote). This is because quite often it is provided to us as part of the operating system installed on our computers. When we purchase a new microcomputer the required communications hardware (LAN adapter or modem) is usually supplied with it. So, at work we have a dedicated LAN connection, and at home, with a computer, modem, and remote access software, we can dial into a remote access server and perform any computer-related functions that we can at work.

Once we dial in, we need additional communications software to perform certain tasks. Internet communications are usually accomplished through free Web browsers, such as Microsoft's Internet Explorer and Netscape's Communicator. To access IBM mainframes, we need 3270 emulation; to access IBM AS400s, we need 5250 emulation. To access UNIX systems and other ASCII-based mini and microcomputers, we need some form of DEC's video terminal emulation (VT). All of these terminal emulators are provided by a number of vendors as integrated packages, which are usually purchased by the organization for which we work.

End user support and file transfer software are also important for a company. For example, a nurse manager, when contacted about a problem by a staff nurse, can access the system and mirror what the staff member does. This is also how a vendor provides assistance to a remote customer. File transfers are becoming part of everyday computer usage. We transfer files over the Internet, over our LAN, to and from our host systems, and to computers at home.

Database Management

A computer database is the electronic counterpart to a file cabinet and its contents. It is used to store data and can be manipulated for information. We can use a microcomputer and a database management system (DBMS) in place of a manual filing system to handle many of our information and record-keeping needs, such as personnel records, education records, budget management, and equipment inventory.

A DBMS allows for the construction of databases through tables. A table is a collection of records composed of data fields that have a common layout. When a data field is defined, its length is set and the type of data that can be stored in it established. Data types can be character or text (allowing letters, numbers, and special symbols), numeric (allowing only numbers), logical (allowing only yes or no, true or false), or date/time (allowing only numbers in a date and time format. Exhibit 13-5 is an example of an employee table definition.

Once a table is created, forms or screens can be established to add, modify, or delete information (see Exhibit 13-6 for an example of a database screen).

EXHIBIT 13-5

Example of an Employee Table Definition

Database:	Nursing.MDB
Table:	Employee
Date:	Wednesday, June 22, 2005

PROPERTIES

Date Created:	6/22/2005 10:25:20	GUID:	Long binary data
Last Updated:	6/22/2005 10:50:08	Name Map:	Long binary data
Order By On:	False	Orientation:	0
Record Count:	0	Updateable:	True

COLUMNS

NAME	TYPE	SIZE	DESCRIPTION
Emp name	Text	30	Employee name. Required, indexed (duplicates OK).
Emp SSN	Text	9	Employee SSN. Required, indexed (no duplicates), primary key. Input mask 000\-00\-0000;;_.
Emp job code	Text	1	Employee job code.
Emp assignment number	Text	3	Employee assignment number.
Emp position number	Text	6	Employee position number. Required.
Emp class code	Text	4	Employee class code.
Emp class title	Text	50	Employee class title.
Emp job status	Text	2	Employee job status.
Emp hire date	Date/Time	8	Employee hire date. Input mask 99/99/0000;0;_.
Emp termination date	Date/Time	8	Employee termination date. Input mask 99/99/0000;0;_.
Emp pay ID	Text	1	Employee pay ID.
Emp license number	Text	20	Employee license number.
Emp license renewal number	Text	20	Employee license renewal number.
Emp license date	Date/Time	8	Employee license date. Input mask 99/99/0000;0;_.
Emp license expiration	Date/Time	8	Employee license expiration date. Input mask 99/99/0000;0;_.
Emp liability insurance	Yes/No	1	Employee liability insurance.
Emp unit	Text	20	Employee unit.
Emp shift	Text	20	Employee shift.
Emp address 1	Text	30	Employee address 1.
Emp address 2	Text	30	Employee address 2.
Emp city	Text	20	Employee city.
Emp state	Text	2	Employee state.
Emp zip	Text	9	Employee zip. Input mask 00000\-9999;;_.
Emp phone	Text	10	Employee phone. Input mask !\(999") "000\-0000;;_.

TABLE INDEXES

NAME	NUMBER OF FIELDS	ORDER
Emp Name	1	Ascending
Emp SSN	1	Ascending
Primary Key	1	Ascending

USER PERMISSIONS

Admin	Delete, Read Permissions, Set Permissions, Change Owner, Read Definition, Write Definition, Read Data, Insert Data, Update Data, Delete Data

GROUP PERMISSIONS

Admins	Delete, Read Permissions, Set Permissions, Change Owner, Read Definition, Write Definition, Read Data, Insert Data, Update Data, Delete Data
Users	Delete, Read Permissions, Set Permissions, Change Owner, Read Definition, Write Definition, Read Data, Insert Data, Update Data, Delete Data

EXHIBIT 13-6
Example of a Database Screen

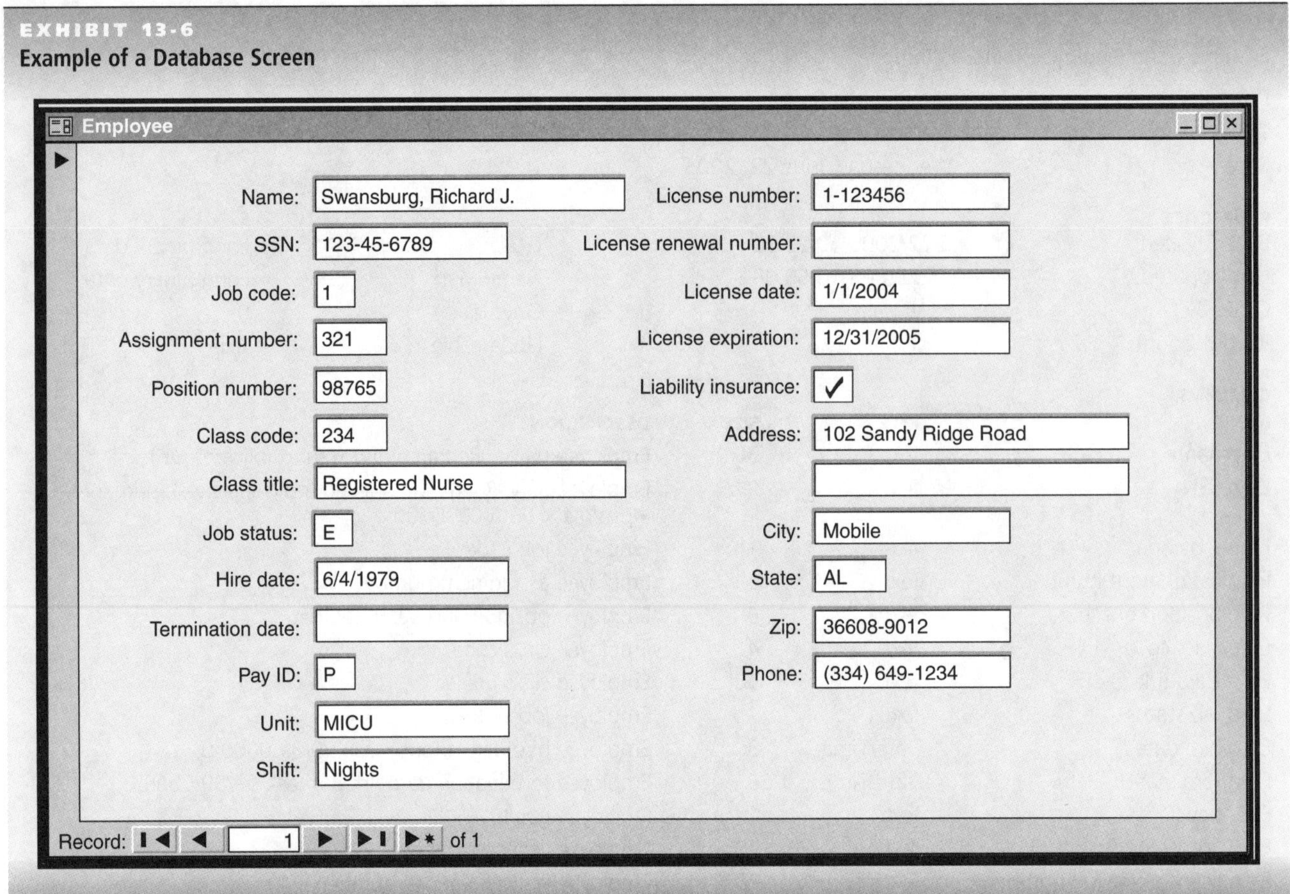
Employee

Name: Swansburg, Richard J.
SSN: 123-45-6789
Job code: 1
Assignment number: 321
Position number: 98765
Class code: 234
Class title: Registered Nurse
Job status: E
Hire date: 6/4/1979
Termination date:
Pay ID: P
Unit: MICU
Shift: Nights

License number: 1-123456
License renewal number:
License date: 1/1/2004
License expiration: 12/31/2005
Liability insurance: ✓
Address: 102 Sandy Ridge Road
City: Mobile
State: AL
Zip: 36608-9012
Phone: (334) 649-1234

Record: 1 of 1

EXHIBIT 13-7
Example of a Database Report

EMPLOYEE LISTING MICU

EMPLOYEE NAME	POSITION	TITLE	HIRE DATE	LICENSE	INSURANCE	PHONE
Adams, Judy M.	97531	RN	7/1/1994	1-468248	Yes	(334) 434-3557
Armstrong, Sabrina T.	85477	US	3/23/1988		No	(601) 631-3357
Conner, Rebecca A.	85547	US	6/1/1992		No	(334) 343-1656
Dawson, John B.	96656	RN	6/15/1998	1-575112	Yes	(334) 457-9888
Gooden, Amanda W.	84544	US	10/21/1991		No	(334) 434-5129
Grimes, Sharon N.	91154	RN	6/3/1986	1-223556	Yes	(601) 631-5451
Hodges, Charles S.	97551	RN	7/10/1982	1-155454	No	(334) 633-6117
Hooker, Mary Beth	81144	US	8/7/1976		No	(334) 457-5721
Inge, Janice M.	84198	US	7/10/1982		No	(334) 434-5199
Johnson, Mary B.	97751	RN	6/6/1972	1-011959	Yes	(334) 633-7413
Jones, Sandra P.	97494	RN	9/12/1988	1-299114	Yes	(334) 457-8745
Morris, Barbara R.	97691	RN	6/9/1999	1-591344	Yes	(334) 633-2424
Nearly, Susan O.	95775	RN	1/15/1997	1-529911	No	(334) 457-8711
Parker, Frank C.	98511	RN	11/11/1991	1-300551	Yes	(601) 632-4685
Reynolds, Sara A.	94417	RN	5/27/1991	1-299911	Yes	(334) 457-9577
Swansburg, Richard J.	98765	RN	6/4/1979	1-123456	Yes	(334) 649-1234
Williams, Gesina S.	91554	RN	6/8/1995	1-449521	Yes	(334) 633-7124

EXHIBIT 13-8
Example of a Database Menu

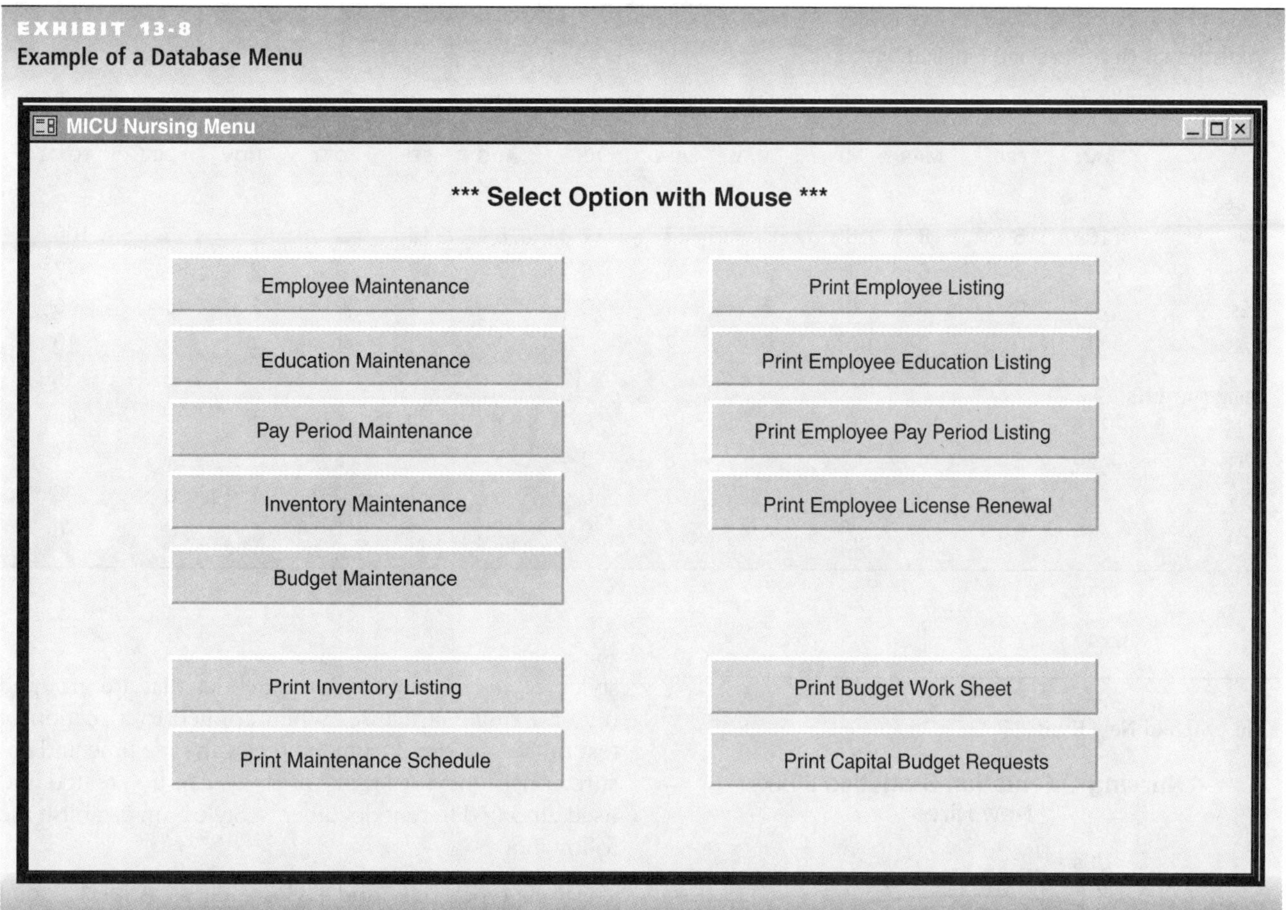

Queries can be established to display the information in various formats or order. Reports can be established to display the information on paper, transparencies, and labels (see Exhibit 13-7 for an example of a database report). Menus with procedures can be created to allow easy access to and execution of these forms, queries, and reports (see Exhibit 13-8 for an example of a database menu). Advantages to database management are the ease in maintaining information, the timely retrieval of information, and the concurrent access of this information by individuals from different locations.

Spreadsheet

A spreadsheet is a tool used to record and manipulate numbers. The original model for the spreadsheet was the paper ledger used for business accounting, such as the recording of debits and credits. An electronic spreadsheet is a piece of software that turns a computer into a highly sophisticated calculator. Huge quantities of numbers can be recorded, manipulated, and stored simply and easily. Nurses can use the information from spreadsheets to maintain statistics (see Exhibit 13-9), create graphics (see Exhibit 13-10), and plan budgets (see Exhibit 13-11).

A spreadsheet is made up of columns and rows of memory cells. These cells can be varied in size to allow for small or very large numbers. In addition to storing numbers, cells can store text and formulas. Text is used for titles, column and row headers, comments, and instructions. Formulas are used to perform the actual mathematical manipulation (addition, subtraction, multiplication, and division) of memory cells and their numbers. Formulas even provide for special financial, math, and statistical functions such as averages and standard deviations. Formulas are what really make a spreadsheet a powerful number-crunching tool. Another important spreadsheet capability is graphing, which allows numbers to be displayed visually. Exhibits 13-12 and 13-13 are examples of bar and line graphs, respectively.

Spreadsheets are the best tool to use in situations that require the management of a lot of numbers. For this reason, they lend themselves particularly well to financial management, speeding up such processes as budgeting, forecasting, and developing tables and schedules.

EXHIBIT 13-9
Statistics for New Hires and Terminations

NURSING ORIENTATION STATISTICS													
	JAN	FEB	MAR	APR	MAY	JUN	JUL	AUG	SEP	OCT	NOV	DEC	TOTAL
HIRES													
RNs	10	6	8	5	7	27	11	8	13	3	3	5	106
LPNs	3	3	6	1	2	11	5	2	7	4	2	1	47
USs	0	0	0	0	2	1	0	0	2	0	1	0	6
NAs	1	0	0	3	0	2	0	1	1	1	1	0	10
TERMINATIONS													
RNs	11	4	10	6	3	17	8	11	9	5	1	5	86
LPNs	2	5	4	1	3	8	3	5	3	5	1	1	41
USs	0	0	0	1	1	1	0	0	2	0	1	0	6
NAs	1	0	0	2	0	2	0	1	1	1	1	0	10

EXHIBIT 13-10
Pie Graph of New Hires

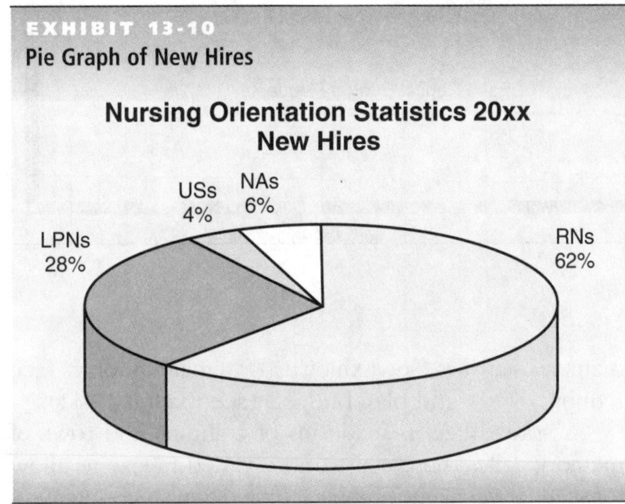

Word Processing and Desktop Publishing

Word processing is the manipulation of words and special characters to produce a printed document. Desktop publishing is the manipulation of text and graphics to produce documents of publication quality. The difference between the two processes used to be vast. Today, each has incorporated aspects of the other. We can, using specialized software, easily produce such documents as memos and letters, policies and procedures, resumes, forms, envelopes and labels, instruction sheets, manuals, posters and signs, books, and newsletters. Exhibits 13-14 and 13-15 show examples.

Word processing and desktop publishing applications have tools for the management of multiple document styles. Styles contain formatting codes that are grouped under a single structure. When applied to a section of text or to an entire document, they can save time and ensure consistency. A library of styles can be created and used among different documents. Styles can establish the following:[11]

- Font type, size, and style, such as Arial 10-point normal, *Times New Roman 12-point italic*, and **Letter Gothic 14-point bold**.
- Spacing between lines and paragraphs.
- Margins, tabs, and text alignment.
- Page headers and footers.
- Numbering and outline formats.
- Form size, type, and orientation.

Other tools that are often included in these programs are a spell checker, a thesaurus, and a grammar checker. The spell checker contains a dictionary to which the text can be compared. Words not in the program's dictionary can be added to a supplement. When the spell checker is used, words that it does not recognize are highlighted. A list of alternative words is generated, along with options to replace, edit, or add a word to the supplement. The thesaurus generates a list of synonyms and antonyms that can be used in place of selected words. The grammar checker is used to check the document for grammar and style errors. It will interpret the presentation of the subject and make recommendations for improvement.

Other utilities are available for performing block functions that operate on words, sentences, paragraphs, or pages within a document. These functions include copying, moving, deleting, formatting, centering, and case conversion. Searching for and replacing particular words

EXHIBIT 13-11
Example of a Departmental Budget

Hospital Information Systems Budget
October 200x–September 200x

Pg 1: Oct 200x–Jan 200x

SUB CODE DESCRIPTION	ORIGINAL BUDGET	BALANCE AVAILABLE	PERCENT USED	OCT 200X CURRENT	YEAR	NOV CURRENT	YEAR	DEC CURRENT	YEAR	JAN 200X CURRENT	YEAR
1600 Student wages	$15,000	$4,084	73	$ 746	$ 746	$ 786	$1,532	$1,145	$2,677	$ 738	$ 3,415
1660 Accrued salaries	$ 0	$ 0	100		$ 0		$ 0		$ 0		$ 0
Salaries	$15,000	$4,084	73	$ 746	$ 746	$ 786	$1,532	$1,145	$2,677	$ 738	$ 3,415
2110 Medical–surgical supplies	$ 250	$ 75	70	$ 21	$ 21		$ 21	$ 23	$ 44	$ 18	$ 62
2130 Drugs	$ 0	$ 0	100		$ 0		$ 0		$ 0		$ 0
Medical–Surgical Supplies	$ 250	$ 75	70	$ 21	$ 21	$ 0	$ 21	$ 23	$ 44	$ 18	$ 62
2320 Office supplies	$ 250	$ 89	64	$ 37	$ 37	$ 7	$ 44		$ 44	$ 15	$ 59
2330 Copying and binding	$ 400	($25)	106	$ 28	$ 28	$ 31	$ 59	$ 33	$ 92	$ 37	$ 129
2340 Printing	$ 0	$ 0	100		$ 0		$ 0		$ 0		$ 0
2400 Housekeeping supplies	$ 100	$ 25	75	$ 11	$ 11	$ 7	$ 18		$ 18		$ 18
2500 Maintenance supplies	$ 100	$ 22	78		$ 0	$ 25	$ 25		$ 25	$ 21	$ 46
2700 Food expense	$ 0	$ 0	100		$ 0		$ 0		$ 0		$ 0
General Supplies	$ 850	$ 111	87	$ 76	$ 76	$ 70	$ 146	$ 33	$ 179	$ 73	$ 252
3110 Travel	$ 4,000	$ 618	85		$ 0	$1,398	$1,398		$1,398		$ 1,398
3140 Local travel	$ 500	$ 13	97	$ 46	$ 46	$ 42	$ 88	$ 38	$ 126	$ 41	$ 167
3160 Workshop and training	$ 1,500	$ 522	65		$ 0		$ 0		$ 0	$ 750	$ 750
Travel–Entertainment	$ 6,000	$1,153	81	$ 46	$ 46	$1,440	$1,486	$ 38	$1,524	$ 791	$ 2,315
3230 Contract labor	$ 0	$ 0	100		$ 0		$ 0		$ 0		$ 0
3290 Computer software	$ 2,500	($204)	108	$ 286	$ 286		$ 286	$ 368	$ 654		$ 654
3360 Equipment maintenance/repair	$ 1,500	$ 244	84		$ 0	$ 128	$ 128		$ 128	$ 227	$ 355
3370 Maintenance contracts	$ 3,500	$ 200	94	$1,500	$1,500		$1,500		$1,500	$1,800	$ 3,300
3410 Equipment rental	$ 0	$ 0	100		$ 0		$ 0		$ 0		$ 0
3650 Telephone base	$ 252	$ 0	100	$ 21	$ 21	$ 21	$ 42	$ 21	$ 63	$ 21	$ 84
3660 Telephone, long distance	$ 0	$ 0	100		$ 0		$ 0		$ 0		$ 0
3720 Books and subscriptions	$ 250	$ 86	66	$ 121	$ 121		$ 121		$ 121		$ 121
Other Expenses	$ 8,002	$ 326	96	$1,928	$1,928	$ 149	$2,077	$ 389	$2,466	$2,048	$ 4,514
5050 Minor equipment (<$500)	$ 3,500	$ 774	78		$ 0		$ 0	$ 771	$ 771	$ 257	$ 1,028
Minor Equipment Expenses	$ 3,500	$ 774	78	$ 0	$ 0	$ 0	$ 0	$ 771	$ 771	$ 257	$ 1,028
Total Expenses	$33,602	$6,523	81	$2,817	$2,817	$2,445	$5,262	$2,399	$7,661	$3,925	$11,586

EXHIBIT 13-12

Example of a Bar Graph

Nursing Orientation Statistics 20xx
New Hires
RNs LPNs USs NAs
30
25
20
15
10
5
0
Jan Feb Mar Apr May Jun Jul Aug Sep Oct Nov Dec

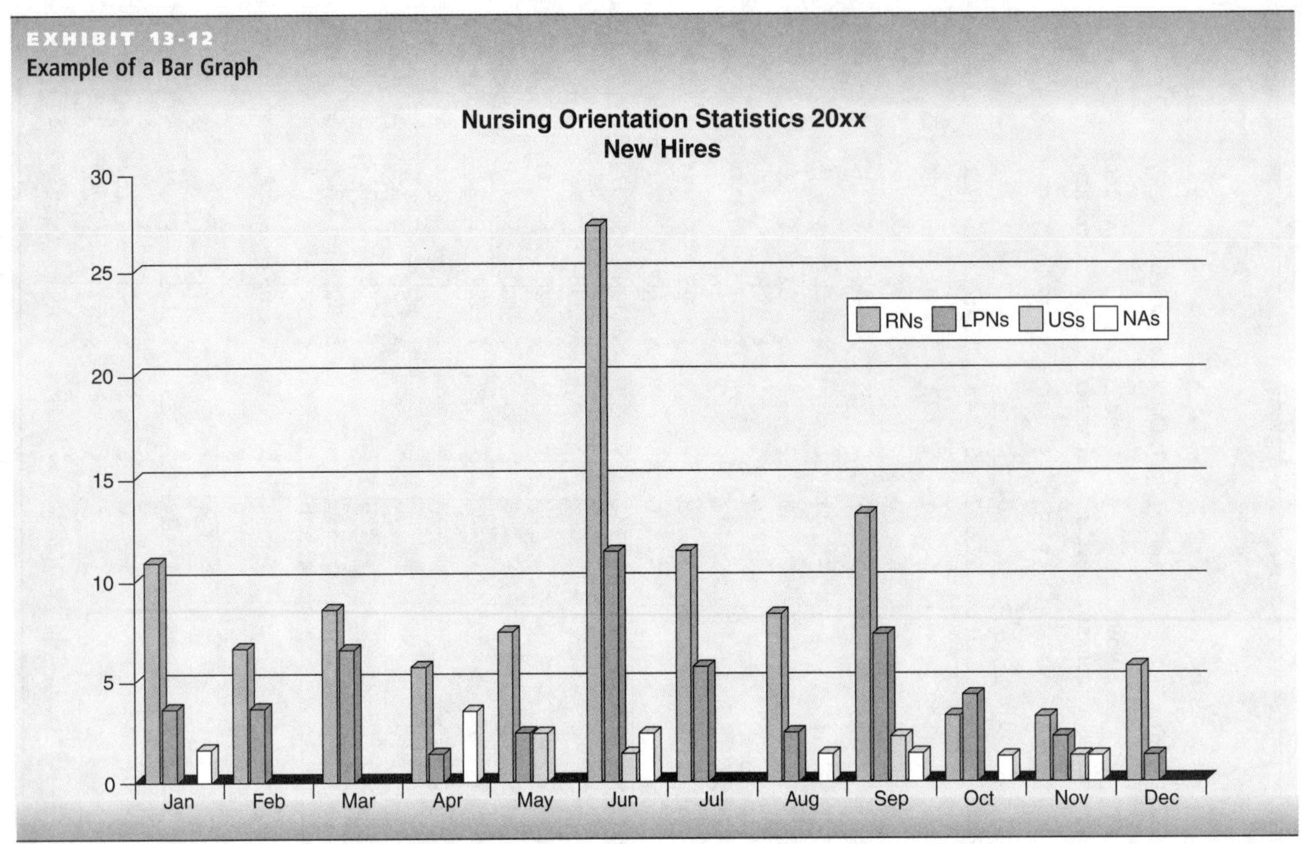

EXHIBIT 13-13

Example of a Line Graph

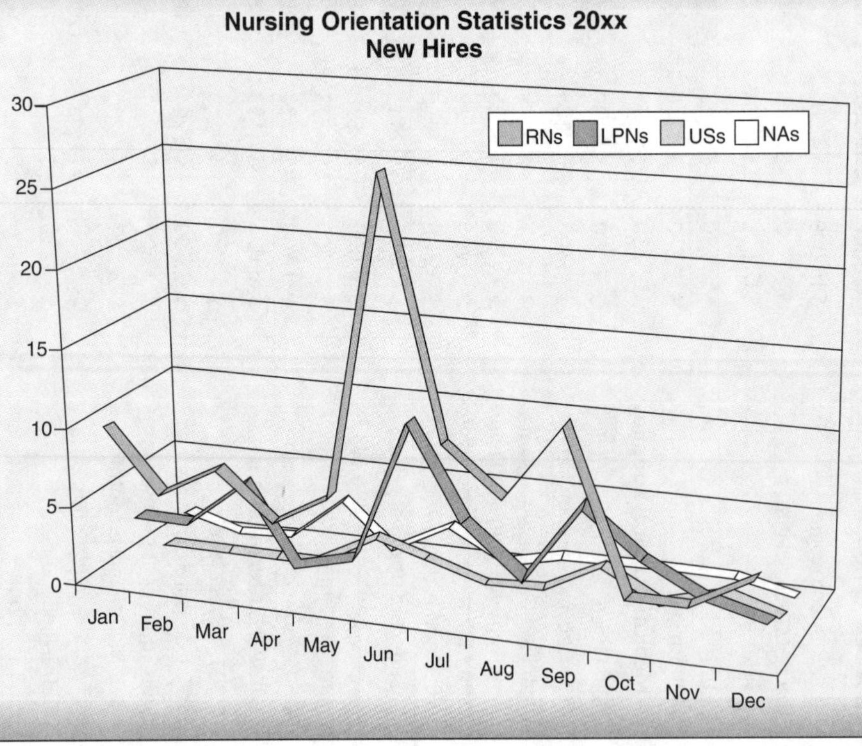

Nursing Orientation Statistics 20xx
New Hires
RNs LPNs USs NAs
30
25
20
15
10
5
0
Jan Feb Mar Apr May Jun Jul Aug Sep Oct Nov Dec

EXHIBIT 13-14
Example of a Policy

Policy Number:	5.11
Effective:	April 2003
Revised:	February 2005
Reviewed:	January 2005
Approved:	
Page:	1 of 1

University Hospitals

SUBJECT: University Hospitals Information System Error Screen Report

I. POLICY STATEMENT:
All error screens displayed on the University Hospitals Information System are to be documented and the report sent to the Information Systems department.

II. PROCEDURE:
When an error screen appears on the computer, the employee should:
1. Make a printout of the Error Screen by pressing "PA1" on the computer keyboard.
2. Beginning with the Master Menu, make printouts of each successive screen that led to the error screen.
3. Highlight each step of the procedure being performed on the screen printouts.
4. Complete the "Information System Error Screen Report," attach all printouts of the screens, and forward to the supervisor.
5. The supervisor will review the information for completeness and forward the report to the Information Systems department.

or phrases can be done by a simple request. Margins can be justified and words automatically hyphenated within set margins. Pages can be automatically defined and numbered.

Shell documents or templates can be created, in which the common content of a document never changes, but some areas are reserved for text that will change each time a new document is created from the template. The best examples of this are in memos and letters. The document and a list of variable information can be created separately and merged for printing.

Personal Information Manager (PIM)

A personal information manager application is an electronic version of the daily appointment book or day planner. It incorporates an address book, a calendar, e-mail, a journal, notes, and tasks. It can also include a groupware capability that allows direct collaboration with other devices that share the same PIM software. Today's PIMs work with two platforms of personal computing: a desktop or notebook computer and a personal digital assistant (PDA). A PDA is a computing device small enough to be carried in the pocket. It offers the same personal information management capabilities as a PIM does on a desktop computer. Often, the PDA includes a tool for synchronizing information between the PDA and the desktop system. This allows calendar or contact information to be entered into one system and then transferred to the other system.

The address book component provides a database for storing information about personal and professional contacts. This would include names, titles, addresses, telephone numbers, e-mail and Web addresses, and various other personal and professional information. The address book is a fundamental part of other PIM components and even other applications, such as word processing and spreadsheet applications. In the calendar, appointments and tasks can be created and scheduled. These can be one-time events or events that recur over a given period of time. When a meeting is scheduled, attendees can be invited directly (via e-mail or the groupware feature) from the address book. When invitees acknowledge their availability, their schedules automatically get updated to show the meeting, and the meeting organizer receives an accepted response. Reminders can be assigned to these events so as to provide notifications to the attendees.

Tasks can be created, scheduled, and assigned in much the same way as appointments can. A task indicates a duty or job that is to be performed. It often includes information related to its priority, start date, due date, percent complete, and status. Notes are brief pieces of information that are recorded. They can be assigned to defined categories and associated with events and tasks. A journal provides for a recorded account of daily events,

EXHIBIT 13-15
Example of a Form

REQUISITION

Requisition No. ____________

Departmental Request No. ____________ Date *June 27, 2005*

UNIVERSITY HOSPITALS
Mobile, Alabama 36608

To: PURCHASING OFFICE
The following order is requested by:

DIVISION *Information Technology Services* DEPARTMENT *Information Systems* ACCOUNT NO. *75150-323*

DELIVER TO *Information Systems* ROOM & LOCATION *Room 212, 2nd Floor*

QUANTITY	ITEM	UNIT	COST
5	Academic Windows 2000 Professional	$78.95	$394.75
PRICES ARE REQUIRED ON ALL REQUISITIONS		TOTAL	$394.75

CHECK HERE IF YOU ESTIMATED PRICE ____ PRICE QUOTED BY ____________

NAMES AND ADDRESSES OF VENDORS IN ORDER OF PREFERENCE (ATTACH ALL QUOTATIONS)

1. GE Capital ITS 3250 Downs Street Mobile, AL 36606 (334) 471-2471	2. Quoted Price ________	3. Quoted Price ________

The authority to issue purchase orders rests solely with the University Hospitals purchasing department. The University Hospitals assumes no obligation except on a previously issued and duly authorized purchase order. Direct orders by departments must show evidence of definite and particular permission.

FOR ACCOUNTING USE		
USE	FUND	AMOUNT

SIGNED ____________ REQUESTOR

APPROVED ____________ DEPARTMENT HEAD

APPROVED ____________ DEAN

APPROVED ____________ CONTROLLER

experiences, and reflections. These may include conversations, meetings, telephone calls, letters, and work performed. A journal and notes can be quite useful in remembering critical information at a later date, and a search tool is usually provided to find specific words or phrases in the subject or contents.

"E-mail is just the latest chapter in the evolving history of human communication."[12] It has become a convenient method of corresponding with others instead of using the telephone, fax, or postal service, and it has become a common part of our personal and professional lives. For this reason, the e-mail component is the cornerstone of today's PIM software. It provides us with services that allow us to send and receive our e-mail within the organizational setting and on the Internet, rules and folders for separating and storing our e-mail based upon sender or content, tools for archiving and retrieving old e-mail, and an easy way to transfer pictures and files with our daily contacts.

EXHIBIT 13-16
Example of Presentation Graphics to Discuss Coronary Disease

Coronary Disease Risk Factors

- Diabetes
- Family history
- High blood pressure
- High blood cholesterol
- Overweight
- Sedentary lifestyle
- Smoking
- Stress

Graphics

Graphics programs can produce images that can be used for presentations, illustrations, and classes. Graphics can be printed, displayed to a monitor, or projected onto a screen for viewing by a large audience. They can also be converted to presentation aids, such as overhead transparencies, videotapes, and slides.

In the past, graphics programs focused on the visual display of numerical data in the form of bar, line, and pie graphs. This was a legacy of the early use of graphics by business and management. Today, graphics systems can be used to illustrate almost anything. Features have been incorporated to display graphics in a slide show or with animation. Such presentation capability can be very helpful to a nurse trying to present information related to various business and clinical subjects. See Exhibits 13-16 and 13-17 for examples.

Graphics can be created as part of the program in association with some numerical data; they can be scanned; the user can create them freehand; or they can be purchased as an add-on to the graphics program.

Information Systems

The demands of working with automation in nursing can be great. Nurses may be asked to interact with specialized and generalized nursing information systems as well as with hospital information systems.

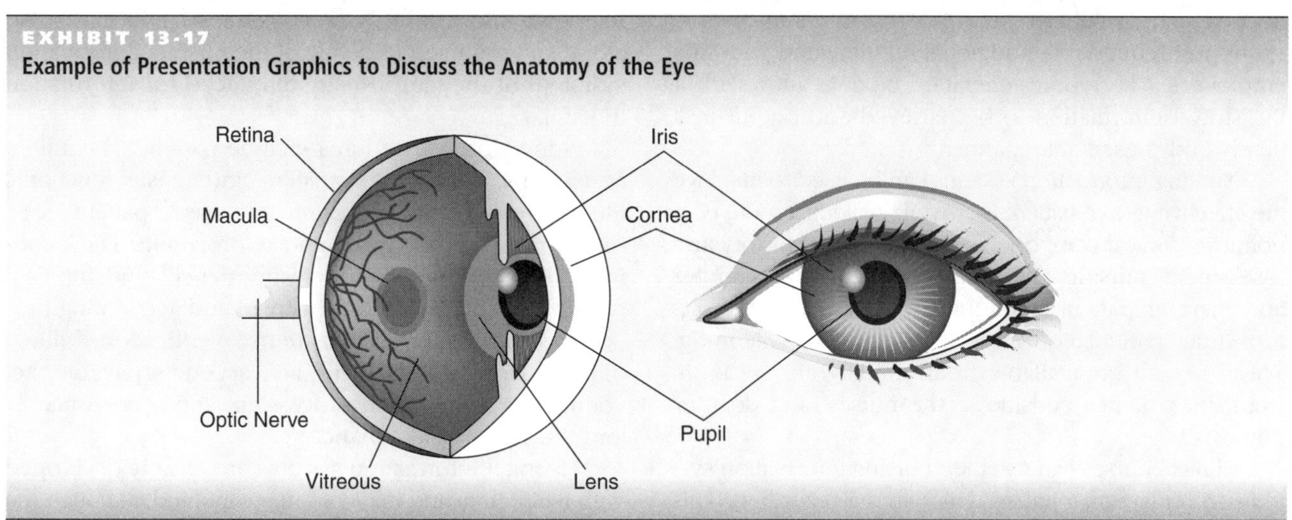

EXHIBIT 13-17
Example of Presentation Graphics to Discuss the Anatomy of the Eye

Nursing Information Systems

Nursing information systems are software packages developed specifically for nursing use. These programs may be explicit to a particular area of nursing application, or they may be general to the support of the nursing services division. Examples of nursing areas that can benefit from unique information systems support include mental health, neonatology, acute care, urology, enterostomal therapy, oncology, maternity, operating room, and infection control.

General nursing information systems have multiple programs, or modules, that are used to perform various clinical, educational, and management functions. Most nursing information systems have modules for classification, staffing, scheduling, personnel management, and report generation. Other modules may be included, such as budget development, resource allocation and cost control, case mix and diagnosis related groups (DRG) analysis, quality management, staff development, modeling and simulation for decision making, strategic planning, short-term demands for forecasting and work planning, and program evaluation.

Modules for patient classification, staffing, scheduling, personnel management, and report generation are often interrelated. Patients are classified according to established acuity criteria. The patient classification information is put into the staffing module, and staffing levels are calculated according to various workload formulas. Actual staffing is also input and a comparison of census, patient acuity, needed staffing, and actual staffing can be made. Schedules are then prepared using the information from the staffing and personnel records modules.

DRG analysis and quality management are done to associate patient acuity, quality of care, and DRG. This is helpful for establishing future guidelines and care needs for patients according to their DRGs. The budget is also supported by the census, patient acuity, and needed staffing patterns. This information is invaluable to support requests for additional full-time and part-time employees. The report generation module allows all of the stored information to be retrieved and output in a timely and presentable manner.

Nursing information systems can be used to improve the effectiveness of patient care while making it more economical. Clinical components include patient history and assessment, nursing care plans, nursing progress notes and charting, patient monitoring, order entry and results reporting, patient education, and discharge planning. These can all be available from virtually any location, from the patient's bedside to the nurses' and doctors' homes.

Clinical nurses can use their nursing information systems to replace manual systems of data recording. This may reduce costs and improve quality of care as well as quality of work life. Clinical nurses can collect and input clinical data and use the computer to analyze it to formulate treatment plans. They can use quantitative decision analysis to support clinical judgments. Automated consultation can be applied to screen for adverse drug reactions, interactions, and preparation of correct dosages. Computers can be programmed to reject orders that could cause problems in these and other areas, thus preventing errors.[13]

Curtin reminds nurses to provide "high-touch" in this high-tech world. Technology, computers, and information systems provide the knowledge to save lives or to prolong them. Nurses can return control to patients and families when they have lost their freedom of action or understanding of events. Nurses can keep control through the exercise of human compassion.[14] High-tech includes the new scientific knowledge of microelectronics, computers, information, sensors, processors, displays, and education. Its objective is the solution of society's total problems, not just those of health care.[15] Helping nurses provide high-touch while using high-tech should be a primary goal of nurse managers.

Hospital Information Systems

Hospital information systems are large, complex computer systems designed to help manage the information needs of a hospital. They are tools for interdepartmental and intradepartmental use. A typical hospital information system will have components for admissions, medical records, patient accounting, nursing, and order entry and results reporting. Other components can exist for virtually any department and for practically any purpose. Divisions such as nursing (the nursing information system), laboratory, radiology, pharmacy, and personnel and payroll may be so large and complex that they have their own information systems. These systems may stand alone and run independently of the hospital information system, but they are usually interfaced for information transfer.

Admissions procedures include patient scheduling, admissions, discharges, transfers, and census functions. Medical records procedures include master patient index functions, abstracting (diagnosis/procedure/DRG coding), transcription and correspondence, and medical record location functions. Business and accounting procedures include patient insurance verification, billing, billing followup, billing inquiry, accounts payable, accounts receivable, cash processing, and service master and third-party maintenance.

Hospital information systems are usually developed with mainframe and minicomputers in mind, although the trend today seems to favor distributed data networks. The advantages and disadvantages of each strategy should be weighed prior to implementation. Selection, development, and implementation of information systems can take years. This time will vary depending on the system and the complexity of its applications. It may actually be a continuous process. The initial cost can be millions of dollars for the hardware and software. Continued yearly maintenance is required and can cost hundreds of thousands or even millions of dollars.

Implementation of Information Systems

Nurse managers should be involved in the implementation and development of information systems and the direction of their users. Implementation of an information system requires preparation of a management plan. The first step is to form an implementation committee to assess the current system and what is wanted from the proposed system. This assessment should lead to a strategic plan, as acquiring an information system requires a significant expenditure of human, material, and financial resources.

The procurement process begins by asking vendors to respond to a request for information (RFI). This provides the implementation committee with valuable information related to system purpose and capability. From this a request for proposal (RFP) is created and sent to selected vendors. The RFP must be accurate and clearly worded to prevent any misinterpretation of the system's requirements. This formal process is important because the only way of being sure that a vendor understands and promises to meet an information system's expectations is to get the requirements on paper.[16]

Once the available systems have been reviewed and priced, a selection must be made based on which system fits the organization's needs and budget. From here the process proceeds to contract development. A properly designed and negotiated contract is crucial for the protection of the purchaser. A good contract does three things:[17]

- It insures that the vendor clearly understands your expectations of the system's capabilities and costs.
- It provides a means for recovery in the event that the system fails or does not perform properly.
- It provides a guarantee for continuous maintenance, support, and system updates needed to protect the investment and stay current with advances in computing.

Once the contract has been signed, the real project implementation begins. A project manager is assigned, a project implementation plan is developed (see Exhibit 13-18), and resources are allocated. Commitment to this process is essential from the bottom level users to executive management. In 1998, only 26% of organizational IT projects were successful: completed on time, on budget, and with all the features as specified.[18]

Finally, after the information system is live it must be evaluated to determine whether it meets the organization's needs as proposed. If it does, payments must be made to the vendor as per the contract. If it doesn't, the contract must be reevaluated, and a new course of action must be planned.

Data Warehousing and Knowledge Management

Information and knowledge are valuable commodities in today's complex and competitive health care environment. Vast amounts of data are stored in various legacy information systems within our health care organizations. These systems were developed to promote throughput and to limit redundancy, not to encourage data analysis and decision support. Data warehousing has become the new means for collecting, structuring, and storing data into repositories that provide for quick retrieval and intuitive analysis. "When designed and used properly, data warehouses lead to more effective business decisions in less time, which can increase a company's competitive advantage."[19]

Information is stored in various hypermedia systems (documents, e-mail, and Web pages) within our health care organizations. These systems require tools to cull, retrieve, and present these buried knowledge assets. "Knowledge management encompasses an overarching business strategy aimed at exposing and taking advantage of a company's information, experience, and expertise to serve customers better and respond quickly to changing market conditions."[20] Knowledge management incorporates data mining (discovering hidden information in data) and ad-hoc query and reporting services that attempt to tie the knowledge together on a common platform.

Decision Support Systems, Expert Systems, and Predictive Technology

A decision-support system (DSS) is software that provides personnel with essential information to substantiate the making of decisions. An expert system is software that uses a knowledge base, rules, and inference to aid in solving problems. An expert system is associated with a particular discipline, and experts in that field develop the knowledge base, rules, and conclusions. Predictive technology refers to the process of using the information content in large, complex databases so as to understand and predict the actions of various entities in health care (patients, providers, and payers). These predictions are used to improve business decisions.[21]

EXHIBIT 13-18

Example of a Project Implementation Plan

ID	ACTIVITY	DURATION	START	FINISH
1	UNIVERSITY HOSPITALS RESULTS REPOSITORY PROJECT STARTUP	2.5d	9/11/00	9/13/00
4	ADMINISTRATIVE	120d	9/13/00	2/28/01
5	Project Status Meetings	115.25d	9/15/00	2/23/01
13	Project Steering Committee Meetings	95.25d	9/20/00	1/31/01
19	Quality Assurance Review Visit	2d	9/13/00	9/15/00
20	Project Supervision	120d	9/13/00	2/28/01
21	PROJECT INITIATION	10d	9/14/00	9/27/00
22	Pre-Implementation Planning	1d	9/14/00	9/14/00
24	Project Planning	2d	9/15/00	9/18/00
28	Adapt Network	5d	9/18/00	9/22/00
30	Project Kickoff	7d	9/19/00	9/27/00
35	HARDWARE AND SOFTWARE	12.5d	9/13/00	9/29/00
36	Hardware/Software Installation	12.5d	9/13/00	9/29/00
39	Software Delivery Validation	9d	9/13/00	9/26/00
43	ANALYSIS	58d	9/28/00	12/18/00
44	Results Repository Surveys/Process Flow/Tables	15d	9/28/00	10/18/00
48	Results Repository Interfaces	20d	10/19/00	11/15/00
51	Results Repository Profiles/Procedures	11d	11/16/00	11/30/00
59	Nursing Assessment Surveys/Process Flow/Procedures	11d	11/27/00	12/11/00
63	Nursing Assessment Master Files	3d	12/12/00	12/14/00
65	Nursing Assessment Reports/Project Scope	2d	12/15/00	12/18/00
68	TRAINING	42d	12/18/00	2/13/01
69	Training Preparation	12d	12/18/00	1/2/01
73	Educate Users	30d	1/3/01	2/13/01
77	LIVE EVENT	28d	1/22/01	2/28/01
78	Live Event Preparation	22d	1/22/01	2/20/01
83	Results Repository Live Event	4d	2/23/01	2/28/01
86	Nursing Assessment Live Event	5d	2/22/01	2/28/01
88	Live Event Support	5d	2/22/01	2/28/01
90	POST-LIVE	10d	3/1/01	3/14/01
91	Evaluation and Feedback to Management	10d	3/1/01	3/14/01
92	Monitor Production System	6d	3/1/01	3/8/01
95				

"Organizations that create a strategy and implement DSS tools to provide decision makers with the critical information they need to face the competition and maintain quality and costs will have the advantage."[22]

Four types of decision makers exist: analytical, intuitive, accommodating, and integrated. Analytical decision makers seek to use quantitative, rational, and logical reasoning. They seek a single, predictable cause to a problem; ignore the unpredictable; and simplify the complex. Intuitive decision makers consider the whole problem using an unstructured and spontaneous approach to its resolution. Accommodating decision makers are either analytical or intuitive, but experience has taught them to adopt the other style when appropriate. Finally, integrated decision makers don't have a dominant style. They reason, analyze, and gather facts that trigger their use of intuition.

A clinical DSS can be implemented to drive the appropriate process improvement activities required to achieve successful care outcomes.[23] Good decision-support systems should blend analytical tools with intuitive heuristics to provide insight about complex factors that can't be built into models. These systems must assist in the modification of analytical results when they contradict what intuition tells us.

DSSs should provide for quick and convenient access to data extraction and analysis tools. They should provide a wide range of models for investigation and summary. They should track experience to factor in past decisions and results. They should allow for the input of values, ethics, morals, and goals. They should help to understand what is known, and to recognize what has been overlooked. They should provide alternatives and their interpretations. In the end, they must be capable of presenting understandable results to the decision makers.[24]

Expert systems encode the relevant knowledge and experience of experts to make them available to less knowledgeable persons. An example would be to take the accumulated knowledge and experience of clinical nurse specialists in neuroscience nursing, encode them in a computer system, and make the system available to clinical nurses working in the neuroscience area. A nurse would identify a situation requiring a decision, the criteria defining the problem, and objectives for handling the situation. The expert system would evaluate the information and provide a list of ways to manage the situation. The nurse would then evaluate the alternatives and make the decision.

Predictive technology provides organizations with a way to identify and exploit behavioral patterns hidden within their data. This technology is capable of learning from experience and improving its predictive capabilities over time. Patient interactions can be analyzed to allow health care providers to determine the preferences, usage patterns, and future needs of the patient. Opportunities to apply predictive technology in healthcare may include the following:[25]

- The detection of fraud and abuse perpetrated by patients and providers.
- The prediction of future clinical outcomes.
- The prediction of future resource use.
- The prediction of complex cases that can benefit the most from case management.

Nursing Management Applications

Many applications are available for nursing management. These include a calendar of events, a nursing management minimum data set (NMMDS), and a human resources information system.

A calendar can be useful in supplying nursing personnel with dates and times of staff meetings, committee meetings, and educational events (see Exhibit 13-19). The calendar could be an Internet-browser-based application that is available on the organization's intranet. This would provide for simple point-and-click access to events and their details from any personal computer, at work or home. Information for the calendar could be linked to and provided from the organization's information systems, such as the human resource system. Through the use of these calendar links, employees could actively schedule themselves for meetings or classes. When they choose an event like an educational class, their names could be added to the class role and automatic notifications could be sent to their nurse managers.

The NMMDS is a research based management data set available from the American Organization of Nurse Executives. It has 17 elements clustered around 3 broad categories of environment, nurse resources, and financial resources. "It is a means by which data about the context and support of direct health care delivery are organized, classified, managed, accessed, and researched. The principle behind the NMMDS is that nurse executives need hard data to make the difficult quality decisions that need to be made in today's operating environment."[26] Implementing the NMMDS empowers nursing management with quality data to answer questions related to outcomes of critical paths, turnover rates of personnel, nurse satisfaction, personnel ratings, budgets, and productivity. It also provides data to compare time periods.[27]

The management of human resources can be a formidable task for health care organizations. The collection and manipulation of information associated with this management can require significant time and manpower. The development and implementation of a human resources information system can be a blessing to the organization and to the professionals who manage these resources.

Front-end components can be established to analyze information related to all of the job applicants who apply to the organization and information related to the advertising and recruitment of these applicants. Some information needs to be retained on each person who applies for any job position. This information can be useful for understanding the professional market and for addressing concerns about equal opportunity hiring practices. Applications analysis can show how many people apply for a position by specific indicators. See Exhibit 13-20 for an example report. Advertising analysis can provide recruitment information related to the method and placement of advertisements. See Exhibit 13-21 for an example report.

Individuals who are hired can be pulled from the applications analysis component and added to the permanent employee database. This database is the central foundation of the human resources system; it maintains

EXHIBIT 13-19
Example of a Nursing Calendar

Nursing Calendar **OCTOBER 20xx**

Monday	Tuesday	Wednesday	Thursday	Friday
2 Nursing Orientation 0800 Nursing Council 1300	**3**	**4** Diabetes Management 1430	**5** Understanding Nutrition 1430	**6**
9 Body Mechanics 0730 Body Mechanics 1930	**10** Annual Education 0800 CPR 1300	**11**	**12** 6th Floor Staff Meeting 1515	**13** Antibiotic Therapy 0730 Antibiotic Therapy 1930
16 ACLS Class 0800 Patient Monitoring 0800 Infusion Pumps 1300	**17**	**18** Understanding ECGs 0730 Understanding ECGs 1930	**19** Quality Improvement 1200	**20** Hospital Picnic 1100
23 Body Mechanics 0730 Body Mechanics 1930	**24** CPR 1300	**25** CCU Staff Meeting 1515	**26**	**27** Antibiotic Therapy 0730 Antibiotic Therapy 1930
30 IV Certification 0900	**31** Halloween Party 1530			

EXHIBIT 13-20
Example of an Applications Analysis Report

APPLICATIONS ANALYSIS REPORT FOR THE MONTH OF SEPTEMBER 200x

POSITION		F	M	AM	AS	BA	CA	HI	PI	DIS	VET	DVET
01412	Registered nurse	3	0	0	0	2	1	0	0	0	0	0
02456	Registered nurse	2	0	0	0	1	1	0	0	0	0	0
02457	Registered nurse	6	2	0	1	2	4	1	0	0	0	0
11923	Licensed practical nurse	7	0	0	0	5	2	0	0	0	0	0
15934	Assistant administrator	3	12	0	0	1	14	0	0	0	0	0
22921	Unit secretary	11	1	0	1	8	3	0	0	1	0	0
23110	Education specialist	5	2	0	0	2	5	0	0	0	1	0

EXHIBIT 13-21

Example of an Advertisement Analysis Report

ADVERTISEMENT ANALYSIS REPORT FOR THE MONTH OF SEPTEMBER 200X

ADD NO.	PLACEMENT	DATE	RN	LPN	PHR	PT	RT	CLK	MG	OTH
1622	Channel 5	09/01/xx	3	2	0	0	1	0	0	5
1633	Channel 10	09/01/xx	1	1	1	0	0	1	0	2
1734	Newspaper	09/03/xx	1	1	1	1	0	0	1	1
1775	Internet	09/03/xx	2	0	2	0	1	0	1	1
1622	Channel 5	09/08/xx	0	0	0	0	1	3	0	1
1633	Channel 10	09/08/xx	2	0	0	1	0	1	0	2
1734	Newspaper	09/10/xx	5	1	1	1	1	0	1	3
1775	Internet	09/10/xx	0	0	0	1	1	0	0	2
1622	Channel 5	09/15/xx	1	1	0	0	2	0	0	7
1633	Channel 10	09/15/xx	0	3	2	0	1	1	0	6
1734	Newspaper	09/17/xx	1	3	3	0	1	4	0	5
1775	Internet	09/17/xx	3	2	1	0	1	0	0	1
1734	Newspaper	09/24/xx	2	0	0	0	1	0	1	0
1755	Internet	09/24/xx	1	0	0	0	1	0	2	0

EXHIBIT 13-22

Example of an Employee Termination Report

EMPLOYEE TERMINATION REPORT FOR THE MONTH OF SEPTEMBER 200X

POSITION	NAME	TITLE	DATE	REASON
00356	Johnson, Mary J.	Registered nurse	09/26/xx	Q
10234	Armstrong, Helen M.	Licensed practical nurse	09/08/xx	Q
16212	Mims, Janet K.	Registered nurse	09/13/xx	F
17335	Baker, Donald M.	Registered nurse	09/05/xx	Q
17366	Smitherman, Carolyn S.	Registered nurse	09/22/xx	R
18549	Jackson, Melanie J.	Unit secretary	09/01/xx	Q
18675	Hanson, Marcus K.	Respiratory therapist	09/29/xx	Q

all of the information related to employees and their positions, from the moment they are hired until they are terminated. (See Exhibit 13-22 for an example of a termination report). The database can be used to maintain information about personnel with special skills or credentials, and it can identify employees facing license renewal deadlines and those who need additional training. Additional components can be integrated into the human resources system to collect and report information on employee education, time, and attendance.

The educational component maintains all of the information associated with the education of employees. (See Exhibit 13-23 for an example of an employee education report.) This information can also meet the reporting needs of the institution as to the requirements of the state board of nursing and the Joint Commission on Accreditation of Healthcare Organizations. Education elements may include the following:

- New employee orientation
- Clinical specialty courses
- Continuing education offerings
- Competency validation of skills
- Nursing station in-service education
- Annual required reviews[28]

The time and attendance component maintains the information associated with employees' work, vacation, holiday, and sick time. The information here produces timesheets. From the human resources system, information can be exported and imported to the hospital and nursing information systems. It may also be exported to general-purpose application software for various purposes.

EXHIBIT 13-23
Example of an Employee Education Report

EMPLOYEE EDUCATION REPORT

EMPLOYEE NAME: JONES, MARY L.
POSITION NUMBER: 353367
NURSING UNIT: MICU

COURSE TYPE	DESCRIPTION	DATE COMPLETE	EVAL CODE	CLASS HOURS	CLINICAL HOURS	CONTACT HOURS
C	Antibiotic therapy	10/27/xx	S			1.0
	Understanding ECGs	10/18/xx	S			2.0
	Subtotal Continuing Education					3.0
I	Patient monitoring	10/16/xx	S	4.0		
	Infusion pumps	10/16/xx	S	1.0		
	Subtotal In-Service Education			5.0		
O	Personnel	10/02/xx	S	2.0		
	Fire and safety	10/02/xx	S	3.0		
	Infection control	10/02/xx	S	3.0		
	Legal issues	10/03/xx	S	4.0		
	Cardiopulmonary resuscitation	10/04/xx	S	4.0		
	Information systems	10/06/xx	S	8.0		
	Unit orientation	10/27/xx	S		120.0	
	Subtotal Orientation			24.0	120.0	
S	IV Certification	10/30/xx	S	3.0		
	Subtotal Skills Competency			3.0		
	Totals			32.0	120.0	3.0

Ethical, Legal, and Security Issues

Certain ethical issues are involved in the use of technology in nursing. *Ethical* means conforming to professional standards of conduct. Romano defines *privacy* as "control over exposure of self or information about oneself and freedom from intrusion. Privacy denotes the right of an individual to decide how much personal information to share. It includes a right to secrecy of information and protection against the misuse or release of this information."[29] *Confidentiality* means being entrusted with the privacy of others that was shared with you in confidence. The relationship of the three terms can be expressed as a patient entrusting privacy to a professional who has an ethical responsibility to maintain the confidentiality of that information.

Legal issues associated with automation may involve the confidentiality of patient information and the risk associated with clinical decision making based upon computerized information. One method of addressing these issues is by maintaining professional standards. Information systems should be designed, developed, and implemented to validate patient outcomes and support professional nursing standards. This means that computer technology for nursing use needs to be based on nursing input from start to finish. This requires the use of expert nurses who have sufficient clinical, theoretical, educational, research, and management expertise to adequately represent professional standards. It also requires a unified nursing profession that can specify clear design criteria and professional standards guidelines.[30]

Nurses should also be capable of assessing and managing the legal risks associated with automated information management. Computer data should be examined, analyzed, interpreted, and appraised. Forced selections and unclear logic should be questioned. Nurses should not hold as fact the belief that clinical decision making based on the use of technology results in better patient care.

The American Nurses Association, the American Health Information Management Association, and the Canadian Nurses Association offer guidelines and strategies for minimizing legal risks associated with automated charting:[31]

- Never give your computer password to anyone.
- Do not leave a computer terminal unattended after you've logged on.

- Follow procedure for modifying mistakes. Computer entries are part of the permanent record and cannot be deleted.
- Do not leave patient information displayed on a screen for others to see. Also, keep track of printed information about patients and dispose of it appropriately when it is no longer needed.
- Follow your institution's confidentiality policies and procedures.

Automation in nursing also involves security issues. *Security* means the level to which hardware, software, and information is safe from abuse and unauthorized use or access, whether accidental or intentional. From a management standpoint, professionals need to be aware that security must be overseen from physical, operational, and ethical viewpoints.

Physical security deals with the control of access to hardware, the assessment and determination of environmental threats, and the prevention of loss. Operational security deals with the threats to information. It includes the assessment and prevention of unauthorized access or use of information, the policies and procedures governing the management of information, and the procedures required for recovery from loss of information. Ethical security deals with the individual's ability to conform to professional standards of conduct. This means that nurses have to respect the privacy of information. They must accept and enforce all guidelines that are imposed for the maintenance of physical and operational security of computer systems.

Nurses should be aware of various security measures that may be built into information systems. One of the first priorities should be the ability to perform auditing: leaving a trail of who did what, where, and when. Logs can record by whom, when, and where the system is accessed. This same information can be captured when vital information is created, modified, or deleted. Standard procedures should be in place for the routine auditing of this information.

A significant amount of security may be associated with an individual's computer ID. Every individual should be assigned his or her own personal ID. This ID should have the person's name, title, department, security level, and menu linked to it. There should be a password that protects the ID and is known only by the user. Procedures should be in place to force users to change their passwords every 30 to 90 days and allow them to change passwords more often as desired. A number of each user's old passwords should be stored for comparison purposes, and the user should not be allowed to reuse these passwords.

The security level should be implemented in a hierarchical manner from administrator to nursing assistant. It can be a range of numbers from largest to smallest that can be tested to determine who can perform particular functions. Menus that determine a user's ability to interact with the system should be developed and assigned based upon departmental and job requirements.

Summary

The intent of this chapter is to provide an overview of nursing and information technology. The computer has become an everyday tool for handling information. In health care, computers provide support for clinical communication and documentation and the management of complicated financial environments.

Computers are used to support and run highly complex information systems that have tremendous capacities for the manipulation and storage of information. Virtually any nursing process can be augmented or implemented through the use of information technology. There are systems that assist nurses in documentation of patient care, order processing, clinical decision making, and patient and professional education. Other general-purpose application software is available for personal productivity enhancement. Nurses have needs for document preparation, number crunching, and record keeping. They also find that graphics, multimedia, and communications applications are invaluable tools for presentations and educational support.

We must also not forget the human side of nursing; we have ethical and moral responsibilities to protect the privacy that patients have entrusted to us. Maintaining the security of information is an active and ongoing duty. As overseers of this information, we must not think of our right to know, but our privilege to know.

APPLICATION EXERCISES

EXERCISE 13-1 Discuss the technologic changes that you have experienced and how you believe they have influenced your life.

EXERCISE 13-2 Discuss the current information technology environment you are working in or are being exposed to in health care. Identify changes that you expect to see in the next 5 years.

EXERCISE 13-3 Which type of computer network(s) do you use within your organization? Identify the various discrete computers (servers with information systems) attached to the network of your organization. Try to develop a graphical representation of the hardware and software environments.

EXERCISE 13-4 What role does the Internet have in the information technology environment of your organization? Identify and discuss the resources available to nursing through the Internet.

EXERCISE 13-5 Identify and discuss information technology used by various nursing personnel (unit secretary, registered nurses, nursing management, and clinical specialists) in your organization. Include personal computer applications, information systems, and diagnostic equipment.

EXERCISE 13-6 Identify and discuss the development of various applications using personal computer applications software. Pick a project and implement it.

EXERCISE 13-7 Identify an area of information management (in your current nursing environment) that is not automated, and develop a proposal for obtaining an information system for it.

EXERCISE 13-8 Discuss your views on ethics, privacy, confidentiality, and security. Which security measures do you interact with in your environment? Is there room for improvement?

NOTES

1. Rutsky, R. L. (1999). Techno-cultural interaction and the fear of information. *Style*, 267.
2. Feretic, E. (2000). Never too old. *Beyond Computing*, 8.
3. Hagland, M. (1997). Buyers and sellers. *Health Management Technology*, *1*, 20–23.
4. *The American Heritage Dictionary of the English Language* (3rd ed.). (1996). Boston: Houghton Mifflin.
5. Welcome to 2010. (2000, March 6). *Business Week*, 102.
6. Blackford, J. (1999). The future of computing: For 500,000 years, technology has advanced while people remained the same. In the next millennium, the human race plays catch-up. *Computer Shopper*, 319.
7. Derfler, F. J., Jr. (2000). Virtual private networks. *PC Magazine*, 146.
8. Coile, R. C., Jr. (2000). The digital transformation of health care. *Physician Executive*, 8–15.
9. Ferry, J. (1999). Virtual doctors on the horizon in Seattle. *Lancet*, 926.
10. Schreiber, C. (2000, April 3). For your eyes only: HHS aims to protect patient confidentiality. *HealthWeek*, 1, 15.
11. *Microsoft Word 2000* (Microsoft Corporation, 1999).
12. Granger, P. (1999, September 20). *Newsweek*, 58.
13. Gottinger, H. W. (1984). Computers in hospital care: A qualitative assessment. *Human Systems Management*, *6*, 324–345.
14. Curtin, L. (1984). Nursing: High touch in a high-tech world. *Nursing Management*, *1*, 7–8.
15. McKenzie-Sanders, P. (1983). The central focus of the information age. *Business Quarterly*, 87–91.
16. Carr, D. F. (2000). Meeting of the minds. *Internet World*, 45.
17. Fischer, R. X. & Singh, S. P. (2000). Checklist for a good contract for IT purchases. *Health Management Technology*, 14.
18. Raths, D. (2000). Managing your three-ring circus–The role of project manager is complex and risky, but getting a grip on your staff and project processes can help ensure success. *InfoWorld*, 93.
19. Steinacher, S. (1999). Organized data boosts corporate IQ: Make effective business decisions in less time by creating a data warehouse. *InfoWorld*, 65.

20. Roberts-Witt, S. L. (2000). Knowledge management: Know what you know. *PC Magazine*, 165.
21. Biafore, S. (1999). Predictive solutions bring more power to decision makers. *Health Management Technology*, 12.
22. Waldo, B. H. (1998). Decision support and data warehousing tools boost competitive advantage. *Nursing Economic$*, *21*, 91–93.
23. Rosenstein, A. H. (1999). Inpatient clinical decision-support systems determining the ROI. *Healthcare Financial Management*, *51*(5).
24. Sauter, V. L. (1999). Intuitive decision-making. *Communications of the ACM*, 109.
25. Biafore, 1999.
26. Simpson, R. L. (1997). What good are advanced practitioners if nobody at the top knows their value? *Nursing Administration Quarterly*, *91*(2).
27. Huber, D., Schumacher, L., & Delaney, C. (1997). Nursing Management Minimum Data Set (NMMDS). *Journal of Nursing Administration*, 42–48.
28. Robinette, J. E. & Weitzel, P. S. (1989). Design and development of a computerized education records system. *Journal of Continuing Education in Nursing*, 174–182; Keenan, G. M., Heath, C., Treder, M., Stocker, J., & Yakel, B. (2003). HANDS: Refining methods to generate comparable nursing data. *International Journal of Nursing Terminologies and Classifications*, 28; Feuerback, R. D. & Panniers, T. L. (2003). Building an expert system: A systematic approach to developing an instrument for data extraction from the literature. *Journal of Nursing Care Quality*, *2*, 129–138.
29. Romano, C. A. (1987). Privacy, confidentiality, and security of computerized systems. *Computers in Nursing*, *2*, 99–104.
30. Woolery, L. K. (1990). Professional standards and ethical dilemmas in nursing information systems. *Journal of Nursing Administration*, *1*, 50–53.
31. Iyer, P. (1993). Computer charting: Minimizing legal risks. *Nursing*, 86.

REFERENCES

Amadio, J. (2000). Share and share alike. *Entrepreneur*, 59.

Ammenwerth, E., Mansmann, U., Iller, C., & Eichstadter, R. (2003). Factors affecting and affected by user acceptance of computer-based nursing documentation: Results of a two-year study. *Journal of the American Informatics Association*, *10*(1).

Andrieu, M. (1999). A better future for work? *OECD Observer*, 53.

Baxter, B. (1997). Exploring newsgroups. *Nursing*, *26*(1).

Braue, D. (1998). Network your business. *Australian PC World*, *72*(5).

Brekka, T. (1995). Select mobile computers tailored to healthcare environment. *Health Management Technology*, *48*(2).

Chernicoff, D. P. (1994). Networking history in a nutshell. *PC Week*, *12*(4).

Cini, A. (1996). The networking bowl. *Digital Age*, *22*(6).

Craft, N. (1996). No touch technique. *British Medical Journal*, *318*(2).

Dash, J. (2000). Users take cautious approach to "E-Health." *Computerworld*, *10*(1).

Domrose, C. (2000, January 24). Virtual nurse: The Internet is expanding health care possibilities. *HealthWeek*, 16.

Hayes, Frank. (1999). 100 years of IT. *Computerworld*, *74*(1).

Howe, Dennis. (1993). *The free on-line dictionary of computing*. Retrieved on July 29, 2005 from http://www.foldoc.org.

Kasoff, J. (2003). Consider this . . . Nursing references at the point of care. *Journal of Nursing Administration*, *33*(1).

Kilgore, C. (2000). Movement toward Internet-based patient records. *Family Practice News*, 65.

Moschella, D. (1999). Ten turning points in the IT industry's history. *Computerworld*, *33*(1).

Muehleman, F. (1999). Computer firsts paved way long before PC became PC. *Triangle Business Journal*, 41.

Park, S. A., Park, J. H., Jung, M. S., Lee, H. J., Joo, M. K., & Park, S. H. (2003). Development of a system for nursing diagnosis and intervention management. *International Journal of Nursing Terminologies & Classifications*, *14*(4).

Rowh, M. (1999). Casting your net. *Office Systems 99*, *11*(1).

Sanborn, S. (1999). Internet milestones. *InfoWorld*, 34.

Satava, R. (1999). Emerging technologies for surgery in the 21st century. *Archives of Surgery*, 1197–202.

Stevens, L. (2000). Health care turns to the Web. *InternetWeek*, 33–37.

Telingator, S. (2000). Merging healthcare and the Internet in the new century. *Health Management Technology*, 42.

Vetter, R. & Kroeker, K. L. (1998). The Internet in the year ahead. *Computer*, *143*(2).

APPENDIX 13-1
Glossary of Commonly Used Computer Terms

ABEND: Abnormal end of task.
Algorithm: A prescribed set of rules for the solution of a problem in a finite number of steps.
Artificial intelligence: The capability of a machine that can proceed or perform functions that are normally concerned with human intelligence, such as learning, adapting, reasoning, self-correction, and automatic improvement.
Batch processing: A system that takes a set of jobs from disk, executes them and returns the results to disk, all without human intervention. Can be scheduled and executed at a later date and time.
Binary: The number system based on the 2 choices of 0 and 1.
Bit: The smallest unit of data, a binary digit of 0 or 1.
Buffer: Intermediate storage, used in input/output operations to temporarily hold data/information.
Bug: A mistake or error in a computer program.
Byte: A set of eight adjoining bits thought of as a unit.
Cache: A storage buffer that contains frequently accessed instructions and data.

(continued)

APPENDIX 13-1 ***(continued)***

Central processing unit (CPU): The part of the computer that controls all of the other parts. It consists of a control unit, an arithmetic and logic unit, and memory (registers and cache).
Character: A letter, digit, or other symbol that is used as part of the representation of data. A byte.
Compact disc (CD): A type of disk storage that uses magneto-optical recording and lasers.
CRT (cathode ray tube): Cathode ray terminal. A display terminal used as an input/output station.
Data: A representation of numbers or characters in the form suitable for processing by a computer.
Database: A collection of files or tables.
Database management system: A specialized type of software used for the organization, storage, and retrieval of data in a database.
Disk: Disc. Round, flat magnetic media used for the storage of data.
Downtime: The elapsed time when a computer is not available for use. It may be scheduled for maintenance or unscheduled because of machine or program problems.
Expert system: An application that contains a knowledge base and a set of algorithms or rules that have been derived from human expertise to provide assistance in decision making.
Extranet: An extension of an organization's intranet, over the Internet, enabling communication between the institution and people with whom it deals.
Field: A unit of data within a record.
File: A collection of related data with a given structure.
Forecasting: Predicting the future by an analysis of data.
GUI (graphical user interface): A user interface to a computer based on graphics.
Hard copy: Printed computer output in the form of reports and documents.
Hardware: The physical computer equipment.
Information systems: Computer systems designed to store and manipulate information for communication and decision support.
Input/Output (I/O): The transfer of data between an external source and internal storage.
Interface: The point at which independent systems or computers interact.
Internet: A worldwide network of computer networks that use the TCP/IP network protocols to facilitate data transmission and exchange.
Intranet: A privately maintained computer network that can be accessed only by authorized persons, especially members or employees of the organization that owns it.
Key: A field or fields within a record that makes that record unique with respect to other records in a file.
Kilobyte (KB): 1,024 bytes.
Local area network (LAN): Two or more computers connected for local resource sharing.
Mainframe computer: A powerful computer capable of being used and interacted with by hundreds of users, simultaneously.
Megabyte (MB): 1,024 kilobytes.
Microcomputer: A small computer built around a microprocessor.
Minicomputer: A midsize computer, smaller and less powerful than a mainframe, but larger and more powerful than a microcomputer.
Modeling: A representation of a complex system used as a basis for simulation to allow for the prediction and understanding of the system's behavior.
Modem: A device that converts digital data from a computer to an analog signal that can be transmitted on a telecommunications line and that converts received analog transmissions to digital data.
Multimedia: The combination of different elements of media, such as text, graphics, audio, video, animation, and sound.
Multitasking: A mode of operation that provides for the concurrent execution of two or more tasks.
Online processing: A system that provides for the immediate, interactive input and processing of data.
Operating system: Software designed to control the hardware of a specific computer system in order to allow users and application programs to use it.
Printer: A terminal or peripheral that produces hard copy or printed output.
Program: A set of computer instructions directing the computer to perform some operation.
Random access: A storage technique whereby a file can be addressed and accessed directly at its location on the media or a record can be addressed and accessed directly within a file.
Record: A group of related fields of data treated as a unit.
Robotics: The science or study of mechanical devices designed to perform tasks that might be otherwise done by humans.

APPENDIX 13-1

Sequential access: A storage technique whereby a file can be addressed and accessed only after all those before it on the media have been or a record can be addressed and accessed only after all those before it in the file have been.
Simulation: Attempting to predict aspects of the behavior of some system by creating an approximate model of it.
Software: A program or set of programs written to tell the computer hardware how to do something.
Spreadsheet: A specialized type of software for manipulation of numbers.
Table: A collection of related records in a database management system.
Trend: A systematic pattern of change over time.
User-friendly: Software considered easier to use for novices.
Voice communication: Interaction with a computer by voice recognition.
Wide area network (WAN): A network of two or more groups of computers or computing devices that are remote from each other and connected by telecommunication equipment.
Word processor: A specialized type of software for the manipulation of words to produce printed material.

CHAPTER 14

Health Policy, Legal, and Regulatory Issues

Linda Roussel, RN, DSN
Mary-Eliese Merrill, RN, MSN

Evolved people respect differing views, understanding that life's meaning is to be found everywhere. They are open, always learning and growing. An evolved person knows that there is only one truth, but many different ways of seeing it.

Lance Secreten

LEARNING OBJECTIVES AND ACTIVITIES

- Describe policy and public policy and its relationship to health care issues.
- Outline a policy process.
- Differentiate among the elements of a risk management program.
- Identify the risks professional nurses face regarding malpractice and other torts.
- Outline a plan for professional nurses to use to reduce the risks of legal actions.

CONCEPTS: Policy, public policy, agenda setting, nurse practice acts, contracts, torts, negligence, malpractice, assault and battery, false imprisonment, slander and libel, liability, wills.

NURSE MANAGER BEHAVIORS: Applies legal principles that manage risks to and reflect the values of the organization and providers of care; assures compliance with regulatory and professional standards.

NURSE EXECUTIVE BEHAVIORS: Applies legal principles that maintain quality nursing care and satisfactory service to customers. This satisfactory service is not only legal but also ethical and moral, reflecting the values of the leader. Fosters empowered decision making, accountability, and autonomy in nursing practice for professional nurses.

Introduction

As health care has evolved throughout history, the interpretation and implementation of principles, standards, and laws governing delivery and services have changed as well. Five significant factors have added to these changes in health care systems:[1]

1. Place (site of delivery)
2. People (who receives care)
3. Preventive model (reward for health, not sickness)
4. Paradigm (quality improvement and customer satisfaction)
5. Process (modern technology)

Exhibit 14-1 makes a comparison of old health care paradigm with the new paradigm. Professional nurses continue to integrate the role of educator, researcher, administrator and political activist and continue to expand their roles. Such adaptation expands the scope of nursing practice by addressing health care issues that are a matter of public interest. "Decisions that affect the public interest are made over time in the policy arena."[2]

As nursing has evolved as a profession, nurses' liability has increased. Assuming authority, responsibility, and accountability for their professional practice, professional nurses increasingly are being subjected to scrutiny by state boards of nursing representing the policing power of the state to protect the public welfare. Nurses are also increasingly being subjected to malpractice lawsuits. When nurses become defendants in legal actions, other nurses serve as expert witnesses both for the defense (representing the practitioner) and the prosecution (representing the plaintiff). Expert witnesses testify to the standard of care required of the health care provider and whether it was met. For these reasons, professional nurses need basic knowledge of the legal aspects of nursing.

EXHIBIT 14-1
Comparison of Old Health Care Paradigm with New Paradigm

OLD PARADIGM	NEW HEALTH CARE PARADIGM
Hospital based, acute care	Short-term hospital: same-day surgery, 23-hour stays; pre-hospital testing and precertification; telehealth/telemedicine; home health; mobile vans; school and mall clinics
Specialty units	Cross-training (multiskilled workers): LDRP, OR/PACU, CCU/telemetry
Hierarchical management	Decentralization (unit budget, scheduling, variance); shared governance; strategic plan
Physician as captain of ship; others are followers	Inter/multidisciplinary team, collaboration; case management (registered nurse/broker)
Nurse as employee; job focused, "refrigerator nurse"	Nurse as professional: career-focused clinical ladder; continuing credentials; tuition reimbursement, paid certification exam
Medical condition; focus on segment	Holistic person in family/community; pastoral care, parish nurse
"Sick" care; focus on cure	Health care, health promotion, prevention programs; focus on cure, care, and continuity of care; complementary health alternatives
Cost containment; focus on billing	Focus on patient and accountability of caregivers/agency; electronic patient record, patient/continuous quality improvement, care maps
Written medical record	Integrated electronic records: smart card, bedside computers
Fee for service	Managed competition (HMO, PPO, IPA)
Physician as employer	Physician as employee; capitation system
One insurance plan	Variety of insurance options ("covered lives"): basic plan, dental, eye, long-term care, cancer, disability
80 to 100 percent	Greater deductible, lower percentage coverage, or copayment insurance

Source: Milstead, J. A. (Ed.). (2004). Health policy and politics: A nurse's guide (2nd ed.). Sudbury, MA: Jones and Bartlett.

Health Policy

Policy can be described as both entity and process. Scholars in political science have defined policy and developed models that are useful for nurses. Public policy serves to direct problems to government and to secure government's response. There is much debate regarding the boundaries and domain of government and the extent of differences between the public and private sectors; however, generally both sectors are affected by public policy. Environmental (hazardous materials, safety standards in the workplace) and defense (testing biological and chemical warfare) policies are two examples that illustrate this point.[3]

Policy as Entity

Policy as entity serves as standing decisions within an organization or agency. "As formal documented directives of an organization, official government policies reflect the beliefs of the administration in power and provide direction for the philosophy and mission of government organizations."[4] These directives or documents can take the form of position statements (state boards of nursing); goals, programs, and proposals; and laws. Laws often reflect the will of society; are made at the international, federal, state, and local levels; and serve to guide conduct. The creation of laws occurs in the legislative branch of government; however, the force of law is handled by presidential vetoes, executive orders, and judicial interpretations. Milstead describes three types of judicial interpretation:[5]

1. Courts interpret the meaning of laws, which may be broad or vaguely written. It is often the intent of lawmakers to address broad situations for greater applicability. These interpretations are generally used by agencies to write regulations that are more specific

and guide implementation of the law. The Americans with Disabilities Act (ADA) is an example.
2. Courts can determine the application of laws. "The court system, especially the federal court system, has been called upon to resolve conflicts between levels of government (state and federal) and between laws enacted by the legislature and interpretation of powerful interest groups."[6] Examples of this type of interpretation include eligibility for participation in various federally sponsored programs and the interpretation of the Constitution.
3. Courts often regulate laws. "Regulations are another type of policy initiative."[7] Laws are often written in general terms, with regulations following with greater specificity to guide their interpretation, administration, and enforcement. The Administrative Procedures Act (APA) was created to provide citizens the right to review and give input throughout the process of developing regulations. This act provides a structure and process that is public and open, which affords the average constituent the ability to participate in the process of public decision making.

Policy as Process

Policy can also be studied as process. The policy process can serve as a model for better understanding public and health care policy making. Milio provides one theoretical perspective in the policy process, and he describes four major stages in decision making related to government policy translation:[8]

1. Agenda setting
2. Legislation and regulation
3. Implementation
4. Evaluation

Formal and informal relationships are developed among members in each stage, both within and outside the government.

Agenda Setting

Agenda setting serves to identify a societal problem or concern, which is then brought to the attention of the government. This is a stage at which professional nurses can get involved, particularly as issues relate to the populations they care for and serve. The many issues surrounding the advent of acquired immune deficiency syndrome (AIDS) is one example. Involvement by health care providers, gay rights activist organizations, and the AIDS Coalition to Unleash Power (ACT UP) was instrumental in influencing the federal government to reconsider the definition of AIDS, broadening it to include persons other than homosexuals. By enlarging the definition and populations served, the government made a greater segment of society eligible for services. Research and funding initiatives followed suit in addressing this national health care crisis.

Government Response

The formal response from governmental sources constitutes the legislative and regulatory stages. Government responses often take three forms:

1. Laws
2. Rules and regulations
3. Programs

Senators and representatives bring bills to the floor of either house and are often flanked by special interest groups that wish to put their agendas forward. Authorization and appropriations processes are different in the legislative processes; professional nurses have the opportunity to influence both. Writing letters, making calls, signing petitions, and being involved in one's professional organization are strategies that can affect these processes. Senators and representatives will often ask the expert opinions of professional nurses to clarify their agenda and make a stronger case for their various bills. The American Nurses Association (ANA) and the American Medical Association (AMA) are often sought out for these opinions, as they are viewed as the professions' "speaking bodies." Administrative rule making often serves as an effort to bring about order within environments that are conflicted and unstable.[9] Rule making can take the form of reinforcing precedent or of breaking new ground and addressing concerns not previously considered. Funding (or lack thereof) is also indicative of an initiative's priority. This can serve as a way to weaken rules that are viewed as too restrictive. Professional nurses should seek ways to contribute or intervene before final rule making. Along with laws, rules, and regulations, programs are concrete manifestations of solutions to problems.[10] The program design serves as a coordination of legislative intent, budgetary expediency, and political feasibility.[11]

Policy and Program Implementation

Policy execution occurs in the implementation stage and is measured against the achievement of goals. This phase includes activities in which legislative mandates are carried out, often through programs. Legislators often look to experts to provide evidence-based information. "If government officials do not know qualified, appropriate experts, then decisions about program planning and design often are determined by legislators, bureaucrats, or staff who know little or nothing about the problem or the solutions."[12] An example of how powerful the professional nurses' voice can be is the outcry of 40 nursing organizations that stood together to oppose the AMA's proposal for a new type of low level health care worker called a registered care technician (RCT). This proposal would have placed patients in jeopardy and created dead-end jobs. Due to the power of those voices raising concerns regarding safe patient care, the RCT proposal did not go further.

Policy and Program Evaluation

During the evaluation stage, the policy performance or program outcomes are appraised. Even when it is outlined in a linear way, the policy process may not necessarily be sequential, linear, or rational. Evaluation is a logical component of the policy process. "Evaluation research is a powerful tool for defending viable programs, and for providing rationale for program failure."[13] Evaluation should begin early on and continue throughout a program in order to avoid fatal flaws. Milstead describes the Tuskegee experiment (1932–1972), in which a group of African Americans was used as a control group and denied antibiotic treatment for syphilis even after treatment was validated as successful. This example underscores the need for vigilant monitoring and evaluation to address moral and ethical concerns as part of the legislative and public policy process.[14]

Nurses and Public Policy

Professional nurses, as the largest group of health care professionals in the country and as providers of the most direct and continuous care to individuals, have a responsibility to be "at the table." Learning the legislative process and understanding strategic positioning to make positive policy changes can aid the professional nurse in this process. The nurse administrator can foster an environment and culture of political awareness and sensitivity to the various public policy issues that confront nurses daily. This is particularly important when considering cost, quality, and access to health care.

Nurse Practice Acts

In 1899, nurse leaders in the United States decided that nursing had reached the stage of acknowledged indispensability as an occupation in the care of the ill and convalescent, and furthermore that this occupation was so intimately bound up with the safety and health of the public that it required regulation and control in the education of those who desired to engage in it[15]. The leaders who inspired the struggle were keenly aware that, since all progress must have a beginning, some effective legislation was better than none at all: time would serve to improve the extent of control, to fill in the gaps, and to remedy the errors. The important thing was to get some law on the books. The first states to enact laws were North Carolina in 1902 and New Jersey, New York, Virginia, Maryland, Indiana, California, Connecticut, and Colorado in 1903.

Nurse practice acts are the policing power of the state. The acts are laws that define nursing, mandate and set standards for licensure, mandate licensure examinations, regulate schools of nursing, set standards for curricula of schools of nursing, require continuing education for licensure renewal, mandate investigation of reports of violation of nursing practice, regulate the discipline of violators of nurse practice laws, and regulate advanced practice nurses. State nursing boards are used to render decisions regarding nursing practice and how it relates to other disciplines and new tasks that nurses are asked to perform. The boards provide decisions as to which tasks may be delegated (not requiring orders or oversight) and which may become independent nurse functions. The state boards may also provide decisions as to which functions professional nurses may delegate to licensed practical/vocational nurses.

Nurse practice acts protect the public against negligence, malpractice, and other torts. Through their boards of nursing, nurse practice acts discipline violators by probation, revocation of license, and referral to criminal courts. Patients injured by professional nurses also may pursue redress through civil courts.

Legal Aspects of Contracts

A contract consists of (1) an offer and (2) an acceptance, which constitute (3) the agreement between (4) two or more parties (5) having legal capacity (6) to do or forbear the doing of (7) a legal act for (8) a price, which in legal parlance is termed *consideration*.[16]

The first legal principle of nursing is that the professional nurse must qualify for and become licensed in a state to meet the legal requirement for the right to practice professional nursing. Every state in the United States has a mandatory nurse-licensing requirement.

Professional nurses make oral and written contracts. They accept or reject offers of employment and make counteroffers. Once an offer is accepted, revocation by either party is a breach of contract. When agents of parties make contracts, the parties to the contract are called principals, and those who made the contracts are called agents. An example of this is when nurse staffing agencies act as agents for nurses and hospitals. Professional nurses negotiate those contract terms that will satisfy them: salary, benefits, and shift differential; hours of work and shift rotation; moving, housing, travel, and education expenses; and payment of malpractice insurance premiums. It is best to have all contract terms written and signed before accepting a job. Legally, both parties to a contract must live up to the terms of the contract or be subjected to the possibility of civil litigation.

Professional nurses are bound by contracts between unions and employers when such contracts exist. When seeking employment, the professional nurse should ask whether there is a union and about the terms of the contract, which would bind him or her.

Principle: A principal of a contract cannot require the other principal to commit an illegal act, which is prohibited by law or violates the spirit of the law.

Advanced practice nurses may enter into contracts with managed care organizations. When doing so, advanced practice nurses should make sure the following contract categories are covered:[17]

1. The parties are clearly identified.
2. The preface includes statements found in the body of the contract.
3. Terms are defined.
4. Provider duties are specified.
5. Payer–contractor duties are specified.
6. Utilization review is specified.
7. Claims management is specified.
8. Medical records are specified.
9. Provider compensation is specified.
10. Patient duties are specified.
11. Liability issues are specified.
12. Quality issues are specified.
13. Marketing is specified.
14. Insolvency protection is specified.
15. Terms of the contract are specified.
16. Termination conditions are specified.
17. Exclusivity is specified.
18. Other general provisions are specified.

When contracting with managed care organizations and other providers, professional nurses need a sound business plan that keeps them solvent and limits their liability. It is wise to consult an attorney on these matters.

Legal Aspects of Torts

Three legal terms that are intertwined are *tort*, *negligence*, and *malpractice*. A tort is a civil wrong that can be redressed in a civil proceeding. This category includes negligence, the doing or not doing of an act that a reasonable person under similar circumstances would or would not do, and which act or failure to act is the proximate cause of injury. A proximate cause is one that in a natural and continuous sequence produces an event that results in an injury. The last person who could have reasonably prevented the injury from occurring is associated with the proximate cause of injury. Malpractice is the unskillful or negligent practice of a professional person whereby the health of a person (patient) is injured (malpractice).

For a malpractice lawsuit to be successful, the following conditions must exist:

1. There must be a duty between the injured party and the person who allegedly caused the injury.
2. There must be a breach of this duty.
3. The breach of duty must be the proximate cause of the injury.
4. The injured party must have experienced damages or injuries recognized as compensable by law.

One of the earliest and most famous cases of negligence by a nurse is the Somera case, reported in *The International Review*, July 1, 1930, pp. 325–334. Lorenza Somera, as the head nurse, was directed by the operating surgeon to prepare 10% cocaine with adrenaline for administration to a patient for a tonsillectomy. Miss Somera repeated and verified the order. A few moments after the injection was given, the patient showed symptoms of convulsions and died. The operating surgeon meant to say 10% procaine. Only Miss Somera was found guilty of manslaughter due to negligence. The negligence consisted of fulfilling an order that the nurse should have known by reason of her training and experience was an incorrect one. Although the physician was negligent, the cause of death was the nurse's negligence.[18]

When in doubt, obtain confirmation and use caution.

Malpractice suits are endemic in the United States, mostly owing to a multitude of alleged errors. Results of the Harvard Medical Practice Study of 1984 found that at least 4% of hospitalized patients suffer an adverse event, two thirds of which are preventable. Thus, estimates are that **one million preventable injuries** and **120,000 preventable deaths** from errors occur annually. In 1998, the cost of these adverse events was estimated at $100 billion, a conservative estimate.

Evidence indicates that most errors are caused by the system and not the provider of care. However, the provider—that is, the individual practitioner—is usually punished by the system for the failure of the system. Punishment results in the provider not reporting errors. Regulatory agencies, employers, and professional organizations are now making efforts to change this punitive culture into one that redesigns systems and prevents errors.[19] This approach is compatible with the theory of quality management of W. Edwards Deming, covered in

Chapter 17 (Quality Management). The Joint Commission on Accreditation of Healthcare Organizations (JCAHO) and other accrediting bodies are looking to health care facilities to formulate systems that promote processes that look at aggregate data, evaluate failures, and implement changes to correct the problems rather than looking for an individual to blame. This is validated in the emphasis put on patient safety by JCAHO. JCAHO publishes the patient safety goals annually and focuses on those areas that have been identified as high risk areas.

Because government functions are performed for the public welfare, it is difficult to sue the government. In 1946, the Congress of the United States passed P.L. 601, Title 4, the Federal Torts Claims Act. This law allows persons to sue the federal government for negligence of its employees. The monetary claims are restricted. Most states do not allow lawsuits against them and are protected by sovereign immunity, that is, the supreme power residing in the people.

Criminal responsibility may ensue from negligence in which the course of conduct is palpably imprudent and unreasonable.

Criminal responsibility may ensue from negligence in which the course of conduct is palpably imprudent and unreasonable.[20]

Assault and Battery

Assault and battery are torts that can involve nurses. *Assault* includes

> (1) a threat or attempt, (2) coupled with an apparent ability to execute the threat or attempt, (3) to put another in fear of an immediate offensive or harmful contact (4) which is intended and which is neither consented to nor privileged.[21]

Battery is

> (1) the execution of the threat or attempt to commit an assault, or the unlawful touching or striking of another (2) by any means, which results in bodily contact (3) that is intended and is neither consented to nor privileged.[22]

Here is an example of assault and battery. The nurse approaches a patient and tells her he is going to give her a bath. The patient, who is mentally sound, tells the nurse she does not want him to bathe her. After conferring with his supervisor, the nurse proceeds to undress and bathe the patient. When the patient's husband arrives, the patient is in emotional turmoil. The husband gathers the facts and writes a letter of complaint to the administrator, who replies that the patient cannot refuse to be bathed by any competent nurse. The husband consults with a professional nurse acquaintance who determines that the husband will settle for a letter of apology that states that his wife will not be forced to accept being bathed by a nursing employee again. Although the letter averts a lawsuit, given the patient's refusal and the nurse's disregard for the patient's choice, the result would be a charge of assault and battery.

Other Torts Applicable to Nurses

Other torts that have the potential for occurring in health care and that nurses should be aware of are false imprisonment; slander and libel; and destruction, injury, or loss of another's property.

False imprisonment occurs when a person is

> (1) confined or imprisoned by any means (2) unlawfully by another, (3) for no matter how short a time, (4) with intention to cause such confinement or imprisonment, (5) of which the one confined or imprisoned has knowledge, and which is neither consented to nor privileged.[23]

A nurse who carries out any nursing intervention without the patient's consent, even if the intervention is beneficial, is potentially guilty of professional misconduct. The nurse may be disciplined by the state board of nursing and could be sued by the patient or face an allegation of battery or civil assault.

A person cannot be confined to a psychiatric facility because he or she exhibits behavior that is annoying to another person. There are reports of instances of improper restraint of institutionalized residents that constitute false imprisonment and assault and battery. This is further reason for careful and thoughtful approaches to the restraint and seclusion policy in any health care facility.

Slander is

> the (1) malicious (2) utterance by speaking of base or defamatory words concerning another's reputation or profession which tend to expose him to contempt, ridicule, or public hatred, (3) are published to another, (4) are intended, and are neither true nor privileged.[24]

Libel is

> the (1) malicious (2) utterance either in writing or printing, or by signs, pictures or caricatures, of base or defamatory words concerning another's reputation or profession which tend to expose him to contempt, ridicule, or public hatred, (3) are published to another, (4) are intended, and (5) are neither true nor privileged.[25]

Privileged Communication

Certain communications are privileged and cannot be used against the accused in a court of law. These include communication between attorney and client, physician and patient, clergyman and member of congregation, members of a household, and prospective and former employers.

A person who defames the character of another and causes a loss of professional reputation must be able to prove the truth of the accusation. Truth is the absolute defense to an action in slander and libel. It is difficult for prominent public figures to sue successfully for slander and libel.

Liability

A person who takes or appropriates another person's property under admittedly wrongful circumstances can be charged with a crime and be subject to civil court action as well. Because nurses are frequently required to handle the property of others, liability for negligence may result if a patient's property is lost or damaged. To avoid a charge of negligence in handling patient's property, the nurse exercises reasonable care and follows the policies and procedures of the employing institution.

Nurses may be asked to witness patient's signatures on legal documents such as wills. The nurse must know the various laws governing witnessing of patient's signatures. Many states have laws defining who can or cannot witness signatures on certain documents. When in doubt, the nurse should not sign and should seek out the institution's legal counsel.

Ignorance of the law is no excuse. When a law exists and the nurse violates it, the nurse is subject to criminal charges.

Nurses with Specialized Knowledge

With the growth of medical malpractice cases there has been a rise in the use of nurses in various health-related cases. One example is the nurse as an expert witness. A nurse may be used as an expert witness if he or she is a professional nurse who can speak with authority on a subject, field, and specialty of nursing. As an expert witness, the nurse is a legal participant in litigation involving malpractice. There is an allegation that a negligent act is committed. The negligent act involves the nurse as expert witness when it is an alleged violation of nursing practice, or sometimes when the nurse reviews the whole medical record and assists the lawyer with finding the correct information necessary to support and present the case. Each side will have an expert witness.

The use of nurses as expert witnesses has led to a broader subspecialty for nurses: the legal nurse consultant or expert witness does the following:

- Reviews records, charts, and depositions of other witnesses. Gives opinions based on expert knowledge of standards of nursing care related to all aspects of the care of the patient at the center of the suit.
- Gives depositions under oath. Is well prepared by the attorney with whom she is working. Must remember questions asked and answers given when the case goes to trial, because the opposing lawyer will try to confuse the expert witness and cause the jury to doubt the expertise and credibility of the opposing side's expert witness.
- Does a literature search for similar cases plus up-to-date articles related to all medical and nursing aspects of the case.

A nurse becomes an expert when someone related to the case suggests or refers the attorney to the nurse. The attorney and the nurse establish a rapport and make a contract. Together the attorney and the nurse establish a theory of the case. Preparation for the deposition and trial must be thorough, with records thoroughly analyzed by both the nurse and the attorney. The expert nurse not only notes records that support his or her case but those entries, or lack thereof, that support the opposition's case.[26] An expert opinion must have evidentiary scientific reliability to be admissible.[27]

Qualifications to become a legal nurse consultant or expert witness include clinical experience, formal education (an advanced degree is preferred, although not required), publication in peer-reviewed journals, ability to speak in terms a jury can understand, good eye contact, a record of accepting cases for plaintiffs and defendants, and participation in professional organizations. The role

EXHIBIT 14-2

Case Study in Which a Legal Nurse Consultant May Be an Expert Witness

An elderly, blind, female resident in a nursing home in Alabama fell and broke her hip. The family sued the nursing home for negligence. The resident's chart indicated that the nursing personnel had planned her care with the resident and arranged the furniture in her room and the position of her bed so she could safely go to her chair and to the bathroom. The nursing personnel had carefully documented repeatedly communicating the plan to the resident, and she followed it without incident for more than two years.

The plaintiff's lawyer charged that the resident should have been restrained in bed with instructions to call nursing personnel before getting up for any reason. The defendant's lawyer and expert witness prepared and presented a theory of the case that showed documented nursing care planning that had given this resident safe freedom of movement for more than two years. The jury believed the expert witness and acquitted the nursing home. Afterward jury members congratulated the expert witness.

of the legal nurse consultant may be greater than the expert witness, as his or her knowledge of legal areas is greater than the area of clinical expertise. In addition, there is a certification as a legal nurse consultant accredited by the American Board of Nursing Specialties. Exhibit 14-2 describes a case in which a legal nurse consultant may be involved as an expert witness.

Risk Management

Risk management can be defined as a process that centers on identification, analysis, treatment, and evaluation of real and potential hazards.[28] Risk management has its beginnings in transportation and industry, particularly in investigations into aviation and traffic accidents. The primary reasons for these investigations were to determine patterns or causative factors in the accidents and then to eliminate, or at least control, as many factors as possible.[29]

Hayden describes risk management as the risk of financial loss. Specifically, she addresses control of financial loss resulting from legal liability. Financial loss and legal liability can be best understood by the following steps:[30]

1. Identifying patterns and trends of risk through internal audits and claims.
2. Reporting individual risk-related incidents and taking steps to reduce the liability related to them.
3. Developing and engaging in product evaluation systems with appropriate informed consent protocols.
4. Vigilant evaluation of patient care settings to determine risks.
5. Preventing those occurrences likely to be a liability to the organization.

Hayden further describes three aspects of risk identification that should be monitored on a continuous basis:[31]

1. Clinical settings, clinical problems, personnel, and specific incidents involving patients, employees, and visitors.
2. Safety management.
3. Procedures for evaluation and followup on identified risks.

In addition, review of pertinent documents such as medical records, incident reports, pharmacy logs, infection control reports, and utilization review reports is paramount to a successful risk management program. Excellent communication skills are essential when interacting with medical and administrative staff and with clients. Substandard communication skills are often the root of a complaint or claim.[32]

The JCAHO recommends the establishment of an integrated risk management–quality assurance program that would provide a more efficient and cost-effective method of evaluation than having two separate functions. Specific emphasis has been on the patient safety goals, which are updated annually and are program-specific. The following parameters are incorporated into the JCAHO model for risk management:[33]

1. Continuing education and in-service training.
2. Use of data from a variety of sources, such as patient surveys and feedback from other providers (referring or referral facilities).
3. Improvement of credentialing protocols for practitioners.
4. Development and enforcement of rules, regulations, policies, and procedures.
5. Establishment of written criteria to evaluate risk factors, including followup on conclusions reached.

Bennett further describes the importance of both quality improvement and risk management, identifying issues associated with quality patient care, collecting and analyzing data, making recommendations, and evaluating outcomes to prevent reoccurrences and upgrade quality. Avoidance of costly malpractice litigation is as important as is providing safe and quality patient care.[34] Five common reasons for malpractice litigation are injuries to patients resulting from the following:[35]

1. Errors or failures in safety of care that result in patient falls.
2. Failure to identify and document pertinent information (omissions of significant data).
3. Failure to correctly perform treatments or nursing care.
4. Failure to communicate significant data to patients or other therapists.
5. Errors in medications.

Adhering to standards of care (general and specialty nursing) can provide a model for risk management. Quality nursing care is concerned, compassionate, and nurturing. It is often within the context of a therapeutic nurse–patient relationship that problems are solved and errors avoided. Effective communication is a cornerstone to a therapeutic relationship and is enhanced by active listening, empathy, understanding, and positive reinforcement. When the patient and family truly feel cared for, errors that do occur are considered in the context of this relationship. In addition, the following primary responsibilities of every nurse are essential in preventing malpractice litigation:[36]

1. Practice safely, that is, deliver quality nursing care to all patients.
2. Incorporate effective patient rapport in nursing practice.
3. Keep accurate and complete records.
4. Act reasonably—as all other professional nurses would in the community, the state, and the nation—to give standard nursing care.

The risk manager uses carefully planned public relations; makes private explanations; apologizes when necessary; and collects, prepares, and presents evidence.[37] The risk manager's job duties are further outlined in Exhibit 14-3.

Process

The following process describes an effective risk management program:[38]

EXHIBIT 14-3
Risk Manager Competencies

1. Keep an up-to-date manual, including policies; lines of authority; safety roles; disaster plans; safety training; procedures; incident and claims reporting; procedures and schedule; and description of retention/insurance program.
2. Update programs with changes in properties, operations, or activities.
3. Review plans for new construction, alterations, and equipment installation.
4. Review contracts to avoid unnecessary assumptions of liability and transfer to others where possible.
5. Keep up-to-date property appraisal.
6. Maintain records of insurance policy renewal dates.
7. Review and monitor all premium and other billings and approve payments.
8. Negotiate insurance coverage, premiums, and services.
9. Prepare specifications for competitive bids on property and liability insurance.
10. Review and make recommendations for coverage, services, and costs.
11. Maintain records and verify compliance for independent physicians, vendors, contractors, and subcontractors.
12. Maintain records of losses, claims, and all risk management expenses.
13. Supervise claim-reporting procedures.
14. Assist in adjusting losses.
15. Cooperate with the director of safety and the risk management committee to minimize all future losses involving employees, patients, visitors, other third parties, property, and earnings.
16. Keep risk management skills updated.
17. Assess the system for causes of errors and adverse events. Fix the system.
18. Use focus groups to identify unreported errors and adverse events. Eliminate punitive organizational culture.
19. Prepare annual report covering status, changes, new problems and solutions, summary of existing insurance and retention aspects of the program, summary of losses, costs, major claims, and future goals and objectives.
20. Prepare an annual budget.

1. Identify areas within the organization that expose it to loss.
2. Evaluate the potential loss those exposures represent.
3. Treat the exposure through two broad categories: risk financing and risk control.
4. Reduce the severity of the loss through risk control strategies such as hospital bill write-offs or early investigations of the event.

Employing these strategies is a joint effort of the risk management department along with health care providers, because it is everyone's responsibility to provide a safe environment for the patient. Such strategies include early warning systems, documentation, informed consent, and patient relations.[39]

Early Warning Systems

Early warning systems include strategies that involve acquiring early information and knowledge of the occurrence of an untoward event. Early warning provides an opportunity to evaluate the incident while the circumstances are still very clear. "Early reporting also allows the organization to secure medical records related to the event and equipment that may have malfunctioned and contributed to the event."[40] With computerization, a formal information system may be put in place, with labels for generic screens or occurrence screens that serve as a set of criteria and list the kinds of "red flag" occurrences that indicate a loss.

The nurse manager and the clinical staff are often the key players in reporting early warnings. Claims management can be included in the early warning systems. It includes analysis of risk for possible loss frequency and severity—that is, the assessment of potential claims based on data analysis. This information (written and verbal reports) is used to investigate potentially compensable events and losses and their causes, thereby determining liability and settlement value.

Documentation

Documentation strategies are essential to an effective risk management program. The medical record generally serves as a means of determining whether a deviation existed in the standard of care. Contradictions, inconsistencies, and unexplained time gaps in the medical records signal potential problems during litigation. It is recommended that documentation take place as soon after the occurrence as possible and that a minute-by-minute recording is done during the emergency. When time is of the essence, brief notes with times, interventions, and other relevant information should be written on a piece of paper and transferred to the medical records as soon as the crisis is over. Any corrections to the medical record should be done with a thin line drawn through the original entry, dated and initialed. Information should be documented as a factual recording, and objectivity should be practiced. Documentation of any instructions given to the patient should also be recorded.

Informed Consent

Informed consent does not involve just the signing of a consent form. This procedure has little relation to the patient's understanding of the procedure to be performed. Informed consent is the provision of enough information to patients to enable them to make a rational decision whether or not to undergo a treatment. The form that is signed, however, indicates that adequate information has been given to the patient and that understanding and consent have been duly explained. Exceptions to the rule are emergency treatments and situations in which such disclosure could potentially adversely affect the patient's medical condition. Informed consent may be sought for diagnosis, nature and purpose of the proposed treatment, risks and consequences of the proposed treatment, and feasible treatment alternatives.

Patient Relations

Patient relations are important; often the deterioration of the professional-to-patient relationship is what leads to malpractice claims. Many large health care organizations employ patient representatives who provide services such as orienting patients and their families to organizational policies, procedures, and services; resolving complaints; making phone calls and mailing letters; and daily follow-up. Volunteers often assist the patient representative.[41]

Incident Reporting

Incident reporting is an effective technique of a good risk management program. The tool itself should be constructed to collect complete and accurate information, including the name, address, age, and condition of the individual involved; exact location, time, and date of the incident; description of the occurrence; physician's examination data; bedrail status; reason for hospitalization; names of witnesses; and extent of out-of-bed privileges.

Use

Incident reports are used to collect and analyze future data for the purpose of determining risk-control strategies. These reports are prepared for any unusual occurrence involving people or property, whether or not injury or damage occurs. Blake describes the use of a multiple causation model in incident report investigation. This theory suggests that causes, subcauses, and contributing factors weave together in particular sequences to cause incidents. An incident may have many concomitant causes; therefore, seeking out as many causes as possible and rating them by their proximate or primary influence on the incident may be useful in reducing the chance of the incident recurring. Proximate causes are often referred to as unsafe acts and conditions and are generally the most apparent and closest cause of the incident. Primary causes are procedural in nature, and such causes are discovered though backtracking from the proximate cause.

Blake identifies six principles of risk management related to incident investigation:[42]

- Principle I: Each cause of an incident reflects a management problem.
- Principle II: One can predict that sets of circumstances will produce incidents. These circumstances can be identified and controlled.
- Principle III: In any given group or array, a relatively small number of items will tend to give rise to the largest proportion of results.
- Principle IV: The purpose of incident investigation is to locate and define the operational errors that allow incidents to occur.
- Principle V: Accountability is the key to effective incident investigation and analysis.
- Principle VI: The past performance of an organization or unit tends to forecast its future performance.

Preparation

The incident report is discoverable by the plaintiff's attorney. It should be prepared by the involved employee(s) in a timely manner to ensure accuracy and objectivity of reporting. It must be complete and factual. The incident report is corrected in the same manner as any other medical record and should not be altered or rewritten. It should contain no comments criticizing or blaming others. To keep the incident report from being discoverable, it must be sent directly from preparer to attorney to ensure confidentiality. Nurse managers frequently insist on reviewing the report, although they can obtain accurate information from the patient's chart and from conversations with the preparer. The incident report should be prepared in a single copy and should never be placed on the patient's medical record. Exhibit 14-4 lists the dos and don'ts of incident reporting.

Attorneys can prepare abstracts of data from collective incident reports. Thus, attorneys can identify the number of occurrences of particular incidents. The information will be used by the risk manager to do his or her job—for example, to do trend analysis to establish patterns and to determine needed education and training of personnel to reduce risks.[43]

It may be institutional policy to send the incident report to the risk manager, but an alternative method of notification is better. The preparer can call the risk manager and nurse manager and give them verbal information on

EXHIBIT 14-4

DOs and DON'Ts of Incident Reporting

DO

- Report any event involving patient mishap or serious expression of dissatisfaction with care.
- Report any event involving visitor mishap or property.
- Be complete.
- Follow established policy and procedure.
- Be prompt.
- Act to reduce fear in the nursing staff.
- Correct in the same manner as any medical record.
- Include names and identities of witnesses; record their statements on separate pages.
- Report equipment malfunctions, including control numbers. Remove equipment from service for testing.
- Keep the report confidential.
- Report to nurse manager.
- Confer with risk manager.
- Work to provide nursing care to meet established standards.
- Attend all staff development programs.
- Confirm all telephone orders in writing.

DON'T

- Place blame on anyone.
- Place report on the patient's chart.
- Make entry about an incident report on the patient's chart.
- Alter or rewrite.
- Report hearsay or opinion.
- Be afraid to consult, ask questions, or complete incident reports. They can be part of your best defense and protection.
- Prescribe in the physician's domain.
- Be cold and impersonal to patients, families, or visitors.

the need to investigate and evaluate deviations from the standard of care and for making corrections. To accomplish this, managers will have to establish a climate of trust that supports incident reporting by nurses. The JCAHO requires that incidents be reported.

Accident Reporting

Incidents involving employees are frequently referred to as accidents. The person preparing the accident report should follow the same principles as those for incident reporting. These principles will usually be covered by institutional policy and procedure. Perceptions vary too much to require personnel to discriminate between an incident and accident. Accidents are incidents, and many incidents are accidents.

Infection Control

A major area for quality control and risk management is infection control. Infections acquired in hospitals are called *nosocomial infections*. Many hospitals will have full-time infection control nurses who investigate all reported nosocomial infections. A source of relevant data is the medical laboratory. It is good policy to have all laboratory reports indicating a positive result for infectious diseases routed to the infection control nurse. The diseases will be investigated and procedures implemented to prevent their spread and future development. Staff development is a major function of infection control. Standards followed are those of the Centers for Disease Control and Prevention.

Other basic principles of law important to nursing include the following:[44]

1. Ignorance of the law is not an excuse for wrongdoing. If a law exists but a person does not know it, that person will not be excused for breaking it.
2. Every person is responsible for his or her own actions. The nurse must know the cause and effect of all actions or will be subject to suit for malpractice when harm occurs to a patient.
3. A nurse will not carry out an illegal order of a physician or any other health care provider. The nurse must know that the order is a legal one before carrying it out.
4. New nurse graduates must not be assigned to duties beyond their competence.
5. An employer hiring a nurse is required to exercise ordinary, prudent policies and procedures.
6. By the "respondent superior" or "master–servant" rule, injury by an employee because of negligence makes both employee and employer equally responsible to an injured party. The injured party may sue both employer and employee. Both may not necessarily be found guilty.
7. Professional nurses should carry malpractice insurance. Even when an employer insures an employee, the licensed employee is usually not covered outside the place of employment.
8. Malpractice lititgation can be reduced by documenting telephone advice to patients, improving communication and listening skills, and effectively obtaining patients' informed consent.

9. Malpractice risks are increased when professional nurses supervise unlicensed employees.
10. Knowledge of state laws, such as mandatory reporting of abuse, is important for nurses.
11. Courts have interpreted ERISA (Employee Retirement Income Security Act) to limit physician autonomy and subordinate clinical decision making to cost-containment decisions made by managed care organizations.
12. Good provider–patient relationships contribute to preventing malpractice suits.
13. Iatrogenic injuries are a significant public health problem that must be addressed by professional nurses.
14. The costs of malpractice litigation can be reduced by managing risks rather than vindicating providers accused of malpractice. Successful risk management techniques include credentialing of professional staff, monitoring and tracking of complaints and incidents, and documenting in the patient's medical record.
15. The medical malpractice field appeared in the United States around 1840 and has been sustained by changing pressures on medicine, adoption of uniform standards, the advent of medical malpractice liability insurance, contingency fees, citizen juries, and the nature of tort pleading.
16. Human errors in clinical nursing practice are common and underreported.
17. With increased credentialing of advanced practice nurses in HMOs, there will be increased liability for their employers and increased need for personal malpractice insurance.
18. The nursing profession appears to hold its licensees to safer standards than does the medical profession; therefore, nurses are disciplined more often and more harshly than are physicians.
19. Personal involvement with patients places the professional nurse in jeopardy of legal action by the state board of nursing.
20. Many charting practices can help decrease the liability risks for nurses.

Tort reform has as its objective reducing the costs of liability insurance premiums for providers and subsequently to the patient. Inherent to this process is the fact that mistakes by providers are withheld from patients even when they result in morbidity and mortality.[45]

Ten rules can help a nurse avoid going to court:[46]

1. Know the law.
2. Document everything.
3. Make no negative comments about the patient.
4. Question authority.
5. Stay educated.
6. Manage risks.
7. Don't hurry through discharge.
8. Be discreet.
9. Use restraints wisely.
10. Be kind.

Summary

Nurse practice acts originated in the United States in 1902, when the first such law was enacted by North Carolina. These acts represent the policing power of the state and protect both patients and nurses. With the advance of knowledge and technology, professional nurses are required to have advanced education and training. Lawsuits against torts, such as negligence, are common and require professional nurses to purchase malpractice insurance. Other torts include assault and battery; false imprisonment; slander and libel; and destruction, injury, or loss of property. In the course of their practice, professional nurses may face civil or criminal charges.

In addition to being a defendant, the professional nurse may be called on to act as an expert witness for either the plaintiff or defendant. Employing institutions protect themselves by maintaining risk management departments.

APPLICATION EXERCISES

EXERCISE 14-1 Interview a risk manager. How do the risk manager's job duties compare with those outlined in Exhibit 14-3? What risk prevention strategies does the manager use? What has been the cost of losses caused by negligence during the past year?

EXERCISE 14-2 Examine the incident reporting program in a health care agency. What are its strengths? Its weaknesses? How can it be improved?

NOTES

1. Venegoni, S. L. (1996). Changing environment of healthcare. In J. V. Hickey, R. M. Ouimette, & S. L Veregoni (Eds.), *Advanced practice nursing: Changing roles and clinical applications* (pp. 77–90). Philadelphia: Lippincott.
2. Milstead, J. A. (Ed.). (2004). *Health policy and politics: A nurse's guide* (2nd ed.). Sudbury, MA: Jones and Bartlett Publishers.
3. Ibid., 15.
4. Ibid., 15.
5. Ibid., 16.
6. Ibid., 16.
7. Ibid., 17.
8. Milio, N. (1989). Developing nursing leadership in health policy. *Journal of Professional Nursing*, *5*(6), 315.
9. Lowi, T. (1989). *The end of liberalism*. New York: Norton.
10. Milstead, 2004.
11. Skocpol, T. (1995). *Social policy in the United States*. Princeton: NJ: Princeton University Press.
12. Milstead, 2004, 27.
13. Ibid., 22.
14. Ibid.
15. Lesnik, M. J. & Anderson, B. E. (1947). *Legal aspects of nursing*. Philadelphia: Lippincott *1*, 25–26.
16. Ibid., 50.
17. Nugent, J. (1995). Managed care contract checklist redux. *PT: Magazine of Physical Therapy*, 34–36.
18. Lesnik & Anderson, 1947, 258.
19. Lesnik & Anderson, 1947, 172.
20. Ibid., 181.
21. Ibid.
22. Ibid., 194.
23. Ibid., 202.
24. Ibid.
25. Ibid.
26. Cady, 2000, 49.
26. *Daubert v. Merrell Dow Pharmaceuticals, Inc.*, 509 U.S. 579, 113 S. Ct. 2786, 125 L. Ed. 2d 469 (1993).
27. Intravenous Nurses Society. (1990). Revised intravenous nursing standards of practice. *Journal of Intravenous Nursing*, *13*(suppl), s91.
28. Rogers, J. T. (1985). *Risk management in emergency medicine*. Dallas: Emergency Medicine Foundation, American College of Emergency Physicians, 2.
29. Hayden, L. S. (1992). Risk management strategies. *Journal of Intravenous Nursing*, 288–290.
30. Ibid.
31. Ibid.
32. Wilkinson, R. & Moore, B. J. (Eds.). (1990). *Quality assurance in ambulatory care* (2nd ed.). Chicago: Joint Commission on Accreditation of Healthcare Organizations, 25.
33. Bennett, B. (1993). Quality care through risk management. *Orthopaedic Nursing*, 54–55.
34. Troyer, G. & Salman, S. (1986). *Handbook of health care risk management*. Germantown, MD: Aspen.
36. Bennett, 1993.
37. Joseph, D. & Jones, S. K. (1984). Incident reporting: The cornerstone of risk management. *Nursing Management*, 22–23.
38. Goldman, T. A. (1991). Risk management concepts and strategies. *Journal of Intravenous Nursing*, 199–204.
39. Ibid.
40. Ibid.
41. Ibid.; QAs pave the way: The quest for quality. (1988). *Hospital Profiles*, *1*, 4–5.
42. Blake, P. (1984). Incident investigation: A complete guide. *Nursing Management*, *1*, 37–41.
43. Poteet, G. W. (1983). Risk management and nursing. *Nursing Clinics of North America*, 457–465; Henry, K. H. (Ed.). (1985). *Nursing administration and law manual*. Gaithersburg, MD: Aspen.
44. Irving, A. V. (1998). Twenty strategies to reduce risk of a malpractice claim. *Journal of Medical Practice Management*, 130–133; Helm, A. (1999). Liability, UAPs and you. *Director*, 15–16, 29; Freed, P. E. & Drake, V. K. (1999). Mandatory reporting of abuse: Practical, moral, and legal issues for psychiatric home healthcare nurses. *Issues in Mental Health Nursing*, 423–436; Jacobson, P. D. & Pomfret, S. D. (2000). ERISA litigation and physician autonomy. *JAMA*, 921–926; Klimo, G. F., Daum, W. J., Brinker, M. R., McGuire, E., & Elliot, M. N. (2000). Orthopedic medical malpractice: An attorney's perspective. *American Journal of Orthopedics*, 93–97; Thomas, E. J., Studdert, D. M., Burstin, H. R., Orav, E. J., Zeena, T., Williams, E. J., et al. (2000). Incidence and types of adverse events and negligent care in Utah and Colorado. *Medical Care*, 261–271; Wilson, L. L. & Fulton, M. (2000). Risk management: How doctors, hospitals and MDOs can limit the costs of malpractice litigation. *Medical Journal of Australia*, 77–80; Mohr, J. C. (2000). American medical malpractice litigation in historical perspective. *JAMA*, 1731–1737; Meurier, C. E., et al. (2000). Understanding the nature of errors in nursing: Using a model to analyze critical incident reports of errors which had resulted in an adverse or potentially adverse event. *Journal of Advanced Nursing*, 202–207; Benesch, K. (1994). Emerging theories of liability for negligent credentialing in HMOs, integrated delivery and management care systems. *Trends in Health Care, Law & Ethics*, 41–42, 28, 45; Flaherty, M. (1998, October 12). Crossing the line: When nurses push the limits. *HealthWeek*, 14–15; Habel, M. (2000, January 24). Documenting patient care, part 1: Requirements, charting systems, and reimbursement. *HealthWeek*, 10–11; Habel, M. (2000, February 21). Documenting patient care, part 2: Limit liability, trends and computer chartering. *HealthWeek*, 10–11.
45. Terhune, C. (1998, March 4). Rules on reporting errors in hospitals cause alarm. *Wall Street Journal*, 11–12.
46. Stein, T. (2000, May 15). On the defensive: More patients are naming nurses in malpractice suits. *HealthWeek*, 1, 18.

REFERENCES

Brent, N. J. (2001). *Nurses and the law: A guide to principles and application*. Philadelphia: W. B. Saunders.

Cady, R. (2000). So you want to be an expert witness? Things you need to know. *MCN: American Journal of Maternal/Child Nursing*, 49.

Castledine, G. (2000). Case 34: Patient consent: Nurse who carried out manual evacuation without consent. *British Journal of Nursing*, *9*(17), 1123.

Davis, G. S. (1996). Learning the ropes of contracting. *Provider*, 32–34.

Ginty, M. J., Golding, P. S., & Jellison, M. B. (1995). The basics of managed care contracting: What every nurse executive needs to know. *Aspen's Advisor for Nurse Executives*, 1, 4–6.

Goldsmith, C. (2000). Blowing the whistle: Laws protect nurses who report healthcare fraud. *NurseWeek*, 16.

Goodroe, J. H. & Murphy, D. A. (1994). The algebra of managed care. *Hospital Topics*, 14–18.

Gunn, I. P. (1999). Regulation of health care professionals, part 2: Validation of continued competence. *CRNA*, *2*, 135–141.

Hogue, E. E. (1994). Contracting with managed care providers. *Journal of Home Health Care Practice*, *1*, 17–23.

Jacobs, L. A. (2000). An analysis of the concept of risk. *Cancer Nursing*, *1*, 12–19.

Jenkins, M. & Torrisi, D. L. (1995). Nurse practitioners, community nursing centers, and contracting for managed care. *Journal of the American Academy of Nurse Practitioners*, *2*, 119–123.

Kinsman, J. (2000). Malpractice liability in health professional education. *Radiology Technology*, *2*, 239–246.

Kroll, M. (1999). Bringing together nursing and law: A fitting combination in today's health care environment. *Health Care Management*, *1*, 48–52.

Lindberg, G. E. (1995). The any-willing provider controversy. *Rehab Economics*, *8*(6), 79–81.

Malugaani, M. (2000, August 21). Nurse interrupted: A disciplinary action can put a wrinkle in your career and tie you up in knots. *HealthWeek*, 1, 18–19.

Osley, M. (1995). Liability risks of the hold harmless clause in managed care. *Journal of Legal Nurse Consulting*, *1*, 12–13.

Pozgar, G. D. (2004). Legal aspects of health care administration (8th ed.). Sudbury, MA: Jones and Bartlett.

Satinsky, M. A. (1996). Advanced practice nurse in a managed care environment. In J. V. Hickey, *Advanced practice nursing* (pp. 26–45), Philadelphia: Lippincott-Raven.

Sheehan, J. G. (1999). Public? Private information sharing in healthcare fraud investigations. *Journal of Health Law*, *8*, 593–620.

Silver, M. S. (1999). Incident review management: A systemic approach to performance improvements. *Journal of Healthcare Quality*, *1*, 21–27.

Varga, K. (1998). How to protect yourself against malpractice. *Revolution*, *1*, 55–57.

Waidley, E. (1999, September). Nursing information systems, name badges. *HealthWeek*, 17.

CHAPTER 15

Collective Bargaining

Linda Roussel, RN, DSN

Do not, I beg you, look for anything behind phenomena. They are themselves their own lessons.

Goethe

LEARNING OBJECTIVES AND ACTIVITIES

- Describe traditional and nontraditional collective bargaining strategies to improve the patient care environment.
- Identify major reasons for greater unionization among professional nurses.
- Discuss the meaning of collective bargaining.
- Discuss the history of collective bargaining in nursing.
- Identify the characteristics of a profession and their relationship to collective bargaining.
- Identify and discuss the issues that lead to unions and collective bargaining.
- Describe the process of collective bargaining.
- Describe a grievance procedure and illustrate how it should work.
- Discuss the processes of arbitration and mediation.
- Discuss the benefits of collective bargaining.
- Discuss the ills of collective bargaining.

CONCEPTS: Collective bargaining, professional employee, grievance, arbitration, supervisory influence, strike, organizational autonomy, mandatory overtime, unions.

NURSE MANAGER BEHAVIORS: Designs human resource management policies to prevent possible union organizing activities; shares knowledge and skills with students, colleagues and others; serves as a mentor and role model.

NURSE EXECUTIVE BEHAVIORS: Designs human resource management policies to make employment satisfying to employees and to facilitate open communication among employees and managers; establishes and facilitates a framework for professional nursing practice based on core ideology, which includes vision, mission, philosophy, core values, evidence-based nursing practice, and standards of practice.

Introduction

Improvement in wages, the primary purpose of collective bargaining in the past, is no longer the focal point of most negotiations. "Much more essential to nurses is assuring they have a safe practice environment free of mandatory overtime and other work issues, and a voice in the resource allocation decisions that affect their ability to achieve quality health outcomes for patients."[1] Control over practice, flexible scheduling, and a collegial environment are viewed as essential to a quality work life for professional nurses. Nurse activists note that finding processes, structures, and methods, such as collective bargaining, may offer nurses control over practice. This control is crucial to the survival of professional nursing in the face of an acute nursing shortage crisis.[2]

Research validates the importance of professional nurses having control of their practice; in fact, for many nurses this control is the deciding factor to remain in one's job and the profession. Peter D. Hart Research Associates found that in 2001, 21% of a sample of 700 nurses in current practice reported the desire to leave their positions due to stress and physical demands of work. Participants further reported that an improvement in staffing ratios would be a primary reason for remaining on the job and in the profession.[3] Nurses who had been in their positions longer than 5 years were asked why they remained. Satisfactory pay and benefits, collegial environment, and flexible scheduling were identified as the top reasons that nurses stayed longer than 5 years in their positions.[4] Additionally, research on shared governance models (which are prevalent in magnet hospitals) found positive patient outcomes; these models were also found to create nursing practice environments that attracted and retained professional nurses. Such structures were described as being conducive to autonomy and control over practice.[5] Recurrent themes are control over professional nursing practice, flexible schedules, and collegial respect.

These themes are also common subjects of collective bargaining agreements, which often cover the following issues:[6]

- Mandatory and voluntary overtime
- Acuity-based staffing systems
- Use of temporary nurses
- Protections from reassignments, work encroachment by nonnurses, and mandated nonnursing duties
- Provisions for work orientation and continuing education
- Whistle-blower protection
- Health and safety provisions, such as free hepatitis B vaccines
- "Just cause" language for discipline and termination
- Provisions for nursing and multidisciplinary practice committees

Collective Bargaining Defined

Collective bargaining is the "process by which organized employees participate with their employers in decisions about their rates of pay, hours of work, and other terms and conditions of employment."[7] Collective bargaining is the process through which the representatives of the employers and employees meet at reasonable times; confer in good faith about wages, hours, and other matters; and put into writing any agreements reached. The duty to bargain is required of both the employer and union.[8]

Collective bargaining is the means by which professional nurses can influence hospital nursing care delivery systems and labor–management relations through a united voice.[9] Collective bargaining is often viewed as a power relationship, either adversarial or cooperative.[10] Executives of firms have learned that employee empowerment and autonomy is good for business. As productivity increases, this knowledge has led to increased training of employees at the production level, elimination of middle management, decentralization of decision making with participatory management at the production level, and an upsurge in the success of the firm. This commitment to sharing power gives employees less reason to resort to collective bargaining.

History in Nursing

Laws

The following is a chronology of collective bargaining laws related to nursing in the United States:

- 1935: The National Labor Relations Act (NLRA), which is sometimes called the Wagner Act, notes that hospitals are "employers." Thus, it protects employees of private, for-profit health care institutions.
- 1947: Under the amendment to the NLRA (called the Taft–Hartley Act), Congress excepts not-for-profit hospitals from coverage, from the right to organize, and from the right to bargain collectively.
- 1960: The National Labor Relations Board (NLRB) excepts proprietary hospitals from coverage by the NLRA.
- 1974: The NLRA amendments repeal exceptions and subject all acute care hospitals to coverage by the act. These amendments make no change in the NLRB's authority to determine the appropriate bargaining unit in each case.
- 1989: The NLRB rules that eight bargaining units are appropriate for each hospital. One such unit will be solely for registered nurses. The ruling is challenged by the American Hospital Association.
- 1991: The US Supreme Court upholds the ruling for eight bargaining units, which include separate units for RNs, physicians, other professionals, technical employees, skilled maintenance employees, clerical employees, guards, and other nonprofessional employees. The exception is units with fewer than six employees.[11]
- 1994: A Supreme Court decision indicates that in any business in which supervisory duties are necessary to the provision of services, personnel who use independent judgments to direct the work of less-skilled employees are supervisors and are not protected by the NLRA. More recently, employers of nurses have used this decision to challenge unions, decrease licensed personnel, and increase assistive, nonlicensed personnel.[12]
- 1995: With the support of the American Nurses Association (ANA), the Michigan Nurses Association argues successfully before the NLRB that nurses are not supervisors, as claimed by the Michigan Hospital Medical Center, and are therefore eligible to bargain collectively.[13]

The National Labor Relations Act of 1947 defines a professional employee as

(a) any employee engaged in work (i) predominantly intellectual and varied in character as opposed to routine mental, manual, mechanical, or physical work; (ii) involving the consistent exercise of discretion and judgment in its performance; (iii) of such a character that the output produced or result accomplished cannot be standardized in relation to a given period of time; (iv) requiring knowledge of an advanced type in a field of science or learning customarily acquired by a prolonged course of specialized intellectual instruction and study in an institution of higher learning or a hospital, as distinguished from a general academic education or from an apprenticeship or from training in the performance of routine mental, manual, or physical processes; or (b) any employee who (i) has completed the courses of specialized intellectual instruction and study described in clause (iv) of paragraph (a), and (ii) is performing related work under the supervision of a professional person to qualify himself to become a professional employee as defined in paragraph (a).[14]

Strauss summarizes the characteristics of professional behavior:[15]

- Specialized education and expertise
- Autonomy
- Commitment
- Societal responsibility for maintenance of standards of work.

Pavalko differentiates between professionals and other workers by stating that professionals have the following:[16]

- A systematic body of knowledge and theory as a basis for work and expertise
- Social ability in times of crisis; the professional is sought out by the public
- Specified training, including transmission of ideas, symbols, and skills
- Motivation for service to clients
- Autonomy, self-regulation, and control by individual practitioners
- A sense of long-term commitment
- A need for common identity and destiny, with shared values and norms
- A code of ethics

Professional nursing organizations have supported the development of nursing theory, the goal of self-regulation, and a code for nurses with interpretive statements. Such a code includes behaviors such as maintaining competency in nursing and participation in activities that contribute to the development of the profession's body of knowledge. When unable as individuals to attain their goals, professional nurses pursue them through collective bargaining.

Nursing Organizations and Unions

The American Nurses Association (ANA) is historically the primary professional organization for American nurses. The following outlines the history of collective bargaining by nursing organizations:[17]

- 1946: ANA becomes active.
- 1970: One third of US work force is organized.
- 1977: 20% of hospital workers are represented by labor unions.
- 1980: 23% of US work force is organized.
- 1982: ANA represents 110,000 nurses, with the goal of controlling and protecting the nursing practice.
- 1985: Ohio Nurses' Association represents nurses in 29 facilities. The Michigan Nurses' Association represents 4000 nurses in 60 bargaining units.
- 1989: 17% of US work force is organized, a decline of 6% since 1980.
- 1990: SNAs represent 139,000 registered nurses, with 841 bargaining units in 27 states. Other unions represent 102,000 RNs. Twelve percent of US work force is organized (according to T. Porter-O'Grady).
- 1991: Within 3 months of the Supreme Court decision allowing all-RN bargaining units, 20 petitions for union elections are filed by nurses in seven states. An estimated 1.12 million nurses do not belong to unions.
- 1992: According to Joel, 20% of health care workers are now organized, an increase of 6% of health care workers since 1980. Approximately 3.6 million hospital employees are protected by collective bargaining.

The difference between the 1977 and the 1992 percentages may relate to the measure of hospital workers versus that of the entire health care industry. In 1992, an additional 10 petitions for RN bargaining units brought the total to 30 petitions, 23 of which were filed by constituent members of the ANA.

Of more than 1.6 million practicing registered nurses, (approximately 67.9% of whom work in hospitals), about 250,000 are represented by collective bargaining. Collective bargaining by the California Nurses Association is more than 50 years old. The pioneers were Shirley Titus, RN, a nurse leader, and J. St. Sure, a labor lawyer, who together built a good public relations image and a solid database. Their work promoted a sense of self-confidence among nurses. Their interest preceded that of the ANA.[18]

In 1999, the ANA House of Delegates passed historic changes in bylaws to better support SNAs in their organizing and collective bargaining efforts. The United American Nurses (UAN) replaced the Institute of Constituent Member Collective Bargaining Programs. The UAN focuses on existing work to organize and represent RNs who want support through collective bargaining to deal with issues such as staffing levels and workplace safety.[19]

The National Labor Assembly of the UAN will elect the seven-member Executive Council. The Council will be composed of a chairperson, a vice chairperson, a secretary, a treasurer, and four directors-at-large. The first Council will be members of the Executive Board of the UAN.[20]

Many nurses are represented by trade unions; the ANA would rather represent them itself. Of the 2.6 million RNs in the United States, 190,000 are members of the ANA. Through the ANA, the SNAs represent 102,000 nurses in collective bargaining.[21]

Issues

Issues that lead to petition for unions develop between employers and employees, usually because employers do not want to share power with employees. Historically, the chief executive officers of firms built bureaucratic organizations to retain power in the management structure. This has been costly for firms and has resulted in their restructuring to eliminate layers of management, empower employees with management knowledge and skills, and improve productivity and profits.

Among the major issues leading to unions and collective bargaining are the following:[22]

- Absence of procedures for reporting unsafe or poor patient care. Quality of patient care is the number one issue.
- Short staffing and improper skills mix to correspond to patient acuity.
- Floating without orientation and training.
- Use of temporary personnel and unlicensed assistive personnel.
- Resistance of employers to accept joint decision making.
- Adversarial relationships between nurses and management and exploitation of nurses by management.
- Lack of respect for employees.
- Lack of autonomy, that is, incursion by management into the scope of practice.
- Lack of promotional opportunities.
- Lack of professional practice committees.
- Lack of staff development and continuing education opportunities.
- Lack of child care and elder care.
- Lack of involvement.
- Poor differentials for shift work, education, and experience.
- Low wages and limited benefits.
- No pension portability.
- Lack of employee assistance programs.
- Poor on-call arrangements and lack of flexible schedules.
- Overwork, mandatory overtime, and shift rotation.
- Low morale.
- Performance of nonnursing duties.
- Poor management and poor communication.
- No ability to take sufficient breaks.
- Fair policies and practices for discipline and dismissal.
- Assurance that patient classification systems have practicing nurse inputs.
- Fair and consistent standards, policies, and practices.
- Adequate health insurance.
- Assurance that competence and qualification are considered with seniority.
- Vacancy posting so that all nurses have an opportunity.
- Lack of a system to apply peer review.
- Lack of career ladders.

The professional nurse works in an environment where human resources are not always valued but are viewed as a commodity. Professional nurses might get fired for such actions as questioning physician authority or refusing to work where they feel they are not qualified. Thus, they often work in a climate of fear that results in poor morale, poor productivity, stifling of creativity, reluctance to take risks, ineffective communication, and reduced motivation.[23] Ultimately, these factors lead to an unbearable level of job stress, which culminates with a letter of resignation.

Kleingartner believes that ANA is working on too many issues simultaneously. She also states that nurses lack economic sophistication, as well as financial resources.[24]

Process

Once nurses have decided to pursue collective bargaining because they believe they have no alternative, the general process is as follows:

1. An organization committee is formed. It should be broad based in structure and representative of the major issues so as to represent all prospective members on all shifts and in all practice areas. Members should be well known and respected.
2. The major campaign issues are identified and discussed.
3. The organizing committee does research to obtain extensive knowledge of all facets of the institution, including history, structure, organization, finances, administration, and culture.
4. A timetable is prepared, delineating the specific organizing activities.
5. Possible employer tactics are identified and discussed, and specific strategies are developed to manage them.
6. A system is established for keeping in constant communication with nurses.
7. A structural plan is made, including adoption of a set of bylaws and election of officers.

8. Recognition occurs by the employer or NLRB certification. Voluntary recognition requires authorization cards signed by a majority of nurses. If the employer will not recognize the action, NLRB certification requires that at least 30% of the nurses sign cards. A majority is best.
9. An election is held in which nurses vote for or against a collective bargaining unit. The NLRB sets the election date by mutual agreement. Notices posted on employee bulletin boards include the date, hours, and places of election; payroll period for voter eligibility; description of the voting unit; a sample of the ballot; and general rules for conduct of the election. With a majority of voting nurses (50% plus 1) voting for it, the NLRB certifies the petitioners as the exclusive bargaining unit. If there is no majority, the NLRB will not accept another petition for 1 year.
10. A bargaining committee is elected by the nurses to negotiate a contract.[25]
11. A contract is negotiated. Members of the bargaining committee should survey the membership to gather data for contract proposals. At the first bargaining meeting proposals are made. The easiest ones should be settled first. Management strategy will be to try to set the tone of the sessions and to package proposals so that they can slip some past the nurses. Their strategies will include flattery, conciliation, anger, astonishment, and total silence. For this reason, nurse members should track all proposals using minutes of the meetings and make index cards listing the proposals of each side. Debriefings at the end of each session are helpful. The nurse team should respond to management with care, spirit, and no unconditional concessions.[26]
12. When all proposals have been fully discussed and agreed on, the contract is written.
13. The contract is then presented to union members who vote to ratify or reject it. If ratified, it is signed by both sides.
14. The contract is enforced through grievance and arbitration procedures. It is reviewed or amended on a regular basis.[27]

Grievance Procedures

A strong grievance procedure increases employee satisfaction, so it is a good human resource management tool, with or without a union. Potential trouble spots are identified early and may include claims for higher wages when jobs are modified. Grievance procedures must be perceived as fair. Their contents should be told to all employees, and managers should be trained to follow them. This training allays managers' fears.[28]

The grievance policy should be communicated as an employee benefit and included in the personnel handbook (see Exhibit 15-1). Peer review should be used in employee appraisals involving grievances and final decisions. Some courts have equated peer review to due process. Peer review builds values of conflict resolution, teamwork, decision making at lower levels, employee empowerment, and ownership.[29]

Eldridge suggests the following points for effective settlement of grievances:[30]

1. Accurate definition of the problem: Does it violate the contract or the law? Is it timely? Documented?
2. Timely presentation: Follows the time limits and steps of the grievance procedure and for notifying appropriate persons.
3. Documentation: Facts; claim adjustment desired; form signed, dated, and given to appropriate persons.
4. All stops are performed with a businesslike attitude to facilitate objectivity and communication.

Nursing is difficult, complex, and requires specialized knowledge. All nurses should commit to a written employment agreement with a grievance procedure. This should be done whether they represent themselves or are represented by a union. When nurses use a labor organization, they should use one with a large membership and a long and successful history.[31] The ANA and some SNAs fall into this category.

Mediation is a process under which an impartial person (the mediator) facilitates communication between parties to promote reconciliation, settlement, or understanding among them. The mediator may suggest better ways of resolving the dispute, but may not impose his own judgment on the issues for that of the parties.[32]

Mediation

Mediation is assisted negotiation. When the negotiating parties cannot reach agreement on an issue during contract negotiations or during a labor dispute unresolved by grievance procedures, the issue is referred to a mediator trained to resolve such disputes. The mediator assists the parties in defining the issues, dissolving obstacles to communication, exploring alternatives, facilitating the negotiations, and reaching an agreement. In law cases, mediation works 80% of the time or more.

Successful mediation involves good faith: all parties are present during the entire mediation session; there is adequate time; the mediator lays ground rules, describes the process, and answers questions; the session is private; the parties are separated into "caucuses" in which their

EXHIBIT 15-1
Sample Employee Grievance Procedure

GRIEVANCES AND DISCIPLINARY ACTIONS

8.1 GRIEVANCE AND APPEAL PROCESS

Metropolitan Medical Center provides a means for you, as a regular employee who has completed the probationary period, to appeal disciplinary actions, including dismissal, suspension, or demotion when used as a disciplinary action, that you feel are unjust or to submit a grievance for any working condition that results in inequities or other situations which have a negative effect on morale. The Medical Center, in its sole discretion, reserves the right to determine whether an action is a management right as outlined in Section 4.5 of this Handbook and, therefore, not subject to grievance and/or appeal. Layoffs and written warnings may not be appealed.

This process may be used in a situation where there are allegations that an individual has been discriminated against based on race, sex, religion, color, national origin, age, disability, disabled veteran, or Vietnam Era veteran status. In such an event, if the individual against whom such allegations have been made is either in the first or second step of the grievance and appeal process, the employee should contact the Department of Human Resources to institute a grievance. This process is available to an employee who alleges such discrimination is related to the issue of sexual harassment.

Employees in their probationary period may only appeal if they feel they have been discriminated against on the basis of race, sex, religion, color, national origin, age, disability, disabled veteran, or Vietnam Era veteran status. Additionally, this process is available to a probationary employee who alleges such discrimination is related to the issue of sexual harassment.

8.1.1 FIRST STEP

If you are considering initiating a grievance or appeal, you should first discuss the matter with your Department Head. You should state your case, in writing, to your Department Head and state the adjustment desired. This should be done within 10 working days of the occurrence.

8.1.2 SECOND STEP

If your grievance is not settled to your satisfaction with your Department Head, you may appeal, in writing, to your Assistant Hospital Administrator within 10 working days of the response to step one.

8.1.3 THIRD STEP

If your grievance is not handled to your satisfaction in step two, you may appeal, in writing, to your Division Head within 10 working days of the response to step two.

8.1.4 FINAL STEP

If your grievance is not handled to your satisfaction in step three, you may request, in writing, the Assistant Vice President of Human Resources to schedule a hearing before the Staff Grievance and Appeal Committee.

A hearing before the committee is a nonadversarial proceeding and attorneys are not allowed to participate on either side. You may select another university employee who is both willing and able to arrange his/her work schedule accordingly to represent you in the grievance/appeal hearing.

The committee's recommendations are presented to the Vice President for Financial Services for a final decision. The Assistant Vice President of Human Resources will advise the concerned parties of the decision and assist in any personnel action required.

8.2 DISCIPLINARY GUIDELINES

Disciplinary guidelines have been established by the Metropolitan Medical Center so that you and other employees will be accorded a process of progressive discipline as set forth in these guidelines. The guidelines on the following pages show example violations and the degree of disciplinary action that may be required for each.

Your supervisor has the authority to determine an appropriate corrective measure through disciplinary action for any other violation of conduct not listed in the guidelines. The Medical Center reserves the right to change the particular type of discipline noted on the listed guidelines, due to the extent and severity of a particular offense. In some instances, even though previous violation of policy has not occurred, the severity of the offense may result in disciplinary action, up to and including dismissal.

So that the safety and productivity of all employees of the Medical Center is insured, a progressive disciplinary program has been established. If you fail to observe the accepted norm of behavior, your supervisor may issue either a verbal or written warning. Written warnings will be made a part of your permanent personnel file. Oral and written warnings may not be appealed. A layoff may not be appealed as it is not a disciplinary action.

(continued)

EXHIBIT 15-1 *(continued)*

8.2.1 FELONY CHARGES

If you, as a regular or temporary employee of the Medical Center, are charged with a felony offense, you shall be suspended without pay pending the outcome of your trial. A temporary or grant-funded employee who is charged with a felony offense shall be suspended without pay pending the outcome of the trial or the ending date of the employee's temporary appointment or grant funding, whichever is earlier. You are responsible for notifying your supervisor if you are charged with a felony offense.

If you are suspended without pay because of a felony charge, and are otherwise eligible for benefits, you may continue to participate in the group medical and life insurance programs. You are responsible for making arrangements with the Payroll Office to pay the total monthly premium costs for these benefits.

If you are convicted of a felony offense, you shall be immediately dismissed.

If you are found not guilty of the felony offense as charged, you shall be reinstated with back pay for the period during which you were suspended without pay pending outcome of your trial with no break in service and you shall retain accrued vacation and sick leave benefits. A temporary or grant funded employee shall be reinstated with back pay until the ending date of the employee's temporary appointment or grant funding, whichever is earlier.

conversations are private; and the mediator shuttles between parties until a settlement is reached. The parties negotiate the settlement.[33]

Arbitration

Whereas a mediator works with the parties in a dispute to get them to resolve their differences, an arbitrator examines the facts and makes a decision that is binding. Arbitration uses as the source of law the express provisions of the contract, past practices of the industry, and the shop (health care and nursing). Past practices must:[34]

- Be unequivocal (clear, consistent, acceptable); be accepted by the people involved as the normal and proper response to the underlying circumstances presented.
- Have longevity; have existed for a sufficient length of time to have developed a pattern.
- Have mutuality; both parties regard the conduct as correct and customary in handling the situation.

Practices that are long-standing and have been accepted by both parties are as binding as if written. Subjects not covered in the agreement are the residual rights of management, including the methods of operation and direction of the work force. Union rights include areas of benefits, wages, and working conditions. Unchallenged customs and practices are considered accepted as part of the agreement by both parties. Arbitrators should effectuate the agreement and contain conflict.[35]

Supervisory Influence

With the power of unions generally declining, goals for unions of professional nurses are best met by multipurpose organizations that can respond and adapt to the particular concerns of nurses, such as "supervisory influence." Generally, employers raise these concerns with relation to who will represent professional nurses. Rank-and-file nurses may be concerned that nurse managers will dominate the bargaining unit through membership in the SNA. The bargaining unit needs some insulation from SNA members who are managers. The issue usually extends beyond legal characterizations to political overtones of power and control within the organization. The California Nurses Association established the legal standard on the issue of supervisory influence in the Sierra Vista case in 1979. This standard is best met by an integrated, multipurpose professional association as a bargaining agent.[36] This agent would include and meet the needs of clinical nurses of all specialties along with nurse managers, educators, and researchers who are members of the SNA.

Advantages of Unionization

Unions view the health care field as a potential pool for membership, which is a threat to hospital leaders. Concrete evidence shows "that collective bargaining, when used effectively, actually facilities delivery of the best care and services."[37]

Collective bargaining has contributed to the high standard of living for the working people of Western countries. Employee compensation levels are higher when they are determined at the bargaining table.[38]

Collective bargaining is viewed by employees as an enforceable way to secure justice in the workplace and a way for them to share power with employers. It provides fundamental protection against arbitrary or unfair treatment in the matter of promotions, remuneration, dismissal, and retirement. The bargaining agreement or contract balances management power with the combined might of all the employees. Protection under collective bargaining is greater than the contract itself. Unfair management authority can be challenged through a grievance system.[39] Contracts with nurses frequently include reference to the ANA code for nurses and standards of nursing practice.[40]

Research indicates that nurses have been reluctant to exercise collective power. Involvement peaks during organizing activity and in times of crisis or conflict. Nurses are more involved with committees related to the nursing product than with those related to bargaining unit affairs.[41]

The Michigan Nurses Association views its members as nurses who have combined the philosophies of professional nursing care and collective bargaining. The goal of this association is protection of patients through protection of nurses' professional and economic rights.[42]

Contracts give nurses input on nursing care standards, policies, and procedures. Unions improve working conditions related to shift rotation, floating, nonnursing duties, flexible staffing, meal breaks, rest periods, time away from work, continuing education, tuition reimbursement, educational leave, grievance and arbitration procedures, maternity/paternity leave, discipline, posting of vacancies, recall from layoffs, peer review, career ladders, joint committees to improve safety and quality of patient care, and adherence to the code for nurses.[43]

The success of unions depends on the quality of the work environment and the credibility and effectiveness of the organization as a bargaining agent and workplace advocate.[44] Outcomes of labor negotiations will depend on employee and employer relationships, attitudes, and philosophies.[45] Researchers estimate that union members average salaries that are 6% higher than those of nonunion workers.[46]

Hannah and Shamian state that the foundation of modern nursing is a professional practice model of nursing. This model can be achieved through collective bargaining and nursing information.

The following are the characteristics of a professional practice model of nursing:[47]

- Multidisciplinary and interdisciplinary collaboration
- Accountability
- Practice based on a sound and discipline-specific scholarly foundation (that is, knowledge, theory, and inquiry)
- Autonomy rooted in a clear understanding of the scope and boundaries of the discipline of nursing
- Awareness of the sociopolitical context of practice
- Self-motivated professional development, including self and peer evaluation, aimed at maintaining currency of practice knowledge

The professional practice model of nursing care can be achieved through functional, team, primary, or case management methodologies. The best environment is a decentralized organizational structure using self-governance.

Collective bargaining environments can be suitable for a professional practice model of nursing that provides for career mobility, advancement, and wage increases using criteria beyond mere seniority.[48]

The purposes of collective bargaining include "facilitating communication between the parties to the contract; establishing and maintaining mutually satisfactory salaries, hours of work, and working conditions; prompt disposition of differences of opinion or grievances; and resolution of disputes."[49] The goal is collaboration. A fully implemented nursing information system provides clinical data quickly; improves nurses' work; and coordinates management activities, physician-delegated tasks, and professional nursing practice. Decision-support systems are information systems designed to provide the information needed to make clinical decisions about patient care. Inputted data (such as history and test results) are processed against stored data to give decision outputs, such as differential nursing diagnosis and suggested therapeutic recommendations.

Source data entry should be conducted from bedside terminals or through two-way radio transmission. Patient discharge abstracts should be expanded to include nursing care delivery information. A nursing minimum data set is available. The collective bargaining unit can be a powerful ally to nursing management in integration of a professional practice model of nursing informatics.[50]

A former union member claims that unionism is a lopsided religion with management as the devil.

Disadvantages of Unionization

Unions cost money and create adversarial relationships. They focus on seniority rather than merit. Before joining a union, the nurse should study its experience or history and its track record. The nurse should talk to union members, tally the annual costs for dues and fees, and read the financial statement.[51]

Because they are elected as are politicians, union officials have a vested interest in maintaining a combative relationship with management. Unions may discourage hard work and personal ambition while encouraging dependence.[52]

Once nurses gain collective bargaining status they exhibit low participation in related activities. A survey of 261 registered nurses employed in voluntary hospitals in New York State and represented by the New York State

Nurses Association for collective bargaining produced the following results:[53]

1. Few nurses attended union meetings regularly, although more did than do blue-collar workers.
2. Only 10.3% of respondents attended union conventions. Excuses included family responsibilities, location, expense, time off, and lack of interest.
3. Members read literature from the bargaining agent.
4. Few nurses submit bargaining demands.
5. Of respondents, 45% voted in local bargaining unit elections and 35% in statewide elections.
6. About two thirds read the bargaining agreement.
7. Few file formal grievances. Of those who did file, 65% filed for professional concerns and 37.5% for economic concerns. One-third knew little about the grievance procedure. They handled grievances informally first.
8. Nurses do not appear prepared to assume leadership roles in bargaining units.
9. College-educated nurses were more aggressive about work stoppages and picketing.

The writer concluded that "nurses who have adopted collective bargaining and who fail to exercise their responsibilities are responsible for the abridgement of their own rights and the success or failure of collective bargaining in their institutions."[54]

Strikes

Strikes are usually a last resort. Striking nurses are frequently portrayed in a negative way by the media. A 1980 content analysis of 893 US newspaper articles presented a more negative image of the nurse than did newspaper articles on other nursing subjects. There were more negative headlines, criticism of nurses, and negative relationships reported in the articles about strikes. A desire for higher salaries was the major strike issue reported by newspapers, conveying the message that nurses were more interested in personal economic gain than in quality of patient care.[55]

Causal factors that may contribute to a strike vote include the following:[56]

1. Perceived lack of responsiveness by nurse administrators in solving everyday problems experienced by nursing staff
2. Fear of change experienced by nursing staff
3. Resistance by nurses to the national trend of using unlicensed, assistive personnel to reduce operating costs
4. Perceived reduction in benefits for the nursing staff
5. Environmental and workplace health and safety concerns
6. Perceived inequities in salaries between the nursing staff and senior executives

Firing striking workers is illegal, but it is standard management strategy for companies to threaten to hire permanent replacements. Companies are then obligated to hire former strikers only as future openings occur. In 1989, approximately 21,000 workers in US companies lost their jobs through permanent replacement policies. Organized labor has been unable to obtain federal legislation banning replacement of employees who strike. In 1938, the Supreme Court ruled that permanent replacements are legal.[57]

Vulnerability

There has been increased interest in collective bargaining among health care workers since the 1991 Supreme Court decision. The long-term goal of the ANA is to "enable the country's two million nurses to achieve control over their own practice and work environment."[58] If nurse administrators wish to avoid dealing with collective bargaining units, they should create the conditions under which nurses have equivalent control.

The signs and symptoms of increased vulnerability to collective bargaining activity are those of an unhealthy environment:[59]

1. Increased nursing staff turnover
2. Increased employee-generated incidents
3. Increased grievances filed
4. Breakdown in communication
5. Sudden changes in staff behavior
6. Increased inquiries about personnel policies and practices
7. Changes in behavior of "problem children"
8. Pro-union, collective bargaining, or professional organization literature, posters, or graffiti
9. Organization of and invitation to off-site meetings for staff members only
10. Formation and submission of petitions
11. Managers' "gut" feelings

Nurse administrators should do a formal assessment of collective bargaining and make a plan for action that prevents it. Some of the activities to consider in this plan of action are training of front-line management in communications, counseling, mentoring, participatory management, shared governance, and addressing quality-of-care issues immediately.[60] Other actions to take include the following:

- Make the nurses feel like stakeholders. This is especially important with advanced, technically trained nurse specialists.
- Make nurses feel connected and invested in their work so they will be creative and productive.

- Prepare nurses to increase their role functions as members of interdisciplinary teams.
- Examine the possibility of new partnership models with nurses: shared ownership, gainsharing, bonuses, pay for performance, outcome pay, per diem contracting, caseload payment structures, benefit smorgasbords, increased autonomy of work, participation, and self-managed teams.
- Work can be redesigned as a result of union leadership and management partnership, with mutually formed mission, goals, and planning for the future.[61]

Collective bargaining is unnecessary when nurses and management communicate well and participate in decision making. It is unnecessary when nurses receive adequate support and appropriate recognition. Nurses should be provided with a voice in decision making, resources to do the job, safeguarding of standards of nursing practice, protection of employment rights, and attractive terms and conditions of employment.[62] These are all aspects of a model of HRM that works and that keeps nurse employees happy.

Good management prevents the need for collective bargaining by nurses. Poor management promotes collective bargaining.

One of the most important benefits of collective bargaining is increased job security. Nurses can be fired for economic reasons and for incompetence, but management should be sure terminations are done only for good and just causes. Laws prevent discrimination on the basis of sex, race, religion, national origin, age, handicap, and for some types of whistle-blowing. The NLRA prevents discrimination on the basis of union activity. Termination should never be related to acts violating public policy or for refusal to perform an illegal practice.[63]

The employer is considered to have the absolute right to determine staffing patterns, ratios, and other personnel requirements. Employers should consider input from nurses in formulating standards of nursing practice; providing education benefits; and ridding nurses of nonnursing work; and for hiring, promotions, and transfers.[64]

Summary

Collective bargaining through unionization is a process whereby employees join together to gain collective power that somewhat neutralizes the power of management. The collective bargaining process has been used in the nursing profession for approximately 50 years. In 1991, the US Supreme Court affirmed the ruling of the NLRB that professional nurses could form a distinctly separate bargaining unit within hospitals.

Issues related to collective bargaining include pay, benefits, and conditions of work related to provision of quality care to patients. Many professional nurses are reluctant to use the process of collective bargaining. Those who do put the safety of patients above their own concerns.

Implementing the theory of human resource management that puts trust in employees by training them to manage themselves is the best management strategy to deter collective bargaining. Nursing and health care leaders who work collaboratively with practicing clinical nurses through decentralization and participatory management prevent collective bargaining. It has been proven time and again that people who manage their own work and who make professional decisions about their practice increase the productivity and profitability of the firm.

APPLICATION EXERCISES

EXERCISE 15-1 Interview a professional nurse who is a member of a union. Determine his or her perceptions of the benefits of collective bargaining. What does he or she perceive as the weaknesses of collective bargaining?

EXERCISE 15-2 Prepare a plan to evaluate the vulnerability of a health care organization to collective bargaining. Use it to assess the organization. Prepare a list of recommendations for decreasing the vulnerability of the organization to collective bargaining. Present the results to the nurse administrator. This exercise may be done by a small group of nurse managers or students.

NOTES

1. Budd, K. W., Warino, L. S., & Patton, M. E. (2004). Traditional and non-traditional collective bargaining: Strategies to improve the patient care environment. *Online Journal of Issues in Nursing*. Retrieved July 24, 2005 from http://www.nursingworld.org/ojin/topic23/tpc23_5.htm.
2. Goodin, H. J. (2003). Collective bargaining. *Journal of Advanced Nursing*, *43*, 335–350; McClure, M. L., Poulin, M. A., Sovie, M. D., & Wandelt, M. A. (2002). Magnet hospitals: Attraction and retention of professional nurses (the original study). In M. L. McClure & A. S. Hinshaw (Eds.), *Magnet hospitals revisited: Attraction and retention of professional nurses*. Washington, DC: American Nurses Publishing.
3. Peter D. Hart Research Associates. (2003). *The nurse shortage: Perspectives from current direct care nurses and former direct care nurses*. Retrieved December 1, 2003, from the American Federation of Teachers Web site: http://www.aft.org/healthcare/downloadfiles/Hart_Report.pdf.
4. Lacey, L. M. (2003). Called into question: What nurses want. *Nursing Management*, *34*(2), 15–17; Lacey, L. M. & Shaver, K. (2004). Retaining staff nurses in North Carolina. *North Carolina Center for Nursing*. Retrieved January 17, 2004, from http://www.nursenc.org/research/retain_staff.pdf.
5. Aiken, L. H. (2002). Superior outcomes for magnet hospitals: The evidence base. In M. L. McClure & A. S. Hinshaw (Eds.), *Magnet hospitals revisited: Attraction and retention of professional nurses*. Washington, DC: American Nurses Publishing.
6. Budd, Warino, & Patton, 2004, 1–20.
7. White, B. (1984). An introduction to collective bargaining. *Oregon Nurse*, 23, 27.
8. Common questions about union organizing and representation. (1985). *Michigan Nurse*, 3; Fulmer, W. E. (1982). *Union organizing: Management and labor conflicts*. New York: Praeger.
9. Hannah, K. J. & Shamian, J. (1992). Integrating a nursing professional model and nursing informatics in a collective bargaining environment. *Nursing Clinics of North America*, 31–45.
10. Beletz, E. E. (1982). Nurses' participation in bargaining units. *Nursing Management*, 48–50, 52–53, 56–58.
11. Cleland, V. S. (1988). A new model of collective bargaining. *Nursing Outlook*, 228–230; Supreme Court affirms eight bargaining units per hospital. (1991). *The Regan Report on Nursing Law*, 1; Easterling, J. F. (1983). Autonomy, professionals, and collective bargaining. *Michigan Nurse*, 86–87; Acord, L. G. (1982). Protection of nursing practice through collective bargaining. *International Nursing Review*, *29*(5), 150–152; Stickler, K. B. (1990). Union organizing will be divisive and costly. *Hospitals*, 68–70; Brenner, P. S. (1983). Labor relations in nursing. *Michigan Nurse*, 2–4; Flanagan, L. (1991). How the bargaining process works. *The American Nurse*, 11–12; Lippman, H. (1991). Expect to hear about unions. *RN*, 57–72; Nurses hail crucial Supreme Court ruling. (1991). *California Nurse*, 1.
12. Markus, K. (1994, December 2). Ruling may change labor relations. *NURSEWeek*, *5*, 12.
13. ANA supports MNA in Lansing NLRB case. (1995). *Michigan Nurse*, 13.
14. Brenner, 1983, 2–4.
15. Strauss, G. (1968). Professionalism and occupational associations. *Industrial Relations*, *2*(3), 7–31.
16. Pavalko, R. (1971). Sociology of occupations and professions. Itasca, IL: Peacock.
17. Easterling, 1983; Brenner, 1983; Acord, 1982; MacLachlan, L. D. (1990). Meeting the challenges of collective bargaining. *California Nurse*, 1, 4–5; Porter-O'Grady, T. (1992). Of rabbits and turtles: A time of change for unions. *Nursing Ecomonic$*, 177–182; Joel, L. (1992). Collective bargaining: A positive force in the workplace. *The Missouri Nurse*, 18–20; Lippman, 1991; Shinn, L. J. (1992). NLRB rulemaking upheld: What's next for hospitals? *Aspen's Advisor for Nurse Executives*, 7–8; "Nurses hail," 1991; Beyond collective action: Individuals can protect their jobs. (1985). *Ohio Nurses Review*, 5–6; Steps to organize and obtain a collective bargaining contract. (1985). *Michigan Nurse*, 2; Hepner, J. O. & Zinner, S. E. (1991). Nurses and the new NLRB rules. (1991). *Health Progress*, 20–22; Stanley, J. (1987). Collective Bargaining Turns 40. *California Nurse*, 1, 3.
18. Ibid.
19. News from ANA: ANA house of delegates approves significant reshaping of the association. (1999). *Nevada Reformation*, 14–15.
20. ANA creates new labor entity. (1999). *Oregon Nurse*, 8.
21. Ibid.
22. Brenner, 1983; Lippman, 1991; Shinn, 1992; Fenner, K. M. (1991). Unionization: Boon or bane? *Journal of Nursing Administration*, 7–8; "Nurses hail," 1991; Hepner & Zinner, 1991; Benton, T. (1992). Union negotiating. *Nursing Management*, *23*(3), 70, 72; Krasnansky, J. A. (1992). Time to stop the debate. *RN*, 116; Holmsted, L. (1991). E & GW annual business meeting. *The Maine Nurse*, 5.
23. Wheaton, D. (1991). Collective bargaining: Confronting the conflicts. *The Maine Nurse*, 10.
24. Kleingartner, A. (1969). Professional association: An alternative to unions? In R. Woodworth & R. Peterson (Eds.), *Collective negotiations for public and professional employees* (pp. 241–245). Glenview, IL: Scott, Foresman.
25. "Steps to organize," 1985; Beletz, 1982.
26. Friedheim, M. K. (1982). Negotiating a union contract. *Medical Laboratory Observer*, 58–63.
27. "Steps to organize," 1985.
28. Eubanks, P. (1990). Employee grievance policy: Don't discourage complaints. *Hospitals*, 36–37.
29. Ibid.
30. Eldridge, I. (1986). Some techniques and strategies of collective bargaining. *Washington Nurse*, 13.
31. Krasnansky, 1992.
32. Brutsche, S. (1990). Mediation cross-examined. *Texas Bar Journal*, 584.
33. Ibid.
34. Dvorak, J. M. (1983). Past practice concepts in collective bargaining. *Michigan Nurse*, 5–7.
35. Ibid.
36. McLachlan, L. D. (1990). Meeting the challenges of collective bargaining. *California Nurse*, 1, 4–5.
37. Flanagan, 1991.
38. Acord, 1982.
39. White, 1984.
40. Easterling, 1983.
41. Beletz, 1982.
42. "Steps to organize," 1985.
43. Ibid.; Acord, 1982.
44. Joel, 1992.
45. Shinn, 1992.
46. Hepner & Zinner, 1991.
47. Hannah & Shamian, 1992.
48. Ibid.
49. Ibid.
50. Ibid.
51. Lippman, 1991.
52. Worsler, R. (1993, September 27). Still fighting yesterday's battle. *Newsweek*, 12.

53. Beletz, 1982.
54. Ibid.
55. Kalisch, P. A. & Kalisch, B. J. (1985). Policy and perspectives on newspaper reports of nurse strikes. *Research in Nursing and Health*, 243–251.
56. Pointe, P. R., Fay, M. S., Brown, P., Doyle, M., Perron, J., Zizzi, L., et al. (1998). Factors leading to a strike vote and strategies for reestablishing relationships. *Journal of Nursing Administration*, 35–43.
57. Levinson, M. & Chideya, F. (1993, July 19). One for the rank and file. *Newsweek*, 38–39.
58. Sparks of union activity. (1991). *Journal of Nursing Administration*, 4.
59. Fenner, 1991.
60. Ibid.
61. Porter-O'Grady, 1992.
62. Joel, 1992.
63. "Beyond collective action," 1985.
64. Cohen, A. (1989). The management rights clause in collective bargaining. *Nursing Management*, 24–26, 28–30.

REFERENCES

Apfer, J., Zabava Ford, W. S., & Fox, D. H. (2003). Predicting nurses' organizational and professional identification: The effect of nursing roles, professional autonomy, and supportive communication. *Nursing Economics*, *21*, 226–232.

Forman, H. & Davis, G. A. (2002). The rising tide of healthcare labor unions in nursing. *Journal of Nursing Administration*, *32*, 376–378.

Reynolds, A. (1992). ANA institute makes great strides for collective bargaining. *Pennsylvania Nurse*, *1*, 17.

Szcepanski, A. (2003a). Just cause: Security for your job. *Michigan Nurse*, *76*(2), 11, 13.

Szcepanski, A. (2003b). Mandatory subjects of bargaining. *Michigan Nurse*, *76*(1), 7.

CHAPTER 16

Evaluation

Linda Roussel, RN, DSN

> The shell must be cracked apart if what is in it is to come out, for if you want the kernel you must break the shell. And therefore, if you want to discover nature's nakedness, you must destroy its symbols, and the farther you get in the nearer you come to its essence. When you come to the One that gathers all things up into itself, there your soul must stay.
>
> Meister Eckhart

LEARNING OBJECTIVES AND ACTIVITIES

- Define the term *controlling*, (or evaluating).
- Describe the relationship of controlling (evaluating) to the other major functions of management: planning, organizing, and directing (leading).
- Describe the use of controls as management tools.
- Describe the use of standards for controlling or evaluating.
- Demonstrate controlling (evaluating) techniques.
- Use a set of standards to evaluate the controlling (evaluating) function of a nursing agency or unit.
- Describe evidence-based management and its relevance to evaluation and control.

CONCEPTS: Controlling, evaluating, standards, Gantt chart, performance evaluation and review technique (PERT), benchmarking, evidence-based management.

NURSE MANAGER BEHAVIORS: Uses legal and accreditation standards to control and evaluate all activities of the organization; promotes implementation of processes that deliver data and information to empower staff in decision making; advocates for and supports a process of participative decision making, promotes the development of policies, procedures, and guidelines based on research findings and institutional measurement of quality outcomes.

NURSE EXECUTIVE BEHAVIORS: Obtains input from representative nursing personnel to develop and implement a master control plan incorporating legal and accreditation standards; supports information handling processes and technologies to facilitate evaluation of effectiveness and efficiency of decisions, plans, and activities in relation to desired outcomes; ensures educational opportunities for staff based on evaluation findings—specific to the population served, professional practice, available technologies, or required skills—to enhance quality in health care delivery.

Introduction

The final element of management defined by Fayol is *evaluation* or *control*, which he defined as "verifying whether everything occurs in conformity with the plan adopted, the instructions issued, and principles established. It has for its object to point out weaknesses and error in order to rectify them and prevent recurrence."[1]

Urwick defines controlling or evaluating as "seeing that everything is being carried out in accordance with the plan which has been adopted, the orders which have been given, and the principles which have been laid down."[2] Urwick refers to three principles of controlling:[3]

1. The principle of uniformity ensures that controls are related to the organizational structure.
2. The principle of comparison ensures that controls are stated in terms of the standards of performance required, including past performance. In this sense, controlling means setting a mark and examining and explaining the results in terms of the mark. This is often called benchmarking.
3. The principle of exception provides summaries that identify exceptions to the standards.

Controlling should be based on facts. When issues arise, people should settle them through direct contact. To stimulate cooperation, employees need to participate from the beginning. Nurse managers can teach employees to cooperate across departmental lines and to let reason and common sense prevail.[4] Management authors, including nurses, have described the controlling process as follows:[5]

1. Establish standards for all elements of management in terms of expected and measurable outcomes. These are the yardsticks by which achievement of objectives is measured.
2. Apply the standards by collecting data and measuring the activities of nursing management, comparing standards with actual care.
3. Make any improvements deemed necessary from the feedback.
4. Keep the process continuous for all areas, including the following:
   a. Management of the nursing division and each subunit.
   b. The performance of personnel.
   c. The nursing process and product.

The controlling process may be expressed as a formula:

$$Ss + Sa + F + C \rightarrow I$$

Where Standards set + Standards applied + Feedback + Correction yield Improvement.

According to Peters, vision, symbolic action, and recognition make up a control system in the truest sense of the word. Peters also states that "what gets measured gets done."[6]

Evaluation as a Function of Nursing Management

Evaluation (control) is "the management function in which performance is measured and corrective action is taken to ensure the accomplishment of organizational goals."[7] Control includes coordination of numerous activities: decision making related to planning and organizing activities, and information from directing and evaluating each worker's performance. Evaluation is also concerned with records, reports, organizational progress toward aims, and effective use of resources. Control uses evaluation and regulation; controlling is identical to evaluation.[8] Koontz and Weihrich defined controlling as "the measurement and correction of the performance in order to make sure that enterprise objectives and the plans devised to attain them are accomplished."[9]

Systems Theory

Feedback and adjustment constitute the control element of nursing management. In the patient care model, output is described or defined in terms of the patient and is measured by quality indicators and outcomes. In case management, these indicators are predicted and met on a timed basis. Discharge planning will take note of them. When the outcomes or indicators fall short, the information is fed back to the clinical nurses, who make adjustments in the case management plan and the process controlled by the critical path. Both the patient and nurse are system inputs, whereas throughput consists of nursing actions related to patient outcomes and managerial actions related to setting goals for nurses' behavior. Quality management is the process by which the nursing product or process is measured and action prescribed to correct deficiencies.

Similarly, systems theory can be applied to performance evaluation of the registered nurse as output. Input is still the patient and the nurse, with throughput the managerial actions related to goals for nurse behavior. A performance results contract between clinical nurse and nurse manager spells out agreed-on performance goals or results. When these goals are not being met, the nurse manager discusses the deficiency with the clinical nurse, and they agree on corrective actions. In an open system the process is continuous.

An effective control system has standards, measuring tools, and a surveillance process culminating in corrective action. A quality control program for measuring patient care will have these same components.[10]

Controlling is the second physical act of administration (the first physical act is directing). It is the fourth and final element of the administrative composite process (ACP), after directing, planning, and organizing. All functions of management—planning, organizing, directing, and controlling—occur simultaneously. Inputs would include resources other than the clinical nurse, such as supplies, equipment, and plant, plus all of the direct and indirect cost elements used in achieving the outputs.[11]

Nurse managers will use staffing reports, budget status reports, and other information to control the functioning system. These reports are both monitoring devices and feedback to the clinical nurses and care managers.

Management Tools: Measurement Issues

In the process of evaluation, policies and procedures are used as standards. Observations, questions, patient charts, patients, and health care team members also serve as sources of data. Corrective actions can be corroborative, disciplinary, or educational.[12] In the process of feedback, a positive experience will stimulate motivation and contribute to the growth of employees.[13]

Controls are management tools for improving performance. Among the controls are rules that let people know what is expected of them and how functions are to be coordinated. Communication as information is essential to control. Self-control is essential to managerial control, because it is the highest form of control. Self-control includes being up-to-date in knowledge, giving clear orders, being flexible, understanding reasons for behavior, helping others improve, increasing problem-solving skills, staying calm under pressure, and planning ahead. Employees should be told the facts in clear, deliberate language. Effective nursing managers set limits and make these limits known to their employees. Then, when a line is crossed, the appropriate disciplinary action can be taken. This is achieved by corrective action that is consistently applied after checking the facts.[14]

Controls can be separated into two elements: mechanical and sociological. There are three stages of control. The first two are mechanical elements and the third is sociological element:[15]

1. A predetermined definition of standards for a level of performance.
2. Measurement of current performance against the standards.
3. Corrective action when indicated.

Nurse managers will avoid the unintended consequence of control, that is, noncompliance. Because control can be perceived as a threat from unwanted power and authority, it can trigger defense mechanisms such as aggression and repression. Lemin advocated the following approaches to control: time, a high degree of mutual trust, a high degree of mutual support, open and authentic communications, clear understanding of objectives, respect for differences, use of member resources, and a supportive environment. These approaches will lead to conflict resolution, changed beliefs and attitudes, genuine innovation, genuine commitment, strengthened management, and prevention of unintended consequences of control.[16]

In a good control system, controls should do the following:[17]

1. Reflect the nature of the activity.
2. Report errors promptly.
3. Be forward-looking.
4. Point out exceptions at critical points.
5. Be objective.
6. Be flexible.
7. Reflect the organizational pattern.
8. Be economical.
9. Be understanding.
10. Indicate corrective action.

The best way to ensure the quality of nursing services provided in the patient units is to establish philosophy, standards of care, and objectives. At least two of these, philosophy and objectives, involve planning—further evidence that the major functions of management take place simultaneously.[18] Controlling mechanisms also include accreditation procedures, consultants, evaluation devices, rounds, reports, inspections, and nursing audits.[19]

Nurses activate the processes of control. This function involves the use of power and should be used by nurse managers to promote openness, honesty, trust, competence, and even confrontation. This function also involves value systems, ethical decision making, self-control, professional self-regulation, and control by an aggregate of professionals. Quality management programs excel in quality of care, including accessibility, beliefs, and attitudes of patients about health care; structure of health care; processes of care; professional competence; outcomes of care; and self-regulation. Audits and budgets are the major techniques of control.[20]

Control functions can be differentiated among levels of managers. For example, the nurse manager of a unit is concerned with short-term operational activities, including daily and weekly schedules, assignments, and effective use of resources. This nurse manager also keeps records of absences and incidents and prepares personnel appraisals, which are control activities subject to quick changes.

Two measurement methods are used to assess achievement of nursing goals: task analysis and quality control. In task analysis, the nurse manager inspects the motions, actions, and procedures laid out in written guidelines, schedules, rules, records, and budgets. Task analysis is a study of the process of giving nursing care. It measures physical support only; a few tools have been developed to do task analysis in nursing. In quality control the nurse manager is concerned with measurement of the quality and effects of nursing care. The American Nurses Association (ANA), the Joint Commission on Accreditation of Healthcare Organizations (JCAHO), and other organizations have developed mechanisms or models for measuring nursing care. Many quality management techniques are referred to as audits.[21]

Standards

A prime element of the management of nursing services is a system for evaluation of the total effort, including evaluation of the management process, the practice of nursing, and all nursing care services. Evaluation requires standards that can be used to gauge the quality and quantity of services. The key source for these standards, which are available for both management and practice, is the ANA, whose publications include *Scope and Standards for Nurse Administrators* and *Standards of Clinical Nursing Practice*. These documents can be of assistance in developing the objectives of the division of nursing and of each unit and clinic. Objectives are developed into operational or management plans, and systematic and periodic review of accomplishment of these objectives will be part of the evaluation system. A management evaluation system can be developed with a similar format. The nurse executive and other nurse managers can effect further evaluation through development of criteria for nursing rounds.

Performance standards can be used for individual performance, and criteria can be developed for collective evaluation of patient care. The latter may include the standards for use during nursing rounds as well as the criteria for the quality management program.

Standards are established criteria of performance, planning goals, strategic plans, physical or quantitative measurements of products, units of service, labor hours, speed, cost, capital, revenue, program, and intangible standards.[22] They have also been defined as "an acknowledged measure of comparison for quantitative or qualitative value, criterion, or norm . . . a standard rule or test on which a judgment or decision can be based." Nursing managers develop, in collaboration with clinical nurses, the "clinical nursing criteria against which to measure patient outcomes and the nursing process."[23] These standards are stated as patient outcomes, nursing care processes, incident reviews, and evidence-based practice.[24]

The following are eight categories of standards:[25]

1. Physical standards. Example: using patient acuity ratings to establish nursing hours per patient day.
2. Cost standards. Example: cost per patient day for supplies.
3. Capital standards. Example: a new program of monetary investment, such as a patient teaching staff.
4. Revenue standards. Example: the revenue per hour of nursing care received by patients.
5. Program standards. Example: a program designed to develop a new nursing service for changing clients' behavior regarding exercise, eating, or other health activities.
6. Intangible standards. Example: Staff development costs in nursing.
7. Goals. Intangible standards are frequently replaced by goals, including those for qualitative measurements.
8. Strategic plans, as control points for strategic control, are also used as standards. As nurse managers increase their involvement in strategic planning, they will need to perform strategic control.

Schoessler describes a process for preparing documentation for a JCAHO visit, including a system for maintaining ongoing documentation that is being adapted to changes in JCAHO standards. Such a system ensures that standards are kept up-to-date and prevents last-minute crisis preparation for JCAHO visits.

Self-study is also a method of meeting JCAHO safety requirements. Employees are held accountable for meeting the standard and are tested to verify competence.[26] Programs are written and distributed by education personnel, and records are maintained on education cards or by computer. Self-study methods can be used to meet other standards.

Measuring productivity is a function of the controlling process. To perform this measure, management establishes a measurement of productivity as the standard for each department and unit. Inputs are reported to appropriate cost-center managers each month. Productivity measurement tools should be developed, with input from the people being measured. This development may be done locally or through consultation. Nursing departments with computerized patient classification systems often have accurate productivity indices and reporting. Tools to evaluate productivity of independent nurse practitioners are available.[27] Exhibit 16-1, Operational Plan, is an example of an evaluation or controlling plan for nursing services.

Controlling Techniques

Specific controlling techniques include planned nursing rounds by nurse managers from all levels, checklists from the ANA *Scope and Standards of Nurse Administrators*, ANA *Standards of Clinical Nursing Practice*, JCAHO *Comprehensive Accreditation Manual for Hospitals,* and other published standards of third-party payers such as those put forth by the Centers for Medicare and Medicaid Services (CMS).

Nursing Rounds

An effective controlling technique for nursing managers is planned nursing rounds, which can be placed on a schedule and can include all nursing personnel. Rounds cover issues such as patient care, nursing practice, and unit management. To be effective, the results should be discussed with appropriate nursing personnel in a follow-up conference. Part of the evaluation process takes place as a result of the communication occurring during the rounds. Exhibit 16-2 shows a protocol for planned monthly nursing rounds.

Nursing Operating Instructions

Nursing operating instructions or policies become standards for evaluation and controlling techniques (see Exhibit 16-3).

EXHIBIT 16-1

Operational Plan

MISSION STATEMENT TO WHICH OBJECTIVE APPLIES

The division of nursing has a stated philosophy and objectives. Personnel of each department or unit within the division will have their own philosophy and will set up their own objectives. The objectives will be continuously evaluated, and a written statement as to progress will be sent to the chair's office each August and February.

PHILOSOPHY STATEMENT TO WHICH OBJECTIVE APPLIES

We believe that a continuous evaluation of the activities of the division of nursing is necessary to assess how effectively the needs of the patients are being met and to take action to improve nursing service when indicated. Research must be performed, and the results must be analyzed, adapted, and implemented to modify nursing procedures and practices for the attainment of more effective patient care.

OBJECTIVE 6

The patient benefits from close nursing supervision of all nonprofessional personnel who give patient care, and the patient benefits from continuous evaluation of the nursing care given and of performances of all nursing service personnel based on professional standards.

PLANS FOR ACHIEVING OBJECTIVE	ACTION AND ACCOUNTABILITY	TARGET DATES	ACCOMPLISHMENTS
1. Plan and execute a system of continuous evaluation and appraisal of nursing services.	1. Make complete rounds throughout the hospital at least once a day from nursing office. Establish a system of formal nursing rounds by chair, assistants, and clinical nursing coordinators monthly.	Apr. 23, 20xx	Being done.
	2. Do a monthly nursing audit. Have committee chair brief the chair of the division of nursing afterward.	Dec. 1, 20xx	Criteria for major nursing diagnosis outcomes completed. Committee combined with other disciplines. Criteria applied to four nursing diagnosis outcomes with retrieval by medical records personnel and corrective actions taken.
	3. Develop standards for patient care. Use ANA *Standards of Clinical Nursing Practice* for evaluating patient care. Obtain copies for all head nurses.	Jan. 1, 20xx	Obtained. Being incorporated into system by committee of staff nurses. Will cross-check with job performance standards.
	4. Develop standards for personnel performance.	Dec. 31, 20xx	Completed for clinical nurses I, II, and III, charge nurse, in-service education coordinator, clinical coordinator, chair and assistants, operating room supervisor and staff nurses, public health nurse, and rehabilitation nurse.
	5. Set up a system whereby managers attend a. Change-of-shift reports. b. Unit conferences. c. Unit in-service programs.	July 1, 20xx	Receiving reports and need to plan for their use. Will discuss with managers.

EXHIBIT 16-1

PLANS FOR ACHIEVING OBJECTIVE	ACTION AND ACCOUNTABILITY	TARGET DATES	ACCOMPLISHMENTS
	6. Review and use ANA *Scope and Standards for Nurse Administrators* to develop an evaluation and inspection checklist.	Dec. 1, 20xx	
2. Study organization.	1. Reorganize as needed. Have organization chart printed.	July 1, 20xx	Done as hospital policy.
	2. Write policy on unit policies and procedures.	July 1, 20xx	Done as nursing operating instruction 160-2-4.
3. Establish a counseling program for all nursing personnel.	1. Program counseling sessions for all head nurses. Have them do the same for those they supervise.	Jan. 1, 20xx	All done once by Jan. 1, 20xx.
	2. Use the job performance standards.		

EXHIBIT 16-2

Protocol for Planned Monthly Nursing Rounds

1. The chair, assistant chair, and other appropriate nursing personnel will make nursing rounds monthly.
2. Time is 10:00 to 11:00 A.M. unless otherwise indicated.
3. Schedule:

UNIT	DAY
1F	1st Tuesday
2A	1st Wednesday
2B	1st Thursday
2F	2nd Tuesday
ICU	2nd Wednesday
4A	2nd Thursday
3A	2nd Friday
3-OB	3rd Tuesday, 10:30 to 11:30 A.M.
3F	3rd Wednesday
4B	3rd Thursday, 11:00 A.M. to 12:00 noon
5A, CCU	4th Tuesday
5B	4th Wednesday

4. All unit nursing personnel are welcome to attend these rounds with their head nurse. Patient care needs come first. The following areas will be covered as rounds are made to each patient's bedside:
   a. Nursing histories
   b. Nursing care plans
   c. Nursing notes
   d. Nurses' signatures on necessary documents
5. Other management areas of note will be discussed after bedside rounds:
   a. Equipment and supplies
   b. Staffing and assignments
   c. Narcotic registers

The ANA *Scope and Standards for Nurse Administrators* can be developed into a checklist for evaluating the management processes of nursing services. Exhibit 16-4 shows a format for converting these standards into a usable control tool.

The ANA *Standards of Clinical Nursing Practice* can be implemented in several ways. One way is to convert the set of standards into a checklist as in Exhibit 16-4. Written protocols should be developed to implement a program for the evaluation process. Another way these protocols may be implemented is by using them to develop the evaluation standards, as in Exhibit 16-5.

Gantt Charts

Early in the twentieth century, Henry L. Gantt developed the Gantt chart as a means of controlling production.

EXHIBIT 16-3
Operating Instructions

1. Special care units will maintain policies and procedures relative to their mission. (These procedures will be reviewed, updated, and signed at least annually.)
   a. Intensive care unit
   b. Critical care unit
   c. Newborn/intensive care unit nursery
   d. Renal dialysis
2. Special care units will maintain a list of equipment needed to achieve their mission.
3. Supplies and equipment
   a. Blount resuscitator will have percent adaptor to increase oxygen concentration.
   b. Ambu resuscitator will have tail on to increase oxygen concentration.
   c. Humidification will not be used with oxygen with Ambu resuscitator.
   d. Trays from Central Sterile Supply will be returned as soon as used so that instruments will not be lost or misplaced.

EXHIBIT 16-4
Format for Converting the ANA *Scope and Standards for Nurse Administrators* into a Usable Control Tool

STANDARD NO. ________ :

Measurement Criteria	Yes	No
(List)		

EXHIBIT 16-5
Standards for Evaluating the Controlling (Evaluating) Function of Nursing Administration of a Division, Service, or Unit

1. An evaluation plan exists and is used for each nursing department, service, or unit.
2. Each evaluation plan is specific to the needs and activities of the individual department, service, or unit.
3. Evaluation findings are given in immediate feedback to subordinate nursing personnel.
4. Standards are accurate, suitable, and objective.
5. Standards are flexible and work when changes are made in plans and when unforeseen events and failures occur.
6. Standards mirror the organizational pattern of the nursing division, service, or unit.
7. Standards are economical to apply and do not produce unexpected results or effects.
8. Nursing personnel know and understand the standards.
9. Application of the standards results in correction of deficiencies.

The chart, which is usually used for production activities, depicts a series of events essential to the completion of a project or program.

Exhibit 16-6 shows a modified Gantt chart that could be applied to a major nursing administration program or project. The five major activities identified are segments of a total program or project. The chart could be applied to a project such as implementing a modality of primary nursing or implementing case management. The following are possible nursing activities for a project:

- Gather data.
- Analyze data.
- Develop a plan.
- Implement the plan.
- Evaluate, give feedback, and modify the plan as needed.

Exhibit 16-6 is only an example. Application of this controlling process by nurse managers would be specific to the project or program, and the time elements for the various activities would vary. Using subcategories of activities with estimated completion times could also modify these five major activities. The nurse manager's goal is to complete each activity or phase on or before the projected date.

Critical Control Points and Milestones

Master evaluation plans should have critical control points: specific points in production of goods or services at which the nurse administrator judges whether the objectives are being met qualitatively and quantitatively. Critical control points tell whether the plan is progressing satisfactorily. They pinpoint successes and failures and their causes. Critical control points tell managers whether they are on target with regard to time, budget, and other resources. Milestones are segments or phases of specific activities of a project or program that are projected to occur within a time frame.

Exhibit 16-7 represents a modified Gantt chart with networks of milestones and critical control points.

The critical path is

1 ➤ 2 ➤ 3 ➤ 4 ➤ 5 ➤ 6 ➤ 7 ➤ 8 ➤ 9 ➤ 17 ➤ 18.

Line 5 represents evaluation of all other nursing actions. This illustration is a simplified version of a control technique. Case management also uses critical paths with milestones and control points. Any major nursing program could have dozens or even hundreds of milestones and critical control points. This system also is known as the program evaluation and review technique (PERT).

Application of the milestone technique involves establishing a network of controllable pieces when planning a project or program. Each piece of the project or program

EXHIBIT 16-6
Modified Gantt Chart

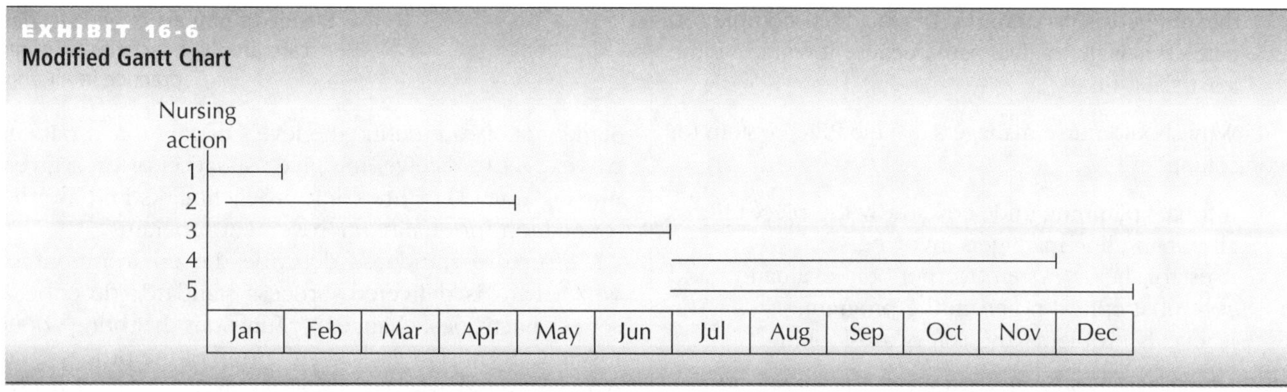

Note: Five nursing actions are needed to complete a program planned to start in January and end in December. In Exhibit 16-7, these five actions are translated into milestones and critical control points.

EXHIBIT 16-7
Milestones and Critical Control Points

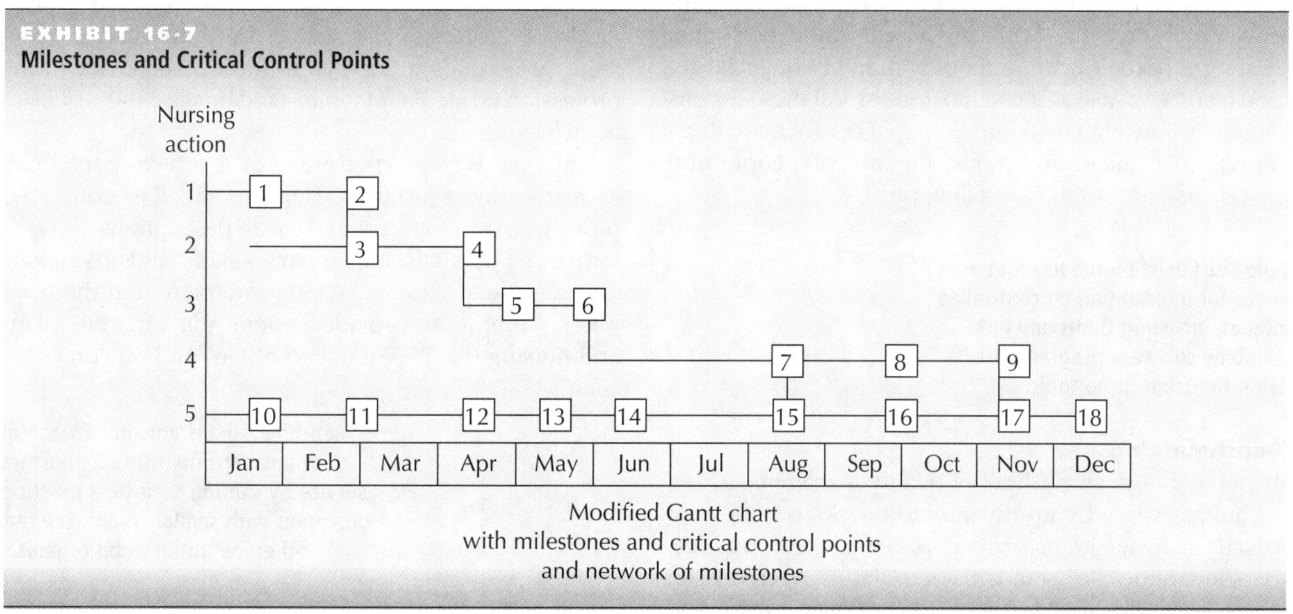

Modified Gantt chart with milestones and critical control points and network of milestones

is also allocated a prorated portion of the total budget. A nurse manager could use this technique to evaluate the actual expenditure amount versus the estimated budget at the end of each step of activity (or monthly) of the project or program. These will be the critical control points, as each would culminate in the achievement of a milestone. Each event may represent a budgeting allocation, a period of time or time span, or a continuum of several or all of these. Bar graphs are frequently used to depict milestone budgeting. Budgeting is a major controlling technique in any of its forms.[28]

Program Evaluation and Review Technique (PERT)

The program evaluation and review technique was developed by the Special Projects Office of the US Navy and applied to the planning and control of the Polaris weapon system in 1958. The PERT system has been widely applied as a controlling process in business and industry.

PERT uses a network of activities, each of which is represented as a step on a chart. A time measurement and an estimated budget should be worked out that include the following:[29]

1. Finished product or service desired.
2. Total time and budget needed to complete the project or program.
3. Start and completion dates.
4. Sequence of steps or activities required to accomplish the project or program.
5. Estimated time and cost of each step or activity.
6. Three paths for steps 4 and 5:
   a. Optimistic time.
   b. Most likely time.
   c. Pessimistic time.
7. Calculation of the critical path, the sequence of the events that would take the longest time to complete

the project or program by the planned completion date. This is the critical path because it will leave the least slack time.

Why should nurse managers use the PERT system for controlling?

- It forces planning and shows how the pieces fit for all nursing line managers involved.
- It establishes a system for periodic evaluation and control at critical points in the program.
- It reveals problems and is forward-looking.

The PERT system generally is used for complicated and extensive projects or programs, such as planning and implementing a system of nursing diagnoses, nursing interventions, and nursing outcomes.

Many records are used to control expenses and otherwise conserve the budget. These include personnel staffing reports, overtime reports, monthly financial reports, and expense and revenue reports. All these reports should be available to nurse managers to help them monitor, evaluate, and adjust the use of people and money as part of the controlling process.[30]

Multiple sites exist on the Internet as resources for information on controlling techniques, including Gantt and PERT charts. Many software programs are available for using these tools.

Benchmarking

Benchmarking, an offshoot of quality management, is a technique whereby an organization seeks out the best practices in its industry to improve its performance. Benchmarking is a standard, or point of reference, in measuring or judging factors such as quality, values, and costs. The following are examples of benchmarks that could apply to nursing:[31]

- Establishing a skill mix of nursing employees to obtain the highest quality of patient care at the lowest cost, which is called vertical leveraging. Horizontal leveraging uses cross-training to boost productivity. If the average for the industry were a ratio of 60% registered nurses to 40% other nursing personnel, the institution would make a decision to meet or exceed this ratio.
- An operating room utilization rate of 80% or higher if the industry rate is 75%.
- An average turnover time between cases of 15 minutes if the industry rate is 20 minutes.
- A reduction of 10% from the average-for-industry cost of supplies per patient day.
- A reduction of 50% from the average-for-industry rate of hospital-acquired infections.

Standards of practice and standards of care are the benchmarks for nursing practice in all domains.

Standards of care define the levels of care that a patient can expect to receive in a given situation or on a given nursing unit. They are clinical benchmarks and are the foundation for quality improvement programs.

Structure standards describe the environment in which care is delivered. Process standards describe a series of activities, changes, or functions that bring about result. Clinical standards, a subgroup of the process and outcome standards, are developed to include clinical issues specific to areas of practice. These include both standards of care and standards of professional practice. According to the ANA, standards of care are authoritative statements describing a competent level of practice. Standards of professional practice are authoritative statements describing a competent level of behavior in the professional role.[32] Outcome standards are the results to be achieved.

Standards of practice are used to structure the quality management program. They are linked to policy and procedure development and to job descriptions and performance appraisals. Implementation of standards is done through use of generic nursing care plans and the computer. Computers provide generic nursing care plans and nursing diagnoses, interventions, and outcomes.[33]

Benchmarking is enhanced when quality teams perform at the highest level of service by sharing their best practices and processes with similar committee teams in other institutions and organizations.

Quality management is a necessary element of benchmarking. The following are some benefits of benchmarking:

- Goals and objectives are set, and full team support to meet them is obtained.
- Performance regarding practices, processes, and outcomes is continually improved.
- Commitment and accountability for excellence exist.
- New approaches are sought out, learned, and adapted to.
- Organizational communication is improved.
- Clinical governance is improved.
- Patient satisfaction is improved.

The benchmarking program includes planning during team meetings, collection of specific data, data analysis to determine gaps, integration through keeping all team members informed, action, and followup and monitoring.[34]

Master Control Plan

To fulfill this important management function, nurse managers can use a master control or evaluation plan. It can be a general plan for all, with each manager adding specific items for his or her own management area. A sample master control plan is depicted in Exhibit 16-8.

Evidence-Based Management

"Evidence-based management means that managers, like their clinical practitioner counterparts, should search for, appraise, and apply empirical evidence from management research in their practice."[35] It is essential that managers document and systematically review their actions and

EXHIBIT 16-8
Master Control Plan

OBJECTIVE 1
Inspect for and identify the presence of written, current, and practical statements of mission, philosophy, vision, and objectives for the division of nursing and each of its component units. The statements should reflect the purposes of the health care organization and give direction to the nursing care program.

Actions

1. The written statements of mission, philosophy, and objectives were current (reviewed or revised within the past year).
2. They existed for the division of nursing and for each department, ward, unit, and clinic.
3. They were written by appropriate nursing personnel, representative of people who will accomplish them.
4. The philosophy reflected the meaning of clinical practice.
5. The philosophy was developed in collaboration with consumers, employees, and other health care workers.
6. The objectives were specified, written in behavioral terms, and achievable.
7. They guided the process of implementing the philosophy.
8. They were used for orientation of newly assigned personnel and were otherwise widely distributed and interpreted.
9. They supported the mission, philosophy, and objectives of the institution.
10. Nursing personnel knew the rights of individuals and served as advocates for these rights.

OBJECTIVE 2
Inspect for and identify the presence of written operational or management plans for accomplishment of the objectives of the division of nursing and each of its component units.

Actions

1. The written operational or management plans were current (entries within past 30 days).
2. They existed for the division of nursing and for each department, ward, unit, and clinic.
3. They included specific actions to be taken to achieve objective, target dates, and names of personnel assigned responsibility for each action.
4. They were used to evaluate progress; accomplishments were listed.

OBJECTIVE 3
Inspect for and identify the presence of an organizational plan for the division of nursing and each of its component units.

Actions

1. The organizational plan was current; it agreed with actual organization when checked.
2. It existed for the division of nursing and for each department, ward, unit, and clinic.
3. It showed the relationships among component parts, spelling out the major functions of each, and it showed relationships with other services.
4. The organizational plan supported the mission assigned to personnel.
5. All nursing functions were managed by the nurse administrator.

OBJECTIVE 4
Inspect for and identify the presence of adequate policies and procedures for guidance of personnel of the division of nursing and each of its component units.

Actions

1. Policies and procedures of the division of nursing and of each department, ward, unit, and clinic were current (reviewed within past year).
2. Policies and procedures did not duplicate those of higher echelons.
3. Policies and procedures were not obsolete, restrictive, or inappropriate in context.
4. Content of location of policies and procedures was known by people who needed this information.
5. Policies and procedures for special care units included.
   a. Function and authority of unit director.
   b. Admission and discharge criteria.
   c. Criteria for performance of special procedures, including cardiopulmonary resuscitation, tracheostomy, ordering of medications, administration of parenteral fluids and other medication, and the obtaining of blood and other laboratory specimens.
   d. The use, location, and maintenance of equipment and supplies.
   e. Respiratory care.

(continued)

EXHIBIT 16-8 *(continued)*

f. Infection control.
g. Priorities for orders for laboratory tests.
h. Standing orders, if any.
i. Regulations for visitors and traffic control.

6. The nursing annex to the disaster plan was current and included.
   a. Recall procedures.
   b. Assignment procedures.
   c. Training plan.

OBJECTIVE 5
Inspect for and identify the presence of job descriptions and job standards for all personnel throughout the division of nursing.

Actions

1. Job descriptions and job standards existed and were current throughout the division of nursing (reviewed within past year).
2. Nursing personnel participated in formulating them.
3. Nursing personnel were classified according to competence, and salaries were commensurate with qualifications and positions of comparable responsibility within the agency and the community.
4. Job descriptions were used for purposes of counseling and helping employees to be productive.
5. They were used for orientation of newly assigned personnel.
6. They described the functions, qualifications, and authority of each position identified in the organizational plan.
7. They were readily available and known to each employee.
8. There was a designated nurse leader for the division of nursing who was a registered nurse with educational and experiential qualifications in nursing practice and the administration of nursing services.

OBJECTIVE 6
Inspect for and identify the presence of a master staffing plan for the division of nursing and each of its component units.

Actions

1. A master staffing plan existed and was current for the division of nursing and each department, ward, unit, or clinic. It showed authorized versus assigned personnel and was reviewed at least monthly.
2. Adequate personnel policies existed to give guidance to nursing personnel in the planning of time schedules and to allow for mobility so that personnel could be matched to jobs.
3. Avenues of communication existed to give input from nursing personnel to the nurse administrator regarding staffing problems.
4. An active plan existed for sponsoring newly assigned personnel and for identifying their special training and experience and their desired assignments.

OBJECTIVE 7
Inspect for and identify the presence of a planned counseling program for all personnel of the division of nursing.

Actions

1. The nurse executive had a planned program for counseling with managers, including charge nurses.
2. Counseling occurred at least every 6 months on a scheduled basis.
3. Charge nurses counseled with individual staff members on a scheduled basis at least once every 6 months.
4. The counseling process included discussion of progress toward personal objectives, and revisions resulted from the sessions. Job standards were reviewed, and special educational and experience goals were discussed and acted on.
5. Records of counseling sessions were available and were reviewed.
6. A career progression plan was operational.

OBJECTIVE 8
Inspect for and identify the presence of a system of evaluation of nursing activities in the division of nursing and each of its component units.

Actions

1. A system for evaluation of the division of nursing and each of its departments, wards, units, and clinics was in operation.
2. Change-of-shift reports and ward conferences were being periodically evaluated (at least once every 6 months).
3. Management plans indicated current evaluation of accomplishment of objectives (within past 30 days).
4. Management personnel, including the nurse executive, made planned ward rounds at least monthly and checked all aspects of department, ward, unit, or clinic management, including the following:
   a. Narcotic registers
   b. Nursing histories
   c. Nursing care plans
   d. Nursing notes
   e. Drug levels and security
   f. Supplies and equipment
   g. Assignment procedures
   h. Patient records

EXHIBIT 16-8

5. The quality assurance program was in effect, and at least one problem per month had been evaluated since June 1.
6. There was provision for inclusion of other health care disciplines and consumers in evaluating the nursing care programs.
7. Results of evaluation were used to assess planning for change.

OBJECTIVE 9
Inspect for and identify the representation of division of nursing personnel on institution-wide and departmental boards, committees, and councils.

Actions

1. The division of nursing was represented on institution-wide boards, committees, and councils whose activities affected nursing personnel directly.
   a. Social actions
   b. Personnel boards such as awards and benefits
2. Nursing service committees had specific objectives.
3. Membership was current and representative of all appropriate segments of the nursing staff.
4. Minutes of meetings reflected progress toward objectives and followup of problems.

OBJECTIVE 10
Inspect for and identify the existence of a working public relations program that serves as a means of communication between personnel of the division of nursing and the community they serve.

Actions

1. Evaluation programs existed to tell consumers of the nursing services available to them and to receive feedback from consumers on the types of services they needed.
2. There was a planned program to publicize nursing activities and recognize contributions and accomplishments of nursing personnel.

OBJECTIVE 11
Inspect for and identify the existence of a planned program for training and continuing education for all divisions of nursing personnel.

Actions

1. Written statements of mission, philosophy, and objectives existed and were current (reviewed within past year).
2. An operational or management plan for the accomplishment of objectives was current (entries made within past 30 days).
3. The plan listed activities, set priorities and target dates, assigned responsibility, and provided for continuous evaluation.
4. The plan provided for identification of training and continuing education needs, including input from participants, translation of needs into objectives, and the accomplishment of objectives.
5. An orientation program existed and included philosophy and objectives of organization and nursing service, personnel policies, job descriptions, work environment, clinical practice policies and procedures, and operational policies and procedures.
6. Supplemental classes were taught to meet on-the-job training needs.
7. Training programs were documented.
8. The program supported career advancement.

OBJECTIVE 12
Inspect for and identify the existence of procedures and policies for providing needed primary nursing care to patients.

Actions

1. Collection of data on each patient was sufficient to permit identification and assessment of the patient's needs and to institute an individual plan of care. Included were admission data and the patient's nursing history.
2. The nursing care plan included the nursing diagnosis, prescription for care, and patient's teaching needs.
3. The plan was used to provide care to the patient, and there was an ongoing reassessment of the patient's needs with appropriate changes made in the plan of care.
4. There was evidence that nursing actions required by physicians' orders, nursing care plans, and hospital policies were accomplished appropriately. Observations of patient's progress and response to actions were made and recorded.
5. There was evidence of interpretation and implementation of the ANA *Standards of Clinical Nursing Practice*.
6. Nursing administration had a plan for reviewing the requirements for giving credentials to individuals and health care organizations and for participating in their implementation.
7. Guidelines existed for assignment of personnel based on level of competence.
8. There were policies to use unit managers and ward clerks to perform clerical, managerial, and indirect service roles.
9. Nursing administration provided resources to accomplish primary nursing care to patient: facilities, equipment, supplies, and personnel.

decisions in such a way as to further add to the evidence base for effective management practices.[36]

Evidence-based management had been limited for a multitude of reasons: poorly indexed practical application, limited training in using evidence in making management decisions, and limited size and resources in some health care organizations to conduct and evaluate applied research.[37] The Institute of Medicine has identified five practices which are believed to provide an agenda for developing greater evidence-based management practices:[38]

1. Balancing the tension between efficiency and reliability.
2. Creating and sustaining trust.
3. Actively managing the process of change.
4. Involving workers in work design and workflow decision making.
5. Creating a learning organization.

Evaluating critical management and operational functions and processes further underscores the need to provide evidence to improve patient and staff outcomes.

Summary

Evaluating is an ongoing function of nursing management that occurs during planning, organizing, and directing activities. Through this process, standards are established and then applied, followed by feedback that leads to improvements. The process is continuous.

Each nurse manager should have a master control plan that incorporates all standards related to these actions. This plan can be applied to obtain immediate feedback and meet the objectives of control established for the unit, department, or division. The plan will verify results, provide instructions, and apply principles of uniformity, comparison, and exception.

Controls include policies, rules, procedures, self-control or self-regulation, discipline, rounds, reports, audits, evaluation devices, task analysis, quality control, and benchmarking. They should reflect the nature of the activity and be forward-looking, objective, flexible, economical, and understandable. Controls should lead to continuous action.

Standards are the yardsticks for evaluation and include ANA *Scope and Standards for Nurse Administrators* and *Standards of Clinical Nursing Practice*. Other standards include management plans, goals, programs, costs, revenues, and capital. Physical standards use Gantt charts, critical control points, milestones, and PERT. Each nurse manager should have a master evaluation plan, including a plan to further evaluate decisions with sound evidence.

APPLICATION EXERCISE

EXERCISE 16-1 With a group of your peers or colleagues, use Exhibits 16-5 and 16-8 to discuss developing a new evaluation plan for a nursing cost center. Incorporate the standards from both exhibits. How can they be measured? Modify them as necessary. Use your final product to evaluate the cost center.

NOTES

1. Fayol, H. (1949). General and industrial management (C. Storrs, Trans.). London: Sir Isaac Pitman & Sons, 107.
2. Urwick, L. (1944). The elements of administration. New York: Harper & Row, 105.
3. Ibid., 107–110.
4. Ibid., 113–117.
5. Koontz, H. & Weihrich, H. (1990). *Management* (5th ed.). New York: McGraw-Hill, 394–395; Hodgetts, R. M. (1990). *Management: Theory, process, and practice* (5th ed.). Orlando, FL: Harcourt Brace, 226–229; Fulmer, R. M. & Franklin, S. G. (1982). *Supervision: Principles of professional management* (2nd ed.). New York: Macmillan, 214–216; Rowland, H. S. & Rowland, B. L. (1997). *Nursing administration handbook* (4th ed.). Gaithersburg, MD: Aspen, 15–16, 35–44; Drucker, P. F. (1973). *Management: Tasks, responsibilities, practices*. New York: Harper & Row, 495–505; Marriner-Tomey, A. (1996). *Guide to nursing management and leadership* (5th ed.). St. Louis: Mosby, 379; Mosley, D. C., Pietri, P. H., & Megginson, L. C. (1996). *Management: Leadership in action* (5th ed.). New York: HarperCollins, 492–512.
6. Peters, T. (1987). Thriving on chaos. New York: Harper & Row, 587, 593.
7. Rowland & Rowland, 1997, 40.
8. Kron, T. & Gray, A. (1987). *The management of patient care: Putting leadership skills to work* (6th ed.). Philadelphia: W. B. Saunders, 100.
9. Koontz & Weihrich, 1990, 393.
10. Barnum, B. S. & Kerfoot, M. (1995). *The nurse as executive* (4th ed.). Gaithersburg, MD: Aspen, 229.
11. Arndt, C. & Huckebay, L. M. D. (1980). *Nursing administration: Theory for practice with a systems approach* (2nd ed.). St. Louis: Mosby, 22–46.
12. Franck, P. & Price, M. (1980). *Nursing nanagement* (2nd ed.). New York: Springer Publishing, 135.
13. Holle, M. L. & Blatchly, M. E. (1982). *Introduction to leadership and management in nursing*. Monterey, CA: Wadsworth Health Services Division, 178–185.
14. Levenstein, A. (1981). *The nurse as manager* (M. J. F. Smith, Series Ed.). Chicago: S-N Publications, 17–33.
15. Lemin, B. (1977). First line nursing management. New York: Springer, 47–51.

16. Ibid.
17. Fulmer & Franklin, 1982, 216–217.
18. Ramey, G. (1976). Setting standards and evaluating care. In S. Stone & D. Elhart (Eds.), *Management for nurses*. St. Louis: Mosby, 79.
19. Donovon, H. M. (1975). *Nursing service administration: Managing the enterprise*. St. Louis, MO: Mosby, 160–169.
20. Beyers, M. & Phillips, C. (1979). *Nursing management for patient care* (2nd ed.). Boston: Little, Brown, 109–141.
21. Douglass, L. M. (1986). *The effective nurse: Leader and manager* (5th ed.). St. Louis: Mosby, 245–278.
22. Koontz & Weihrich, 1990, 394–395.
23. Ganong, J. M. & Ganong, W. L. (1980). *Nursing management* (2nd ed.). Gaithersburg, MD: Aspen, 191.
24. Rosswurm, M. A. & Larrabee, J. H. (1999). A model for change to evidence-based practice. *Image: The Journal of Nursing Scholarship*, *31*(4), 317–322; Matthews, P. (2000). Planning for successful outcomes in the new millennium. *Topics in Health Information Management*, 55–64; Silver, M. S. (1999). Incident review management: A systemic approach to performance improvements. *Journal of Healthcare Quality*, *1*, 21–27.
25. Koontz & Weihrich, 1990, 396–398; Harrington, C., Kovner, C., Mezey, M., Kayser-Jones, J., Burger, S., Mohler, M., et al. (2000). Experts recommend minimum nurse staffing standards for nursing facilities in the United States. *Gerontologist*, *1*, 5–16.
26. Haggard, A. (1992). Using self-studies to meet JCAHO requirements. *Journal of Nursing Staff Development*, *4*, 170–174.
27. Kearnes, D. R. (1992). A productivity tool to evaluate NP practice: Monitoring clinical time spent in reimbursable patient-related activities. *Nurse Practitioner*, 50, 52, 55.
28. Koontz & Weihrich, 1990, 424; Hodgetts, 1990, 243; Beyers & Phillips, 1979, 134–135; Rowland & Rowland, 1997, 36; Fulmer & Franklin, 1982, 221–227; http://www-mmd.eng.ac.uk/people 9/17/2004; http://gracie.santarosa.edu, 9/17/2004.
29. Koontz & Weihrich, 1990, 424–428; Hodgetts, 1990, 240–242; http://www.criticaltools.com, 9/17/2004; http://www.infosystems.eku.edu, 9/17/2004.
30. Ganong & Ganong, 1980, 257.
31. Patterson, (1993). Benchmarking study identifies hospitals' best practices. *OR Manager*, 11, 14–15.
32. American Nurses Association (ANA). (1991). *Standards of clinical nursing practice*. Washington, DC: Author.
33. McAllister, M. (1990). A nursing integration framework based on standards of practice. *Nursing Management*, 28–31.
34. Murray, J. A. & Murray, M. H. (1992). Benchmarking: A tool for excellence in palliative care. *Journal of Palliative Care*, *8*(4), 41–45; Woomer, N., Long, C. O., Anderson, C., & Greenberg, E. A. (1999). Benchmarking in home health care: A collaborative approach. *Caring*, 22–28; McGowan, S., Wynaden, D., Harding, N., Yassine, A., & Parker, J. (1999). Staff confidence in dealing with aggressive patients: A benchmarking exercise. *Australia New Zealand Journal of Mental Health Nursing*, 104–108; Voyles, C. R. & Boyd, K. B. (1999). Criteria and benchmarks for laparoscopic cholecystectomy in a free-standing ambulatory center. *JSLS*, 315–318; Gardner, D. & Winder, C. (1998). Using benchmarking to improve organizational communication. *Quality Assurance*, 201–211; Nurse staffing law may herald benchmarks. (1999). *Healthcare Benchmarks*, 137–138; Johnson, B. C. & Chambers, M. J. (2000). Foodservice benchmarking: Practices, attitudes, and beliefs of foodservice directors. *Journal of the American Dietetic Association*, 175–182; Bucknall, C. E., Ryland, I., Cooper, A., Coutts, I. I., Connolly, C. K., & Pearson, M. G. (2000). National benchmarking as a support system for clinical governance. *Journal of Royal College of Physicians London*, 52–56.
35. Axelsson, R. (1998). Towards an evidence-based health care management. *International Journal of Health Planning and Management*, *13*, 307.
36. Walshe, K. & Rundall, T. (2001). Evidence-based management: From theory to practice in health care. *The Milbank Quarterly*, *79*(3), 429–458.
37. Page, A. (Ed.). (2004). *Keeping patients safe: Transforming the work environment of nurses*. Washington, DC: National Academies Press, 2004.
38. Ibid.

REFERENCES

American Nurses Association (ANA). (1995). *Scope and standards for nurse administrators*. Washington, DC: Author.

Balle, M. (1999). Making bureaucracy work. *Journal of Management in Medicine*, *13*(2–3), 190–200.

Coombs, C. R., Doherty, N. F., & Loan-Clarke, J. (1999). Factors affecting the level of success of community information systems. *Journal of Management in Medicine*, *13*(2–3), 142–153.

Dreachslin, J. L. (1999). Diversity leadership and organizational transformation: Performance indicators for health services organizations. *Journal of Healthcare Management*, *8*, 427–439.

Institute of Medicine. (2003). *Health professions education: A bridge to quality: Quality chasm series*. Washington, DC: The National Academies Press.

Jones, L. (1991). Integrating research activities, practice changes, and monitoring and evaluation: A model for academic health. *Quality Review Bulletin*, *8*, 229–239.

Kurec, A. S. (1999). Recruiting, interviewing, and hiring the right person. *Clinical Laboratory Management Review*, *8*, 251–261.

Patient satisfaction measures more meaningful with new standardized surveying system. (1999). *Data Strategic Benchmarks*, *7*, 149–153

Swansburg, R. C. (1976). *Management of patient care services*. St. Louis: Mosby.

Walker, J., Brooksby, A., McInerny, J., & Taylor, A. (1998). Patient perceptions of hospital care: Building confidence, faith and trust. *Journal of Nursing Management*, *5*, 193–200.

Ziegler, J. C. & Van Ellen, N. K. (1992). Implementation of a national nursing standards program. *Journal of Nursing Administration*, *1*, 40–46.

CHAPTER 17

Quality Management

Beverly Blain Wright, RNC, CNA, CPHQ

LEARNING OBJECTIVES AND ACTIVITIES

- Differentiate between quality management and total quality management.
- Discuss Deming's 14 points of management theory.
- Discuss Deming's seven deadly management theory diseases.
- Identify nursing's external and internal customers.
- Identify and discuss seven components of a quality management program.
- Differentiate between quality management tools and describe when they should be used.

CONCEPTS: Quality management (QM), total quality management (TQM), quality control (QC), Shewhart Cycle, internal customer, external customer, Theory Z, quality circles, structure, process, outcome.

NURSE MANAGER BEHAVIORS: Develops a quality management program demonstrating integration of standards. Selects elements of TQM theory to improve staff productivity.

NURSE EXECUTIVE BEHAVIORS: Demonstrates theory of TQM in development of quality management program that meets or exceeds accreditation requirements.

Introduction

A master control plan is needed to evaluate the efficacy of any nursing department or service. A critical component of such a plan will be the *quality management* (QM) program.

Effective quality management should be founded on the philosophy that group behaviors can be transformed into a desirable culture. As costs, client expectations, and other aspects of health care become more demanding, it becomes more important that quality management consider and build upon *total quality management* (TQM) principles. In TQM, quality is a state of mind; it is a work ethic involving everyone in the company,[1] and it involves *participative management*, the process of making decisions at lower levels within the organizational hierarchy. TQM gives every employee the opportunity to make management contributions, thereby reducing or eliminating adversarial relationships.[2]

Nursing *quality assurance* (QA) programs began in hospitals in the 1960s with the voluntary implementation of audits. QA programs were designed to set standards for nursing care delivery and to establish criteria by which to evaluate these standards. An integral part of assuring quality involved management, resulting in the evolution of the term QA to QM.

The Joint Commission on Accreditation of Healthcare Organizations (JCAHO) reports that in order to assure quality, continuous improvement must be demonstrated. Hence synonyms for QM programs have emerged, such as quality improvement (QI), continuous quality improvement (CQI), and performance improvement (PI). *Quality control* (QC), an aspect of QM, is concerned with sustaining conformance to standards.

Accreditation mandates that many aspects of health care must be incorporated into QM programs. Divisional or departmental programs must support an organization's mission. QM plans now incorporate customer satisfaction and patient rights. Dependent upon leadership, QM programs may or may not incorporate TQM philosophy.

Total Quality Management Gurus

W. Edwards Deming

W. Edwards Deming is considered by many to be the pioneer in quality management. An advocate for the principle of management for quality, he found that 80%–85% of problems are with the system; only 15%–20% are with workers. Workers should be told this and and should be given the freedom to speak and contribute as thinking, creative human beings. Deming's theory of management includes 14 points (see Exhibit 17-1). Deming also warned against the seven "deadly diseases" that decrease productivity and profitability because they destroy employee morale (see Exhibit 17-2).

Total quality management and benchmarking should be an integral part of strategic and operational planning.[3] TQM does not compromise organizational effectiveness; it improves it and contributes to an enterprise, increasing the market share of a business.[4]

Application of Deming's Theory

According to Piczak, General Douglas McArthur summoned W. Edwards Deming to set up quality circles for the Japanese in 1950.[5] When Deming presented the quality methods to 45 Japanese industrialists, they applied the methods. "Within six weeks, some of the industrialists were reporting gains of as much as 30% without purchasing any new equipment."[6]

Using Deming's methods managers and workers have a natural division of labor: the workers do the work of the system, and the managers improve the system. Thus the potential for improving the system never ends. Because workers know where the potential for improving the system lies, consultants are not needed. Managers know that the system is subject to a great variability and that problem events occur randomly. The common language for managers and workers is elementary statistics, which all workers learn.[7]

Variation

Deming advocated the use of the language of statistics to identify which problems are caused by workers and

EXHIBIT 17-1

Deming's 14 Points

1. Create constancy of purpose toward improvement of product and service. Everyone should have a clear goal every day, month after month. Satisfy the customer and reduce variation so all employees do not have to constantly shift their priorities.
2. Adopt a new philosophy by learning how to improve systems in the presence of variation, thus reducing variation in materials, people, processes, and products. End tampering and overreacting to variation.
3. Cease dependence on inspection to achieve quality by thoroughly understanding the sources of variation in processes and working to reduce variation.
4. End the practice of awarding business on the basis of price tag alone. Instead, minimize total cost by working with a single supplier.
5. Improve constantly and forever every process for planning, production, and service. Everyone uses PDCA (plan-do-check-act) cycle.
6. Institute training on the job. Know methods of performing tasks and standardize training. Accommodate variation in ways people learn.
7. Adopt and institute leadership. Work to help employees do their jobs better and with less effort. Learn which employees are within the system and which are not. Support company goals, focus on internal and external customers, coach, and nurture pride in workmanship.
8. Drive out fear, including fear of reprisal, fear of failure, fear of providing information, fear of not knowing, fear of giving up control, and fear of change. Fear makes accurate data nonexistent.
9. Break down barriers among staff areas, between departments. Promote cooperation. What is the constant, common goal?
10. Eliminate slogans, exhortations, and targets for the work force. Improvement requires changed methods and processes. Leaders change the system.
11. Eliminate numerical quotas for the work force and numerical goals for management. All people do not work at the same level of speed. There will be variation. Use realistic production standards. Eliminate management by objectives and use a system that rewards people's efforts toward improvement.
12. Remove barriers that rob people of pride of workmanship. Eliminate the annual rating or merit system.
13. Institute a vigorous program of education and self-improvement for everyone. This can be any education that improves self-esteem and potential to contribute to improvements in existing processes and advances in technology.
14. Put everyone in the company to work to accomplish the transformation.

Source: Reprinted from *Out of the Crisis* by W. Edwards Deming by permission of MIT and The W. Edwards Deming Institute. Published by MIT, Center for Advanced Engineering Study, Cambridge, MA 02139. Copyright 1986 by The W. Edwards Deming Institute. Dr. Deming rejected the concept of TQM, saying it was undefined.

EXHIBIT 17-2
Deming's Seven Deadly Diseases

1. Lack of constancy of purpose.
2. Emphasis on short-term profits.
3. Evaluation of performance, merit rating, or annual review.
4. Management by use of only visible figures.
5. Mobility of management.
6. Excessive medical costs.
7. Excessive costs of liability.

which by the system. The most-used statistical tool is that of variation, which measures whether an activity is under control or, if it is not, to what degree it is out of control. Statistics enable workers to control variation by teaching them to work more intelligently. The common language of statistics may enhance discussion between participants of quality circles.[8] Variation is the concept that distinguishes normal routine changes in a process from unusual, abnormal changes that can be attributed to specific causes. Variations in performance are mostly attributable to the system. In some examples, Deming found 400% variation in performance attributable to the system.[9]

According to Deming, Shewhart, and others, there are chance (common) causes and special (assigned) causes of variation. *Chance causes* are common causes that are the fault of the system. They are system variations such as process input or conditions that are ever present and cause small, random shifts in daily output. They occur in 90% of cases and require fundamental system change by management. Chance causes are controlled causes. A system totally influenced by controlled variation or common causes is said to be in statistical control.

A *special*, or assigned, *cause* is specific to a particular group of workers, an area, or a machine. It is uncontrolled variation resulting from assignable causes or source. Special causes occur in less than 10% of cases. They require identification of the source and preventive action. Special causes require timely data to effect changes that will prevent bad causes and keep good causes happening. (See Exhibit 17-3.)

Management by action uses the Deming (Shewhart) cycle. The cycle should be kept in constant motion and used at all levels of the organization. Reports should conform to the new system.[10]

Training in statistical process control takes the guesswork out of what is really happening in an operation. Statistical process control aims to prevent errors by identifying where they occur. The process is then tightened to improve the outcome. In looking at safety systems, Smith indicated that 85–90% of problems have common causes (the system) while only 10–15% of problems have special causes (employees). Using control charts to determine whether the causes of accidents are common or special can lead to development of methods to prevent accidents. Employees can then set goals to reduce the special causes.[11]

Variation is a part of everything—of the supplies used by nurses, employee performance, and much else. Causes exist other than common and special causes. One such cause is tampering or making unnecessary adjustments to compensate for common-cause variation. Another is structural variation caused by seasonal patterns and long-term trends.[12]

According to Deming, we should "measure the variations in a process in order to pinpoint the causes of poor quality." Quality improves as variability decreases.[13] Statistical charts are used to plot variations from the ideal in the production process and determine the right course to correct those variations.

Joseph Juran

To Juran, quality means fitness to serve, correct service the first time to meet customers' needs, and freedom from deficiencies. Quality necessitates employee involvement, with management leading the effort in planning, control, and improvement so that requirements are met. Quality requires identification of customers and their needs in a product-by-product and step-by-step process.[14]

Juran applies quality management to all functions at all levels of the enterprise and incorporates the exercise of personal leadership and participation by top managers. In Juran's ideal workplace, all managers would be educated in quality management techniques. There would be a sense of unity, in which every employee knows the direction of the new course and is stimulated to go there. Resisting forces are multiple functions, levels in hierarchy, and product lines.[15] All of these resisting forces are prominent in health care agencies.

Juran's philosophy of quality is based on three major premises: quality planning, quality control, and quality improvement. According to Juran, this quality trilogy can be grafted onto the strategic planning process. (See Exhibit 17-4.)

Philip B. Crosby

Crosby earned his reputation as a quality guru at International Telephone and Telegraph (ITT). He defines quality by four absolutes.[16] (See Exhibit 17-5.)

Culture and climate are important to achieving Crosby's absolutes. A climate of innovation is created because continuous innovation keeps customers coming back. The organizational culture often must be changed to raise every person's basic expectations. A small group of people may be used to uphold ethics and integrity.

EXHIBIT 17-3

Application of the Deming (Shewhart) PDCA Cycle to Total Quality Management

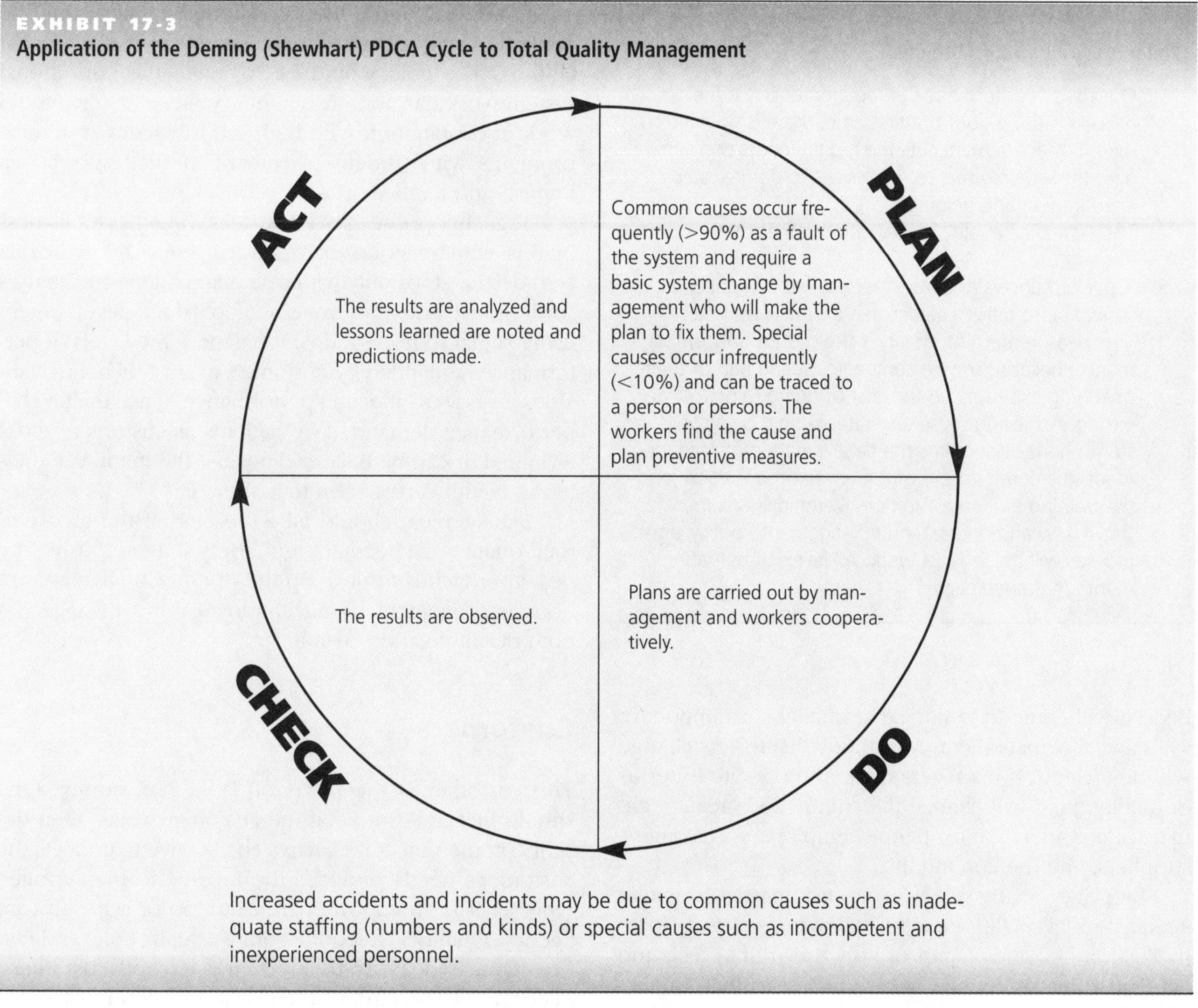

Increased accidents and incidents may be due to common causes such as inadequate staffing (numbers and kinds) or special causes such as incompetent and inexperienced personnel.

EXHIBIT 17-4

Juran's Quality Trilogy

1. *Quality planning* creates a process for meeting goals under operating conditions.[17]
   - Identify customers, both internal and external
   - Determine customer needs
   - Develop product features that respond to customer needs
   - Set goals that meet needs of customers and suppliers
   - Develop process to produce the product features
   - Prove process meets quality goals during operations
2. *Quality control*, the second activity of the quality process, is performed by operations personnel who put the plan into effect by identifying deficiencies, correcting them, and monitoring the process. Quality control includes the following:[18]
   - Choose what to control
   - Choose units of measurement
   - Establish measurement
   - Establish standards of performance
   - Measure actual performance
   - Interpret the difference
   - Take action on the difference
3. The third and final premise of the Juran philosophy is *quality improvement*, which should be purposeful and in addition to quality control. Quality improvement includes the following:[19]
   - Prove the need for improvement
   - Identify projects for improvement
   - Organize to guide the projects
   - Diagnose to find the causes
   - Provide remedies
   - Prove remedies are effective under operating conditions
   - Provide for control to hold the gains

EXHIBIT 17-5
Philip B. Crosby's Four Absolutes

1. Quality is "conformance to requirements." If the process is done right the first time, there is no need to redo it. Management sets the requirements and supplies the wherewithal to employees to do the job by encouraging and helping.
2. The system of quality is prevention rather than appraisal.
3. A performance standard of zero defects. A policy should be to deliver defect-free products on time.
4. The measurement of quality is the cost of nonconformance, because service companies spend half of their operating expenses on the cost of doing things wrong. Achieving these absolutes should be a constant priority. It requires the determination of management, the commitment of the entire organization, and the training and education of all employees. When they know and understand management's policy, employees will make TQM work. All levels of management are trained early.

People will come to believe that quality is as important as financial management. An attitude that fosters change will be created. If managers think and operate in terms of quality, they will change the culture and create a climate of consideration for people, employees, customers, suppliers, and the community.

By policy, every department and unit has a quality strategy and a quality function. All managers participate in TQM; it becomes a part of how they think, feel, and act. Nurse managers may want to use Crosby's Quality Management Maturity Grid to measure QA aspects of their department or unit and then expand use to other areas (see Exhibit 17-6).

Genichi Taguchi

The Taguchi method focuses on "robust quality" of service to meet customer performance expectations every time, even under severe operating or environmental conditions. Taguchi's approach to quality control involves complicated mathematical formulas.[20]

The theory of robust quality could be applied to the nursing process in a research and development project. Variance in the application of the nursing process (using various nursing modalities, nursing diagnoses, and nursing care standards, including interventions and outcomes) could be studied using the theory of robust quality. The object of this theory is to reduce the things that can go wrong in applying the theory of nursing and to minimize variations around the customer's (patient's) performance requirements.

In education, the theory of robust quality could be applied to eliminate state board failures as well as course failures. The goal would be to make the educational system work harmoniously. Thus, college faculty would work in cooperation with high school faculty to reduce problems with student placement in such subjects as English and mathematics.

Taguchi opposes zero defects, saying that robustness begins with meeting exact targets consistently, while zero defects stops only within a certain tolerance. He uses "orthogonal array," a system of product development using signal-to-noise ratios. It balances the levels of performance demanded by customers against the many variables, or noises, affecting performance. Once the level of performance demanded by patients as customers is determined, it can be balanced against the many variables in the health care system that affect it.[21]

Management should take the best of the theory of total quality management and apply it assiduously. The best approach is to develop the philosophy that continuous improvement by all employees and managers is both desirable and possible.

Customers

The customer is the focus of TQM philosophy. One should first find out what the customer wants, then describe it, then meet it exactly. The service that meets the customer's needs provides the income to the supplier, whether it is an educational institution or a health care agency. Quality is freedom from waste, trouble, and failure. One endeavors to meet and exceed customers' needs and expectations, then continues to improve.[22]

While total quality management techniques have not always produced significant change in organizational performance, customers demand an enhanced focus on continuous quality improvement.[23] Many failures of TQM result from the failure of managers to understand the complexity of making changes in organizations with multiple subcultures and interests.[24] Covance Laboratories achieved cultural change through quality assurance practices that improved efficiency, productivity, and customer and employee satisfaction.[25] An unrelenting effort toward continuous improvement in health care will result in unflinching customer loyalty, sustainable growth, and impressive performance.[26]

EXHIBIT 17-6
Quality Management Maturity Grid

MEASUREMENT CATEGORIES	STAGE ONE: UNCERTAINTY	STAGE TWO: AWAKENING	STAGE THREE: ENLIGHTENMENT	STAGE FOUR: WISDOM	STAGE FIVE: CERTAINTY
Management understanding and attitude	No comprehension of quality as a management tool. Tend to blame quality department for "quality problems."	Recognize that quality management may be of value but not willing to provide money or time to make it all happen.	While going through quality improvement program, learn more about quality management; becoming supportive and helpful.	Participating. Understand absolutes of quality management. Recognize personal role in continuing emphasis.	Consider quality management an essential part of company system.
Quality organization status	Quality is hidden in manufacturing engineering departments. Inspection probably not part of organization. Emphasis on appraisal and sorting.	A stronger quality leader is appointed but main emphasis is still on appraisal and moving the product. Still part of manufacturing or other.	Quality department reports to top management, all appraisal is incorporated, and manager has role in management of company.	Quality manager is an officer of company; effective status reporting and preventive action. Involved with consumer affairs and special assignments.	Quality manager is on board of directors. Prevention is main concern. Quality is a thought leader.
Problem handling	Problems are fought as they occur; no resolution; inadequate definition; lots of yelling and accusation.	Teams are set up to attack major problems. Long-range solutions are not solicited.	Corrective action communication established. Problems are faced openly and resolved in an orderly way.	Problems are identified early in their development. All functions are open to suggestion and improvement.	Except in unusual cases, problems are prevented.
Cost of quality as percentage of sales	Reported: Unknown Actual: 20%	Reported: 3% Actual: 18%	Reported: 8% Actual: 12%	Reported: 6.5% Actual: 8%	Reported: 2.5% Actual: 2.5%
Quality improvement actions	No organized activities. No understanding of such activities.	Trying obvious "motivational" short-range efforts.	Implementation of the 14-step program with thorough understanding and establishment of each step.	Continuing the 14-step program and starting Make Certain.	Quality improvement is a normal and continued activity.
Summation of company quality posture	"We don't know why we have problems with quality."	"Is it absolutely necessary to always have problems with quality?"	"Through management commitment and quality improvement we are identifying and resolving our problems."	"Defect prevention is a routine part of our operation."	"We know why we do not have problems with quality."

Source: B. J. Deutsch. "A Conversation with Philip Crosby." *Bank Marketing* (April 1991), 25. Reprinted with permission from the Bank Marketing Association.

Internal and External Customers

There are both internal and external customers, all of whom should be given service. In nursing management, the external customers are patients, employers, and the community. These customers will be satisfied by quality care that produces a patient improved to the point of being discharged and able to get on with his or her life. A patient facing death wants a quality of care to make his or her remaining time peaceful. The employer wants knowledgeable and skilled workers; the community wants a productive citizen.

Internal customers are those who interact with each other within and among departments and disciplines, such as nursing, pharmacy, radiology, and medical laboratory. Clinical nurses are customers of nurse managers, admission services, and others. The customer should be satisfied quickly and economically if nurse managers are to stay in business. This core of customers includes those who generate a profit and inspire nurses to their best ideas and highest motivation.[27]

The focus of TQM is harmony, not competition or adversarial relations, and satisfying such customers, not confronting them. The continual quest for improvement would reduce variation, adversarial relationships within and among departments, and disharmony. This can be done by developing information and using statistical tools to analyze it.[28]

Quality is not a program but a philosophy and a way of life. It is a survival issue. Traditional management is out. Quality management is customer-oriented, decentralized, empowering, and quality-focused.[29] Quality nurses aim for a world-class quality of care. This entails learning to deal with the most difficult patients and families. Nurse managers should facilitate the capability of clinical nurses to deal with difficult customers.

Nurse managers and practitioners identify customers of their services at the following input points: definition, production, delivery, and followup.

Cross-functional teams and an open, trusting, cooperative relationship are essential. Self-managed teams perform multiple functions and schedule their own work, develop budgets, and deal directly with customers. They will be trained to develop needed relationships, do networking, deal with vendors, and manage projects.[30]

To make TQM effective requires appropriate development of a responsive and supportive organizational environment, change in management culture, teamwork, focus on customers, and continuous feedback to staff.[31] Among the processes that have affected enterprises positively are fundamental changes that stress teamwork and customer over turf and hierarchy.[32]

Successful customer relations requires constant training and education programs. The need for staff development will continue to increase as nursing deals with improved technology, greater product reliability, a customer-service orientation, and flexibility in adapting to change. Nurse managers will continue to move decisions down the chain of command to all associates or team members. An educated and well-trained work force is a nursing imperative. Every team member will need the skills of reading, understanding math, and conveying ideas.[33]

Techniques that leaders can use to improve relationships with suppliers, customers, and other partners include: (1) a company-wide negotiation infrastructure to apply the knowledge gained from forging past agreements to improve future ones (managed care contracts especially), (2) broadened measures to evaluate negotiators' performance beyond matters of cost and price, (3) drawing a clear distinction between elements of an individual deal and the nature of the ongoing relationship between the parties, and (4) making negotiators feel comfortable walking away from a deal when it's not in the company's best interests.[34]

Culture and Climate

TQM requires a favorable environment for total quality behavior in which values are shared as worthwhile or desirable and beliefs as truth. All employees in such an environment, including top management, believe in focusing on customers, both internal and external.[35]

This promotes a warm, friendly climate in which employees feel good about themselves, others, and their work. Employees in such a culture trust managers who facilitate their work and treat them as equals. Fear has been driven out through leadership that has promoted teamwork, respect, and trust. Rites and rituals that may be changed in a total quality culture include the abolition of reserved parking and the increased visibility of managers throughout the workplace.

Linkow suggests changing the culture through a total quality culture matrix tool (see Exhibit 17-7) that follows these steps:

1. Describe the current culture through group brainstorming and interviewing.
2. Establish seven core total quality values and beliefs.
3. Correlate core values and beliefs with current culture.
4. Determine the strength of the current culture.
5. Identify targets for culture change. These will be core values and beliefs with negative or nonexistent correlation or that are low in strength.

EXHIBIT 17-7
Total Quality Culture Matrix

Cultural Media	Current Culture Examples	Customer Focus	Employee Focus	Teamwork	Safety	Candor	Total Involvement	Process Focus	Symbols
		Core Values/Beliefs							
Heroes	Employee who got out of a hospital bed for important meeting with a client	●	Δ	Δ	Δ				
	Person who left his family on vacation to work with client	●	Δ	Δ					
	Understudy steps in at last minute for sick "star" and makes resoundingly successful presentation to tough clients	●		○					● = highly correlated
Myths and Artifacts	No titles on business cards		○	○			○		
	Stories of failures with clients are told with relish		○			●			○ = correlated
	Employees do whatever it takes to satisfy the client	●	Δ						Δ = negatively correlated
Rites and Rituals	Anyone may be interrupted at any time		Δ	○			○		
	When a problem is identified a list of solutions is brainstormed by a group			●			○		
	CEO walks through headquarters many afternoons asking, "What are you working on?"		○	●			○		

Strength of Culture	Customer Focus	Employee Focus	Teamwork	Safety	Candor	Total Involvement	Process Focus	Symbols
Thickness	●	Δ	○	Δ	○	○	Δ	● = high
Extent of Sharing	●	○	●	Δ	●	○	Δ	○ = medium
Clarity of Ordering	●	○	●	Δ	○	○	Δ	Δ = low

Source: Reprinted with permission of P. Linkow, Interaction Associates, Cambridge, Massachusetts.

6. Use the group to change culture.
7. Use external threats to mobilize internal forces of change.[36]

Nursing organizations within institutions should have ideals, vision, and values.

Like other sectors of the economy, health care organizations must have sound business plans that attack the status quo and entrenched players, and they must find new technologies that improve or replace earlier ones. "The economic, social, and cultural factors underlying the new economy are rock solid."[37]

Theory Z Organizations

Theory Z organizations focus on consensual decision making. The leadership style of such organizations is a democratic one that includes decentralization, participatory management, employee involvement, and an emphasis on quality of life. Leaders are managers who concentrate on developing and using their interpersonal skills. This theory has been attributed to William Ouchi.[38]

Using Theory Z management, an "organization can significantly benefit from facilitating the creative ideas and input of the members of that organization."[39]

Theory Z management and TQM are closely interrelated. Both start with planning that includes emphasis on staff development to improve quality of staff and their work. They start with a statement of philosophy that embodies the elements of both theories, and they proceed to the training of managers. Theory Z and TQM both require a long-term relationship between the organization and the employees. The organization invests in the employee by caring, by focusing on career needs, and by assisting employees to integrate their work and home lives through child care centers, wellness programs, recreation, shift options, counseling, and opportunities for career development. Results have included production of generalists who can do more than one job, reduction of turnover rate from 30% percent to 4%, unity because of the greater independence of nurses, reduced interdepartmental conflicts, reduced costs, improved risk management, and improved quality.[40]

Quality Circles

Quality circles are a participatory management technique that uses statistical analyses of activities to maintain quality products. The technique was initiated in Japan after World War II through Deming's teaching. The concept is to use statistical analysis to make quality improvements. Workers are taught the statistical concepts and use them through trained, organized, structured groups of 4 to 15 employees, called quality circles. Group members share common interests and problems and meet on a regular basis, usually an hour a week. They represent other employees from whom they gather information to bring to the meetings.[41]

Employees are trained to identify, analyze, and solve problems. Involved in the process, they make solutions work because they identify with ownership. As a result of being recognized, they develop good will towards their employers.

Quality circles are effective when facilitators, leaders, and members are trained in group dynamics and quality circle techniques. Leaders act as peers to generate ideas to improve operations and eliminate problems. In the process all quality circle members reach consensus before decisions are recommended or implemented. Training occurs during subsequent meetings.[42]

The objects of quality circles are participation, involvement, recognition, and self-actualization among clinical nurses caring for patients. Output from these objects of quality circles contributes to the knowledge base of human behavior and motivation, which is important to the development of nursing management theory. This theory will be learned and used by nurse managers concerned with developing job satisfaction of professional nurses in delivering quality nursing care.

Quality circles should meet successful group design guidelines, including the following:[43]

1. Participation groups process or have access to the necessary skills and knowledge to address problems systematically. All actors in the process receive training. Support people participate only as needed.
2. Formalized procedures enhance the effectiveness of the group. Systematic records are kept, and formal schedules of meetings adhered to.
3. To promote communication, participation groups are integrated horizontally and vertically with the rest of the organization. Accomplishments are publicized through award dinners and publicity in in-house newspapers. Organized higher-level support groups hear the ideas of lower-level groups. All are limited by usual formal and informal communication mechanisms and routes.
4. Groups are a regular part of the organization and not a special or extra activity. They are composed of members of natural work groups. Results are measured in terms of ongoing organizational objectives and goals.
5. Normal accountability processes operate using the same skills, habits, and expectations as general organizations.
6. Groups manage themselves and are assisted by leaders and facilitators who are peer group members.
7. Participation occurs in such areas as decisions about job enrichment; hiring; training in problem-solving skills, management skills, and business conditions; pay based on skill mastery; gain sharing; and union management relationships based on mutual interests.

Research indicates that productivity and morale improve strongly when employees participate in decision making and planning for change. It is important that participation include goal setting, because participation will lead to higher levels of acceptance and performance of these goals. Research also shows that highly nonparticipatory jobs cause psychological and physical harm.

It is an ethical imperative to prevent harm by enabling employees to participate in work decisions.

Quality circles may use Pareto analysis, histograms, graphing techniques, control charts, stratification, scatter diagrams, brainstorming, cause-and-effect diagrams, run analysis, and conflict resolution. Success factors of quality circles include management commitment and involvement, labor union involvement, training, and patience. Tangible benefits include improved quality, increased productivity, and increased efficiency. Intangible benefits include improved worklife quality, safety, morale, and job satisfaction.[44]

Quality circles should have themes. Participants should know how to select or recognize the themes they will work on, then assist with implementation of the solution.[45]

The health care industry in the United States will solve its problems by producing a higher quality product more efficiently.[46] Total quality management techniques combined with motivational management techniques and critical-thinking strategies provide a conceptualization of clinical teaching and learning.[47]

Components of a Quality Management Program

A quality management program is composed of the following components:

1. Clear and concise written statements of purpose, philosophy, values, and objectives.
2. Standards or indicators for measuring the quality of care.
3. Policies and procedures for using such standards for gathering data. These polices define the organizational structure for the program.
4. Analysis and reporting of the data gathered, with isolation of problems and variances.
5. Use of the results to prioritize, plan action, and correct problems and variances.
6. Monitoring of clinical and managerial performance and ongoing feedback to ensure that problems stay solved.
7. Evaluation of the quality management system.

These components may be conceptualized in many different ways. One component builds on another. Batalden and Stoltz describe a framework for the continual improvement of health care (Exhibit 17-8), which incorporates underlying knowledge, policy for leadership, tools and methods, and daily work applications.[48] The mission, vision, guiding principles, and integration of values are critical to the policy for leadership. "For the continual improvement of health care, tools and methods are available that can accelerate building and using knowledge and communicating that understanding to others."[49] Tools and methods can be grouped into four major categories: process and system, group process and collaborative work, statistical thinking, and planning and analysis. Daily work applications include developing models for testing change and making adjustments as well as review of the improvements. Conceptualizing quality management principles provides the nurse with tools for assisting the nursing department with the overall QM process.

Statements of Purpose, Philosophy, and Objectives

The initial planning of a quality management program includes the development of clear and concise statements of purpose, philosophy, and objectives. The program's purpose and philosophy go hand in hand with the organizational purpose and philosophy and should be interwoven with the organization's values. The JCAHO gives specific guidelines designed to assess and improve

EXHIBIT 17-8

The Framework for the Continual Improvement of Health Care

UNDERLYING KNOWLEDGE	POLICY FOR LEADERSHIP	TOOLS AND METHODS	DAILY WORK APPLICATIONS
Professional knowledge: • subject • discipline • values	Mission, vision, and quality definition Guiding principles	Process, system Group process and collaborative work	Models for testing change and making improvement Review of improvement
Improvement knowledge: • system • variation • psychology • theory of knowledge	Integration with values	Statistical thinking Planning and analysis	

Source: P. B. Batalden and P. K. Stoltz. "A Framework for the Continual Improvement of Health Care: Building and Applying Professional and Improvement Knowledge to Test Changes in Daily Work." *Joint Commission Journal on Quality Improvement* (October 1993), 426. Oakbrook Terrace, IL: Joint Commission on Accreditation of Healthcare Organizations, 1993, p. 426. Reprinted with permission.

quality of client care. Quality improvement theories—such as those of Deming, Crosby, Juran, and Senge—are recommended to health care organizations to better conceptualize the entire quality management program.[50] An organization need not limit itself to one theory and may incorporate concepts from a wide variety in order to develop a framework that best fits the organization's purpose, philosophy, and objectives. Every quality management program needs well-articulated objectives, and every study a purpose.

Standards for Measuring the Quality of Care

Standards define nursing care outcomes as well as nursing activities and the structural resources needed. They are used for planning nursing care as well as for evaluating it. Outcomes include positive and negative indexes. Standards are directed at structure, process, and outcome issues and guide the review of systems function, staff performance, and client care. A number of health care organizations issue indexes. The Centers for Medicare & Medicaid Services (CMS) annually disclose projected and actual hospital select indicator rates by diagnostic-related groups.

On January 1, 2004, JCAHO's National Patient Safety Goals (NPSGs) went into effect for all accreditation programs. The program-specific goals and objectives mandate implementation, measurement, and evidence of performance without negotiation. For updates on NSPGs, see the JCAHO Web site (http://www.jcaho.org).

For hospitals, the JCAHO has issued accreditation performance measures involving the following functions:

1. Patient-focused functions: ethics, right, and responsibilities; provision of care, treatment, and services; medication management; infection control.
2. Organization functions: improving organizational performance; leadership; management of the environment of care, of human resources, and of information.
3. Structures with functions: medical staff, nursing.

JCAHO also requires measurement of Core Measures, one of the first steps in focusing on key treatment populations. The future scope of Core Measure will expand relation to other clinical areas of interest. The initial core measures (2004) are acute myocardial infarction, heart failure, community-acquired pneumonia, and pregnancy-related conditions. These measures comprise precisely defined data, elements, calculation algorithms, and standardized data collection protocols. An organization's results as well as national results for select core measures may be found on JCAHO'S Web site.

JCAHO requires hospitals to proactively identify risks to patients, initiate actions to reduce risks (Failure Mode Effect and Analysis), and investigate unanticipated adverse "sentinel" events (Root Cause Analysis). The Failure Mode Effect Analysis (FMEA), initiated proactively, involves documenting the ways a process can fail (e.g., a flow chart), why this failure would occur (e.g., a cause and defect diagram), and how a redesign of the process may prevent failure (e.g., a flow chart). Hospitals are required to select annually one high-risk process based in part on JCAHO'S published Sentinel Event Alert. Hospital leaders are to provide education and resources to conduct proactive activities to reduce risk to patients.

Root Cause Analysis is conducted to understand how and why an adverse sentinel event occurred and to prevent its reoccurrence. A *sentinel event* is an unexpected, unwanted occurrence involving death or serious physical injury. It is called "sentinel" because it signifies immediate attention. Root Cause Analysis includes assignment of a team to assess the event as soon as possible (within 72 hours). The team should include staff of all levels closest to the specific case, including those with decision-making authority. The process involves review of events, process failure, action plans, implementation of plans, and followup review.[51]

Other organizations collecting data for quality measurement are the American Hospital Association, Voluntary Hospitals of America, National Committee for Quality Health Care, and the National Association of Health Data Organizations. These organizations will gather, analyze, and publish data on quality of health care for consumers, employers, and the federal government. The standards will include performance standards for providers. The objectives are to achieve improvement in the health status of clients, reduce unnecessary use of health care services, and meet specifications of clients and purchasers. These standards will address improvement of health care quality, functions, and processes that must be carried out effectively to achieve good patient care outcomes, patient care, governance, and management. Quality management theory has been applied in the form of identifying common causes and special causes of performance variation.[52] Outcomes or indexes serve as measures of the value, rank, or degree of excellence (see Appendix 17-1).

Policies and Procedures

The third element of a quality management program is the development of policies and procedures for using standards or indicators for gathering data to measure the quality of care. Batalden and Stoltz describe guiding principles that reflect the organization's assumptions about the responsibilities and desired actions of leaders that will create a positive work environment. It is essential to integrate the leadership policy with the values common to health professionals and underlying health care work; this contributes to shared ownership of the policy by everyone in the organization.[53] The policies and procedures define the organizational structure for the quality management program and prescribe the tools for gathering data.

Data Collection

Data collection tools may be in the form of questionnaires, rating scales, and interviews. Reliability and validity are important concepts in determining the worth of instruments used to measure variables in a study. Reliability is the extent to which an experiment, test, or measurement procedure yields the same results on repeated trials. For example, a scale that measures a person's weight as 100 pounds one minute and as 160 pounds the next would be considered unreliable. Interrater reliability refers to the degree to which two raters, operating independently, assign the same ratings for an attribute being measured. Validity is the degree to which an instrument measures what it is intended to measure. Content (face) validity is the degree to which an instrument adequately represents the universe of content.[54]

The content of measure (standard, indicator, process step) could be written out with options to check "yes," "no," "NA"—and to allow comments. Ideally this could be done electronically (with a hand-held device) and downloaded into a database if resources are available.

Nursing Audits

A basic form of quality data collection is the nursing audit. An *audit* is essentially an examination, a verification or accounting of predetermined indicators. There are three basic forms of nursing audits: structure audits, process audits, and outcome audits.

Structure Audits

Structure audits focus on the setting in which care takes place. They include physical facilities, equipment, caregivers, organization, policies, procedures, and medical records. A checklist that focuses on these categories measures standards or indicators. Structure can include such content as staff knowledge and expertise in addition to policies and procedures for nursing practice. Content related to specific nursing care to meet established standards are included in nursing process audits.

Process Audits

Process audits implement indicators for measuring nursing care to determine whether nursing standards are met. They are generally task-oriented. Process audits were first used by Maria Phaneuf in 1964 and were based upon the seven functions of nursing established by Lesnick and Anderson. The Phaneuf audit is retrospective, being applied to measure the quality of nursing care received by the client after a cycle of care has been completed and the client discharged. The Phaneuf audit has seven subsections:[55]

1. Application and execution of physicians' legal orders
2. Observations of symptoms and reactions
3. Supervision of the client
4. Supervision of those participating in care
5. Reporting and recording
6. Application and execution of nursing procedures and techniques
7. Promotion of physical and emotional health by direction and teaching

The Phaneuf model uses a Likert scoring system. It does not evaluate care recorded.

The Quality Patient-Care Scale (Qual PacS) is a process audit that measures the quality of nursing care concurrently with the cycle of care being given. It has six subsections:

1. Psychosocial–individual
2. Psychosocial–group
3. Physical
4. General
5. Communication
6. Professional implications

In this audit the nurse is evaluated by direct observation in a nurse–client interaction. A 15% sample of nurses on a unit is considered adequate.

Both the Phaneuf and the QualPacS process audits use the performance of the first-level staff nurse as a standard for safe, adequate, therapeutic, and supportive care.[56]

Other open system audits include the Commission for Administrative Services in Hospital (CASH) Scale and the Medicus Corporation Nurses' Audit. They also measure or monitor intervention, assessment, and clinical skills.

Outcome Audits

Outcome audits can be either concurrent or retrospective. They evaluate nursing performance in terms of establishing client outcome criteria. The National Center for Health Services developed an outcome audit based on Orem's description of nine categories of self-care requirements:

1. Air
2. Water and fluid intake
3. Food
4. Elimination
5. Rest, activity, and sleep

6. Social interaction and productive work
7. Protection from hazards
8. Normality
9. Health deviation

These categories are evaluated in terms of the following evidence:[57]

1. Evidence that the requirement is met
2. Evidence that the client has the necessary knowledge to meet the requirement
3. Evidence that the client has the necessary skill and performance abilities to meet the requirement
4. Evidence that the client has the necessary motivation to meet the requirement

Outcome criteria are set for populations. They can evaluate specific aspects of nursing care for particular groups, such as neonates, school-age children, oncology, trauma, forensics, or long-term care. Client care goals should reflect an individual's optimal functioning given his or her current condition and resources for continued care. QA outcome indicators would capture if the goals, or *outcome*, were met or obtained.

The outcome variables as described by Evans and Ruff have face validity as outcomes of functional utility, and their value can be reliably assessed using descriptive statistics. These variables are considered important rehabilitation outcomes by clients, family members, and financial providers and have an impact on long-term functioning.[58]

Morbidity, disability, and mortality during and following provision of health care services are nationally recognized outcomes of health care. Nursing assessment and intervention may make a significant difference in the outcome variables, such as nosocomial infection rates in high-risk clients.[59] McCormick illustrates the direction of outcomes that patients can take related to the assessment and treatments carried out.[60]

Another method of developing outcome criteria includes grouping of items for efficiency: DRGs, specific protocols for treatment, life stages, and like standards. A determination is made as to whether the outcomes are met. If outcomes are not satisfactorily met, deficiencies are identified, corrected, and followed up.

Quality Management Tools

Statistical Techniques

Statistical techniques include measures of central tendency, measures of variability, tests of significance, and correlation. Central tendency refers to the middle value and general trend of the numbers. The three most common measures of central tendency are the mean, the median, and the mode. Measures of variability look at the dispersion of the measures. Three common measures of variability are the range, the standard deviation, and interpercentile measures. The most common measure of interpercentile variability is the interquartile range, which is determined by ranking the order of the measures and then dividing the array into quarters. The range of scores comprising the middle 50% is the interquartile range. The t-test, regression analysis and chi-square tests are tests of statistical significance.[61] Correlation refers to the extent to which two variables are related. The Pearson product–moment correlation coefficient of determination (r^2) is a method whereby cause and effect, or relationships, may be evaluated. This statistical analysis tool may be found in various computer software programs and is used with scatter diagrams. The coefficient of determination (r^2) is helpful in determining the percentage of variance on one variable that can be predicted by the variance on another variable.[62]

Data Analysis

Data analysis tools may be divided into three types: decision-making tools, data analysis charts, and relational charts. Brainstorming and multivoting are types of decision-making tools that involve groups or teams.

With a degree of skill in the use of these tools and methods, workers can obtain and analyze data to validate their ideas about potential improvements and later test the results of changes implemented.[63]

Brainstorming

Brainstorming is a free-flowing generation of ideas. This approach has the potential to generate excitement, equalize involvement, and result in original solutions to the problem. There is no discussion of ideas as they are generated, but the team can build upon the ideas of others. It is very important that no judgments are made concerning an idea's worth or its feasibility. This discussion comes at a later point in the process.
When to use:

- When a list of possible ideas is needed. This technique works well to generate ideas for such tools as the cause and effect diagram.

How to conduct:

1. Define the topic of brainstorming.
2. Give everyone a few minutes to think about the topic and write down ideas.
3. Have the team members call out their ideas. This can be free-flowing, or a structure can be used (such as going around the table with each person giving one idea each time around).
4. As the ideas are generated, one person should write them on a flipchart.

Multivoting

Multivoting is a method to determine the most popular or important items from a list, without a lot of discussion or difficulty. This method uses a series of votes to cut the list in half each time, thus reducing the number of items to be considered.
When to use:

- After a brainstorming session to identify the key items on which the group will focus.

How to conduct:

1. Generate a list of items and number them.
2. If the group agrees, combine items that seem to be similar.
3. If necessary, renumber all items.
4. Each member lists on a sheet of paper the items he or she considers the most important.
5. Tally the votes beside each item on the list.
6. Eliminate those items with the lowest scores.
7. Repeat the above process until the list is narrowed down to an appropriate number for the group to focus on, or until the item with the top priority is identified.

Nominal Group Technique

This is a group decision-making process for generating a large number of ideas in which each member works by himself or herself. This technique is used when group members are new to each other or when they have different opinions and goals. This approach is more structured than that of brainstorming or multivoting.
When to use:

- When the team members are new to each other.
- When dealing with a controversial topic.

How to conduct:

1. Define the task as though you were brainstorming.
2. Write the question to be answered for all to see. Be sure to clarify the question as needed by the group.
3. Give each member 4 to 8 cards or pieces of paper.
4. Members write one selection from the list on each card and assign a point value to each item (i.e., if there are 4 cards, the most important card is numbered 4, next important 3, etc.).
5. The cards are collected and the votes are tallied; mark each item on the list with the value on the cards for that item.
6. The item with the largest number becomes the group's selection.

The Delphi Method

The Delphi method is a combination of the brainstorming, multivoting, and nominal group techniques. This tool is used when the group is not in one location, and it is frequently carried out through mail or e-mail. After each step in the process, the data are sent to one person, who compiles the data and sends out the next step to the participants for completion.

Prioritization Matrix

A prioritization matrix organizes tasks, issues, or actions and prioritizes them by agreed-upon criteria. The tool combines the tree diagram and the L-shaped matrix diagram, displaying the best possible effect. The prioritization matrix is often used before more complex matrices are needed. The matrix applies options under discussion to priority considerations.
When to use:

- When issues are identified and options must be narrowed down.
- When options have a strong relationship.
- When options all need to be done, but prioritization or sequencing is needed.

How to construct:

1. Create L-shaped matrix as depicted in Exhibit 17-9.
2. Prioritize and assign weights to the list of criteria.
3. Prioritize the list options based upon each criterion.
4. Prioritize and select the item(s) across all of the criteria.

Run Chart or Trend Chart

Run charts are graphic displays of data points over time. Run charts are control charts without the control limits. Their name comes from the fact that the user looks for trends in the data or a significant number of data points going in one direction or to one side of the average.

Trends generally indicate a statistically important event that needs further analysis. Resist the tendency to see every variation in the data as significant by waiting to interpret the results until at least 10 (or even better, 20) data points have been plotted.
When to use:

- To display variation.
- To detect the presence or absence of special causes.
- To observe the effects of a process improvement (observe the effects of experiments on a process).

See Exhibit 17-10 for an example of a run chart.

Control charts

Control charts are run charts to which control limits have been added above and below the mean. Generally, upper and lower control limits (UCL and LCL) are statistically determined by adding and subtracting three standard deviations from the mean. Assuming a normal distribution and no special cause variation, a majority of the data points are expected to fall within the UCL and LCL. Variance within the control limits results from aggregate *common causes*, and one should not tamper with the

EXHIBIT 17-9
Prioritization Matrix

	LOW COST	HIGH STRATEGIC PRIORITY	MEETS ACCREDITATION STANDARDS	MD CONCERN	STAFF CONCERN	TOTALS
Repair of roof	3	4	2	3	4	16
Purchase new X-ray machine	5	2	6	1	5	19
Develop Skilled Nursing Unit	4	1	6	2	2	15
Develop better communication with Home Health	2	3	1	4	3	13
Develop a staff newsletter	1	5	3	5	1	15

Key:
1 Strongly feel best choice
2 Feel best choice
3 Uncertain
4 Feel not good choice
5 Strongly feel not good choice
6 Not related at all
Least amount of points is the highest priority; highest amount of points is lowest priority.

process performing as expected. As discussed earlier with regard to Deming's variance, *special cause* variance (data points outside the control limits) occurs in less than 10% of cases and requires evaluation.

When to use:

- To distinguish variation from common and special causes.
- To assist with eliminating special cause variation.
- To observe effects of a process improvement.

EXHIBIT 17-10
Example of a Run Chart

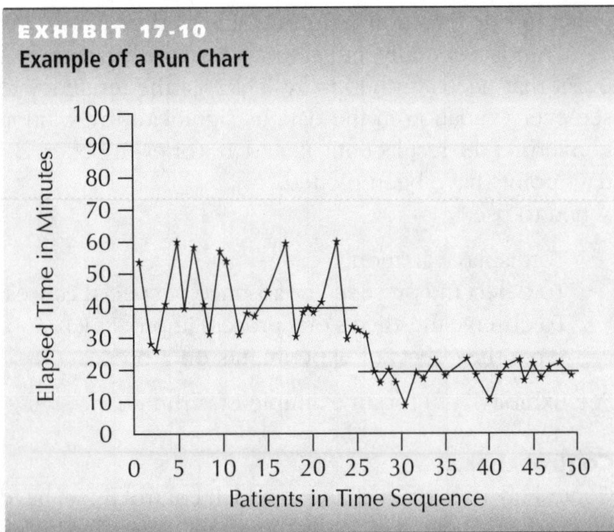

Source: P. B. Batalden and P. K. Stoltz. "A Framework for the Continual Improvement of Health Care: Building and Applying Professional and Improvement Knowledge to Test Changes in Daily Work." *Joint Commission Journal on Quality Improvement* (October 1993), 436. Oakbrook Terrace, IL: Joint Commission on Accreditation of Healthcare Organizations, 1993, p. 436. Reprinted with permission.

How to construct (see Exhibit 17-11):

1. Construct as you would a run or trend chart.
2. Calculate control limits according to the appropriate statistical formula or with a computer program.
3. Plot the control limits on the chart and examine the data for variation.

Process Flow Chart

The process flow chart is a graphical display of a process as it is known to its authors or team. The flow chart outlines the sequence and relationship of the pieces of the process. Through management of the data and information, the team comes to a common understanding and knowledge concerning the process. Information is discussed on the structure (who carries out the specific step in the identified process), what activity is occurring, and finally the outcome or the results.

How to construct (see Exhibit 17-12):

1. Select the process to study.
2. Determine the beginning and the end or the boundaries of the process being studied.
3. The beginning or first step is put inside an oval symbol.
4. Each of the next steps is put into a rectange.
5. When a step in the process involves a decision, the step is inscribed in a diamond. A "yes" and a "no" path or line is drawn from the diamond.
6. Each decision loop reenters the process and is pursued to a conclusion.
7. The ending step, like the beginning step, is put inside an oval.

EXHIBIT 17-11
Statistical Control Chart

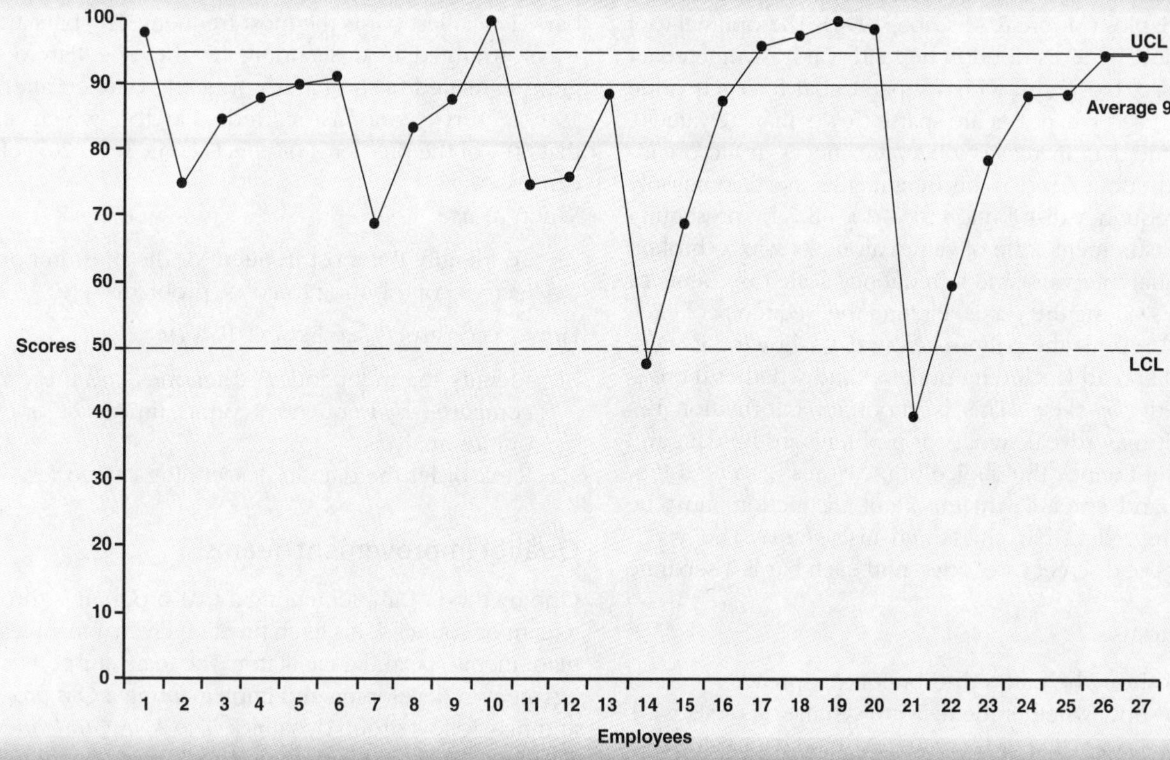

Scores
Employees
UCL
Average 90.3
LCL

EXHIBIT 17-12
Process Flow Chart

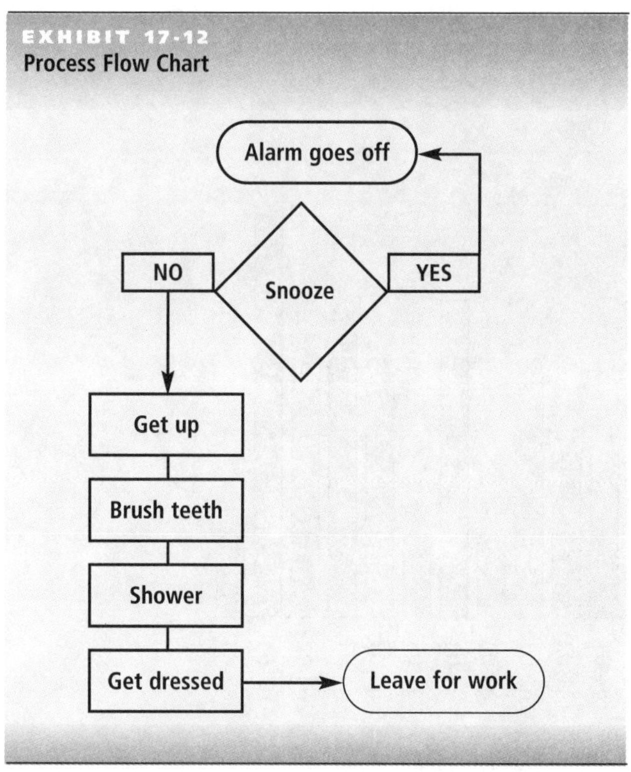

Fishbone Cause and Effect Diagram

A cause and effect diagram is used to analyze and display the potential causes of a problem or the sources of variation. There are generally at least four categories in the diagram. Some of the common categories involve the four Ms—manpower, methods, machines, and materials—or the five Ps—patrons (users of the system), people (workers), provisions (supplies), places (work environment), and procedures (methods and rules).

When to use:

- To identify and organize possible causes of the problem.
- To identify factors that will lead to success.

How to construct:

1. Determine the effect for the diagram and put it on the far right side of the diagram.
2. Draw a horizontal line to the left of the effect.
3. Determine the categories (the 4 Ms or the 5 Ps)
4. Draw a diagonal line for half of the categories above the line and half below the line.
5. Brainstorm the list for each of the categories.
6. Organize each of the causes on each bone.
7. Draw branch bones to show the relationship.

Histogram or Bar Chart

Before further analyzing a set of measured data, one should first review the distribution of values for each of the variables (Moore & McCabe, 1993). The optimal tool for reviewing a distribution depends on how much data there is. A bar graph with a separate bar for each value may be used when data are sparse (fewer than 12 values), but as the data increases it becomes necessary to organize and summarize. A histogram, the most commonly used frequency distribution tool, does this by presenting the measurement scale of values along its *x*-axis (broken into equal intervals) and a frequency scale (as counts or percents) along the *y*-axis. Plotting the frequency of each interval reveals the pattern of the data showing its center and spread (including outliers) and whether there is symmetry or skew. This is important information because it may reveal signals of problems in the data and should influence the choice of measures of central tendency and spread. An important distinction must be made regarding bar charts and histograms. The *x*-axis consists of discreet categories, and each bar is a separate group.

When to use:

- To show the data's distribution or spread.
- To show whether the data are symmetric or skewed.
- To show whether there are extreme data values.

How to construct: See Exhibit 17-13.

Pareto Chart

A Pareto diagram displays a series of bars in which the priority can easily be seen by the varying height of the bars. The tallest bar is the most frequent. The bars are always arranged in descending height. The Pareto diagram is related to the Pareto principle (named after the 19th-century economist Vilfredo Pareto), which states that 80% of the problems or effects come from 20% of the causes.

When to use:

- To identify the most frequent or the most important factors contributing to costs, problems, etc.

How to construct (see Exhibit 17-14):

1. Identify the independent categories and the way to compare—by frequency (count), time, cost, or other unit of analysis.
2. Rank-order the data in descending categories.

Quality Improvement Teams

One method of implementing a QM program is through a team or council. This team functions with a team leader, team members, and a facilitator. The team supports management in developing and implementing a QM program and may follow group dynamics. The ANA *Guidelines for Review of Nursing Care at the Local Level* is pertinent in today's evaluation of outcomes environment.

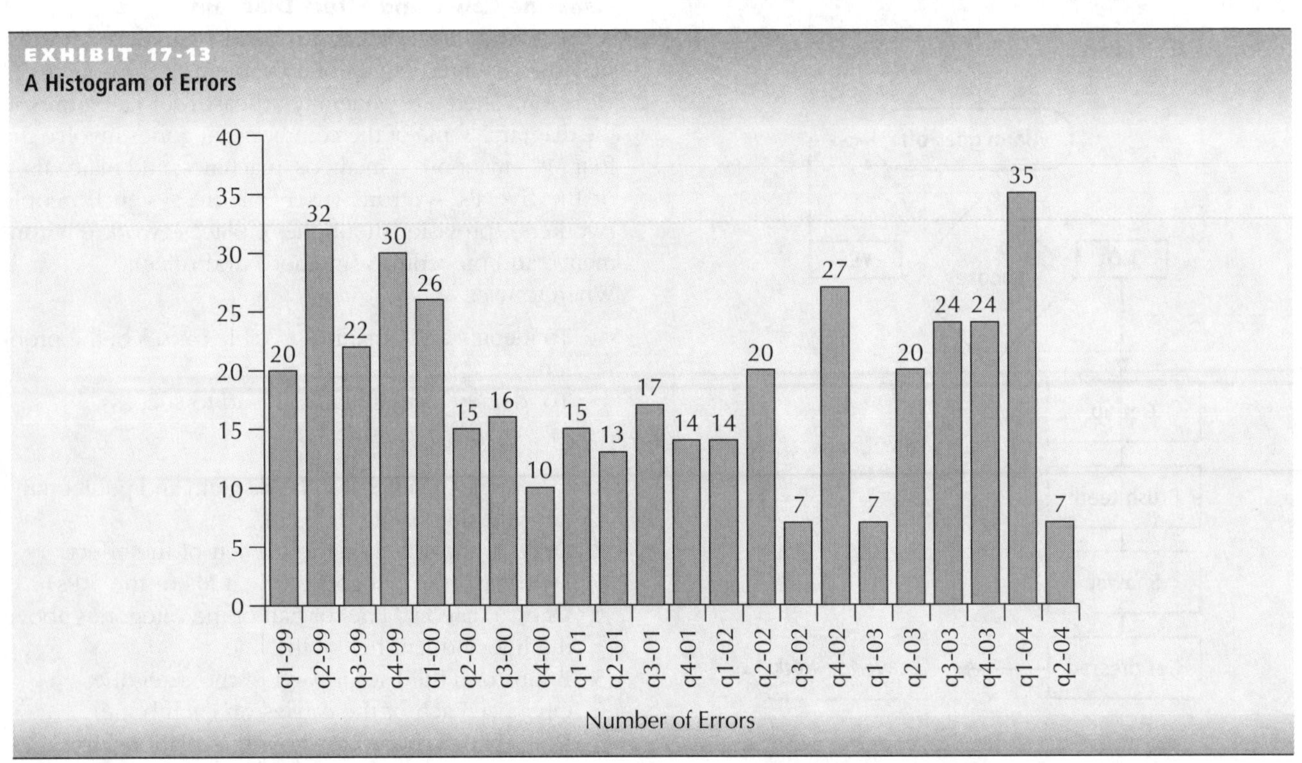

EXHIBIT 17-13
A Histogram of Errors

EXHIBIT 17-14

Generalized Pareto Diagram

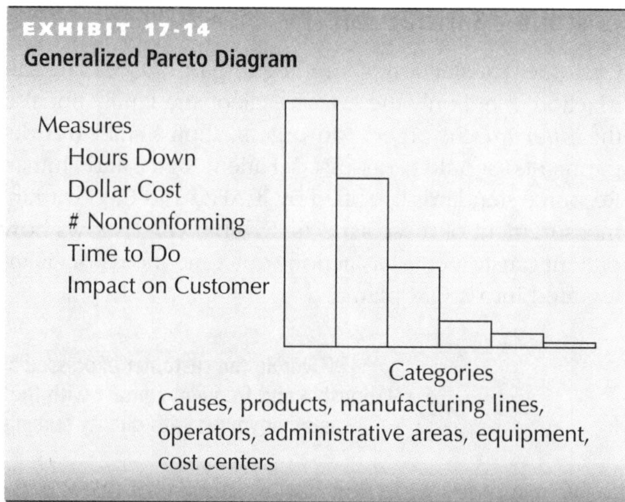

Source: J. T. Burr, Center for Quality and Applied Statistics, Rochester Institute of Technology, One Lomb Memorial Dr., P. O. Box 9887, Rochester, NY 14623-9887. Reprinted with permission.

Problem Identification

Analysis and reporting of the data gathered from the evaluation process lead to problem identification and isolation. Evidence comes from primary sources, such as the client and nursing personnel, and from secondary sources, including the client's chart and family. Active client and family participation should be part of the process. Quality management addresses current problems. Nurses look for patterns or trends of deviation from normal. They also identify deficiencies relating to other departments that affect nursing care. If one takes a systems approach, problem identification is a team approach, with the client and family as major team players.

Problem Resolution

Once problems have been defined and isolated, plans are made to solve them on a priority basis. Those problems that are critical are addressed first, and plans are immediately made and implemented to resolve them. Those involving the safety and welfare of the client take first priority. Other factors used in determining priority will include severity, frequency, benefit, cost-effectiveness, elimination, reduction, association with professional liability, and impact on accreditation. The first consideration is always based on the impact on client care.[64]

In one study, nurses with formal QA experience were more likely to want to write standards for their specialty, participate in peer review, and be on QA committees. They were more interested in QA associated with direct patient care. [65]

Solutions and corrective action for problems will be assigned to appropriate nursing departments, services, and units. The need is to resolve problems, not just evaluate them.

Monitoring and Feedback

The quality management process is cyclic and requires monitoring of clinical and managerial performance and feedback to ensure that problems stay solved. Followup can be expensive and difficult. Its breadth should determine what should be covered. Problems of a multidisciplinary nature, such as those involving occupational therapy, physical therapy, speech pathology, and nursing, can be one consideration.

The cyclic process will continue to set standards of care, take measurements according to those standards, evaluate care from multiple sources, recommend improvements, and, above all, ensure that improvements are carried out.

Accountability for nursing practice is still diffused by the employment environment, and this fact must be addressed and corrected by nurses.

Involvement of Practicing Nurses

Practicing nurses can be stimulated to increase their positive attitudes about quality management by direct behavioral experience. Nurse managers should find out reasons these nurses view QM unfavorably. Negative connotations may exist due to lack of executive administrative support, views that the process is futile without changes in practice and lack of physician involvement. Changing a negative viewpoint may be accomplished by the following strategies:

1. Having practicing nurses identify areas needing improvement.
2. Providing release time for practicing nurses to participate in QM activities, including attendance at committee meetings and time for QM audits.
3. Providing rewards, such as performance results achievement records, that can lead to pay raises, promotions, educational opportunities, or special assignments.
4. Targeting QM to patient care outcomes, the very essence of nursing practice.
5. Involving clinical nurses in management through such techniques as quality circles, employee involvement programs, participatory management, decentralization, "adhocracy," and quality of work life.

6. Establishing a peer review program involving nursing staff at all levels of patient care. Such a program's expectation is to identify outcome criteria based on established standards for nursing practice. Peers determine if outcomes have been met based on ongoing and retrospective audits. Corrective action is determined by peers based on the outcome being adequately met.

Efficiency

Efficiency is concerned with the cost/benefit ratio. Can the appropriate standard be met with a cost acceptable to both consumer and provider?[66] The computer is a labor-saving device for developing and conducting a QM program. Nurse managers will use it and teach other practicing nurses to use it.

Standards will be kept up-to-date and accessible to all units in paper or electronic files. Standards should be cross-referenced.

Charts can be labeled so as to be easily retrieved for nursing QM evaluation. In addition, the long-term care minimum data set (MDS) can be an efficient QM tool for nursing homes. The MDS is a collection of baseline data (physical, social, and psychological factors) that can be used to assess, analyze, and plan care for residents in nursing homes. The 1987 Omnibus Budget Reconciliation Act mandated its specific elements.[67]

The following are some elements of efficiency and effectiveness:

1. Identification of the impact of nursing care on the health of the patient, that is, results or outcomes measured in terms of the patient's health status. Do the notes meet such a standard?
2. A program practical enough to be used in all clinical nursing settings.
3. Random, unannounced samples.
4. Nursing personnel who serve on committees long enough to be proficient.
5. Grading by each person administering criteria.
6. Higher patient acuity combined with shorter hospital stays.
7. Interdisciplinary programs so nurses will not do the work of other disciplines. Nursing is ethically and operationally interdependent with other groups and organizations.
8. Planning for uncertain future by blueprinting scenarios for managing the future, changing the culture of nursing organizations, developing interpersonal skills, and making a creative response to risk taking.[68]
9. Each nurse should be held responsible for self-improvement and for delivering a high standard of patient care.

Customer Satisfaction

Customer satisfaction is an integral part of QM. The satisfaction of not only the *external* client and family but also the *internal* customers (an organization's staff and departments) should be assessed. Patient Rights and Human Resource standards specified by JCAHO and CMS warrant measurement of these aspects. Exhibit A17-1 shows how patient (customer) satisfaction (outcome indicator) is integrated into a QM plan.

Overall, the customer expressed a close relationship and frequent contact with the nurse as synonymous with quality nursing care.

Consumer satisfaction as an outcome of QM can be assessed through methods such as patient, family, and nurse interviews or surveys and observation checklists of nurse–patient interactions.[69]

Quality in the health care marketplace is defined by employers, employee benefit consultants, physicians, and consumers—not by providers (even though physicians are providers, as are hospitals, nurses, and other caregivers). The reason physicians determine quality is that they have control over all orders for diagnosis and treatment procedures. Only one half of consumers, employers, and employee consultants ever differentiate between high- and low-quality hospitals. Two thirds of physicians do.[70]

Good employee relations and consumer relations programs are necessary for success in the health care marketplace, and their good quality must be communicated. Consumers want quality factors in this order:[71]

1. Warmth, caring, and concerns.
2. Expert medical staff that are concerned, thorough, and successful.
3. Up-to-date technology and equipment.
4. Specialization and scope of services available.
5. Outcome.

Training and Communication

Training and communication are important elements of a total quality program. Training includes interpersonal skills, stress management, and conflict management. Learning is a cyclic or continuous process. Nurse managers who play educator roles develop self-awareness by applying learning principles to their own behaviors. Patient education requires an interdisciplinary team approach.

Communication of QM findings, including problems, resolution of problems, and results, must be clear. Both physicians and nursing employees need to be kept up-to-date. Quality must be provided and communicated to be successful. This means that providers as well as consumers will know the status of the quality of care being rendered.

Research and quality management complement each other.

Research and Quality Management

Nursing QM programs can be combined with research programs. Nursing research is being done in clinical settings to improve patient care outcomes. Research can be desirable to nurse managers because it provides prestige, advanced knowledge for nursing professionals, and a database for clinical nursing practice.[72]

Nursing research can be used to evaluate management issues such as staffing, cost management, and staff retention. It produces new knowledge of the relationship between process and outcome. Combining quality management with research makes efficient use of personnel and other resources to link research with a mandatory process, to increase the probability that research will relate to patient care, and to increase sharing of successful quality management programs with others outside the institution.[73]

Summary

Quality management programs assure that quality control standards are maintained and that care delivery continues to evolve toward improvement. QM requires careful planning, development, data collection, resource allocation, and evaluation. Ideally, QM programs should be founded upon TQM, a proven theory waiting for broad application. Leadership is paramount for successful integration of TQM into quality management programs. It is leadership that will change culture and climate to give workers the training they need to affect planning and productivity. Through effective use of quality management tools, the efficiency of nursing interventions or actions can be demonstrated. Quality management programs may lend efficacy of results to research in support of establishing best practice for nursing.

APPLICATION EXERCISES

EXERCISE 17-1 Using a team that represents both nursing leaders within the organization and customers, construct a questionnaire for measuring external customer satisfaction. If such a questionnaire is currently available, review it and make changes only if changes are needed. Use the questionnaire to measure external customer satisfaction with nursing. Analyze the results using appropriate QM tools, and plan for changes to improve external customer satisfaction.

EXERCISE 17-2 Using a team representing nursing leaders within the organization, discuss abolishing the current performance appraisal system. Use brainstorming to generate ideas for pros and cons, then use multivoting to select the first choices from the list.

EXERCISE 17-3 Using a team representing nursing leaders within the organization, identify a major problem. Decide on the data to be measured. Proceed to gather and analyze data and solve the problem using Deming Shewhart cycle or other QM methodology.

EXERCISE 17-4 Using a team representing nursing leaders within the organization, describe the culture of the organization. Discuss how quality management may be incorporated into research. How could best practice be identified and set standards?

EXERCISE 17-5 Make a plan for a quality circle using the guidelines described in this chapter.

EXERCISE 17-6 Examine the quality management program of a health care agency. How does it support the overall mission, vision, and values of the organization?

NOTES

1. Kaufman, J. J. (1989). Total quality management. *Ekistics, 336*, 182–187.
2. Konstam, P. (1992, March 1). Quality should begin at home. *San Antonio Light*, p. D1.
3. Yasin, M. M., Meacham, K. A., & Alavi, J. (1998). The status of TQM in healthcare. *Health Marketing Quarterly*, *15*(3), 61–84.
4. Yasin, M. M. & Alavi, J. (1999). An analytical approach to determining the competitive advantage of TQM in health care. *International Journal of Health Care Quality Assurance Inc Leadership Health Service*, *12*(1), 18–24.
5. Piczak, M. W. (1988). Quality circles come home. *Quality Progress*, *1*, 37–39.
6. Tritus, M. (1988). Deming's way. *Mechanical Engineering*, 28.
7. Ibid., 26–30.
8. Ibid.
9. Duncan, W. J. & Van Matre, J. G. (1990). The gospel according to Deming: Is it really new? *Business Horizons*, 3–9.
10. Francis, A. E. & Germels, J. M. (1989). Building a better budget. *Quality Progress*, *21*, 70–75.
11. Smith, T. A. (1989). Why you should put your safety system under statistical control. *Professional Safety*, 31–36.
12. Joiner, B. L. & Gaudard, M. A. (1990). Variation, management, and W. Edwards Deming. *Quality Progress*, *1*, 29–39.
13. Heinzlmeir, L. A. (1991). Under the spell of the quality gurus. *Canadian Manager*, 22–23.
14. Heinzlmeir, T. R. (1991). Quality can't be delegated. *Supervision*, 6–7.
15. Juran, J. M. (1989). Universal approach to managing for quality. *Executive Excellence*, 15–17.
16. Vasilash, G. S. (1981). Crosby says get fit for quality. *Production*, 51–52, 54; Heinzlmeir, 1991; Oberle, J.; Deutsch, B. J. (1991). A conversation with Philip Crosby. *Bank Marketing*, 22–27; Crosby, P. B. (1984). *Quality without tears: The art of hassle-free management*. New York: McGraw-Hill.
17. Juran, 1989.
18. Ibid.
19. Ibid.
20. O'Neal, C. R. (1991, March 4). It's what's up front that counts. *Marketing News*, 9, 28; Port, O. (1987). How to make it right the first time. *Business Week*, 142–143.
21. Taguchi, G. & Clausing, D. (1990). Robust quality. *Harvard Business Review*, 65–75.
22. Schrage, M. (1992, March 16). Fire your customers. *Wall Street Journal*, p. A12.
23. Friedman, L. H. & White, D. B. (1999). What is quality, who wants it, and why? *Management Care Quarterly*, 40–46.
24. Bloor, G. (1999). Organizational culture, organizational learning and total quality management: A literature review and synthesis. *Australian Health Review*, *22*(3), 162–179.
25. Centanni, N., Monroe, M., White, L. & Larson, R. (1999). Quality beyond compliance. *Quality Assurance*, *7*(1), 17–35.
26. Scheuing, E. E. (1999). Achieving excellence—Creating customer passion. *Hospital Materials Management Quarterly*, 76–87.
27. Schaaf, D. (1991). Beating the drum for quality. *Quality*, 5–6, 8, 11–12.
28. Rex Bryce, G. (1991). Quality management theories and their application. *Quality*, 15–18.
29. What's next on the quality agenda? (1991). *Quality*, 42.
30. Peters, T. (1991, November 12). Family gives 'teams' plenty of experience. *San Antonio Light*, p. E3.
31. Isouard, G. (1999). The key elements in the development of a quality management environment for pathology services. *Journal of Quality Clinical Practice*, 202–207.
32. Hammer, M., & S. Stanton. (1999). How process enterprises really work. *Harvard Business Review*, 108–118, 216.
33. Konstam, P. (1992, January 1). Making productivity grow takes work. *San Antonio Light*, p. 1E.
34. Ertel, D. (1999). Turning negotiation into a corporate capability. *Harvard Business Review*, 55–60, 62–70, 213.
35. Linkow, P. (1989). Is your culture ready for total quality? *Quality Progress*, 69–71.
36. Ibid.
37. Sahlman, W. A. (1999). The new economy is stronger than you think. *Harvard Business Review*, 99–106, 216.
38. Ouchi, W. G. (1981). *Theory Z*. Reading, MA: Addison-Wesley.
39. Adair, M. N. & Nygard, N. K. (1982). Theory Z management: Can it work for nursing? *Nursing & Health Care*, 489–491.
40. Ibid.
41. The theory of quality circles was actually developed by Frederick Herzberg and W. Edwards Deming of the United States approximately 50 years ago. Johnson, S. (1985). Quality control circles: Negotiating an efficient work environment. *Nursing Management*, 34A–34B, 34D–34G; Goldberg, A. M. & Pegels, C. C. (1984). *Quality circles in health-care facilities*. Gaithersburg, MD: Aspen.
42. Ibid.
43. Morhman, S. A. & Ledford, G. E., Jr. (1985). The design and use of effective employee participation groups: Implication for human resource management. *Human Resource Management*, 413–428.
44. Piczak, 1988.
45. Schaaf, 1991.
46. Haughom, J. L. (2000). Transforming US health care: The arduous road to value. *Topics in Health Information Management*, 1–10.
47. Massarweh, L. J. (1999). Promoting a positive clinical experience. *Nurse Educator*, 44–47.
48. Batalden, P. B. & Stoltz, P. K. (1993). A framework for the continual improvement of health care: Building and applying professional and improvement knowledge to test changes in daily work. *Joint Commission Journal On Quality Improvement*, 424–450.

49. Ibid.
50. Deming, W. E. (1986). *Out of crisis*. Cambridge, MA: MIT Press; Crosby, P. B. (1984). *Quality without tears*. New York: McGraw-Hill; Juran, J. M. (1988). *Juran on planning for quality*. New York: The Free Press; Senge, P. M. (1990). *The fifth discipline: The art and practice of the learning organization*. New York: Doubleday.
51. Batalden & Stoltz, 1993.
52. *Comprehensive accreditation manual for hospitals*. (1994). Oakbrook Terrace, IL: JCAHO, 219–266.
53. Batalden & Stoltz, 1993, 434.
54. Measurement tools for analysis. (1997). *NAHQ guide to quality management* (7th ed.). Glenview, IL: NAHQ, 81–105.
55. Curtis, B. J. & Simpson, L. J. (1985). Auditing: A method for evaluating quality of care. *Journal of Nursing Administration*, 14–21.
56. Ibid.
57. Ibid.
58. Evans, R. W. & Ruff, R. M. (1992). Outcome and value: A perspective on rehabilitation outcomes achieved in acquired brain injury. *Journal of Head Trauma*, 24–36.
59. Larson, E., Oram, I., & Hedrick, E. (1988). Nosocomial infection rates as an indicator of quality. *Medical Care*, 676–684.
60. McCormick, K. A. (1991). Future data needs for quality care monitoring, DRG considerations, reimbursement and outcome measurements. *Image: Journal of Nursing Scholarship*, 29–32.
61. Measurement tools for analysis, 1997.
62. Pyrczak, F. (2003). *Making sense of statistics: A conceptual overview* (3rd ed.). LA: Pyrczak Pub, 44–66.
63. Batalden & Stoltz, 1993, 434–438.
64. Rowland, H. S. & Rowland, B. L. (Eds.). Quality assurance. *Hospital Legal Forms, Checklists, and Guidelines*. Gaithersburg, MD: Aspen, 26:1–26:14.
65. Edwardson, S. R. & Anderson, D. I. (1983). Hospital nurses' evaluation of quality assurance. *Journal of Nursing Administration*, 33–39.
66. Rowland, H. S. & Rowland, B. L. (1997). *Nursing administration handbook*, 424.
67. Spuck, J. (1999). Using the long-term care minimum data set as a tool for CQI in nursing homes. In J. Dieneman (Ed.), Nursing administration: Managing patient care (2nd ed., 95–105). Stamford, CT: Appleton & Lange.
68. Allio, R. (1986). Forecasting: The myth of control [Interview with Donald Michal]. *Planning Review*, *1*, 6–11.
69. Taylor, A. G., Hudson, K., & Keeling, A. (1991). Quality nursing care: The consumers' perspective revisited. *Journal of Nursing Quality Assurance*, *1*, 23–31.
70. Coddington, D. C., & Moore, K. D. (1987). Quality of care as a business strategy. *Healthcare Forum Journal*, *1*, 29–34.
71. Ibid.
72. Larson, E. (1983). Combining nursing quality assurance and research programs. *Journal of Nursing Administration*, *1*, 32–34.
73. Ibid.

REFERENCES

Arikian, V. L. (1991). Total quality management: Applications to nursing service. *Journal of Nursing Administration*, 46–50.

Bauerhaus, P. I. (1996). Creating a new place in the competitive market. *Nursing Policy Forum*, 13–20.

Cohen, S. S. (1995). National Committee for Quality Assurance. *Rehab Management*, 13, 109.

Cole, R. (1988). What was Deming's real influence? *Mechanical Engineering*, 49–51.

Dobyns, L. & Crawford-Mason, C. (1991). *Quality or else: The revolution in world business*. New York: Houghton Mifflin.

Duncan, R. P., Fleming, E. C., & Gallati, T. G. (1991). Implementing a continuous quality improvement program in a community hospital. *Quality Review Bulletin*, 106–112.

Eddy, D. M. & Billings, J. (1988). The quality of medical evidence: Implications for quality of care. *Health Affairs*, 19–32.

Eubanks, P. (1992). The CEO experience: TQM/CQI. *Hospitals*, 24–36.

Ferketish, B. J. & Hayden, J. W. (1992). HRD & quality: The chicken or the egg? *Training & Development Journal*, 39–42.

Gitlow, H.S., Gitlow, S. J., Oppenheim, A., & Oppenheim, R. (1990). Telling the quality story. *Quality Progress*, 41–46.

Hutchins, B. (1996). Managing cost and quality. *Rehab Management*, 25–26.

Joint Commission on Accreditation of Healthcare Organizations (JCAHO). (1990). *Primer on indicator development and application: Measuring quality in health care*. Oakbrook Terrace, IL: Author.

Kaluzny, A. D., McLaughlin, C. P., & Simpson, K. (1992). Applying total quality management concepts to public health organizations. *Public Health Reports*, 257–263.

Konstam, P. (1992, March 1). 'Quality' should begin at home. *San Antonio Light*, p. D1.

Ludeman, K. (1992). Using employee surveys to revitalize TQM. *Training*, 51–57.

Maciorowski, L. J., Lar, E., & Keane, A. (1985). Quality assurance: Evaluate thyself. *Journal of Nursing Administration*, *1*, 38–42.

Mackelprang, R. & Johnson, P. B. (1995). Managed care: Balancing costs, quality, and access. *SCI Psychosocial Access*, *4*, 175–178.

Mathews, J. & Katel, P. (1992, September 7). The cost of quality. *Newsweek*, 48–49.

McCabe, W. J. (1992). Total quality management in a hospital. *Quality Review Bulletin*, *3*, 134–140.

McCormick, V. E. (1991). Software helps with hard decisions. *Training*, *1*, 23–24.

McLaughlin, C. P. & Kaluzny, A. D. (1990). Total quality management in health: Making it work. *Health Care Management Review*, *15*(3), 7–14.

Meisenheimer, C. (1991). The customer: Silent or intimate player in the quality revolution. *Holistic Nurse Practitioner*, *1*, 39–50.

Moore, K. F. (1996). Cost or quality when selecting a health plan? *National Policy Forum*, 24.

Nelson, M. F. & Christenson, R. H. (1995). The focused review process: A utilization management firm's experience with length of stay guidelines. *Journal of Quality Improvement*, *9*, 477–487.

Spicer, J. G., Craft, M. J., & Ross, K. C. (1988). A systems approach to customer satisfaction. *Nursing Administration Quarterly*, *1*, 79–83.

Towers, J. (1996). What do you know about NCQA? *Nursing Policy Forum*, 30.

Ubell, E. (1997, September 14). You can get quality care in an HMO world. *Parade Magazine*, 10–11.

Walton, M. (1987). Deming's parable of the red beads. *Across the Board*, 43–48.

Williams, R. (1991, November 4). Putting Deming's principles to work. *Wall Street Journal*, p. A18.

Wolff, G. M. (1986). Systems management: Evaluating nursing departments as a whole. *Nursing Management*, *1*, 40–43.

Woods, M. D. (1989). New manufacturing practices—New accounting practices. *Production and Inventory Management Journal*, *1*, 8–12.

APPENDIX 17-1

Quality Assessment and Improvement Program

MEMORIAL HOSPITAL
DEPARTMENT OF NURSING

QUALITY ASSESSMENT AND IMPROVEMENT (QAI) PROGRAM

I. POLICY STATEMENT

The Memorial Hospital Department of Nursing will monitor the provision of nursing care and the results of nursing care in an ongoing and systematic manner following the Quality Assessment and Improvement Program for the Department of Nursing. This program is designed to improve care based on the monitoring and evaluation of structure, practice (process), and care (outcome) standards, and is consistent with the Quality Assessment and Improvement Plan for Memorial Hospital.

Nursing quality assessment and improvement activities are reported to the QAI Executive Committee of Memorial Hospital.

II. PURPOSE

1. To ensure that the quality of patient care is optimal through a unified program.
2. To provide the process by which the provision of nursing care and end results (patient outcomes) are measured and evaluated against Standards for Nursing.
3. To integrate efforts of physicians and nurses in Special Care Units to continuously improve patient care.
4. To maintain quality care in current use.

III. GENERAL INFORMATION

Structure Standards describe the environment in which safe, effective, and appropriate care takes place, i.e., organization, management, resources, care delivery, productivity, and turnover rate. Structure standards are a form of productivity reporting and are used for management information. Nurse Managers receive daily productivity/variance reports from Nursing Information Systems to assist in monitoring and evaluating structure standards.

Standards of Practice describe the nature and sequence of health care activities and are based on identified important aspects of care. Policies and procedures describe how important aspects of care are carried out.

Standards of Care describe nursing care results for the major patient populations and those patients who receive high-risk, high-volume nursing care.

Care Plans define and describe individual patients' nursing care and expected results.

Quality Care Framework (Exhibit A17-1) clarifies Integration of Standards for Nursing into Quality Assessment and Improvement.

Nursing staff members participate, by way of the Nursing Practice Committee and unit meetings, in the identification of the important aspects of care, identifying the indicators, planning action to improve care, and evaluating the results. All nursing departments participate on CQI teams as assigned.

Each nursing department develops and follows an annual plan for QAI that is maintained on each unit and copies of which are located in the office of Nursing Administration. The JCAHO 10-step process is the method used to accomplish improvements. Each unit plan is assisted by a matrix—used to simplify and clarify information pertinent to each indicator. (See Exhibit A17-2.)

IV. PROCEDURE

Responsibility. The Nurse Manager is responsible for ensuring the completion of QAI activities.

Scope of Care. This is a 406-bed, level I trauma center that provides nursing care by RNs, LPNs, and NAs 24 hours a day to patients requiring emergency services, interfacility transportation, aeromedical transportation, surgical services, postanesthesia care, labor and delivery, obstetrics, intensive care nursery, neonatal transportation, premature nursery, newborn nursery, medical–surgical nursing, burn center, neurotrauma intensive care, surgical intensive care, renal dialysis, medical intensive care, coronary intensive care, and intermediate nursing care. Medical–surgical pediatric patients are located on 6th and 5th South nursing units. Pediatric patients also receive nursing care in the Burn Center, in CCU, and, less frequently, in SICU/NTICU. The scope of care is based on the needs and expectations of the high-risk and high-volume patient who is admitted (Special Care Units) or discharged from each nursing unit. High volume is determined by annual review of diagnoses (DRGs) and by categorizing the diagnoses according to similar patient needs. The largest categories or patient populations having similar needs based on diagnoses are designated as high volume. Patients identified as at-risk are determined by the history of complications within certain groups of patients or for individual patients. In addition to the needs and expectations of the major patient populations, subcategories are identified to reflect those patients who receive problem-prone nursing care and those at risk for developing complications due to their biophysical status.

Important Aspects of Care are identified in addressing the high-volume and/or problem-prone (present a risk

APPENDIX 17-1

EXHIBIT A17-1
Integration of Standards for Nursing into QAI

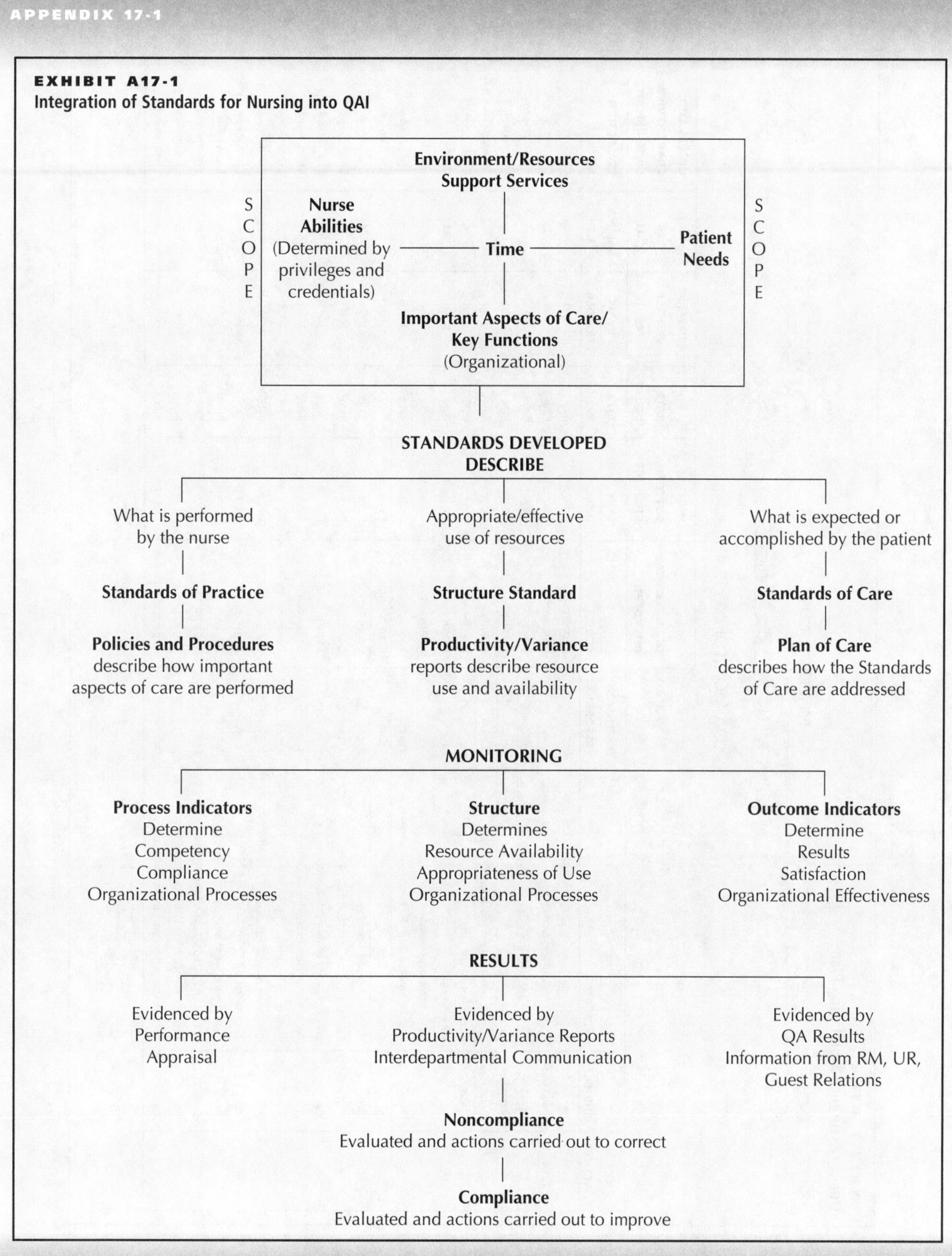

(continued)

APPENDIX 17-1 *(continued)*

EXHIBIT A17-2
Quality Assurance Monitoring Plan

MEMORIAL HOSPITAL

DEPARTMENT: 5th Floor Medical Surgical

QA MONITORING PLAN

				DEPARTMENTAL INTERDEPT.	*PROCESS OUTCOME STRUCTURE*	*RATE* COUNT	<100%; >0 BENCH # TREND	5% 30 ALL	OBSERVATION CHART REVIEW LOGS; REPORTS
KEY FUNCTION	**SUBJECT**	**INDICATOR**	**DIMENSION PERFORM**	**SCOPE**	**TYPE INDIC**	**TYPE INDIC**	**EVAL. TRIGGER**	**SAMPLE SIZE**	**COLLECTION METHOD**
TX/IM	Restraint	Appropriate restraint documentation (12 criteria)	Res	Departmental	Process	Rate	Trend	All	Chart review
PI/TX	Blood Use	Correct transfusion procedure	Safe	Interdepart.	Process	Rate	Trend	5%	Obs/chrt review
TX	Med Use	Medication errors	Safe/Cont	Interdepart.	P/O	Rate	>0	All	Rep/Chrt review
IC	Stand Prec	Handwashing	Appro	Interdepart.	Process	Rate	Trend	5%	Observation
IC	Stand Prec	Correct handwashing procedure	Effec	Interdepart.	Process	Rate	Trend	5%	Observation
IC	Stand Prec	Appropriate glove use	Appro	Interdepart.	Process	Rate	Trend	5%	Observation
EC	Fall	Patient falls	Safe	Departmental	Process	Rate	Trend	All	Obs/Rep
RI	Satisfac	Patient satisfaction/nursing care	Res	Interdepart.	Outcome	Rate	Trend	10/mo	Questionnaire
TX	Plan	Multidisciplinary Goals/Problem form present	Avail	Interdepart.	Process	Rate	<100%	5%	Chart review
TX	Plan	Goals measurable	Appro	Departmental	Process	Rate	<100%	5%	Chart review
TX	Plan	Patient problems individualized	Appro	Departmental	Process	Rate	<100%	5%	Chart review
TX	Plan	Priorities for care identified each shift	Appro	Departmental	Process	Rate	<100%	5%	Chart review
TX	Plan	Priorities based on goals/problems	Appro/Cont	Departmental	Process	Rate	<100%	5%	Chart review
TX	Provide	Focus note relates to priorities each shift	Appro/Cont	Departmental	Process	Rate	<100%	5%	Chart review
TX	Provide	Problem/goal summary each shift	Appro/Cont	Departmental	Process	Rate	<100%	5%	Chart review
TX	Provide	Evaluation of goal attainment each shift	Appro/Cont	Departmental	Process	Rate	<100%	5%	Chart review
PF	Plan	Knowledge deficit on Goal/Problem form	Appro	Departmental	Process	Rate	<100%	5%	Chart review
PF	Provide	Teaching related to goal documented on MPEP	Appro	Departmental	Process	Rate	<100%	5%	Chart review
RI	Edu	Patient instructed on plans for care & expectations	Res	Departmental	Process	Rate	Trend	5%	Chart review
PE	Fall	Patient assessed for fall risk upon admission	Safe	Departmental	Process	Rate	Trend	5%	Chart review
PE	Pain	Patient assessed for pain upon admission	Res	Departmental	Process	Rate	Trend	5%	Chart review

EXHIBIT A17-2 *(continued)*

				DAILY WEEKLY MONTHLY	*MONTHLY* QUARTERLY	DEPT. GROUP	DEPT. GROUP	DEPT. GROUP TITLE	AA; COMMITTEE EXTERNAL GROUP OTHER DEPT.
KEY FUNCTION	**SUBJECT**	**INDICATOR**	**DIMENSION PERFORM**	**COLLECTION INTERVAL**	**REPORT INTERVAL**	**COLLECT BY**	**AGGREGATE BY**	**REPORT BY**	**REPORT TO**
TX/IM	Restraint	Appropriate restraint documentation (12 criteria)	Res	Daily	Quarterly	Staff	QM	QM	AA
PI/TX	Blood Use	Correct transfusion procedure	Safe	Daily	Quarterly	Staff	QM	QM	Bld Use Com
TX	Med Use	Medication errors	Safe/Cont	Daily	Quarterly	Staff	QM	QM	Med Use Com
IC	Stand Prec	Handwashing	Appro	1 Mo/Qtr	Quarterly	Staff	IC	IC NM	IC Committee
IC	Stand Prec	Correct handwashing procedure	Effec	1 Mo/Qtr	Quarterly	Staff	IC	IC NM	IC Committee
IC	Stand Prec	Appropriate glove use	Appro	1 Mo/Qtr	Quarterly	Staff	IC	IC NM	IC Committee
EC	Fall	Patient falls	Safe	Daily	Quarterly	Staff	QM	QM	AA; EC Com
RI	Satisfac	Patient satisfaction/nursing care	Res	Daily	Quarterly	Staff	Satisf Com	Satisf Com	AA
TX	Plan	Multidisciplinary Goals/Problem form present	Avail	Monthly	Quarterly	Nur	DH/QM	DH/QM	AA
TX	Plan	Goals measurable	Appro	Monthly	Quarterly	Nur	DH/QM	DH/QM	AA
TX	Plan	Patient problems individualized	Appro	Monthly	Quarterly	Nur	DH/QM	DH/QM	AA
TX	Plan	Priorities for care identified each shift	Appro	Monthly	Quarterly	Nur	DH/QM	DH/QM	AA
TX	Plan	Priorities based on goals/problems	Appro/Cont	Monthly	Quarterly	Nur	DH/QM	DH/QM	AA
TX	Provide	Focus note relates to priorities each shift	Appro/Cont	Monthly	Quarterly	Nur	DH/QM	DH/QM	AA
TX	Provide	Problem/goal summary each shift	Appro/Cont	Monthly	Quarterly	Nur	DH/QM	DH/QM	AA
TX	Provide	Evaluation of goal attainment each shift	Appro/Cont	Monthly	Quarterly	Nur	DH/QM	DH/QM	AA
PF	Plan	Knowledge deficit on Goal/Problem form	Appro	Monthly	Quarterly	Nur	DH/QM	DH/QM	AA
PF	Provide	Teaching related to goal documented on MPEP	Appro	Monthly	Quarterly	Nur	DH/QM	DH/QM	AA
RI	Edu	Patient instructed on plans for care & expectations	Res	Monthly	Quarterly	Nur	DH/QM	DH/QM	AA
PE	Fall	Patient assessed for fall risk upon admission	Safe	Monthly	Quarterly	Nur	DH/QM	DH/QM	AA
PE	Pain	Patient assessed for pain upon admission	Res	Monthly	Quarterly	Nur	DH/QM	DH/QM	AA

KEY FUNCTION:
PI = Improving Organizational Performance
EC = Environment of Care
IM = Information Management
IC = Infection Control
RI = Patient Rights/Organizational Ethics
PE = Assessment of Patients
TX = Care (Planning/Providing; Anesthesia; Med Use; Nutrition; Op/Invasive; Rehab; Special Tx)
PF = Patient/Family Education

DIMENSION OF PERFORMANCE:
Right thing: Efficacy; Appropriateness
Right thing well: Availability; Timeliness; Effectiveness; Continuity; Safety; Efficiency; Respect and Caring

(continued)

APPENDIX 17-1 *(continued)*

to the patient or nurse) nursing care activities. From the important aspects of care, standards are developed: Standards of Practice, Concurrent Process, Retrospective Process, Standards of Care, Concurrent Outcome, and Retrospective Outcome. Policies and procedures are based on standards determined by the requirements of the major patient populations.

The following generic key functions are important to patient care at Memorial Hospital:

Assessment/Reassessment
Care Plan
Implementation/Evaluation
Continuity of Care
Safety/Universal Precautions/Infection Control
Appropriateness
Teaching/Emotional and Spiritual Support
Medication Administration/Treatments
Discharge Preparation
Confidentiality
IV Therapy

Each Nursing Unit has identified aspects of care related to generic standards for quality assessment and improvement.

Indicators. Elements of the high-volume, problem-prone nursing activities that provide evidence as to whether the care provided is of quality are developed into statements called Indicators for each nursing unit. The Indicator Development Form (Exhibit A17-3) is used to operationalize indicators as needed.

Process Indicators measure how well departments and individuals meet stated standards for practice, use the nursing process, and document care.

Outcome Indicators measure specific patient outcomes and direct departments in needed action and changes toward meeting standards of care.

Evaluation Trigger. A value is placed on the results of each indicator to assist in determining whether opportunity for improvement exists. When counting events (0, 1, 2, 3, . . .), the evaluation trigger may be >0, signifying that each event is evaluated and action is taken to eliminate the type of occurrence. When using rate-based indicators (numerator–denominator), the evaluation trigger could be stated as <100%, signifying that no less than 100% is expected and actions are taken to correct deficiencies. Another type of evaluation trigger is the benchmark. The *benchmark* is a measure of best practice for like populations from other organizations. *Trends* in results may also be used as evaluation triggers. Trending involves at least three consecutive points of data. The goal is to always show improvement. Therefore, actions should be taken for the evaluation of "no trend," "decreasing performance," or "results staying the same."

Collection and Organization of Data. The Nurse Manager or designee sets up an annual Quality Assessment and Improvement Matrix that specifies the sequence and the data to be collected for monitoring. (See Exhibit A17-2.) Data sources include patient charts and questionnaires. Process monitoring may involve staff observation/interview, and outcome monitoring may involve patient/family interview/observation.

Special Care Nursing Units (SICU/NTICU, CCU/MICU, Burn Center, ICN) and medical staff of Special Care Units monitor joint aspects of care and patients, integrating efforts to improve patient care. Nursing concurrently monitors patients applicable to the chosen joint aspect and supplies the medical record number to the medical staff Quality Assurance Coordinator for physician review. Department heads and medical directors discuss findings and opportunities to improve via the Critical Care Committee.

Documentation review classes will be held on Committee Day, the first Tuesday of each month. RNs will be assigned to participate in retrospective review of documentation. Generically, Nursing will monitor 5% of patient admissions for appropriate documentation.

Concurrent monitoring is performed on each nursing unit each month as part of assignments to the nursing staff. Results of monitoring and any adverse effects to the patient as a result of individual performance are addressed and followed up through Nurse Credentialing as part of the Performance Appraisal.

The staff nurse follows Staff Nurse Guidelines for Quality Monitoring (Exhibit A17-4) in using a quality review worksheet or concurrent data sheet for monitoring.

Evaluate. The data is initially evaluated by the Nurse Manager who further involves the staff in evaluation through staff meetings and Nurse Practice Committee Meetings. Evaluation may consist of more intensive review of specific cases or continued monitoring. Concurrent monitoring is advantageous in that the staff nurse who takes corrective action at the time of review is involved in the initial evaluation.

Actions to Improve Care. Methods to resolve problems and improve care identified through monitoring include staff meetings, individual counseling, education,

APPENDIX 17-1

EXHIBIT A17-3
Indicator Development Form

I. Indicator Statement: ______________________________

____

II. Definition of Terms: ______________________________

____

III: Type of Indicator: Rate based ________ Process ________

Sentinel event ________ Outcome ________

IV: Rationale

A. Why useful? ______________________________

B. Supportive references: ______________________________

C. Components of quality assessed: ______________________________

V. Description of Indicator Population

A. (Numerator) / (Denominator) : ______________________________

B. Subcategories: ______________________________

VI. Indicator Data Collection Logic

Data Elements | Data Source

VII. Underlying Factors

A. Patient factors: ______________________________

B. Practitioner factors: ______________________________

C. Organization factors: ______________________________

Source: Joint Commision Primer on Indicator Development and Application. *Measuring Quality in Healthcare*, 1990. JCAHO, One Renaissance Blvd., Oakbrook Terrace, IL, p 914–916.

problem solving with other departments, developing standards, modifying documentation tools, changing departmental/organizational process and related policies, and revision of Quality Assessment. Actions taken will specify who will do what and when.

Specific problems may be referred to standing committees within the department. Problems identified by any staff member that involve any department or activity are documented on a Quality Assurance Problem Reporting Sheet (Exhibit A17-5) and attached with follow-up to the monthly narrative analysis report.

Assess Actions and Document Improvement. A time frame for assessing effectiveness for action is determined. Subsequent findings are reviewed at that time, and further recommendations for action are made if necessary. The QAI Report Grid is completed quarterly for all indicators monitored during the report interval. The Nurse Manager or designee uses the Performance Improvement Report Form to complete the report.

Communicate Relevant Information. Information obtained from staff nurse data collection is communicated

(continued)

APPENDIX 17-1 *(continued)*

EXHIBIT A17-4
Staff Nurse Guidelines for Quality Monitoring

Quality Assurance (QA) monitoring is documented on unit-specific data retrieval sheets by the assigned staff nurse each month. The data retrieval sheets are located on each nursing unit in a QA notebook or in the employee file for QA.

The data retrieval sheets monitor two different aspects of nursing: (1) Standards of practice are monitored by process indicators. Practice/process measures what the nurse does (nursing practice, nursing process) and is stated in terms of "The nurse will. . . ." (2) Standards of care are monitored by outcome indicators. Care/outcome measures the final picture of the patient as a result of nursing/interdepartmental care and is stated in terms of "The patient will . . ." or "The patient can expect. . . ."

The staff nurse retrieves the QA data sheets from the book or file and monitors a patient/chart according to the indicators during a month specified by the Nurse Manager or designee.

The staff nurse uses the column beside the indicator to designate the results of the patient/nurse/chart that is monitored. Each time the indicator is monitored, the adjacent column is used. The month in which the monitoring takes place is written at the top of the page.

The result of monitoring is documented using the following key:

+	Results are compliant
–	Results are not compliant
J	Results are not compliant but are justified
N/A	Results do not apply

When justification (J) is used, the justifier must be written below the standard to which it applies.

> *Example:* The patient was not wearing an identification band because of injuries to the extremities—BUT, *the I.D. band was taped to the head of the bed.*

> *Example:* The nurse did not document confirmation of the enteral feeding tube insertion because M.D. inserted it and started feedings—BUT *the M.D. documented in the progress notes the confirmation of the feeding tube.*

Not applicable (N/A) is used when a specific indicator does not apply for that patient. Examples would be a patient who has no IV tubing to be changed because the patient has an INT, or the patient is discharged without medications needed at home. In these instances, indicators for IV tubing changed or verbalizing understanding of discharge medications would be N/A.

The staff nurse should seek out the patient populations for which the Standard of Care applies versus monitoring one patient for all outcome indicators.

> *Examples:* An abdominal surgery patient is found to monitor the outcome for abdominal surgery patients; a seizure patient is monitored for outcome of seizure patients; a cardiac patient is found to monitor outcome of cardiac patients; a patient with an IV is found to monitor outcomes for IV therapy; a patient who has been discharged, or is in the process of being discharged, is monitored for discharge criteria and discharge teaching.

This process ensures that the standards are applicable in the majority of situations.

At the end of each month the Nurse Manager or designated staff nurse compiles the information from each data sheet and then returns this sheet to the file or QA book. Indicators are monitored every month until they reach quarterly compliance. At that time another standard and/or indicators may be added by the Nurse Manager or designated staff nurse, depending on problems identified.

The staff nurse participates in identifying standards and indicators by way of staff meetings, the Nursing Practice Committee, or one-to-one conferences with the Nurse Manager or designated staff nurse.

appropriately as per the established communication system.

Monitoring results of Special Care Units are communicated through the Critical Care Committee and signed by the Medical Director. All nursing units forward monthly QA reports to the Clinical Administrator for Nursing Practice.

Each quarter the Clinical Administrator for Nursing Practice summarizes each unit's specific report into a Division Report that is signed by the Director of Nursing and the Assistant Administrator for Nursing. Signed original quarterly reports are maintained in the office of Nursing Administration and copies are maintained by the hospital QAI Department.

V. ANNUAL EVALUATION

Quality Assurance for the Department of Nursing and Standards for Nursing are reviewed at least annually

APPENDIX 17-1

EXHIBIT A17-5
Quality Assurance Problem Reporting Sheet

Department: ______________________ Date: ______________________

Initiated by: ______________________ To: ______________________

Problem or concern studied:

____

____

____

How identified and why important (data sources) impact on patient care:

____

____

____

____

Contributing factors:

____

____

Quality goal (after study is completed):

____

____

____

____

Departments involved:

____

____

Referred to department: ______________________ Action taken: ______________________

____

____

____

____

Follow-up plan or recommendations:

____

____

____

Please respond by: ______________________ To: ______________________

Thank you very much. ______________________________________ (signature)

(continued)

APPENDIX 17-1 ***(continued)***

and revised as needed by the Nurse Practice Committee and Nurse Managers. Review and revision of Standards considers:

1. Patient requirements and the effectiveness of the staffing plan.
2. Ability to attract and retain the numbers and types of nursing personnel required.
3. Variance reports that indicate the staffing plan's adequacy or inadequacy to meet patient needs.
4. Monitoring information that relates to the staffing plan.
5. The consistency for the provision of nursing care between units based on Standards.
6. The staff's ability to pursue activities to promote innovation and/or improvement of nursing care.

The annual report will identify any opportunities to improve care, care that improved, and revisions to the plan.

VI. CONFIDENTIALITY STATEMENT
Quality assessment and improvement documents and activities are privileged and confidential for the MH Quality Management Program and are prepared and maintained pursuant to the Code of Mississippi 200x: 6-5-333, 22-21-8, and 34-24-58.

CHAPTER 18

Performance Appraisal

Linda Roussel, RN, DSN
Russell C. Swansburg, PhD, RN

> The illiterate of the 21st century will not be those who cannot read and write, but those who cannot learn, unlearn, and relearn.
>
> Alvin Toffler

LEARNING OBJECTIVES AND ACTIVITIES

- Define *performance appraisal*.
- Describe the purposes of performance appraisal.
- Differentiate among the standards for performance appraisal.
- Describe training approaches for performance.
- Distinguish among performance appraisal methodologies.
- Describe performance appraisal problem areas.
- Distinguish among the major types of pay for performance.
- Identify the criteria used in a pay-for-performance plan.
- Discuss the design of a pay-for-performance plan.

CONCEPTS: Performance appraisal, performance standards, job analysis, job description, job evaluation, feedback, work redesign, peer ratings, self-ratings, pay for performance, merit pay, gain sharing.

NURSE MANAGER BEHAVIORS: Maintains a system of probationary and annual performance appraisals based on job descriptions as standards, bases all pay increases on a merit pay system, seeks constructive feedback regarding his or her own practice, takes action to achieve plans for improvement, and participates in peer review as appropriate.

NURSE EXECUTIVE BEHAVIORS: Develops a system of performance appraisal that uses a combination of supervisor, peer, and self-ratings. Feedback is provided based on input from the nursing staff. Human resource personnel use job analysis, job evaluation, and work redesign techniques to improve employee productivity. Employs a variety of pay-for-performance compensation plans as a part of the annual budget. Identifies industry trends and competencies in nursing administration and nursing practice. Engages in self-assessment of role accountabilities on a regular basis, identifying areas of strength as well as areas for professional and practice development. Evaluates accomplishment of the strategic plan and the vision for professional nursing.

Introduction

Performance appraisal (PA) is a control process in which employees' performances are evaluated against standards. Pay-for-performance incorporates the principles of PA. The literature on PA is voluminous, indicating its value to management. Considerable research has been done on various aspects of the PA process.

Neither employees nor managers like PA. Some employees view PA as being more valued by top management than by themselves and their supervisors. Some managers do not like to do PA because it makes them feel guilty: "Did I do justice by the employee?" As writers of PAs, managers are concerned that they may "cast something in stone" that is inaccurate, be criticized on written grammar and spelling, say something illegal about the ratee, or be unable to substantiate their comments.[1] Other managers are afraid of employees' reactions to ratings. PA requires careful planning, information gathering, and an extensive formal interview, all of which is a time-consuming process. Managers perform activities of short duration, attend ad hoc meetings, perform nonroutine behavior, and focus on current information, all of which are short-term activities compared with the ongoing PA process.[2] The process is usually not interactive, moves slowly, is passive, is isolated, and is not people-oriented.[3]

Measurement of performance is imprecise. Often the focus is on the format, not the people. In some organizations, the human resource (HR) department sends the rating forms to the departments shortly before the end of the fiscal year. The forms must be completed immediately and are done with little or no training or preparation of the rater or ratee. The result is distrust by employees and dread by managers.

A survey of Fortune 1300 companies (1000 industrial and 300 nonindustrial) indicated that 29% of hourly workers are not evaluated by a formal appraisal system; 39% of respondents indicated that where used, PA systems are "extremely effective" or "very effective." PA systems are underappreciated.[4]

Performance appraisal systems require top management commitment. They can be tied to the planning cycle by being related to personnel budgets or included as a management plan. PA systems are most helpful when managers commit to using them for purposes beneficial both to employees and to the organization.

Research in PA domains has little effect on the process or the outcome. Some suggest that research and practice focus on fair and accurate PA as a process before attempting to use it to improve performance.[5]

Performance appraisal literature indicates the following ten results:[6]

1. US industry has used PA systems for an average of 11 years. PA systems had little input from line managers, employees, and customers.
2. Most formats use management by objectives for executives, managers, and professional employees. Trait-based rating scales are the norm for nonexempt employees. Behavioral-anchored rating scales (BARS), forced-choice scales, or mixed standard scales are seldom used. Executives and hourly employees are least likely to be evaluated.
3. Supervisor ratings are most common. Self, peer, and subordinate ratings are seldom used.
4. Very few organizations allow decisions about PA policies or practice to be made at the level at which they are executed.
5. Some raters receive rater training; however, employees' training has seldom been welcomed.
6. Only 25% of raters are held accountable for managing the appraisal process.
7. Few employee opinions about the appraisal process are solicited.
8. Managers are concerned with fairness, justice, and future performance.
9. Of an organizational work force, 60% to 70% is rated in the top two performance levels.
10. A more comprehensive theory of the PA process is needed.

Research indicates that high levels of organizational politics relate to the conscientious job performance of workers.[7]

Purposes of Performance Appraisal

Performance appraisal may be a nurse manager's most valuable tool in controlling human resources and productivity. The PA process can be used effectively to govern employee behavior in order to produce goods and services in high volume and of high quality. Nurse managers can also use the PA process to govern corporate direction in selecting, training, doing career planning with, and rewarding personnel. The Fortune 1300 survey indicated that 80% used appraisal systems to justify merit increases, provide feedback, and identify candidates for promotion, all of which are considered short-term goals. These goals were linked to long-term goals of performance potential for succession planning and career planning but could be much more useful in strategic planning. Of these companies, 58% used PA to identify strengths and weaknesses, whereas 39% used PA for career planning; 89% used PA for general guidelines for salary increases, whereas only 1% used PA for forced distribution of bonuses. Forced distribution sets a limit on the number of high-level ratings.[8]

In addition to being used for promotions, counseling, training and development, staff planning, retention, termination, selections, and compensations, performance monitoring has been found to make employees effective. It is a managerial tool that can facilitate performance levels that achieve the company's mission and objectives.[9]

Appraisal systems are needed to meet legal requirements, including those for standardized forms and procedures, clear and relevant job analysis, and trained raters. When they do not meet such requirements, disciplinary actions, including termination, do not stand up in court.[10]

Motivation

A goal of PA is to stimulate motivation of the employee to perform the tasks and accomplish the mission of the organization. Promotions, assignments, selections for education, and increased pay are some goals that stimulate this motivation.

Salary Problems

Performance evaluation is used to determine and provide equitable salary treatment. Jobs within groups of professionals, such as engineers, physicians, chemists, physicists, and nurses, have the same basic characteristics. Differences exist in the complexity of jobs. One could say that the job of a nurse assigned to a special care unit is more complex than is that of a nurse assigned to an intermediate care unit. Contrast this with the complexity of managing the care of an active intermediate care unit of 20 to 45 patients. The complexity of providing nursing care to many patients, who have differing problems and are being treated by many physicians, in addition to directing many medical care plans and many nonprofessional workers, appears to be equivalent to the complexity of intensive nursing care. In fact, some nurses want to be assigned to special care units not because of the dynamics of the situation but because their sphere of operations is limited. Is a nurse in one of these units entitled to a higher salary than a nurse in the other? The job analysts say yes, if special training is required, complicated specialized equipment is being used, and the nurse is required to make more independent and critical judgments.

The jobs of all professionals can be evaluated using conventional PA techniques. However, arguments abound regarding the relationship of PAs to salaries and promotion. Some writers recommend not performing PAs in times of salary increases and promotions.[11] According to a survey of 875 companies, 32% experimented with some form of performance-based pay.[12]

Kirkpatrick recommends separating appraisals for merit salary increases from appraisals for performance improvement. Appraisals used for merit salary increases look backward at past performance, look at total performance, compare one individual with others doing the same job, are subjective, and are done in an emotional climate. Appraisals used to improve performance look ahead; are concerned with detailed performance; are compared with what is expected regarding standards, goals, and objectives; and are conducted in a calm climate.[13]

For performance reviews related to salary administration, nurse managers should explain to subordinates the basis of decisions. The reviews should be fair and should be totally understood by the managers, who should allow employees to react even to the point of discussing the reviews with higher management. When a high salary increase results, the nurse manager communicates the good news to the employee. Three months should elapse between appraisals for salary administration and those for improved performance.[14]

Expectancy theory states that "the greater a person's expectancy (i.e., subjective probability) that effort expenditure will lead to various rewards, the greater the person's motivation to work hard."[15] Rewards of high value should be obtainable and related to job performance. Employees will repeat rewarded behavior and will be retained, thus maintaining productivity.

Research indicates that productivity increased from 29% to 63% with output-based pay plans versus time-based pay plans. Individual incentive plans are better than group incentive plans.[16]

Adequate pay is the most powerful motivator of performance, and people will not work without it. Other financial incentives, such as shift differentials, education pay, and certification pay, are positive motivators. Research has shown that productivity actually drops with time-based rewards and hourly wages. Good employees will leave rather than work with poorly performing ones. Rewards should be related to job performance. The results can be seen by correlating rewards across individual performances. There should be substantial differences in the rewards.

Kopelman suggests a mixed-consequence system: rewards for good performance, deductions for poor performance. The latter requires coaching, training, counseling, reassigning, or terminating. Important job responsibilities and behaviors deserving of high rewards can be determined from job analysis and should be related to difficult performance standards or goals.[17]

The Xerox Experience

Before 1983, Xerox had a traditional appraisal system, tying merit pay increases to performance rating. Employees were dissatisfied with the lack of an equitable rating distribution. Of employees, 95% were at the level three or four in a four-level rating system. Forced distribution was used to control the numbers of employees above or below a specific level. There were no planned objectives, and the focus was on the summary rating. A task force was used to develop a performance feedback and development process with the following characteristics:[18]

1. Objectives were set between manager and employee.
2. The evaluation was documented and approved by a second-level manager.
3. An appraisal review was held at the end of six months, with review and discussion of objectives and progress. Both manager and employee signed the written report.
4. A final review was held at one year.
5. The process emphasized performance feedback and improvements.
6. A merit increase discussion was held one to two months later.
7. There was agreement on personal goals related to communications, planning, time management, human relations, and professional goals (specialty and job).
8. There were financial and human resource management objectives.
9. Managers were trained in the process.

Regular surveys of the Xerox system indicated that 81% of employees understood their work group objectives better, 84% considered the appraisals to be fair, 72% understood how merit pay was determined, 70% met personal and professional objectives, and 77% favored the system.

Other Purposes

An effective appraisal generates understanding and commitment, leading to productivity. Career development and PA support each other if they share objectives, recognition, concern, and communication. Usually, nurse managers take charge of PA and nurses take charge of career development. They can come together for mutual benefits.

Talent development can be a mutual goal and benefit of the two programs. Performance input supports future options and paths for growth and development of employees.[19]

Accreditation and professional standards may require or suggest the use of performance evaluation.

Performance appraisals can also be used to confirm hiring decisions, particularly when new employees have a probationary period before becoming permanent. This period is crucial because employees can be terminated without the extended termination process. Effective nurse managers will use this period to counsel and coach the employee to perform effectively. The PA will document the process.

Performance appraisal has multiple purposes. Management should determine purposes that fit organizational needs.[20] Perhaps the ultimate purpose of PA is to measure accountability and improve practice standards. In nursing, the delivery of care is a major area to be evaluated. Evaluation addresses strengths and weaknesses, new or altered policies, and the need for more knowledge. Feedback increases self-awareness and professionalism.[21]

Developing and Using Standards

Performance Standards

Performance standards are derived from job analysis, job descriptions, job evaluation, and other documents detailing the qualitative and quantitative aspects of jobs. Performance standards are established by authority, which may be the agency in which they are used or a professional association, such as the American Nurses Association (ANA). They are measuring sticks for qualitative and quantitative evaluation of the individual's performance. These standards should be based on appropriate knowledge, and they should be practical enough to be attained. Like other documents, they must be kept up-to-date.

Job or performance standards for the nurse manager may be developed using the ANA *Scope and Standards for Nurse Administrators*. Performance standards for a job are written and used to measure the performance of the individual filling the job. Employees should know that these standards are being used and know what they are. They may be asked to bring copies of the standards to their supervisor for scheduled counseling. Employees also may be asked to list their accomplishments in relation to the standards. Doing so makes performance counseling less of a threat and allows employees to recognize and discuss their accomplishments. Employees may be guided to recognize areas in which their performance falls short and may be encouraged to voice goals for improvement in these areas. This method of using performance standards has been found to be effective.

The ANA Congress for Nursing Practice has developed and published standards of practice in several specialty areas. The ANA *Standards of Clinical Nursing Practice* can be used in the development of performance standards. Exhibit 18-1 is an example of performance standards for a clinical nurse.

The nurse manager controls nursing productivity with standards that measure nursing performance. Standards are based on history or past experience and "gut-level appraisal by the person in charge."[22] They include establishment of criteria, planning goals, and physical or quantitative measurements of products, units of service, labor hours, speed, and the like.[23]

A standard is "a unit of measurement that can serve as a reference point for evaluating results."[24] In collaboration with clinical nurses, nurse managers develop the units of measurement as both process (intervention) and outcome criteria.

Accuracy and fairness of PA come from having an objective, standards-oriented PA plan. The plan should have objectively defined task standards that can be measured in terms of output and observable behavioral change. These performance standards will relate to both quantity and quality—that is, the who, how, when, where, and what of the work. They will include production standards.[25]

Performance evaluation includes standards for experience, complexities of the job, level of trust, and understanding of work and mission. Friedman recommends developing job standards based on four to eight core responsibilities. For nurse managers, these core responsibilities could be in the major management functions of planning, organizing, directing (leading), and controlling (evaluating). They could also be related to the roles of clinician, teacher, administrator, consultant, and researcher. Finally, these core responsibilities could be related to self-development. Desired behaviors, outputs, or results under each core responsibility are then developed as performance objectives. Objectives are related to or combined with behaviors as standards for performance evaluation.[26] Job analysis, job descriptions, and job evaluations are important sources of standards for performance evaluation.

EXHIBIT 18-1

Performance Standards—Clinical Nurse

PERFORMANCE STANDARDS

1. *Type of work*: Nursing care of patients
   Major duty: Performs the primary functions of a professional nurse (50% of working hours).
   a. Obtains nursing histories on all newly admitted patients.
   b. Reviews nursing histories of all transfer patients.
   c. Uses nursing histories to make nursing diagnoses determining patients' needs and problems. Using this information:
   d. Initiates a nursing care plan for each patient.
   e. Lists goal(s) for each nursing need or problem.
   f. Writes nursing prescription or orders for each patient to meet each need or problem and goal.
   g. Applies the plan of care, giving evidence of knowledge of scientific and legal principles.
   h. Executes physicians' orders.
2. *Type of work*: Management of nursing personnel
   Major duty: Plans nursing care of patients on a daily basis (14% of working hours).
   a. Rates each patient according to number and complexity of needs and goals.
   b. Knows abilities of each team member.
   c. Makes a daily assignment for each team member.
   d. Discusses assignment with each team member at the beginning of each shift.
      i. Listens to taped report with team members.
      ii. Sees that team members review physicians' orders and nursing care plans.
      iii. Answers questions arising from these activities.
   e. Confers with charge nurse and ward clerk periodically to ascertain whether there are any new orders.
   f. Plans for a team conference at a specific time and place and tells team members.
   g. Incorporates division and unit philosophy and objectives into team activities.
   h. Assists with assignment of LPN and RN students, including them as active team members according to their backgrounds and learning needs.
3. *Type of work*: Management of nursing personnel
   Major duty: Supervises team activities (10% of working hours).
   a. Makes frequent rounds to assist team members with care of patients. At the same time, talks to and observes patients to determine:
      i. New needs or problems.
      ii. Progress. Confirms these observations with patient if possible.
   b. Conducts 15- to 20-minute team conference using a specific agenda that has been made known to team members at previous day's conference.
      i. Involves all team members.
      ii. Solicits comments on new problems or special problems of patients and updates selected nursing care plans as needed.
      iii. Assigns roles for next day's team conference.
   c. Writes nursing progress notes and updates remaining nursing care plans.
      i. Assists technicians with writing notes as needed for training. Otherwise reads and countersigns their notes. Writes own notes.
      ii. Updates those nursing care plans not done at team conference. Recognizes this is a professional nurse's responsibility.
      iii. Reads notes of LPNs and RNs.
   d. Communicates nursing service and hospital policies to team members on a daily basis through referral to information such as daily bulletins, minutes of meetings, and changes in regulations.
4. *Type of work*: Management of equipment and supplies
   Major duty: Identifies needs; plans and submits requests for new and replacement equipment and supplies to charge nurse (1% of working hours).
   a. While working with team members, identifies malfunctioning equipment and supply shortages and reports same to charge nurse and ward clerk on a daily basis.
   b. Submits requests for new equipment and supplies to charge nurse on a quarterly basis.
5. *Type of work*: Training
   Major duty: Identifies training needs of team members and plans activities to meet needs (5% of working hours).
   a. Identifies specific training needs of individual team members through daily observation of their performance and interviews.
   b. Evaluates performance through use of performance standards. Makes these standards known to each team member, and holds each responsible for meeting standards.
   c. Plans counseling and guidance of each team member on an individual basis and at least quarterly.
   d. Plans and conducts unit in-service education programs at least monthly. Involves team members.
   e. Recommends team members for seminars, short courses, college programs, and correspondence courses.
   f. Thoroughly orients all new team members. Conducts skill inventory during initial interview and plans on-the-job training for those needed skills in which team member is not proficient.
   g. Annually submits budget requests for training materials and programs to charge nurse.
   h. Makes reading assignments and allows time for team members to use library resources.

(continued)

EXHIBIT 18-1 *(continued)*

6. *Type of work*: Planning patient care
   Major duty: Coordinates nursing resources essential to meeting each patient's total needs and goals (5% of working hours).
   a. Consults with patients' physicians daily.
   b. Requests consultations of clinical nurse specialists. This may include clinical nurse specialists in pediatrics, mental health, medical/surgical, radiology, public health, and rehabilitation.
   c. Consults with other personnel as needed, including chaplain, social worker, recreation worker, occupational therapist, physical therapist, pharmacist, and inhalation therapist. Coordinates with physicians and charge nurse as needed.
   d. Supports philosophy of having ward clerks assume nonnursing activities by assisting with their training as needed on a daily basis to help them become proficient in their duties.
   e. Aggressively pursues having ward clerks do administrative tasks and nursing team members perform the primary functions of nursing. The latter most commonly occurs at patients' bedsides.
7. *Type of work*: Teaching patients
   Major duty: Teaches patients to care for themselves after discharge from the hospital (5% of working hours).
   a. Plans teaching as a major rehabilitation goal for each newly admitted patient. Includes it as part of nursing assessment and enters it on the nursing care plan.
   b. Reviews and updates teaching plans daily.
   c. Involves resource people in teaching program.
   d. Refers cases to visiting nurse for followup.
   e. Makes followup appointments for assessment of progress toward nursing goals with a clinical nurse.
   f. Involves families in teaching as indicated.
8. *Type of work*: Evaluation of care process
   Major duty: Conducts audits of nursing care (3% of working hours).
   a. Audits nursing records on a daily basis.
   b. Performs bedside audit on a weekly basis.
   c. Audits closed charts of discharged patients monthly.
   d. Reviews patient questionnaires.
   e. Discusses results of all audits with team members as a group and on an individual basis.
9. *Type of work*: Personnel administration
   Major duty: Rates performances of team members (2% of working hours).
   a. Writes performance reports.
   b. Discusses reports with individuals to learn their personal goals.
10. *Type of work*: Self-development
   Major duty: Pursues a program of continuing education activities (5% of working hours).
   a. Sets own goals for self-development, including a reading program and a set of educational goals for short courses, conventions, workshops, college courses, and management courses.
   b. Participates in division and departmental in-service education programs.
   c. Participates in nursing service committee activities.
   d. Participates in research projects.
   e. Participates as a citizen in the community through involvement in professional organizations and service projects.
   f. Assumes responsibility for knowledge of, progress in, and utilization of community resources such as:
      i. Health groups
      ii. Civic groups
      iii. General education groups
      iv. Nursing recruitment
      v. Others

Standards will include the dimensions of evidence-based nursing practice, measurable outcomes, and accountability.[27]

Job Analysis

Edwards and Sproull list objective performance dimensions developed by management and employees as a necessity for effective performance appraisal. These performance dimensions are developed from job analysis. "Performance criteria should be: (1) measurable through observation of behaviors of the job, (2) clearly defined, and (3) job-related." Nurse managers and nursing employees would agree on the meaning and priority of each measurement. These standards need not be quantifiable but must be keyed to observable behavior:[28]

Observable behavior ➤ Job analysis ➤ Job standards

Basing performance appraisal on job analysis makes it more relevant and establishes content validity.[29] Job analysis systematically gathers information about a particular job. It "identifies, specifies, organizes, and displays the duties, tasks, and responsibilities actually performed by the incumbent in a given job."[30] Job analysis begins with identification of the domain of content to be measured. The domain of content may be stated in terms of the tasks to be performed, the knowledge base required, the skills or abilities needed for the work, or personal characteristics deemed necessary.[31]

Job analysis will reveal overlaps among jobs so that they can be modified. It can be used to improve efficiency and proficiency by identifying skills certification, altering staffing levels, reassigning staff, selecting new employees, altering management, establishing training objectives and standards, developing career ladders, and improving job satisfaction.[32]

A procedure for doing job analysis is as follows:[33]

1. Name the job specifically, for example, nurse manager–oncology.
2. Go to the workplace, identify the target nurses working in the job family, and talk to them. Ask these questions:
   a. What are the characteristics of a good nurse manager?
   b. What are the characteristics of a poor nurse manager?
   c. How does a good nurse manager differ from a poor nurse manager?
   d. How does a good nurse manager perform tasks better than others?
   e. Give examples of effective performance by a nurse manager.
   f. Why is this nurse manager effective?
   g. Give examples of ineffective performance by a nurse manager.
   h. Why is this nurse manager ineffective?
   i. Describe a nurse manager who performs the job better than anyone else. Why?
   j. Which job skills would you look for if you had to hire someone to be a nurse manager? Why?
   k. Describe the prior training or experience needed to effectively perform as a nurse manager. Why is this so?
3. Have the job incumbents list all duties, tasks, and responsibilities (DTRs) that they perform. Cover a specific time period.
4. List on index cards all DTRs that the job incumbents perform. Do this by observation for a specific time period that coincides with the period covered in item 3 above. DTRs can be listed one to each index card.
5. Compare the two lists, and aim for a consensus between job incumbents' lists and yours.
6. State the duties, tasks, and responsibilities in specific, clear, behavioral terms.
7. Determine the four to eight categories of job tasks to be used, such as managerial, direct care, maintenance, and interpersonal.
8. Classify each DTR into the four to eight core job categories.
9. List the DTRs by priority, and use consensus to improve efficiency.
10. Evaluate DTRs for specificity, indicating how and when they will be performed.
11. Review DTRs with the team, eliminating those with low priority. Rewrite items as needed, making each a unique job skill stated in understandable language.
12. Set standards of performance, including the percentage of time each is to be done.
13. List constraints: educational, experiential, physical, and emotional.
14. Write a summary of the unique facets of the job.
15. Prepare a job analysis questionnaire and administer it to all personnel with the same job title.

Research on job analysis information has shown no significant differences between effective and ineffective retail store managers. Research also has shown no significant differences among police officers between high-job-performers' perceptions of the demands of their jobs compared with low-job-performers' perceptions. Because these research studies are few, and inconclusive in relation to the literature on the subject, nursing researchers should do research in these areas. The described method of developing a master inventory of knowledge, skills, and abilities could be used to develop job analysis for other jobs.[34]

Recent downsizing and demassing of organizations have caused managers to plan and restructure the work of remaining employees. This includes eliminating, simplifying, and combining steps, tasks, or jobs to make work easier and more enjoyable. One goal is to reduce stress by eliminating unneeded rules, procedures, reviews, reports, and approvals.

Oryx, a Dallas-based oil and gas company, used teams to eliminate 25% of internal reports and reduced signatures for capital expenditures from 20 to 4. It reduced the annual budget time from 7 months to 6 weeks and saved $70 million in operating costs in 1 year.

Another goal is to redesign physical work by analyzing jobs using the overall process described by Denton: observe and understand the current decision-making process; use a flow chart to document decisions; evaluate each decision-making step, both current and proposed; implement the change; and evaluate the results after a reasonable time has passed. Money is saved by eliminating ineffective bureaucracy. Sometimes money is saved by adding employees and slowing the production process to improve quality.[35]

Motorola uses these six steps to achieve statistical process control:[36]

1. What do I do?
2. For whom do I work?

3. What do I need to do my work better?
4. How can I specifically design my work?
5. How can I do my work better?
6. Do benchmarking: Measure, analyze, and control the improvement process.

Job analysis is used to establish board certification in nursing specialties, ergonomic criteria for shift workers, licensure examination for registered nurses (NCLEX-RN), job descriptions for nurse editors, compensation systems, redesigns for effective and efficient systems of care, and interviewing techniques for hiring the right applicants.[37]

Job analysis leads to a job description of the work expected by the institution, which can be used for PA.

Job Description

Job Description as a Contract

A job description is a contract that should include the job's functions and obligations and specify the person to whom the employee is responsible. It is a written report outlining duties, responsibilities, and conditions of the work assignment. It is a description of a job and not of a person who happens to hold that job. In 1966, Berenson and Ruhnke wrote:

> That many executives recognize the importance of obtaining good position descriptions is reflected in a survey made several years ago by the American Management Association. In this study, seventy firms reported a median fee of $20,000 paid to management consultants for preparation of their job descriptions. Most significantly, 95 percent of the respondents reported that the expenditure was "definitely worthwhile." In two instances the fee paid for this service approached $100,000.[38]

Most formats for job descriptions include a job title, statements of basic functions (one sentence), scope, duties, responsibilities (areas in which achievements are measured), organizational relationships (for communication), limits of authority, and criteria for performance evaluation. Job descriptions should be one to two pages long.[39]

Use of Job Descriptions

Job descriptions are used for many purposes, including the following:

- Establishing a rational basis for the salary structure.
- Clarifying relationships among jobs.
- Helping analyze employees' duties.
- Defining the organizational structure and support.
- Reassigning and fixing functions and responsibilities in the entire agency.
- Evaluating job performance.
- Orienting new employees.
- Assisting with hiring and placement.
- Establishing lines of promotion.
- Identifying potential training needs.
- Critically reviewing the existing work practices within the agency.
- Maintaining continuity of all operations.
- Improving the workflow.
- Providing data about proper channels of communication.
- Developing job specifications.
- Serving as a basis for planning staffing levels.

Many changes in the dynamic environment of a health care agency (such as changes in personnel, departmental or agency objectives, budget, and technology) create the need for periodic review and revision of job descriptions. Time should not be wasted preparing job descriptions that will not be put to use. Job descriptions should be available to all personnel so that they will know the dimensions of their jobs, who in the agency can help them in their work, how their performances will be evaluated, and the opportunities for advancement. To make the data more useful, numerical values may be assigned to the important elements of the specific duties, as in Exhibit 18-1.

To avoid bias, data for job descriptions should be gathered from several sources. Data may be collected by interviewing the job incumbent, having an incumbent keep a log of duties performed during a specific time period, observing the person, and having the person fill out a questionnaire (job analysis).

Role development of nurse specialists is defined in evolving job descriptions of practice from novice to expert. This role development is being shaped by health care policy, particularly that related to managed care; available resources; increased job complexity; and relationships between job satisfaction and organizational climate. The new career models are founded on self-responsibility, entrepreneurial aptitude, vision, and personal empowerment. The case manager nurse of the 21st century is forward-thinking, flexible, and solution-oriented.[40]

The person preparing the job descriptions should determine the uses that will be made of them so the needed information may be included. It is probably best to introduce job descriptions during a time of favorable economic outlook, when this action will be less threatening to employees. Job descriptions should be introduced to the staff registered nurses first. Managers may fear increased workloads and grievances. It is important to consult with all employees and allow them to discuss, comment on, and recommend changes in the job descriptions for positions. Doing so makes development of job descriptions a cooperative venture, leading to consensus, effective management, and effective performance appraisal. Language used in the job descriptions should be simple and understandable.

Because job descriptions are guides, rigid application of them can result in negative behavior.

Job descriptions should define minimum standards for effective job performance and employment and should not be too detailed. The catch-all phrase "performs other duties as directed" is evasive and should not be put in a job description.

A format is needed for quality and thoroughness of job descriptions. Kennedy recommends the following 11 elements:[41]

1. Header: job title, name and location of incumbent, immediate superiors.
2. Principle purpose or summary; overall contribution of incumbent.
3. Principal responsibilities, including percentage of time spent on each.
4. Job skills: knowledge, skills, and education.
5. Dimension or scope: quantifies areas such as the budget, size of reporting organizations, and impact on the bottom line.
6. Organizational chart.
7. Problem-solving examples.
8. Environment.
9. Key contacts.
10. References guiding the incumbent's actions.
11. Supervision given and received.

Job descriptions can be written to comply with some legal, regulatory, and accrediting requirements, and used to do the following:[42]

1. Meet the licensing laws of the state, rules of accrediting agencies, and Medicare and Medicaid regulations.
2. Determine job ratings and classifications.
3. Determine whether jobs are exempt or nonexempt.
4. Recruit, select, evaluate, and retain employees.

Exhibit 18-2 presents a job description for a bedside nurse in a US hospital around 1887. Exhibit 18-3 is a current job description for a generalized clinical nurse.

Performance Appraisal and Job Descriptions

Tom Peters in *Thriving on Chaos* has a low opinion of job descriptions."[43] "Performance appraisal should be ongoing, based on a simple, written 'contract' between the

EXHIBIT 18-2
1887 Job Description

In its publication, *Bright Corridor*, Cleveland's Lutheran Hospital published this job description for a bedside nurse in a US hospital in 1887.

In addition to caring for your fifty patients, each bedside nurse will follow these regulations:

1. Daily sweep and mop the floors of your ward; dust the patient's furniture and window sills.
2. Maintain an even temperature in your ward by bringing in a scuttle of coal for the day's business.
3. Light is important to observe the patient's condition. Therefore, each day fill kerosene lamps, clean chimneys, and trim wicks. Wash the windows once a week.
4. The nurse's notes are important in aiding the physician's work. Make your pens carefully; you may whittle nibs to your individual tastes.
5. Each nurse on day duty will report every day at 7:00 A.M. and leave at 8:00 P.M., except on the Sabbath, on which day you will be off from 12:00 noon to 2:00 P.M.
6. Graduate nurses in good standing with the director of nursing will be given an evening off each week for courting purposes, or two a week if you go regularly to church.
7. Each nurse should lay aside from each payday a goodly sum of [her] earnings for her benefits during her declining years, so that she will not become a burden. For example, if you earn $30 a month you should set aside $15.
8. Any nurse who smokes, uses liquor in any form, gets her hair done at a beauty shop, or frequents dance halls will give the director of nurses good reason to suspect her worth, intentions, and integrity.
9. The nurse who performs her labors, serves her patients and doctors faithfully and without fault for a period of 5 years will be given an increase by the hospital administration of $.05 a day, providing there are no hospital debts that are outstanding.

EXHIBIT 18-3
Position Description

TITLE: GENERALIZED CLINICAL NURSE (GCN)

General Description. The GCN is a professional nurse with academic preparation at the BSN level or above who provides expert nursing care based on scientific principles; delivers direct patient care and serves as a consultant or technical advisor in the area of health professions; and serves as a role model in the leadership, management, and delivery of quality nursing care by integrating the role components of clinician, administrator, teacher, consultant, and researcher.

Qualifications

1. Educational
   a. Graduation from an accredited school of nursing.
   b. Bachelor of Science in Nursing degree required.
2. Personal and professional
   a. Current state professional nursing license.
   b. Knowledge of and experience in preventive care (screening and teaching).
   c. Demonstrated knowledge and competence in nursing, communication, and leadership skills.
   d. Ability to analyze situations, recognize problems, search for pertinent facts, and make appropriate decisions.
   e. Ability to coordinate orientation and continuing education of clinic staff utilizing appropriate teaching strategies.
   f. Ability to apply principles of change, organizational theory, and decision making.
   g. Membership and participation in professional organizations desirable.
   h. Recognition of civic responsibilities of nursing.
   i. Ability to communicate effectively both in writing and verbally.
   j. Evidence of professional manner and conduct.
   k. Optimum physical and emotional health.

Organizational Relationships. The GCN is administratively responsible and accountable to the nurse administrator. He or she is responsible for assessing, teaching, coordinating, providing appropriate care, and making referrals when necessary.

Activities

1. Clinician
   a. Give direct patient care in selected patient situations and serve as a behavioral model for excellence in practice.
   b. Assist the nursing personnel in assessing individual patient needs and formulation of a plan of nursing care; write nursing orders, when appropriate, for implementation of nursing plan; assist the nursing personnel in documenting the effectiveness of the individualized care.
   c. Set, evaluate, and reevaluate standards of nursing practice; communicate these standards to the nursing personnel; change standards as necessary.
   d. Evaluate nursing care given to patients within the clinical area (assessing and teaching); when appropriate, make recommendations for improvement of that care.
   e. Function as a change agent; identify the barriers to more comprehensive health care delivery, modify behavior, and introduce new approaches to patient care.
   f. Collaborate with other health care providers and make appropriate referrals when necessary.
2. Teacher
   a. Provide an atmosphere conducive to learning.
   b. Teach appropriate preventive measures to clients.
   c. Direct the orientation of new staff and student nurses to ease their role transition and improve their skills, attitudes, and practices.
   d. Consider the needs of the adult learners (nursing personnel) as well as the clinicians' knowledge and expertise when planning continuing education to the clinical practice.
   e. Initiate or assist with the planning, presenting, and evaluating continuing education programs for clinic staff.
   f. Guide and assist staff and nursing students as they assume the responsibility of patient teaching.
3. Administrator
   a. Function as a change agent and appraise leadership, communication, and change processes in the organization and assist with direct strategies for change as necessary.
   b. Work collaboratively with hospital personnel and other health care providers in planning care and making referrals.
   c. Make recommendations relative to improving patient care and staff and student requirements to the appropriate administrative personnel.
   d. Support and interpret the clinical policies and procedures.
4. Self-Development
   a. Assume responsibility for identifying own educational needs and upgrade deficit areas through independent study, seminar attendance, or requesting staff development programs.
   b. Evaluate own nursing practice and instruction of others and the effect these have on the quality of patient care.
5. Consultant
   a. Conduct informal conferences with nursing personnel concerning patient care of specific health problems,

EXHIBIT 18-3

the problem patient, or other pertinent problems related to nursing as suggested by the staff.

b. Assist personnel to develop awareness of community agencies/resources available in planning patient care.
c. Serve as a resource person to patients and their families.

6. Researcher
   a. Determine research problems related to preventive care, nursing clinics, and so on.
   b. Conduct research studies to upgrade independent nursing practice.
   c. Demonstrate knowledge of the current research applicable to the clinical area, and apply this knowledge in nursing care when appropriate.
   d. Research clinical nursing problems through the development and testing of relevant theories, evaluation, and implementation of research findings for nursing practice.
   e. Promote interest in reading and reviewing of current publications dealing with the delivery of preventive care to ambulatory patients.

person being appraised and his or her boss. Limit objectives to no more than three per period (quarter, year). Eliminate job descriptions."

Performance appraisal, the setting of objectives, and job descriptions are control devices. As such, Peter's claims, they are increasingly bureaucratic, run by "experts," and out of touch with the world of human relations, because they promote stability at the expense of flexibility. Most job descriptions are not read or adhered to by successful workers. The alternative is coaching and teaching values.[44]

Job Evaluation

Job evaluation is a process used to measure exact amounts of base elements found in a job. Laws require men and women to be paid equally for equal work requiring equal skill, knowledge, effort, and responsibility under similar working conditions. This factor is important in the fight to achieve pay equity for women and hence for nurses.[45]

Job evaluation rates jobs within a given agency. Although several job evaluation systems exist, The Hay Job Evaluation System is the best known. It was developed in 1951 by the Hay Group, a Philadelphia-based consulting firm, to approve managerial, technical, and professional positions.[46]

The Hay System attempts to measure exact amounts of base elements found in all jobs, including know-how, problem solving, and accountability. Know-how includes practical procedures, specialized techniques, scientific disciplines, managerial knowledge, and human relations skills. Problem solving includes the thinking challenge created by the environment. Accountability includes freedom to act, input of the job on the corporation, and the magnitude of the job. Observations of use of the Hay System indicate that the percentage of specialized know-how decreases with high-level positions, making problem solving and accountability the real payoff factors.[47]

Work Classification

Helton reports a system for work classification to improve white-collar work. The system includes four categories: specialist, professional, support, and clerical. Professional and specialist jobs involve a significant amount of cognitive effort, are not routine, and are challenging. Criteria used to classify white-collar work are work range, work structure, control, and cognitive effort. Applied to nursing, the nurse with a master's degree would be a specialist; the nurse with a baccalaureate degree a professional, the nurse with a diploma, an associate degree, or a licensed practical nurse a support person; and aides and clerks equivalent to clerical workers. It would be economical to develop or integrate aides and clerks into one job classification.[48]

Some people believe that autonomy and bureaucracy are incompatible; however, bureaucratic activities that support professional nurses' autonomy are desirable.

Job redesign uses job enlargement and job enrichment. Job enlargement uses horizontal loading to add tasks of equal difficulty and responsibility to jobs. Job enrichment uses vertical loading to add tasks that increase the difficulty and responsibility of jobs. Job enlargement and job enrichment have beneficial results, including increased productivity. In 32 experiments involving job redesign, 30 indicated impact; the median increase in productivity was 6.4%. Employee satisfaction increased in 20 cases and was tied to more pay for increased work, less supervision, and more worker autonomy.

To make job redesign effective, nurse managers need to make accurate diagnosis and real job changes. They need to address technological and personnel system constraints; support autonomy; have a bureaucratic climate; have union cooperation and top management and supervising management support; have individuals ready to fill the jobs; and have contextual satisfaction with pay, supervision, promotion opportunities, and coworkers.[49]

Work Redesign

Work redesign needs to encompass the entire nursing care system. Work redesign should incorporate cultural issues, management structure, practice patterns, task and operating system alignment, and commitment to continuous quality improvement. Work redesign is serious work.[50]

A hostile internal culture fostering competition depresses performance because players tend to attempt to beat rivals rather than perform tasks well. The weaker party may give up, whereas the stronger one feels dangerously invincible. Friendly competition is replaced by mistrust, suspicion, and scorn. Change this type of environment to one of cooperation and higher performance. Outside competition can stimulate employees.[51]

Other suggestions for work redesign include the following:[52]

- Define the existing culture; identify the desired culture. Identify gaps, and plan to close them in a manner consistent with the vision and strategies of the health care system.
- Change structures to those that facilitate autonomy, multidisciplinary teams, new work designs, and participation in reward and risk.
- Change unwanted patient outcomes by identifying and changing practices and processes that create them.
- Because treatment design drives work redesign, gather and analyze data about treatment types and number.
- Redesign operating policies, systems, and jobs. Assess all of them using teams of practitioners who decide which to eliminate, modify, or add. Assess everything.
- Create a customer–supplier model of quality improvement to provide quality and quantity of products and services that customers want. Consider all of these as management work.

Training

Nurse managers should be educated to do effective PAs that will maintain employee productivity. Training will entail coverage of subjects such as motivational environment, appropriate job assignment, proper supervision, establishing job expectancies, appropriate job training, interpersonal relationships, providing feedback, interviewing, coaching, counseling, and PA methods.

Training raters makes PA work. The goal of such training is improved productivity. A training program can give nurse managers a conceptual understanding of PA as a management system for transmitting, reinforcing, and rewarding the behaviors desired by the organization. Raters need to know how PAs will be used. Research indicates that raters have been found to vary ratings depending on their use. Refresher training is recommended after one year. PA training can be conducted with other management development programs.[53]

An effective appraisal system will have an objective, reliable method to evaluate whether raters are qualified. Training of raters should focus on specific evaluating errors. Research indicates that rater training decreases accuracy because the raters become more sensitive to typical rating error and change their responses, thus creating new errors. Training programs should be designed to increase awareness of this fact and correct for it. Raters will be trained to capture all components of an individual's contribution to the organization, including qualitative behavior. All behavior does not reduce to quantitatively measurable performance.[54]

Training based on feedback is specific. Train the raters in behavior observation, documentation of critical performance incidents that support the consensus of a team evaluation, sensitivity to employees in legally protected categories, and performance criteria.[55]

Feedback

An analysis of 69 articles reporting 126 experiments in which feedback was applied indicated that feedback with goal setting, behavioral consequences, or both was much more consistently effective than was feedback alone. Daily and weekly feedback produced more consistent effects than did monthly feedback. Also, feedback accompanied by money or benefits of food and gasoline produced improvements in behavior more often than did praise. Graphs were used to illustrate feedback results, demonstrating the highest proportion of consistent effects. The conclusion is that feedback graphically presented at least weekly along with tangible rewards yields effective work performance.[56]

Training will include providing specific feedback to raters on timeliness, completeness, rating errors, and quality and consistency of ratings. Training methods include case studies, role plays, behavioral modeling, discussion, and writing exercises that evaluate actual appraisals, relating them to job descriptions.[57]

Feedback closes the loops by tying together the appraisal process. Feedback informs the ratee of achievements compared with expectations. It must be timely, constructive, and objective, and it must ensure that the ratee knows and can respond. The goal is to have good results continue by eliminating frustrations, which lead to lowering of goals and performance.[58]

Rater feedback from team evaluation consensus addresses systematic inconsistencies, including unlawful bias. Correction by feedback creates improved accuracy of the system, improved morale, increased worth, and increased productivity. Team evaluation consensus identifies inaccurate raters for directed training or elimination as raters.[59]

Feedback can be provided through coaching, counseling, and interviewing.

Coaching

The appraisal rater is a leader and a coach. Coaching for job performance is similar to coaching for athletic performance. As a coach, the rater does continuous reinforcement of tasks done well and helps with other tasks. In addition, the rater uses knowledge of adult education to train the employees to accomplish assigned work, does two-way communication, and has the necessary resources to do the job.

Coaching can include observing and listening for examples of work, good or bad. The rater coach praises the good and helps improve the bad with a joint action plan. Coaching makes performance evaluation useful.[60]

Coaching is yearlong evaluation and discussion of performance, which eliminates surprises. Progress discussions can be brief, regular, frank, open, and factual and can include the employee's viewpoint. The rater does not try to achieve truth but tries to discuss perceptions. The coach also removes obstacles to satisfactory performance. If the consequences are not working to improve unsatisfactory performance, the coach changes them. The ultimate step is to transfer or terminate the employee.[61]

Progressive discipline protects the employer from unwarranted liability resulting from discrimination charges and lawsuits, but it fails to bring about behavioral change in employees to make them fully functioning, committed team members. Employees already perceive PA to be evaluative and judgmental, not developmental. Progressive discipline combined with performance evaluation results in compliant employees. Effective leaders are coaches who gain commitment from employees. Today's employees will put forth effort if stimulated, challenged, and recognized for their efforts. They do not want to be managed; therefore, managers must manage, lead, and coach.

Coaching prevents discipline. The nurse manager as coach is available to observe behavior, provide feedback, and encourage employees to do their best. Coaching is done on a regular basis and is nonjudgmental. Employees believe the coach manager is supporting them to do better, to be successful, to excel.

The following are some actions of an effective manager–coach:[62]

- Listens.
- Views the employee as a person.
- Cares about the employee and helps with personal problems.
- Sets a good example.
- Stretches the employee.
- Encourages the employee.
- Helps get the work done.
- Keeps the employee informed.
- Praises the employee for a job well done, and provides criticism in a forthright manner.

An employee, who can do the job effectively, may not need coaching. Coaching is personal. It is a process that involves time, interviews, observation, feedback, and help to make employees successful. The process may be repeated as necessary.

A written coaching plan is helpful. It should be positive and upbeat. The manager writes the suggestions to be used for employee improvement. These suggestions should not be overstated but should describe behaviors, not characteristics. Appropriate alternative behaviors should be included in all coaching plans and sessions. The rater observes and gives feedback to correct wrong behavior or reinforce improvements by praise, factoring him or herself into the problem as a possible contributor to it. Coaching should be done frequently and feedback given immediately with incremental changes so that employees are not stretched to the breaking point. The goal is to build a relationship that helps an employee do a good job or move on.[63]

Counseling

Counseling can be the most productive function of supervision. Counseling interviews are for the purpose of advising and assisting an individual to grow and develop self-direction, self-discipline, and individual responsibility. The counseling interview is a helping relationship involving direct interaction between the counselor (rater) and the counselee (ratee). In a counseling interview, a personal face-to-face relationship takes place. One person helps another recognize, accept, examine, and solve a certain problem.

Nurse managers can use the counseling interview to offer support and to:

- Help workers develop realistic pictures of themselves, their abilities, their potential, and their deficiencies.
- Explore courses of action.
- Explore sources of assistance.
- Accept incontestable limitations and learn to live with them, whether physical, emotional, or intellectual.
- Make choices and improve capabilities.

Unless they have had special training, most nurse managers are not qualified for in-depth, extensive counseling in areas involving personality structure or analysis of psychological or emotional conditions. Nurse managers must be wary of tampering with the psyche of the worker. In such cases, nurse managers should know and be able to recommend sources of help.

Although counseling interviews are conducted to promote desirable behavior, the term *counseling* should not be used synonymously with the term *reprimand*. Reprimands belong more properly in the progress and informational type of interview.

One often hears supervisors say, "I have counseled him on what will happen if he does not improve." This is not counseling; this is informing a worker of the consequences of certain types of behavior or performance.

Three approaches can be used for the counseling interview: directive, nondirective, and elective. When using the directive approach, the interviewer knows in advance what will be discussed. In this approach, the interviewer gives advice, makes suggestions, helps the individual make meaningful decisions, and may even take action on some of the decisions made. This approach can be quite successful in career counseling.

The nondirective approach starts with the individual being counseled on strengths and weaknesses, potential, and problems. The individual takes responsibility for solving the problems; the counselor aids by listening. This approach is ideal for personal counseling but requires skill. The person being counseled says what he or she wants and freely expresses feelings; the interviewer must hide personal feelings and not express personal ideas. The counselor is a mirror only, reflecting the thoughts, ideas, and emotions of the counselee. This technique gives the individual an opportunity to think through problems out loud. Usually the employee will come up with some kind of answer or course of action. In using the nondirective approach, it is most important that there be no interruptions or advice on a course of action.

With the exception of the preemployment interview, it is advisable to keep notes during the interview and write a summary afterward. The summary should indicate any decisions made during the interview and any followup action required. A comment should be made in terms of how well the interview accomplished its purpose. No notes should be taken during the preemployment interview, although a summary of the interview and the decision reached should be written up immediately afterward. Taking notes during the interview discourages the applicant and makes it difficult to obtain the information needed.

Career progression depends on present and past duty performance, personal initiative, motivation, professional development, and growth potential. Performance counseling of subordinates is vitally important so they will know where they stand, how well they are doing, and where they can improve. The goal of this counseling is to improve present and future performance, not to make a critical examination of the past. Informal, day-to-day performance counseling dealing with current activities and immediate performance is important and must be continuous; however, it is not enough. Planned, careful performance counseling, scheduled at regular intervals, is needed to encourage self-improvement and to further development. During the counseling interview, the supervisor and subordinate work together to set targets in response to the job description requirements and targets for future job progression. The targets are put into writing, and progress is reviewed at the next session.

Performance counseling results from observation and evaluation of performance based on job standards. Anecdotal records may be kept and will yield facts to support written ratings or reports.

When counseling employees on performance problems, the rater uses a problem-solving approach. Such an approach includes reaching agreement that a problem exists, discussing alternative solutions, agreeing on a solution, and following up on progress.[64]

Interviewing

Interviewing is covered more fully in Chapter 8, Managing a Culturally Diverse Work Force. For appraisal interviews, the problem-solving approach is also more effective than are the tell-and-see and tell-and-listen methods. High ratee participation produces high rater satisfaction. The problem-solving rater has a helpful and constructive attitude, does mutual goal setting with the ratee, and focuses on solutions to problems. The rater also acts with the knowledge that being very critical does not improve behaviors.[65]

Good performance appraisal interviews follow these basic guidelines:[66]

- They are based on detailed, specific notes that address accomplishments and shortcomings.
- They produce no surprises from the coach.
- The drafted appraisal is discussed with the ratee and then finalized.
- Work is started and ended with positive accomplishments.
- Needed changes are specified.
- Criticism is respectful.
- Written responses are allowed.
- Staff members are invited to assess the manager's performance.

Topics for performance appraisal review include the following:[67]

- Regular job duties (based on job description).
- Special assignments and miscellaneous projects.
- Service and professional development.
- Working relations.
- Communication skills.

Peer Ratings

Research has shown that an individual's peers, that is, those people the individual works with from day to day, are a more reliable source for identifying the capacity for leadership than are the person's superiors. The armed services have found that peer nominations for leadership are significant predictors of future performance, a finding that could be tested in the nursing population. Democratic procedures, that is, having peers select the person to be promoted, would probably be threatening to many nurse managers. It has been found that peer selection differs little from selections by superiors. Occasionally, peers see a member of their group as a leader when superiors do not. Peer rating is valid when the group members have sufficient interaction and when group membership is reasonably stable over time. Peer rating is also valid if the position is important within the organization. Peer rating does help to identify potential leaders who go unnoticed by superiors. When several individuals are equally qualified for a position, peer ratings may single out the one with the highest informal leadership status.[68]

Peer evaluation may begin in high school with the Peer and Self-Evaluation System (PSES).[69] Peer rating is the professional model of appraisal used by physicians and is gaining interest and use among professional nurses. Peer rating is advocated as part of a system to make PAs more objective, the theory being that multiple ratings will give a more objective appraisal. Ratings can be obtained from multiple managers, project leaders, peers, and even patients.[70]

Peer review is a PA process among persons with similar competencies who are in active practice. These persons critically review the practice of others using established standards of performance.[71] Peer review is self-regulation and supports the principle of autonomy.[72] It consists of colleagues examining the goal-directed care of colleagues with standards that are specific, critical indicators of care written by colleagues.[73]

The purposes of peer review are to measure accountability, evaluate and improve delivery of care, identify strengths and weaknesses, develop new or altered policies, identify a worker's need for more knowledge (competence), increase workers' self-awareness from feedback (critical reflection), and increase professionalism.[74]

Implementation of a peer review rating or evaluation system includes the following:[75]

- Planning by management and clinical nurses. It may be a steering committee representing these categories of nurses plus those from the domains of research and education.
- Having a shared governance type of environment.
- Defining the peer review process and who is a peer.
- Setting goals.
- Outlining the process through consultation with management, HR personnel, and a labor attorney. A decision is made as to who gathers the data. It can be the employee, with a clinical nurse specialist as coordinator. Decisions are also made as to when and how often the interview will be done and how the outcome will be handled.
- Developing a tool using the job description.
- Obtaining multiple inputs: peer reports, self-reports, and coach reports. The manager acts as coach and counselor.

The peer review process may be developed using three distinct phases of establishing a peer review program: familiarization, utilization, and internalization.[76] Phase 1, familiarization, is characterized by the development of trust, talking through the process, and establishing that the performance, not human worth, is being evaluated. Phase 2, utilization, is defined as trial-and-error responses in which objectives are refined; the peer review process takes a sharper focus. Phase 3, internalization, occurs when there is complete actualization of the entire peer review process; onsite, hands-on evaluations are conducted and findings are acted upon.

A new performance evaluation system is needed for flattened organizations with only one manager for 30 to 100 employees. Peer evaluation meets this need and, when done within a team, should be anonymous. Peers are more knowledgeable about each other's performance than is the manager. Peer review can improve teamwork. Rigg recommends using one rating category of overall capability, with a bell-shaped curve ranking criteria. Written comments are made for only those results falling outside the range.[77]

Peer review can be taught using videotapes developed locally. Studies of peer review indicate that professional nurses view it favorably, although some consider it a threat to friendship, time-consuming, and artificially inflated. It does not always change the level of staff satisfaction with PAs. Because nurses are more often directly accountable to their employers than to their customers, peer review requires strong management support.[78]

A survey of advanced practice nurses indicated peers evaluated only 17.5% of their job performance, with the most frequent evaluation parameters being appropriateness of care, patient satisfaction, patient outcomes, and patient volumes. Patient outcomes fell into four categories: clinical end points, complications, compliance, and functional status.[79]

Self-Rating

Self-rating is another method of performance appraisal that is seldom used. In the Fortune 1300 study, immediate supervisors did 96% of appraisals.[80] Problems with self-raters are the same as with supervisor raters, indicating the need for training of both.[81]

Employee-developed PAs have been found to be tougher than those of supervisors. Employees are the subject-matter experts and do wider coverage of their jobs. Proactive, they establish expectations beforehand. Appraisal interviews are done after self-evaluation, with a common agenda and without surprises; therefore, conversations are more productive. Objectives are under the employee's control. Because they come from employees and supervisors, the job elements and performance indicators are legally defensible and broad in perspective, and they elicit employee commitment.[82]

Self-evaluation can be developed by using small groups. Having a good job description facilitates development of good behavioral expectation appraisal forms that become customized for each position. The HR department can provide a facilitator and other support. The following questions will facilitate performance indicators:[83]

- Think of who has been most effective at this element or task. What behaviors and results can you cite to support your choice?
- Think of the behaviors or results that made you say to yourself, "It would be good if everyone did that." What are they?
- What are the tricks of the trade related to this task or element?
- Think about times when you perform this task well and other times when you are not as successful. What causes the difference?
- How is the average performer different from the excellent one?
- If you were training someone, what would you emphasize?

Self-rating has been found to be threatening because the employee must place him or herself in view of others. Self-rating is a participatory management approach supported by research. Employees who view the organization as being open are more favorable to participating in PAs.[84]

Employees can be trained to research their own performance and the work environment. They can do self-assessments of and then analyze goals and expectations. Employees can also be trained to influence management communication skills to obtain information and advice, express their needs, and learn the style of influence to use on the manager. Thus, employees become protégés of proactive performers.[85]

Although self-appraisals increase employee understanding of performance feedback and provide unique information, they are seldom used. To be effective, self-evaluation should measure similar attitudes as do evaluations by supervisors. Self-appraisals should measure actual performance, relate to same time period as the criterion, be done by individuals who are experienced in self-evaluation, and be tied to a criterion group (coworkers).

Somers and Birnbaum studied a sample of 198 staff nurses in a large urban hospital. They found "no evidence of leniency error or restriction of range in self-appraisal job performance." Convergence between self- and supervisory ratings was also evident and was interpreted as an effect of halo error, that is, a tendency to rate all employees as outstanding. Self-rating requires that employees be trained in its use and focus on core job skills to make it work.[86]

A two-part format for self- and peer evaluation can be used in a peer review evaluation process. The objective of an emergency medical services unit that used this format was to determine competence. Qualification for peer evaluation included the amount of time peers worked together. Results indicated the following:[87]

- Peers rated partners higher than partners rated themselves in intubation, ECG recognition, advanced cardiac life support, skills as an emergency medical technician (EMT)–paramedic, and skills as an EMT–ambulance.
- Self-ratings were higher than were peer ratings in communication, scene management, trauma, patient assessment, and report-rating skills, which are more subjective areas.
- Both peer and self-ratings indicated that patients who were system abusers received the lowest quality of care and that the higher the socioeconomic group, the better the care received.

Research indicates that employee ratings do not differ by age; however, supervisors may view the capabilities of younger employees more positively than those of older employees.[88]

Peer and supervisor ratings have been found to be relatively highly correlated; self–supervisor and self–peer ratings are only moderately correlated. In an assessment center study, peer evaluations were better predictors of subsequent job advancement than were other ratings, including self-ratings. Peer and self-ratings predicted management potential. Behavioral information was important to peer and self-evaluation.[89]

Other Rating Methodologies

Other rating methodologies are less common than are supervisor, peer, and self-ratings. They include team evaluation consensus (TEC), behavior-anchored rating scales (BARS), and task-oriented performance evaluation system (TOPES). These methodologies measure job-related behaviors.

Team Evaluation Consensus (TEC)

Team evaluation consensus uses multiple raters, a method claimed to minimize rater bias and inaccuracies. TEC uses peers, managers, and immediate supervisors for a total of two to eight raters. Direct comparisons are made with other employees or with performance benchmarks of "outstanding" or "consistently exceeds."[90]

Behavior-Anchored Rating Scales (BARS)

Behavior-anchored rating scales list specific descriptors of good, average, and poor performance for each of several to many job aspects. Extensive analysis is required to develop these descriptions, making them time-consuming and difficult to develop. Returns are small.[91]

Descriptions of particular jobs are used to identify key job elements. Key job elements are used to develop descriptive statements of good and bad behavior. An individual's behavior is rated by closeness to behavior descriptions for key job elements (performance dimensions). Job elements, in turn, lead to behavior descriptions for each category of excellent, good, average, poor, and unacceptable, and finally lead to rating of an individual's behavior.

Raters and ratees develop the description list. Personnel time makes BARS expensive to develop. There is no composite performance score. The system is defensible in court. There have been favorable employee response and performance improvement. The results of BARS are more realistic because this system is less threatening than are most PA systems.[92]

Task-Oriented Performance Evaluation System (TOPES)

The task-oriented performance evaluation system concentrates on job tasks rather than behavior, although it is behaviorally based because it measures task accomplishments. TOPES is also legally defensible because it relates directly to the job. Job tasks are weighted for a composite performance score. Employees can be compared across jobs. TOPES is more objective than are other methodologies because it can be used to measure quantifiable performance. Task elements are evaluated by statements that support an excellent, good, average, weak, or unacceptable rating. The score on each task is multiplied by its weight, and scores are added for a composite score.[93]

Problem Areas in Performance Evaluation

It is largely assumed that merit-rating systems of performance evaluation help to develop subordinates and attest to their readiness for pay increases, promotions, selected assignments, or penalties. When such systems have been scrutinized, three main problem areas have been found:[94]

1. Subordinates have not been motivated to want to change.
2. Even when people recognize a need for change, they are unable to make that change.
3. Subordinates become resentful and anxious when the merit system is conscientiously implemented.

Effectiveness

Contrast two situations in which the same job standards are applied. In the first situation, the subordinate is handed a completed rating form and is told to read and sign it. He or she does so but immediately appeals to the next highest level of supervision. The subordinate says that this rating is the lowest received in his or her 15-year career and that he or she has never been told the quality of his or her performance was slipping. Although the situation is resolved in favor of the subordinate, he or she is no longer satisfied with working for the supervisor and must be transferred.

In the second situation, the job standards are discussed with the subordinate before they are used. The subordinate is asked to identify those performance factors and responsibilities that are really important to the success of the unit. He or she is asked also to write out the goals of his or her job as they are seen. The goals are fully discussed by the supervisor and subordinate. Progress is discussed at the request of the subordinate and at stated intervals. As a result, the subordinate is assisted in planning educational activities that will be accomplished in preparation for the career desired.

Which of the two situations meets the criteria of an effective PA?

Weaknesses

Many pitfalls and deficiencies exist in the PA process. Many managers defend PA as a system for improving performance. As used, it probably has negative influences because most people know their shortcomings better than does a supervisor. Criticisms by people who have not been adequately trained to manage an appraisal system cause employees to be anxious and frustrated, to see themselves as failures, and, in some cases, to withdraw.

The rater is influenced by the most recent period of performance, an influence that may be positive or negative. Without objective measurements and records, raters tend to focus on the few outstanding activities that are vivid in their minds. Personal feelings can influence raters, causing positive "halo" or negative "horns" effects. In many instances, the performance is appraised without clear job definitions, job descriptions, and job standards. The employee seldom knows the yardsticks by which performance is being measured. Raters are either lenient or tough, causing a great variance in value judgments. Attitudes about whether the employee deserves a pay increase influence the rater. Some managers believe that all employees are average, and they project their beliefs by rating everyone the same.[95]

Other rating errors include the following:

- Leniency/stringency error. The rater tends to assign extreme ratings of either poor or excellent.
- Similar-to-me error. The rater rates according to how he or she views him or herself.
- Central tendency error. All ratings are at the middle of the scale.
- First impression error. The rater views early behavior that may be good or bad and rates all subsequent behaviors similarly.

Other problems of PA include racial bias, focus on longevity, and complacency of managers. In their usual form, PAs are intrinsically confrontational, emotional, judgmental, and complex. A survey of 360 managers in 190 corporations on the PA process indicated the following:[96]

- 69% viewed objectives as unclear.
- 40% saw some payoff.
- 29% saw minimal benefits.
- 45% were only partially involved in setting objectives for their own performance.
- 81% said regular progress reviews were not conducted.
- 52% said guidelines for collecting performance data were haphazard or nonexistent.
- Only 19% viewed PA as properly planned.
- Only 37% viewed meetings as highly productive.
- 30% saw no worthwhile results.

Performance appraisals are extrinsically affected when format is improper due to lack of manager preparation, confusion about objectives, once-a-year activity, and overreliance on forms. There are also the extrinsic areas of inappropriate values and attitudes: avoidance of conflict to avoid unpleasantness; lack of respect by failing to take the appraisal seriously; and misuse of power, causing the ratee to be beaten down, resentful, and uncommitted.[97]

The Future of PA

Deming advocated the abolition of PAs. PA is the deadliest of Deming's "deadly diseases" that stand in the way of quality management. According to Deming, PAs embody a win-lose philosophy that destroys people psychologically and poisons healthy relationships. A win–win philosophy emphasizes cooperation, participation, and leadership, directed at continuous improvement of quality.[98]

Deming's system provides for three ratings for PA using process data. Using the statistic of variation, ratings will fall within the system, outside the system on the high side, or outside the system on the low side. If the rating is within the system, pay corresponds to seniority; if outside the system on the high side, pay should be based on merit; and if outside the system on the low side, the employee should be coached or replaced.[99]

Effective Management of Performance Appraisals

How do we overcome these pitfalls or deficiencies? First, we must be aware of them. Second, we can learn the management-by-objectives approach and treat people as people. As a result, employees will know by which yardsticks they will be measured. The PA will be a joint project. It will be a helpful situation for rater and ratee. If the situation is working correctly, ratees usually will push themselves.

A complex and lengthy evaluation form has not proved effective in rating personnel. Many managers have reduced their rating system to a limited checklist and a write-up that asks for strengths and weaknesses, with specific examples to justify each. Many managers will agree to the following principles for a rating system:

1. The system should be simple, effective, efficient, and administratively feasible.
2. The procedures and uses of the system should be understood and agreed on by line management and the employees being rated.
3. Factors to be rated should be measurable and agreed on by managers and subordinates.
4. Raters should understand the purpose and nature of the performance review. They should be taught to use the system, observe, and write notes, including a critical incident file; organize notes and write evaluations that include examples of evidence; edit their reports; and conduct effective review interviews.
5. Raters should understand the meanings of the dimensions rated, including the dimensions' relative weights. Managers are reported to be able to distinguish among only three levels of performance: poor, satisfactory, and outstanding.
6. Criticism should promote warmth and the building of self-esteem for both ratee and rater.
7. The process should be organized and used to manage employees on a daily basis according to their needs to be coached.
8. Praise or suggestions for improvement should be done at the time of the event.
9. Standards of performance should be set and modified at the time of the event.
10. Performance standards should be valid, reliable, and fair.
11. Managers should be rewarded for good performance evaluation skills.
12. Professionally accepted procedures should be used for job analysis, development of job-related observable performance criteria, and job classifications. Fairness is ensured when processes are applied systematically and uniformly throughout the organization.
13. A fair employment posture committed to equal opportunity should be used. A conscientious and equitable appraisal system reduces lawsuits and ensures fairness and confidence. Such a system should be congruent with administrative and legal guidelines.
14. Work output, not habits and traits such as loyalty, should be measured unless the habits or traits are described by specific examples of observed behavior.
15. Quality, constant innovation, and functional barrier distraction should be emphasized.
16. Appraisal should be less time-consuming through time management: daily feedback, preparation time for annual or semiannual evaluation, execution time that is spread out, and group time for consultation and coordination of appraisal criteria with peers. The last provides for fairness and equity throughout the organization.
17. The number of performance categories should be small, and no forced ranking should be used. Raters should keep it simple: 10% to 20% of the total, superior (bonus × 2); 70% to 85%, satisfactory (bonus); and 5% to 10%, questionable or unsatisfactory (no bonus).
18. The form and process should be kept simple: a one- to two-page written contract drafted with the subordinate and containing one to two specific annual or semiannual objectives; one to two personal, group, or team growth or career-enhancement objectives; one to two objectives to improve skills; and one objective related to the team's strategic theme (such as quality improvement). The manager should use open-ended prose as the format, do formal reviews bimonthly or more often, and be able to recall the content of each contract.
19. Performance goals should be straightforward, emphasizing the manager's desired results and considering what is important to the continuing success of the business.
20. Pay decisions should be made public. No one will be embarrassed if there is equity.
21. Formal appraisal should be made a small part of overall recognition that includes listening, recognition, pay, and involvement.
22. Multiple ratings, including those of ratees' subordinates, should be used.[100]
23. To get employees to buy into performance improvement, managers should create a relationship to individual and organizational performance improvement and, in turn—to add value to the success of each individual—the department and the organization; identify a measurement for each critical point in the process; and present reports and celebrate monthly at staff meetings.[101]

Evaluating performance can be challenging with the differing conceptual models offered as well as tools to be used to document tasks and roles. Paying for performance is a method that has been successful and rewards value-added behaviors and activities in the workplace.

Pay for Performance

Pay for performance is based on equity theory, expectancy theory, the law of effect, and psychological fulfillment. Equity theory indicates that people want to be treated equally and fairly by employers. Expectancy theory says that people believe they can achieve certain levels of performance and, if they do, they expect to be rewarded. The law of effect states that behavior will be rewarded when repeated. Equity theory, expectancy theory, and the law of effect, individually or combined, apply when the employee says, "I believe that when I increase my efforts or inputs to produce sustained greater outputs my employer will increase my rewards." Increased pay that is linked as a reward to increased employee inputs and outputs is pay for performance. When used effectively, the compensation system rewards superior, excellent, and satisfactory performance. People perceive an imbalance in this theory when they put forth greater effort than others but receive the same rewards. They perceive compensation to be inequitable, and pay becomes a dissatisfier.[102] Pay for performance is an incentive program that links pay to employee or corporate performance.[103]

Performance, not longevity, is fast becoming the basis for pay increases in institutions of all sizes. This may apply only to the managerial staff, or it can apply down to the lowest-paid employees in an organization.[104]

Since the recession of 1982, pay for performance has become the mode for pay increases in business and industry. Of 1080 Canadian companies surveyed in 1990, 64% indicated they would use a merit-only pay increase in 1991; 32% would use a general-plus-merit system for pay increases.[105] A 1990 survey of 250 manufacturers indicated that 76% had incentive-based programs.[106] A 1993 survey of 2000 US companies indicated that 6% used pay for performance.[107]

Results of longitudinal research conducted by the Italian National Health Service indicate that performance-related pay for health service professionals requires a careful implementation process to be a powerful tool at management's disposal to increase employees' performance and commitment.[108]

Expected Outcomes

Expectancy theory postulates that individuals will choose among alternatives in a rational manner to maximize expected rewards. A study designed to test subjects' choice of a pay plan from among piece rate, fixed rate, and bonus concluded the following:[109]

- Pay choice has a strong impact on subjects' behavior.
- High-ability individuals choose a piece-rate plan or a bonus plan over a fixed-rate plan.
- Individuals tend to choose a pay plan that maximizes their expected rewards.
- Pay choice results in higher pay satisfaction.

Studies of managers and administrators show a positive relationship between pay-for-performance perception and pay satisfaction. A pay rate higher than that of the outside market also results in greater employee satisfaction. Pay system fairness is a function of factors that pertain to organizational justice, such as participation in pay system development, perceived fairness of allocation procedures, and greater understanding of the pay system.[110]

A company's ability to compete and its company–employee relations are improved by creatively managed compensation systems. Performance-based pay affects profitability, with profits increasing when high or good performance is rewarded with pay incentives. Variable pay affects profitability more than does base pay.[111]

There may be a limit to the ratio of pay for performance. A study of 75 college students that related performance to 0%, 10%, 30%, 60%, or 100% of base pay as incentive indicated that whereas 0% produced no significant incentive, "the productivity of subjects in the 10%, 30%, 60% and 100% incentive groups did not differ. They all produced significant incentive."[112]

Compensation is a part of business strategy. A direct link exists between compensation and achievement of established goals. Increased compensation is an incentive for employees to do well. An employee will work to achieve predetermined goals if there are predetermined rewards.[113]

The following are some reasons for basing pay on performance:[114]

1. Increases job satisfaction. Subordinates who are involved in developing a work plan feel ownership of the process; as a result, they will work harder to make their plan successful.
2. Reduces absenteeism.
3. Increases productivity. Workers will perform clearly identified behaviors that are rewarded. (Mediocrity should not be rewarded.)
4. Decreases voluntary turnover, which says, "I believe I am worth more. Other employers will pay me more."
5. Improves the quality of the employee mix. This system attracts and keeps higher-level performers.

Zenger reported on a study of 984 engineering employees of two large US high tech companies. The study found that offering pay incentive awards confirmed that "extremely high and moderately low performers are likely to remain in firms offering these contracts while moderately high and extremely low performers are likely to depart." The contracts with these companies aggressively rewarded extreme performance and largely ignored moderate performance limits. To correct this, the employer can design a system to retain above-average performers and reduce turnover for only the extremely low performers.[115]

Pay for performance rewards what is valued by the employer, which may be time-in-grade and longevity. In a competitive business environment, however, employers are more apt to value new job skills and new knowledge by paying more for performance that demonstrates their use than for longevity.[116]

Types of Compensation Programs

Exhibit 18-4 lists the major types of compensation programs.[117]

Pay-for-Performance Process

The following are elements of a pay-for-performance process.[118]

1. Compensation should be part of the strategic planning process. When done with employees or their representatives as part of a task force, the compensation plan is more apt to be perceived as fair and to elicit employees' trust.

   Company mission, philosophy, objectives, vision, values, and business plans can be guides to developing a compensation plan. Decisions are made on how to link compensation to employee or company performance and hence to individuals versus groups. It is best to use more than one kind of incentive. The plan should be customized to the organizational culture and core values of a pay system. An obvious link exists between effort and performance and the need for rewards. The organization should consider the need for change and the level(s) of organizational participation. The current compensation system should be assessed for gaps, holes, and overfunding. Potential plan types should then be assigned to close the gaps.
2. Goals should be carefully set. They should be achievable to avoid system errors. When goals are set with employees, they assume ownership of the goals. Organizational performance goals may relate to improving employee motivation, engendering a culture of employees who genuinely care about organizational effectiveness, and tying labor costs to the organization's ability to pay specific amounts. Goals should be made job-specific. Consideration of costs of the plan, consistency with plant and division objectives, and fitting the culture of the organization is taken when developing the plan.
3. Standards for measurement should be precise because they are the benchmarks against which

EXHIBIT 18-4

Major Types of Pay-for-Performance (Compensation) Programs

TYPE	CHARACTERISTICS
Merit Pay	Probably most common. Usually a percentage of base pay. Sometimes part of a pay raise—a percentage for merit and a percentage for longevity. Pay raises are established for each job or group of jobs. Progression at fixed intervals is based on observation of performance. Standards of employees' success are not established a priori. When given as a merit bonus, it is not added to base pay. An individual incentive plan.
Gain Sharing	A profit-sharing plan, usually a group incentive plan. A specific share of the organization's profits is distributed to a group of employees based on production measures, financial performance, and quality of service.
Cash or Lump Sum Bonuses	Usually a share of the profits. Also a group incentive. May be a uniform bonus paid to all or most employees organizationwide.
Pay for Knowledge	Pay is linked to learning new skills and being able to work at a higher level or at more than one specialty.
Employee Stock Ownership Plans	Profit-sharing plan. Some pay cash from interest and dividends. Most are deferred plans. Risky link (ESOPs) between pay and performance for these plans. The direct pay contingency is typically quite small and linked to company performance.
Individual Incentive	Compensation is paid for individual performance.
Small Group Incentive	Each member of a group is compensated for achieving predetermined objectives.
Instant Incentive	Individual compensation for noteworthy achievements.
Recognition Programs	Performance awards to individuals or groups. May be money, educational programs, vacation/travel, certificates, or other symbolic award.

performance is met. Participants should be able to influence standards. Standards may include the following:

- Quality standards related to total quality management or continuous quality improvement for eliminating defects or errors.
- Safety standards related to all customers, internal and external.
- Attendance standards such as pay for unused sick time or paid days off.
- Productivity standards related to volume of inputs versus outputs.
- A pay-for-performance matrix.
- Job descriptions that include specific objectives of each position and measure the accomplishments of those objectives. Job descriptions can be developed with input from incumbents. When job descriptions are related to pay for knowledge, new technology may require help from experts and outside vendors. End results of these job descriptions include items such as "trained and motivated crew" and "safety." Each end result has one to three or four measures of accomplishment, such as "responsiveness to customer's needs" and "number of machine breakdowns." Preparation to meet pay for knowledge includes massive training efforts that may be done in cooperation with vendors, consultants, and educational institutions. An extensive set of training modules can be developed so that training is directly related to the job description.
- Organizational performance: profitability and financial performance.
- Management by objectives.
- Critical incidents: innovation, new products and services, market penetration, and targets.
- Economic value added (EVA). Some companies are awarding bonuses and stock options to managers on the basis of EVA, which is a way of increasing a company's real profitability. EVA equals the operating profits minus taxes minus the total annual cost of capital. The cost of capital includes interest paid on borrowed capital (less the deductible tax) plus equity capital, the money provided by the shareholders. Equity includes investment in human capital. A positive EVA means wealth is being created, whereas a negative EVA means that capital is being destroyed. EVA can be used for service businesses. EVA can be raised by using less capital and giving shareholders higher dividends. Stock prices go up.
- Cooperation among individuals or groups.
- Specific competencies, such as communication, customer focus, adaptability, interpersonal skills, team relationships, and leadership.
- Cultural diversity.

4. An objective performance appraisal system needs to be established that measures the achievement of the standards as employee outputs. The following are some examples:
   - Completion of specific education and training programs.
   - Absence or reduction (including prevention) of accidents, injuries, and illnesses, and measurably reduced pollution.
   - Specific problems solved.
   - Reduced supply inventories and supply use.
   - Reduced patient stays.
   - Increased responsibility.
   - Reduced costs.
   - Demonstrated mastery of knowledge, skills, and abilities.

   Supervisors should be trained to use the (PA) system effectively. The PA system must be objective. Some companies separate PAs from salary reviews. During PAs career development—improvement, job skills, and career growth—is the focus. During the salary review, the focus is on worth—objectives and potential to learn new skills.

   Performance standards should not be confused with results or accomplishments. If cultural diversity is a standard that is measured and rewarded, it will be accomplished.
5. A plan needs to be chosen (see Exhibit 18-4). The structure should be tailored to the performance dimensions of the job.
6. Necessary policies and procedures for implementing the plan must be written and communicated to the participants. All employees need to understand the system, that is, what it is and how it works.
7. The plan is then implemented and monitored.
8. The effectiveness of the plan is evaluated.

Group Versus Individual Plans

Group Plans

Group incentive plans include small groups or work units to which rewards are allocated for group performance exceeding predefined standards, productivity improvement plans, and profit-sharing plans. These plans are designed to encourage teamwork and cooperation with shared profits, information, responsibility, accountability, and participation in decision making.

Group variable pay is used for meeting goals based on collaborative performance and teamwork and thus encourages communication. Quality can become a team sport and a win–win situation. Group variable pay is flexible and can respond to multiple goals and measures and to change. Group variable pay should be funded independently of other pay plans.[119]

Most compensation plans tend to be indecisive. People expect to be rewarded when they increase their output because of work redesign. Managers act as their coaches and facilitators in the process.[120]

Teams, not individuals, increasingly are being rewarded for good work that results in innovation, increased cost control, and higher morale. Team leaders or managers set up worthwhile goals that are easy to measure. Everyone from plant manager on down receives the same annual raise for achieving or exceeding goals. The percentage of pay is set by goals that may be divided between those of the unit and organization. Employees are involved in designing team-based incentive programs. A trusting work relationship is needed. Some companies have teams of 25 to 50 employees who supervise themselves; they have no time clock and no foreperson. After a 3-month probation period, teams take over evaluation. When employee performance is substandard, the team recommends improvement programs, probation, or termination. The team helps hire new employees. Team members identify free riders and layabouts.[121]

Individual Plans

Individual merit pay can create internal competition for pay raises and the withholding of information from each other by competing employees. It encourages individuals to try to improve the system on their own, a difficult job to accomplish. Individual merit pay also uses individual quality outcome measures, which are difficult to develop meaningfully. It encourages a microfocus, decreases flexibility, and produces anxiety.[122]

Competency Model

Individual accomplishments are temporary and variable, whereas competencies and salaries are additive over time. Competency reflects individual performance; accomplishments can result from individual or group efforts. A value-added pay system combines base salary to employee competency and rewards individual or team accomplishment with one-time lump-sum awards. Employees are paid and rewarded for actual accomplishments, and fixed payroll costs are reduced. As employees move through competency levels, the salaries are planned to reflect this. Thus, employees are paid what they are worth to the organization. Employees who exceed goals add value to their positions. The value-added compensation approach is motivational and controls costs.[123]

Benner's research, using the Dreyfuss Model of Skills Acquisition, could be used as the competency model for a pay-for-performance system. Base pay would mirror the five levels of proficiency: novice, advanced beginner, competent, proficient, and expert. A nurse who bettered the time line for achieving a higher level of proficiency could be paid a lump-sum bonus for the accomplishment.[124]

Peer Review

The subjectivity of pay for performance can be partially eliminated by peer review. At one Motorola plant, employees work on peer review for pay. In the early stages, peer review represented 20% of annual pay, with a goal of 50%. Employees vote on one another's performance, putting enormous pressure on fellow workers to perform better. Under the Motorola pay system, all factory workers reach a maximum base pay after 39 weeks on the job. The rest of their pay is based on their individual performance.[125]

Pay Designs

Many employees are willing to risk fat bonuses for superb results. The risk is that bonuses go down with recession. Bonuses hold down fixed costs; merit raises increase costs, driving up retirement benefits.[126]

A study by Schwab and Olson produced a number of findings. These findings included the implementation of a conventional merit system achieved a considerably better link between pay and performance than did a bonus system. A bonus system without periodic adjustments in base wages also performed less well than a conventional merit system, because merit systems benefit from the consistency of true performance over time. One surprising finding was that even a very substantial error in the measurement of performance had only a modest effect on the pay–performance correlation.[127]

Rewards should be consistent, fair, timely, and related to work. They should also be ample.[128] In a pay-for-performance system, the outcomes include increased productivity from "overpaid" performers and rewards for underpaid performers.[129]

Money to fund programs sometimes comes from senior managers who give up their bonuses. Companies also use money from attrition.[130]

The Quaker Oats pet food plant at Lawrence, Kansas, paid employees 5% to 10% above market to attract and retain above-average employees and remain nonunion.[131] To achieve maximal effect on employees, base pay must be kept at a level at or above the industry average. Also, labor costs must be reduced by using incentives not added into base pay.

How to Do a Merit Pay Increase

Merit is a term that is becoming increasingly associated with performance and pay increases for nurses. Merit means that employees receive what they deserve. Pay and rewards are based on the degree of competence employees demonstrate in performing their jobs. Merit systems can include both rewards and punishments. The general goal of a merit performance and pay system is to reward people on an incremental scale so that the top achievers or performers are paid the highest salaries. A merit pay system must have four components:

1. Individual performance standards
2. Measurement scales
3. A budget
4. An award procedure

Merit pay increases are an employee incentive program. Employees who have their competencies developed, encouraged, and recognized have better attitudes about their work and their employers. These employees will work to achieve organizational objectives that support their personal objectives. Merit rewards or punishments are extrinsic. The reward or punishment can be in the form of promotion, praise, recognition, criticism, social acceptance or rejection, or benefits.[132]

Many of these rewards or punishments are activated with a total merit pay system. Extrinsic rewards need to be associated with the intrinsic rewards that come from employees' participation in making decisions about their work and the conditions under which they will perform their work. Professional nurses want control of their nursing practice. They want to participate in management decisions about how they will accomplish this. As a result, they will receive intrinsic rewards from having made the organization successful, because they have contributed to that success.

EXHIBIT 18-5

Policy and Evaluation of Employee Performance

All nursing service employees will have a criteria-based performance evaluation as follows:

1. Initiated on nursing service employee orientation.
2. At the end of the probationary period (3 months).
3. Annually (to be initiated during the following evaluation period for all employees). The annual performance evaluation will be cosigned by the head nurse or supervisor and employee, and filed in the employee's personnel file.
4. When an employee terminates employment or transfers, there will be an evaluation conference. A completed performance results contract will be cosigned by the employee and head nurse/supervisor, then placed in the personnel file.

Conferences and renegotiations concerning the criteria-based performance evaluation may occur as often as the employee/supervisor deems necessary.

Performance Standards

Individual performance standards are written criteria developed by the supervisor in conference with the individual to be evaluated. They evolve from an established, more generalized set of job performance criteria, the job description. These performance standards are tailored to the individual's abilities and goals and to the common expectations of the individual and that person's supervisor. These standards should be measurable, and they should be objectively applied. The supervisor and employee can both observe or know that the standards have been met. These standards can be written in the format of a performance results contract related to the job description. Exhibit 18-5 represents a division of nursing policy. The procedure for implementing this policy involves use of a job description and a performance results contract. (See Exhibit 18-6.)

Measurement Scales

The weights assigned to each key results area can be in terms of units or percentages. It is more practical to assign up to 1.0 unit to each key results area and determine the percentage of achievement at the annual or final conference. Doing so allows objectives to be added, modified, or deleted without readjusting the percentage weight. In Exhibit 18-7, the weights are the numbers assigned to each key results area. The total of these is 100. If the employee achieves 90, then the percentage of achievement for merit pay purposes is 90%. This percentage is used to allocate budgeted wage and salary increases.

Budget

Personnel pay increases are usually projected in the operational budget represented by the excerpt in Exhibit 18-7. They can be related to increases in the consumer price index, to the marketplace, or to the financial status of the institution. The financial status must be a major consideration. The human resources department usually prepares a cost analysis by position (Exhibit 18-8). This cost analysis is the bridge for merit pay increases for the total nursing division.

Award Procedure

Nurse administrators take all performance results contracts for each category of nursing personnel and add up the percent totals for all persons (for the nurse in Exhibit 18-7, this was 90%.). The total for registered teaching nurse II (RTN II) was 1.911%. This number is divided into the total budgeted dollars for RTN II, which was $19,263 (the sum of the amounts for filled and vacant positions labeled "Cost" in Exhibit 18-8). For each percent, each person in this category will be allocated $10.08. A person who receives a 90% merit pay increase will receive 90 × $10.08 = $907.20 (see Exhibit 18-9). This amount is transferred to a personnel action memorandum and processed through payroll. Each employee is told by the supervisor how much merit pay he or she will receive.

The Process

- Step 1. Employee and supervisor have a conference at an appointed time to establish the key results (objectives) that the employee will accomplish over an agreed-on period of time. These results will include organizational objectives from the supervisor and personal objectives of the employee. Each will come to the conference table prepared to present the objectives in an atmosphere of mutual trust and cooperation. At this conference the wording of the key results areas will be negotiated, weights will be assigned to each, time frames will be established, controls or reporting authority will be established, and the approximate date will be set for the next evaluation conference.

EXHIBIT 18-6

Sample Performance Results Contract

1. SCOPE OF RESPONSIBILITY

As clinical nurse consultant, assumes responsibility to improve the quality of health care received by the patient in the defined clinical area of expertise through role modeling, teaching, consultation, and research. The consultant assists nursing personnel to achieve their full potential and satisfaction in providing effective, efficient, and individualized care to patients and their families. The clinical nurse consultant is self-directed, determining the priorities of the role through inter- and intradisciplinary collaboration. Evaluates own practice based on the attainment of individual objectives. Responsible to the director of nursing for staff development.

2. KEY RESULTS AREAS

PERFORMANCE RESULTS	INDIVIDUAL'S PERFORMANCE
a. Schedule monthly meetings with head nurse of each unit to discuss needs and to plan for utilization of clinical consultant in meeting those needs.	I would like to see more assertive behavior in this area. Meetings were often put off and not enough consistent followup—head nurses to set a time. 8%
b. Present in-service for each area as contracted with head nurses.	Observations and needs should be made by both parties in setting up classes. This area has improved since January in some units. 7%
c. Work with department members to evaluate and revise nursing orientation program.	Done. New schedule completed. Meeting held—head nurses of 5th, 6th, 7th, and 8th floors. 10%
d. Orient new staff to orientation program.	Worked with [Name]. 10%
e. Coordinate nursing orientation program with Staff Development, Personnel Relations, and Nursing Service.	Continuous need for smooth coordination and double-checking on dates. 9%
f. Review and revise medication exam as necessary.	Recommendation made to [Name]. 10%
g. Assist in teaching CPR as directed.	Class taught as scheduled. 10%
h. Continue to coordinate and present Drug Update.	Aminoglycoside (antihypertensive agents, penicillin—March). Series started in September—was delayed in starting. Need for assertion in meeting this objective. 9%
i. Present classes based on needs survey.	Equipment Fair done. Coordinated with [Name]. 10%
j. Participate in critical care course—present emergency reinsertion of tracheostomy tube.	Content approved by Alabama Board of Nursing. Very poor evaluations from second class, with many negative comments written and verbalized. 7%

(continued)

EXHIBIT 18-6 *(continued)*

COMPLETE FOR TERMINAL EVALUATION ONLY

	EXCELLENT	GOOD	FAIR	POOR
Attendance				
Initiative				
Quantity of work				
Cooperation				
Eligible for rehire ____ Yes____ No				

3. AUTHORITY CODES

A. Does without reporting
B. Does and reports
C. Gets approval before doing
D. Participates in
E. Recommends to supervisor
F. Assists supervisor under direction

SUMMARY

[Name] has been flexible in coming in for in-service programs on 7–3 and 11-7 shifts. Has completed most of the areas on the performance contract satisfactorily. Is generally well received by new employees and helpful in their orientation to Metropolitan Medical Center.

I would like for [Name] to take more initiative and to be more assertive in identifying needs with the head nurses of the clinical units and in addressing those needs promptly and consistently. [Name] has been active in emergency admission unit and I would like to see more activity on 7th and 8th floors and the NITU.

I would also ask [Name] to address concerns and questions to me directly.

Director Staff Development — May 8, 20xx

Source: Courtesy of the University of South Alabama Medical Center, Mobile, AL.

EXHIBIT 18-7

Calculating Monetary–Merit Increase for RTN II Positions

Percent	Amount	Percent	Amount
100	$1,008	71	$716
99	998	70	706
98	988	69	696
97	978	68	685
96	968	67	675
95	958	66	665
94	948	65	655
93	937	64	645
92	927	63	635
91	917	62	625
90	907	61	615
89	897	60	605
88	887	50	504
87	877	40	403
86	867	30	302
85	857	20	202

- Step 2. A definitive date is established, and the next conference is held. At this conference the supervisor and employee discuss progress in accomplishment of key results areas. The supervisor and employee modify objectives by negotiation, discard those they agree are no longer relevant, add new ones as needed, and discuss and record progress in the accomplishment of each objective. This conference and all succeeding ones can be scheduled at earlier dates on supervisor or employee request.
- Step 3. Conferences are scheduled at 1- to 3-month intervals until the probationary period is completed, the annual rating is required, or the employee transfers or terminates. At these times the contract is summarized, signed by employee and supervisor, and filed in the employee's personnel folder. The weights assigned by negotiated discussion are totaled, and a number is assigned. This number is used in allocating the merit pay increase.

EXHIBIT 18-8
Budget for 4% Merit Pay Increase

NURSING POSITIONS						
POSITION CLASSIFICATION	FTE FILLED	TOTAL CURRENT SALARIES	COST	FTE VACANT	TOTAL CURRENT SALARIES	COST
Licensed practical nurse	84.50	$1,108,339	$44,334	9.00	$110,021	$4,401
RTN I—clinical level I	249.00	4,607,379	184,295	18.00	312,794	$12,512
RTN I—clinical level II	14.00	292,921	11,717	1.00	20,255	810
RTN I—clinical level IIII	1.00	22,755	910	0.00	0	0
RTN I (working supervisor)	45.00	893,820	35,753	0.00	0	0
Registered teaching nurse II	20.00	443,126	17,725	2.00	38,438	1,538
Nursing service supervisor I	11.50	266,910	10,676	2.00	40,228	1,609
	425.00	$7,635,250	$305,410	32.00	$521,736	$20,869
Total cost: Annual			$305,410			$20,869
Monthly			$25,451			$1,739

EXHIBIT 18-9
Standards for Evaluation of Pay-for-Performance Programs

1. There are pay-for-performance programs.
2. They were developed with input from employees.
3. They are based on company philosophy, goals, objectives, and vision.
4. They have policies and procedures.
5. The goals are job-specific.
6. There are standards for measurement.
7. They are linked to an objective performance appraisal system.
8. Rewards are linked to effort and performance.
9. Employees are informed about the programs.
10. Employees trust the programs.
11. Managers are well trained and skilled in administering the programs.
12. The programs are funded or budgeted.
13. An evaluation program is in place to monitor the programs.
14. Productivity and performance outcomes are being measured.
15. The plans are accomplishing the stated objectives.

Merit pay is a difficult procedure to accomplish because employees may not agree with the outcome. Also, supervisors are hesitant to make decisions that give employees variable pay increases. Some experts suggest that merit PA for pay be separated from PA done for other purposes. We have found that the two can work together when planned, communicated, and fairly applied.

Summary

Performance appraisal is a major component of the evaluating or controlling function of nursing management. Both raters and ratees dislike it. If used appropriately and conscientiously, the PA process will govern employee behavior to produce goods and services in high volume and of high quality. Pay for performance integrates concepts from PA to enhance further this evaluation process.

Performance appraisal is a part of the science of behavioral technology and should be viewed as part of that body of knowledge. Nurse managers need this knowledge to manage the clinical nurse effectively and efficiently as a human resource.

When used for merit pay increases, a retrospective use, PA should be separated from appraisal that looks to the future. Output-based pay plans are more effective than are time-based pay plans.

Performance appraisal should be done as a system with:

1. Clearly defined performance standards developed by rater and ratee.
2. Objective application of the performance standards, with both rater and ratee measuring the ratee's performance against the standards.
3. Planned interval feedback with agreed-on improvements when indicated.
4. A continuous cycle. (Raters and ratees should trust each other.)

Teams are effective in implementing pay-for-performance plans.

Job analysis and job description are essential instruments of behavior technology used in PA that provide objectivity and discriminate among jobs.

Coaching, counseling, and interviewing are skills of an effective PA system. In addition to supervisor ratings, PA can include peer ratings, self-ratings, TEC, BARS, and TOPES.

The purposes or uses of PA are multiple. In nursing, PA is used to motivate employees to produce high-quality patient care. The results of performance appraisal are often used for promotion, selection, and termination, and to improve performance. Incentive programs are very common in organizations. The trend is to link pay to employee or corporate performance. Doing so motivates employees to increase productivity, especially when tied to operational measures such as attendance, quality, and safety. The most common individual performance-based pay plans are merit, awards, piece rates, and commissions.

A pay-for-performance plan should be communicated well, have measures that can be influenced by participants, be consistent and fair, provide ample and timely rewards, and be trustworthy.

Participants in a pay-for-performance plan often risk the choice of earning less for the chance to earn more later through higher retirement benefits. Pay for performance starts with reduced wages and salaries, although the base should equal or slightly exceed the industry standard.

Equity theory, expectancy theory, and the law of effect are the basis for pay for performance. People expect equal pay for equal work and increased rewards for increased output.

Problems with PA systems (as well as pay-for-performance plans) include poor preparation of raters and ratees, problems of recency, halo and horns effects, lack of use of standards, leniency/stringency errors, similar-to-me errors, central tendency errors, and first impression errors.

A simple, well-planned PA system can be devised. It will be successful when understood by employees and will require considerable supervisory effort using nursing management theory.

APPLICATION EXERCISES

EXERCISE 18-1 Determine the extent to which a nurse manager exhibits coaching behaviors. Apply these coaching behaviors to yourself or have a group of peers apply it to themselves, and use the results for discussion.

EXERCISE 18-2 With a group of peers, discuss whether the performance appraisal system is too complicated. If it is, how can it be simplified and still meet accreditation and legal requirements? Are these requirements keeping the system too complicated? If so, how?

EXERCISE 18-3 With a group of peers, discuss how the job descriptions can be modified in a manner that is consistent with the vision of the organization. The goal is to make them objective and usable.

EXERCISE 18-4 Use Exhibit 18-9 to evaluate the pay-for-performance programs in a health care organization. These may be individual awards, such as merit awards, piece rate, or individual commissions, or they may be group awards, such as gain sharing, profit sharing, stock options, or bonuses.

How can the programs be improved? Make a management plan for improving them and present it to your supervisor and the director of human resources.

EXERCISE 18-5 If a pay-for-performance program does not exist in your organization, prepare a proposal for one. Present it to your supervisor and the director of human resources. You may want to do this as a group exercise.

Results of longitudinal research conducted by the Italian National Health Service indicate that performance-related pay for health service professionals requires a careful implementation process to be a powerful tool at management's disposal to increase employees' performance and commitment.

NOTES

1. Krantz, S. (1983). Five steps to making performance appraisal writing... *Supervisory Management*, *1*, 7–10.
2. Zemke, R. (1985). Is performance appraisal a paper tiger? *Training*, *1*, 24–32.
3. Krantz, 1983.
4. Fombrun, C. J. & Land, R. L. (1983). Strategic issues in performance appraisal: Theory and practice. *Personnel*, *1*, 23–31.
5. Moroney, B. P. & Buckley, M. R. (1992). Does research in performance appraisal influence the practice of performance appraisal? Regretfully not! *Public Personnel Management*, *4*, 185–195.
6. Bretz, R. D., Milkovich, G. T., & Read, W. (1992). The current state of performance appraisal research and practice: Concerns, directions and implications. *Journal of Management*, *8*, 321–352.
7. Hochwarter, W. A., Witt, L. A., & Kacmar, K. M. (2000). Perceptions of organizational politics as a moderator of the relationship between conscientiousness and job performance. *Journal of Applied Psychology*, *9*, 472–478.
8. Fombrun & Land, 1983.
9. Schneier, C. E., Geis, A., & Wert, J. A. (1987). Performance appraisals: No appointment needed. *Personnel Journal*, *1*, 80–87.
10. Zemke, 1985.
11. Levenstein, A. (1984). Feedback improves performance. *Nursing Management*, *1*, 65–66.
12. Zemke, 1985.
13. Kirkpatrick, D. L. (1986). Performance appraisal: When two jobs are too many. *Training*, 65, 67–69.
14. Ibid.
15. Kopelman, R. E. (1983). Linking pay to performance is a proven management tool. *Personnel Administrator*, 60–68.
16. Ibid.
17. Ibid.
18. Deets, N. R. & Tyler, D. T. (1986). How Xerox improved its performance appraisals. *Personnel Journal*, 50–52.
19. Jacobson, B. & Kaye, B. L. (1986). Career development and performance appraisal: It takes two to tango. *Personnel Magazine*, 26–32.
20. Kelly, K. J. (1990). Administrator's forum. *Journal of Nursing Staff Development*, 255–257.
21. Jambunathan, J. (1992). Planning a peer review program. *Journal of Nursing Staff Development*, 235–239.
22. Fulmer, R. M. & Franklin, S. G. (1982). *Supervision: Principles of professional management* (2nd ed.). New York: Macmillan, 214–215.
23. Koontz, H. & Weihrich, H. (1988). *Management* (9th ed.). New York: McGraw-Hill, 490–494.
24. Ganong, J. M. & Ganong, W. L. (1980). *Nursing management* (2nd ed.). Gaithersburg, MD: Aspen, 191.
25. Blai, B. (1983). An appraisal system that yields results. *Supervisory Management*, 39–42.
26. Friedman, M. G. (1986). 10 steps to objective appraisals. *Personnel Journal*, 66–71.
27. Rambur, B. (1999). Fostering evidence-based practice in nursing education. *Journal of Professional Nursing*, 270–274; Aliotta, S. L. (2000). Focus on case management: Linking outcomes and accountability. *Topics in Health Information Management*, 11–16; Frankel, A. J. & Heft-LaPorte, H. (1998). Tracking case management accountability: A systems approach. *Journal of Case Management*, 105–111.
28. Edwards, M. R. & Sproull, J. R. (1985). Safeguarding your employee rating system. *Business*, 17–27.
29. Price, S. & Graber, J. (1986). Employee-made appraisals. *Management World*, 34–36.
30. Ignatavicius, D. & Griffith, J. (1982). Job analysis: The basis for effective appraisal. *Journal of Nursing Administration*, 37–41.
31. Dienemann, J. & Shaffer, C. (1992). Faculty performance appraisal systems: Procedures and criteria. *Journal of Professional Nursing*, 148–154.
32. Markowitz, J. (1987). Managing the job analysis process. *Training and Development Journal*, 64–66.
33. Ignatavicius & Griffith, 1982; Markowitz, 1987; Prien, E. P., Goldstein, I. L., & Macey, W. H. (1987). Multidomain job analysis: Procedures and applications. *Training and Development Journal*, 68–72.
34. Coaly, P. R. & Sackett, P. R. (1987). Effects of using high—versus low—performing job incumbents as sources of job analysis information. *Journal of Applied Psychology*, 434–437.
35. Denton, D. K. (1992). Redesigning a job by simplifying every task and responsibility. *Industrial Engineering*, 46–48.
36. Ibid.
37. Turner, J. G., Kolenc, K. M., & Docken, L. (1999). Job analysis 1996: Infection control professional. *American Journal of Infection Control*, 145–157; Burgel, B. J., Wallace, E. M., Kemerer, S. D., & Garbin, M. (1997). Certified occupational health nursing. Job analysis in the United States. *AAOHN Journal*, 581–591; Costa, G. (1998). Guidelines for the medical surveillance of shift workers. *Scandinavian Journal of Work Environment Health*, *24* (suppl 3), 151–155; Chornick, N. L. & Yocom, C. J. (1995). NCLEX job analysis study: Questionnaire development. *Journal of Nursing Education*, 101–105; Chornick, N. L. & Wendt, A. L. (1997). NCLEX-RN: From job analysis study to examination. *Journal of Nursing Education*, 378–382; Blancett, S. S. (1997). Nursing journalism leadership. *Nursing Administration Quarterly*, 16–22; Wolfe, M. N. & Coggins, S. (1997). The value of job analysis, job description and performance. *Medical Group Management Journal*, 42–44, 46–48, 50–52; Conn, V. S., Davis, N. K., & Occena, L. G. (1996). Analyzing jobs for redesign decisions. *Nursing Economics*, 145–150.
38. Berenson, C. & Ruhnke, H. O. (1966). Job descriptions: Guidelines for personnel management. *Personnel Journal*, 14–19.
39. Webb, P. R. & Cantone, R. J. (1993). Performance evaluation: Triumph or torture? *Journal of Home Health Care Practice*, 14–19.
40. Kleinpell, R. M. (1999). Evolving role descriptions of the acute care nurse practitioner. *Critical Care Nursing Quarterly*, 9–15;

Quaal, S. J. (1999). Clinical nurse specialist: Role restructuring to advanced practice registered nurse. *Critical Care Nursing Quarterly*, 37–49; Nemeth, L. (1999). Leadership for coordinated care: Role of a project manager. *Critical Care Nursing Quarterly*, 50–58.

41. Kennedy, W. R. (1987). Train managers to write winning job descriptions. *Training and Development Journal*, 62–64.
42. Rowland, H. S. & Rowland, B. L. (Eds.). (1987). Hospital legal forms, checklists, and guidelines. Gaithersburg, MD: Aspen, 23–28.
43. Peters, T. (1987). *Thriving on chaos*. New York: Harper & Row, 596–597.
44. Ibid.
45. Waintroob, A. (1985). Comparable worth issue: The employers side. *The Hospital Manager*, 6–7.
46. TNA's Professional Services Committee. (1985). Nurses and the comparable worth concept. *Texas Nursing*, 12–16.
47. How to establish the comparable worth of a job: Or one way to compare apples and oranges. (1982). *California Nurse*, 10–11; TNA's Professional Services Committee, 1985.
48. Helton, B. R. (1987). Will the real knowledge worker please stand up? *Industrial Management*, 26–29.
49. Kopelman, R. G. (1985). Job redesign and productivity: A review of the evidence. *National Productivity Review*, 237–255.
50. Bolster, C. J. (1991). Work redesign: More than rearranging furniture on the Titanic. *Aspen's Advisor for Nurse Executives*, 4–7.
51. Kanter, R. M. (1990). *When giants learn to dance*. New York: Simon & Schuster, 75–82.
52. Bolster, 1991.
53. Martin, D. C. & Bardol, K. M. (1986). Training the raters: A key to effective performance appraisal. *Public Personnel Management*, 101–109.
54. Edwards & Sproull, 1985.
55. Ibid.
56. Balcazar, F., Hopkin, B. L., & Suarez, Y. (1985). A critical, objective review of performance feedback. *Journal of Organizational Behavior Management*, *1*, 65–89.
57. Martin & Bardol, 1986; Friedman, 1986.
58. Ratcliffe, T. A. & Logsdon, D. J. (1980). The business planning process: A behavioral perspective. *Managerial Planning*, 32–38.
59. Edward & Sproull, 1985.
60. Schneier, Geis, & Wert, 1987.
61. Lachman, V. D. (1984). Increasing productivity through performance evaluation. *Journal of Nursing Administration*, *1*, 7–14.
62. Frankel, L. P. & Ofuzo, K. L. (1992). Employee coaching: The way to gain compliance. *Employment Relations Today*, *5*, 311–320.
63. Ibid.
64. Lachman, 1984.
65. Martin & Bardol, 1986.
66. Wilbers, S. (1993, May 23). Performance reviews can be easier. *San Antonio Express-News*, p. 3G.
67. Ibid.
68. Booker, G. S. & Miller, R. W. (1966). A closer look at peer ratings. *Personnel*, *1*, 42–47.
69. Strom, P. S., Strom, R. D., & Moore, E. G. (1999). Peer and self-evaluation of teamwork skills. *Journal of Adolescence*, *9*, 539–553.
70. Friedman, 1986.
71. Jambunathan, 1992.
72. Jurf, J. B., Ecoff, L., Haley, W., Keegan, P. .L., & Williams, P. A. (1992). First steps toward peer review. *Journal of Nursing Staff Development*, 184–186.
73. Jacobs, M. E. & Vail, J. D. (1986). Quality assurance: A unit-based plan. *Journal of the Association of Nurse Anesthetists*, 265–271.
74. Ibid.; Jambunathan, 1992.
75. Jacobs & Vail, 1992; Jurf et al., 1992; Jambunathan, 1992.
76. Ibid.
77. Rigg, M. (1992). Reasons for removing employee evaluations from management control. *Industrial Engineering*, 17.
78. Jambunathan, 1992; Jurf et al., 1992.
79. Gregg, A. C. & Bloom, K. C. (1999). Performance evaluation and patient outcomes monitored by nurse practitioners and certified nurse–midwives in Florida. *Clinical Excellence in Nursing Practice*, 279–285.
80. Fombrun & Land, 1983.
81. Zemke, 1985.
82. Price, S. & Graber, J. (1986). Employee-made appraisals. *Management World*, 34–36; Andrusyszyn, M. A. (1990). Faculty evaluation: A closer look at peer review. *Nurse Education Today*, 410–414.
83. Ibid.
84. Lovrich, M. P. (1985). The dangers of participative management: A test of unexamined assumptions concerning employee involvement. *Review of Public Personnel Administration*, 9–25.
85. Jacobson & Kaye, 1986.
86. Somers, M. J. & Birnbaum, D. (1991). Assessing self-appraisal of job performance as an evaluation device: Are the poor results a function of method or methodology? *Human Relations*, 1081–1091.
87. Ballinger, J. & Ferko, J., III. (1989). Peer evaluations. *Emergency*, 28–31.
88. Van der Heijden, B. I. (2000). Professional expertise of higher level employees: Age stereotyping in self-assessments and supervisor ratings. *Tijdschr Gerontol Geriatr.*, 62–69.
89. Shore, I. H., Shole, L. H., & Thornton, G. C., III. (1992). Construct validity of self- and peer evaluation of performance dimensions in an assessment center. *Journal of Applied Psychology*, 42–54.
90. Edwards & Sproull, 1985.
91. Zemke, 1985; Edwards & Sproull, 1985.
92. Bushardt, S. C. & Fowler, A. R., Jr. (1988). Performance evaluation alternatives. *Journal of Nursing Administration*, 40–44.
93. Ibid.
94. Fox, W. M. (1969). Evaluating and developing subordinates. *Notes and Quotes*, 4.
95. Coyant, J. C. (1973). The performance appraisal: A critique and an alternative. *Business Horizons*, 73–78.
96. Lofton, R. E. (1985). Performance appraisal: Why they go wrong and how to do them right. *National Productivity Review*, 54–63.
97. Ibid.
98. Moen, J. T. (2004). Performance appraisal systems. *Public Personnel Management*, *5*, 243–248.
99. Mainstone, L. E. & Levi, A. S. (1987). Fundamentals of statistical process control. *Journal of Organizational Behavior Management*, *9*(1), 5–21.
100. Krantz, 1983; Martin & Bardol, 1986; Logan, C. (1985). Praise: The powerhouse of self-esteem. *Nursing Management*, 36, 38; Friedman, 1986; Schneier, Geis, & Wert, 1987; Edwards & Sproull, 1985; Breeze, E. Y. (1968). The performance review. *Manage*, 6–11; Dienemann & Shaffer, 1992; Peters, 1987.
101. MacFalda, P. A. (1998). Performance improvement: How to get employee buy-in. *Radiology Management*, 35–44.
102. Appelbaum, S. H. & Shapiro, B. T. (1992). Pay for performance: Implementation of individual and group plans. *Management*

Decision: Quarterly Review of Management Technology, 86–91.

103. Grossmann, J. (1992). Pay, performance and productivity. *Small Business Reports*, 50–59.
104. Browdy, J. D. (1989). Performance appraisal and pay for performance start at the top. *Health Care Supervisor*, 31–41.
105. Appelbaum & Shapiro, 1992.
106. Grossmann, 1992.
107. Tully, S. (1993, November 1). Your paycheck gets exciting. *Fortune*, 83–84, 88, 95, 98.
108. Adinolfi, P. (1998). Performance-related pay for health service professionals: The Italian experience. *Health Service Management Research*, 211–220.
109. Jiing-Lih Farh, Griffith, R. W., & Balkin, D. B. (1991). Effects of choice of pay plans on satisfaction, goal setting, and performance. *Journal of Organizational Behavior*, *12*, 55–62.
110. Miceli, M. P., Jung, I., Near, J. P., & Greenberger, D. B. (1991). Predictions and outcomes of reactions to pay-for-performance plans. *Journal of Applied Psychology*, 508–521.
111. Milkovich, G. & Milkovich, C. (1992). Strengthening the pay–performance relationship: The research. *Compensation & Benefits Review*, 53–62.
112. Frisch, C. J. & Dickinson, M. A. (1990). Work productivity as a function of the percentage of monetary incentives to base pay. *Journal of Organizational Behavior Management*, *11*(1), 13–33.
113. Berger, S. & Moyer, J. (1991, August 19). Launching a performance-based pay plan. *Modern Healthcare*, 64.
114. Parnell, J. A. Performance appraisals and paying for excellence. *Journal of Organizational Behavior*, *10*, 48–52.
115. Zenger, T. R. (1992). Why do employers only reward extreme performance? Examining the relationships among performance, pay, and turnover. *Administrative Science Quarterly*, 198–219.
116. Williamson, R. M. (1992). Reward what you value and reach new maintenance performance levels. *Plant Engineering*, 113–114.
117. Appelbaum & Shapiro, 1992; Grossman, 1992; Conte, M. A. & Kruse, D. (1991). ESOPs and profit-sharing plans: Do they link employee pay to company performance? *Financial Management*, 91–100; Schwab, D. P. & Olson, C. A. (1990). Merit-pay practice implications for pay–performance relationships. *Industrial and Labor Relations Review*, 237S–255S; Jones, D. W. & Hanser, M. C. (1991). Putting teeth into pay-for-performance programs. *Healthcare Financial Management*, 32, 34–35, 40, 42.
118. Grossmann, 1992; Appelbaum & Shapiro, 1992; Guthrie, J. P. & Cunningham, E. P. (1992). Pay for performance for hourly workers: The Quaker Oats alternative. *Compensation & Benefits Review*, 18–23; Meng, G. J. (1992). Using job descriptions, performance and pay innovations to support quality: A paper company's experience. *National Productivity Review*, 247–255; Performance reviews key in pay for performance and pay. (1993, May 10). *Wall Street Journal*, p. B1; Milkovich & Milkovich, 1992; Berger & Moyer, 1991; Tully, S. (1993, September 20). The real key to creating wealth. *Fortune*, 38–39, 44–45, 48, 50; MacLean, B. P. (1990). Value-added pay beats traditional merit programs. *Personnel Journal*, 46, 48–50, 52; Greenwald, J. (1991, April 15). Workers: Risks and rewards. *Time*, 42–43; Thornburg, L. (1992a). Pay for performance: What you should know. *HR Magazine*, 58–61; Thornburg, L. (1992b). How do you cut the cake? *HR Magazine*, 66–68, 70, 72; McNally, K. A. (1992). Compensation as a strategic tool. *HR Magazine*, 38–40; Browdy, 1989.
119. Zingheim, P. K. & Schuster, J. R. (1992). Linking quality and pay. *HR Magazine*, *1*, 55–59.
120. Harris, C. (1992). Work redesign calls for new pay and performance. *Hospitals*, *1*, 56, 58, 60.
121. Sixel, L. M. (1994, July 24). Team incentives gain popularity as reward method. *San Antonio Express-News*, 8H.
122. Zingheim & Schuster, 1992.
123. MacLean, B. P. (1990). Value-added pay beats traditional merit programs. *Personnel Journal*, *1*, 46–52.
124. Benner, P. (1984). From novice to expert. Menlo Park, CA: Addison Wesley.
125. Swoboda, F. (1994, July 24). Motorola tests peer review of performance for pay. *San Antonio Express-News*, p. 8H.
126. Tully, 1993.
127. Schwab & Olson, 1990.
128. Thornburg, 1992b.
129. Appelbaum & Shapiro, 1992.
130. Goff, L. (1992). Working harder to get the same raise, *Computerworld*, 76.
131. Guthrie & Cunningham, 1992.
132. McGregor, D. *Leadership and motivation*. Cambridge, MA: The MIT Press, 203–204.

REFERENCES

Anthony, C. E. & del Bueno, D. (1993). A performance-based development system. *Nursing Management*, 32–34.

Ballengee, N. B. (1990). Developing a performance appraisal system. *Management Accounting*, 52–54.

Barker, P., Jackson, S., & Stevenson, C. (1999). The need for psychiatric nursing: Towards a multidimensional theory of caring. *Nursing Inquiry*, 103–111.

Barnett, J. & Anderson, G. (1987). Performance appraisal revived. *Senior Nurse*, 20–22.

Bernarden, H. J., Cooke, D. K., & Villanova, P. (2000). Counseling and performance improvement. *Journal of Applied Psychology*, 232–236.

Brooks, B. A. & Madda, M. (1999). How to organize a professional portfolio for staff and career development. *Journal of Nurses Staff Development*, 5–10.

Carson, K. P., Cardy, R. L., & Dobbins, G. H. (1992). Upgrade the employee evaluation process. *HR Magazine*, 88–92.

Chu, N. L. & Schmele, J. A. (1990). Using the ANA standards as a basis for performance evaluation in the home health care setting. *Journal of Nursing Quality Assurance*, 25–33.

Davis, D. S., Greig, A. E., Burkholder, J., & Keating, T. (1984). Evaluating advance practice nurses. *Nursing Management*, 44– 47.

Ernst, E. & Resch, K. L. (1999). Reviewer bias against the unconventional? A randomized double-blind study of peer review. *Complement Therapy Medicine*, 19–23.

Ethridge, J. R. (1990). Criteria for evaluating performance: An empirical study for nonprofit hospitals. *Health Care Supervisor*, 49–56.

Findley, H. M., Giles, W. F., & Mossholder, K. W. (2000). Performance appraisal process and system facets: Relationship with contextual performance. *Journal of Applied Psychology*, 634–640.

Fouracre, S. & Wright, A. (1986). New factors in job evaluation. *Personnel Management*, 40–43.

Goodale, J. G. (1992). Improving performance appraisal. *The Business Quarterly*, 65–70.

Goodson, J. R. & McGee, G. W. (1991). Enhancing individual perceptions of objectivity in performance appraisal. *Journal of Business Research*, 293–303.

Hagenstad, R. (1995). Integrating values into the interviewing and selection process. *Seminars in Nurse Management*, 16–26.

Herbert, G. R. & Doverspike, D. (1990). Performance appraisals in the training needs analysis process: A review and critique. *Public Personnel Management*, 253–270.

Hough, L. M. & Oswald, F. L. (2000). Personnel selection: Looking toward the future—Remembering the past. *Annual Review of Psychology*, *51*, 631–664.

Idaszak, J. R. & Drasgow, F. (1987). A revision of the job diagnostic survey: Elimination of a measurement artifact. *Journal of Applied Psychology*, 69–74.

Keuter, K., Byrne, E., Voell, J., & Larson, E. (2000). Nurses' job satisfaction and organizational climate in a dynamic work environment. *Applied Nursing Research*, 46–49.

King, G. B. (1990). Performance appraisal on the automated environment. *Journal of Library Administration*, 195–204.

Kirby, P. (1992). An aberration: Supervisors who like performance appraisal? *Supervision*, 14–17.

Klimaski, R. & Inks, L. (1990). Accountability forces in performance appraisal. *Organizational Behavior and Human Decision Processes*, 194–208.

Lawler, F. E., III. (1986). What's wrong with point factor job evaluation? *Management Review*, 44–48.

Lee, M. A. (1987). How to use job analysis technique. *Restaurant Management*, 84–85.

Longnecker, C. O. & Goff, S. J. (1992). Performance appraisal effectiveness: A matter of perspective. *SAM Advanced Management Journal*, 17–23.

Mann, L. M., Burton, C. F., Presti, M. T., & Hirsch, J. E. (1990). Peer review in performance appraisal. *Nursing Administration Quarterly*, 9–14.

Manshor, A. T. & Kamalanabhan, T. J. (2000). An examination of raters' and ratees' preferences in process and feedback in performance appraisal. *Psychology Reports*, 203–214.

Martin, D. C. & Bectal, K. M. (1991). The legal ramifications of performance appraisal: An update. *Employee Relations Law Journal*, 257–286.

Martin, R. K. (1999). The role of the transplant advanced practice nurse: A professional and personal evolution. *Critical Care Nursing Quarterly*, 69–76, 86.

Mathes, K. (1992). Will your performance appraisal system stand up in court? *HR Forum*, 5.

McCarthy, J. P. (1991). A new focus on achievement. *Personnel Journal*, 74–76.

McCloskey, J. C. & McCain, B. (1998). Nurse performance: Strengths and weaknesses. *Nursing Research*, 308–313.

McGee, K. G. (1992). Making performance appraisal a positive experience. *Nursing Management*, 36–37.

Meyer, A. L. (1984). A framework for assessing performance problems. *Journal of Nursing Administration*, 40–43.

Mossholder, K. W., Giles, W. F., & Weslowski, M. A. (1991). Information privacy and performance appraisal: An examination of employee perceptions and reactions. *Journal of Business Ethics*, 15–26.

Murphy, K. R. (1991). Criterion issues in performance appraisal research behavioral accuracy versus classification accuracy. *Organizational Behavior and Human Decision Processes*, *50*, 45–50.

Murphy, K. R., Gannett, B. A., Herr, B. M., & Chen, J. A. (1986). Effects of subsequent performance on evaluation of previous performance. *Journal of Applied Psychology*, 427–431.

Nathan, B. R., Mohrman, A. M., Jr., & Milliman, J. (1991). Interpersonal relations as a context for the effects of appraisal interviews on performance and satisfaction: A longitudinal study. *Academy of Management Journal*, 352–369.

Neuman, G. A. & Wright, J. (1999). Team effectiveness: Beyond skills and cognitive ability. *Journal of Applied Psychology*, 376–389.

Odiorne, G. S. (1984). *Strategic management of human resources*. San Francisco: Jossey-Bass.

Parlish, C. (1987). A model for clinical performance evaluation. *Journal of Nursing Education*, 338–339.

Pelle, D. & Greenhalgh, L. (1987). Developing the performance appraisal system. *Nursing Management*, 37–40, 42, 44.

Philp, T. (1992). Getting down to some serious work on staff appraisal. *CA Magazine*, 26, 28.

Reed, P. A. & Kroll, M. J. (1985). A two-perspective approach to performance appraisal. *Personnel*, 51–57.

Ramsey, P. G., Carline, J. D., Blank, L. L., & Wenrich, M. D. (1996). Feasibility of hospital-based use of peer ratings to evaluate the performances of practicing physicians. *Academic Medicine*, 364–370.

Richmond, B. (1992, December 12). Teachers must stand up to school board group. *San Antonio Light*, p. F5.

Rotarius, T. & Liberman, A. (2000). Objective employee assessments: Establishing a balance among supervisory evaluations. *Health Care Management*, 1–6.

Schnake, M. G. & Dumler, M. P. (1985). Affective response bias in the measurement of perceived task characteristics. *Journal of Occupational Psychology*, 159–166.

Schwarz, J. K. (1999.) Assisted dying and nursing practice. *Image Journal of Nursing Scholarship*, *31*(4), 367–373.

Strickland, D. & O'Connell, O. C. (1998). Saving your career in the 21st century. *Journal of Case Management*, 47–51.

Thomas, P. A., Gebo, K. A., & Hellmann, D. B. (1999). A pilot study of peer review in residency training. *Journal of General Internal Medicine*, 551–554.

Waldman, D. A. & Kenett, R. S. (1990). Improve performance by appraisal. *HR Magazine*, 66–69.

Weingard, M. (1984). Establishing comparable worth through job evaluation. *Nursing Outlook*, 110–113.

Williams, S. L. & Hummert, M. L. (1990). Evaluating performance appraisal instruments dimensions using construct analysis. *Journal of Business Communication*, 117–133.

Wren, K. R. & Wren, T. L. (1999). Legal implications of evaluation procedures for students in healthcare professions. *AANA Journal*, 73–78.

Zawackie, R. A. & Norman, C. A. (1991). Breaking appraisal tradition. *Computerworld*, 78.

CHAPTER 19

The Nurse Manager of Staff Development

Lynn P. Norman, RN, MSN

Nursing students and nurses are adults whose learning is based on principles of critical thinking.

LEARNING OBJECTIVES AND ACTIVITIES

- Distinguish among the characteristics of the adult learner.
- Explain the staff development process.
- Describe the roles of staff development educators.
- Describe an andragogical approach to program design.
- Differentiate among the characteristics of learning.
- Describe the role of the teacher in adult education.
- Describe the role of the learner in adult education.
- Use evaluation procedures in adult education.
- Apply the Critical Thinking–Learning Model in staff development.

CONCEPTS: Staff development, andragogy, Critical Thinking–Learning Model of Staff Development, facilitator, preceptorship, evaluation.

NURSE MANAGER BEHAVIORS: Maintains a staff-development staff to meet the legal and accreditation requirements for personnel competency.

NURSE EXECUTIVE BEHAVIORS: Assesses learning needs of nursing staff and implements the Critical Thinking–Learning Model of Staff Development. Coordinates learning experiences for nursing staff and students.

Introduction

Professional nurses are educated in a variety of ways. There are inconclusive findings regarding the effects of different educational paths to RN licensure on nurse performance and patient outcomes. The research described takes into account characteristics, abilities, and work assignments of nurses with and without baccalaureate degrees; however, it does not effectively examine quality of care provided, including patient safety.[1] The National Sample Survey of Registered Nurses (NSSRN) does analyze educational preparation and years of experience in the nursing work force; it notes that baccalaureate-prepared nurses appear to stay in the work force longer and accumulate more years of work experience than do those not prepared at that level.[2] Thus staff development becomes an even greater responsibility.

Staff development educators are challenged to provide creative and consistent high-quality education to adult learners who practice nursing in an environment of rapid advances in technology, budget constraints, and sophisticated performance improvement techniques.[3] Through downsizing and merging of clinical agencies, the role of staff development continues to evolve.

Staff development departments vary in structure, size, roles, and administration. Nurse managers frequently perform the staff development role, sometimes as director of nursing in a small health care organization, as nurse manager, or from other management positions.

Staff development is based on a philosophy of adult education that uses teaching and learning principles and concepts that apply to people who have a combination of responsibilities, including family and financial obligations, employment commitment, and identified areas of interest or specialization. Nurses are adult learners who combine many of these traditional adult responsibilities with the demands of increasingly complex societal and health care provider roles. Consideration of employees' learning style as well as level of motivation should be a factor in planning staff development programs.

Philosophy of Adult Education

Staff development programs are designed to motivate adult learners to consider the learning process as a natural part of living. People are born into society without knowledge. From the day they are born until the day they die, they are part of a society whose institutions are constantly changing. People are capable of learning during this entire life span. Cross believes that "lifelong learning means self-directed growth. It means acquiring new skills and powers, the only true wealth, which you can never lose. It means investment in yourself. Lifelong learning means the joy of discovering how something really works, the delight of becoming aware of some new beauty in the world, the fun of creating something, alone or with other people."[4]

Lifelong learning is essential in nursing because of the rapid changes in the health care delivery system and the changing roles of nursing within that system. Knowledge acquired in basic nursing education programs quickly becomes obsolete. Nursing is influenced by public policy, technology, and societal and economic changes.

Technology, which continually increases in complexity and scope, and innovations in health care are major forces motivating nurses to pursue lifelong learning. Nurses must adjust quickly to the demands associated with high-tech skills in many areas. Effective staff development programs respond to the needs of nurses practicing under increased demands.

Educators and nurse managers planning staff development programs consider that nurses also have lifelong learning needs related to the processes of physical, cultural, political, psychosocial, and spiritual maturation. One of the weaknesses of staff development programs has been their narrow emphasis on the major field of study. Continuing education that focuses on education of the whole person will promote the development of free, creative, and responsible nursing personnel. Staff development programs to educate the whole person are aimed at building competencies for performing various roles in life, which were identified by Malcolm Knowles (1978) as friend, citizen, individual (self), family member, worker, and leisure-time user.[5] For example, nurses are adult citizens of the communities in which they live. It is appropriate that educational systems provide them with skills to enhance their participation in social institutions and to assist in the assumption of responsibilities, rights, and privileges within their communities and larger sociopolitical structures. Motivation may be defined as the energy that causes adults to strive toward competence in matters that they hold to be important. A common culture is created when the staff development educator values and engages the needs of adults. "Adult learners have never been more diverse and we as teachers must be attuned to the influence of diversity and culture on motivation and hence on learning."[6]

Roles of Staff Development

The most notable role of staff development is the focus on developing nursing skills and knowledge within a comprehensive program that includes orientation, in-service education, continuing education programs, and job-related counseling. Orientation introduces employees to new situations and includes content related to philosophies, goals, policies, procedures, personnel benefits, role expectations, and physical facilities. Staff development includes assigning preceptors or mentors as part of the orientation process. Employees need orientation each time their roles change. Staff development also includes job-related counseling, which involves promoting the professional growth of employees by assisting them to deliver their best job performance. Counseling also includes promotion possibilities and assistance in obtaining formal training. In-service education provides learning experiences in the work setting for the purpose of refining and developing new skills and knowledge related to job performance. These learning experiences usually are narrow in scope and brief because they are aimed at only one competency or knowledge area. Continuing education programs are planned and organized around learning experiences in a variety of settings that are intended to build on the educational and experiential bases of the nurse. As a basis for state license renewal, state-board-approved continuing education offerings give nurses new approaches to health care delivery and enhance practice, education, administration, research, and theory development.[7] Examples include workshops, conferences, self-learning modules, and seminars.

A learning experience might be developed to introduce nursing staff in cardiac care to a new, more sophisticated monitoring device.

Expanded roles of staff development also include coordination with schools of nursing to provide optimal student clinical experiences through a preceptorship while maintaining a safe, effective care environment for the client. The preceptorship experience allows students to develop a one-on-one relationship with a nurse, who socializes the students to the nursing role.[8] School of nursing faculty, the preceptor, and staff development educators collaborate to identify learning needs of the nursing student based on clinical learning objectives. The role of preceptor includes being teacher, role model, and evaluator of student learning.[9] Staff development educators create a positive climate and join with nurse managers to prepare the preceptor for the role. Staff development managers, along with nursing faculty, can facilitate this role by offering programs on the role of a preceptor.

The Staff Development Process

Philosophy

The organization needs a statement of beliefs about how it will accomplish its staff development program. The staff development philosophy should relate to the mission and philosophy of the organization of which it is a part. The statement of philosophy should be written by a representative group, not by an individual, and be accepted by staff and administrators.

In writing a philosophy for staff development for health care professionals, the group needs to address its beliefs with regard to the following areas:

1. How learning takes place
2. Teaching methods
3. Employees' responsibility for their own learning
4. Organizational responsibility for providing staff development
5. Clients' right to health care

Organization

A staff development program can function under many organizational models, depending on the philosophy of the agency. A centralized model would have an agency wide staff development department, and the educational staff might consist of nurses or educators who are not nurses. In this model, all departments collaborate in determining and planning the job needs of their staff. The centralized model facilitates scheduling and use of equipment and may prevent duplication of effort. The main criticism of this model is separation of educational staff from nursing staff and perpetuation of the us-against-them attitude.

In a decentralized model, the nursing department has its own organized in-service or staff development department. The nursing staff development department may then adopt a centralized or decentralized model. The strength of a decentralized model is that specific needs can be addressed. The major areas of concern in decentralization are the use and scheduling of classrooms, potential duplication of effort, and the cost of providing multiple small programs. The trend toward decentralization of as many functions as possible in health care organizations makes it easier to expand the roles of staff development.

Personnel

Depending on the governance of staff development, nursing service administrators may be responsible for staff development to promote quality client care. The following are among their responsibilities:

- Providing financial and human resources.
- Establishing policies for staff development.
- Providing release time, finances, or both for staff to attend continuing education offerings.
- Motivating employees to assume responsibility for their own professional development.
- Providing mechanisms to identify staff growth needs.
- Evaluating the effects of staff participation in continuing education offerings on quality of client care.

The manager of staff development is an administrator and an educator who is able to communicate and establish trust, has knowledge and skills in adult education, has knowledge of training resources and subject matter, and understands the program planning process. As an administrator, the manager understands organizational theory and has skills in budgeting, personnel management, and group process. As an educator, the manager has educational skills in diagnosing learning needs, developing learning objectives and lesson plans, selecting and using appropriate teaching techniques, and evaluating the effectiveness of the program.

The professional development staff is selected by the staff development manager to work on planning, implementing, and evaluating staff development programs. The size of the staff depends on the size of the agency. In small agencies the coordinator may be the only staff member. These personnel may be totally decentralized to the unit level. Having support staff that is qualified and in adequate numbers is essential for effective staff development.

Advisory Committees

An advisory committee can be useful for identifying needs and resources and for planning programs. Members of the committee should represent all fields of practice in the agency. Other members may include people with needed expertise. Committee members may increase participation because they can communicate the purpose of staff development programs directly to the people they represent. This committee is important regardless of the size of the agency and governance of staff development.

Budgets

The manager of staff development is responsible for developing and implementing the budget with input from staff. The amount of monies allocated for staff development depends on staff size, the number of new employees that is anticipated, and the resources that are already in existence. The agency administration will demonstrate a commitment to staff development by allocating adequate funds for salaries, staff time for training, periodicals, books, software, audiovisuals, and outside educational resources.

Andragogical Approach to Program Design

The characteristics of adult learners require an andragogical approach to curricular development and teaching in staff development programs. *Andragogy*, defined by Knowles, is the art and science of helping adults learn (in contrast to pedagogy, the teaching of children). The andragogical approach assumes that the learners themselves are the facilitators who create a climate that motivates their own achievement.[10] When staff development programs are designed for nurses, the shift from the traditional teacher-centered approach, in which the focus is on information giving and the teacher, to a student-centered approach, in which the focus is on active learning and the student, requires a fundamental change in the role of the teacher. The didactic (information-giving) teacher is replaced by a facilitator of learning, and the creation of an environment for student learning becomes the new prerequisite. These changes have major implications in terms of staff development; this environment is unlikely to be effective if teachers are not able to take on new roles.[11] The flexibility or level of structure is also important in program design. Cavanagh suggested that tightly structured training programs are incongruent with an andragogical approach. Basic learning principles of cardiopulmonary resuscitation programs are examined in this study, which find that a rapid loss of practical skills and knowledge follows these highly structured training programs.[12]

It is evident that traditional pedagogical approaches to staff development are less effective than is an individual approach based on professional career development.[13] However, programs that teach highly specialized, concrete skills tend to use a more pedagogical approach than do programs that emphasize intellectual exploration. This tendency may need to be addressed in the early planning phase of program design by putting compensatory measures in place.

Mutual Diagnosis of Learning Needs

Effective staff development programs begin with a needs assessment of the learners. Adults are interested and motivated when they enter educational programs because of perceived needs they have identified. Adult learners have a perception of the level of competency they want to achieve and the knowledge they need for better performance in their personal lives or work settings. If adult learners' needs differ from those perceived by staff development program planners, participation in the educational offerings would be decreased or nonexistent. A training program is a waste of time and money if it does not increase the efficiency and effectiveness of workers.[14] As a result, educational needs assessment is the first step in adult education programming.

A common mistake of staff development planners is to assume they know what adults need to learn. This assumption may lead to an unsuccessful educational program.

Needs Assessment Methods

Staff development program planners decide on a method of assessment that will meet their purposes. The following factors should be considered before designing a needs assessment survey:

1. Target population
2. Development time
3. Cost
4. Financial and human resources
5. Analysis time
6. Anonymity
7. Objectivity

The needs survey should address content, design of learning activities, and learners' background. Content relates to the specific topics of interest to the learners. Design of learning activities covers areas such as planning when individuals can attend courses and the types of learning options (such as workshops or modules) that would best facilitate their learning.[15] When considering a method of assessment, it is important to address the needs of the organization and learner. Organizational needs are influenced by factors such as the standards of the Joint Commission on Accreditation of Healthcare Organizations (JCAHO), the American Nurses Association (ANA) Standards for Continuing Education, consumer needs, standards of practice, and the philosophy and objectives of the institution. If staff developers ignore these needs, they may lose the support of the sponsoring organization.

Questionnaire or Survey

A questionnaire is perhaps the most frequently used method for assessing needs. Questions on the survey tool may be either forced choice, which allows selection of one of several categories of context needs, or open-ended, which allows more freedom of response. An example of an open-ended question is: "If I could learn more about stress management, I would like to learn . . ." The survey tool should be designed with a combination of the two types of questions.

A pilot test of the survey is done to ensure that questions are clear and that the data gathered are complete and relevant. Individuals completing the pilot survey are asked to comment on whether they understood the questions, how long it took them to complete the questionnaire, and whether other areas should be added. Their responses are then analyzed by a group, and necessary changes are made to the questionnaire. The advantages of the questionnaire include ease and convenience of administration and ease of computing the results. Disadvantages include the cost of data collection and analysis. Also, if a mailed questionnaire yields a low return, the data may not result in a representative sample. Exhibit 19-1 is one example of a broad-scale questionnaire.

Observation

When used with other methods, observation is an effective way to assess needs. A nurse manager or clinical specialist can observe personnel and perhaps identify learning needs. The effectiveness of this technique is increased when a standardized observation guide is used. A disadvantage of this method is that observations are subjective and can produce incomplete data. For instance, a nurse observed to be charting incorrectly might be doing so because of lack of time, not because of faulty knowledge of the procedure.

Interview

Interviewing a sample representing the target population is a method that can be used to gather valuable

EXHIBIT 19-1
Broad-Scale Questionnaire

How can Staff Development help meet your needs over the next year? Please answer the following questions. This is an anonymous survey.

Check most appropriate.

1. I am:
   ______ a. RN
   ______ b. LPN
   ______ c. NA
   ______ d. WC
2. I work in the following type of nursing area:
   ______ a. Medical
   ______ b. Surgical
   ______ c. Orthopedic/Neuro
   ______ d. Obstetrical
   ______ e. Pediatric
   ______ f. Neonatal
   ______ g. Emergency room
   ______ h. Operating room
   ______ i. Other (specify)______
3. I have worked in my nursing area for:
   ______ a. less than 3 months
   ______ b. 4 to 11 months
   ______ c. 1 to 3 years
   ______ d. 4 to 6 years
   ______ e. over 6 years
4. What is the best time of day for you to attend in-service programs?
   ______ a. mornings
   ______ b. afternoons
   ______ c. evenings
5. What is the best day for you to attend in-service programs?
   ______ a. Monday
   ______ b. Tuesday
   ______ c. Wednesday
   ______ d. Thursday
   ______ e. Friday
   ______ f. Saturday

Circle the most appropriate response, according to your interest, for the following in-service education programs:

4 = I am highly interested.
3 = I am interested.
2 = I am somewhat interested.
1 = I have no opinion or don't know.
0 = I have no interest.

6. 4 3 2 1 0 Respiratory care
7. 4 3 2 1 0 Wound management
8. 4 3 2 1 0 Stress management
9. 4 3 2 1 0 Nursing and the law
10. 4 3 2 1 0 Communication skills
11. 4 3 2 1 0 Nursing process
12. 4 3 2 1 0 Use of computers in nursing
13. 4 3 2 1 0 Death and dying
14. 4 3 2 1 0 Body image
15. 4 3 2 1 0 Cost care
16. What other topics would you like included in in-service education programs? ______
______
______

information about needs. Interviews can clarify ambiguous data gathered through surveys. Respondents often feel more comfortable expressing feelings verbally than in writing. A disadvantage is that data collected are difficult to sort, measure, and report.

Open Group Meetings

Learning needs can be assessed in group discussions when a resource person is available with questions to focus the group on the topic. The resource person should be skilled in the group process technique so that all group members can be aided in expressing their learning needs clearly. This method can be time-consuming and of limited value if group members are hesitant about speaking out.

Analysis of Professional Literature

A systematic review of the previous 6 to 12 months of pertinent journals is an excellent way to identify trends and compare national information with the leader's own setting. This method is inexpensive and can be present- or future-oriented. On the negative side, a review of literature is time-consuming because it involves analyzing and synthesizing many articles to find trends. Also, a time lag is involved in publication, meaning some information may no longer be current.

Competency Model

A competency model is a valuable means for discovering the needs of an individual. In building a competency model, a series of statements is developed that identifies expected performance or behavior. After the competencies are refined to small units that reflect only single behaviors, individuals can compare their performance with each behavior. Staff developers can help individuals identify gaps between their level of competence and the desired level. Individuals can then participate in learning activities to close any gaps.

Employee Performance Appraisals

The performance appraisal can be an effective method for identifying needs if it is done in a positive way. Appraisals should offer constructive criticism. People should be encouraged to state their own hopes and aspirations and identify their learning needs. The rater and the ratee have a clear picture of duties and demands of the job and current abilities and level of performance. The rater and ratee then identify gaps between the desired and the actual levels of performance. Staff development programs are then designed to improve performance or prepare the employee for a new position.

Mutual Planning

Once needs are identified and priorities set, appropriate learning experiences are designed. Adult learners are able to help plan the educational offerings. Professional nurses are more committed to an activity when they have been involved in the decision-making process. Nurses see themselves as self-directed and may resist a staff development program that is imposed on them by the establishment. A committee that represents all subgroups is one mechanism for mutual planning. The nursing service administrator or the education coordinator is responsible for appointing the planning committee.

Translating Learning Needs into Goals

The planning committee should be involved in setting goals for the learning experience. Because developing goals is often a difficult part of the planning process, the staff development program planner will assist the committee. Goals provide intent and direction for movement.[16] Goals are important in providing a basis for planning learning activities, selecting methods and materials, and defining and organizing content. For goals to serve as workable tools, certain guidelines should be followed:

- Goals should be centered on the learner, not the teacher. For example, "The student will understand selected concepts of shock," should replace "The instructor will present selected concepts of shock."
- Goals do not dictate specificity but may simply indicate a general aim. Goals may be inexact and imprecise as long as intent is provided.
- One overall goal may be sufficient for a training program if it is stated broadly. For example, an appropriate goal for a program on care of patients with gastrostomy tubes could be: "The learner will employ care and critical thinking in addressing specific human needs of the patient and family dealing with a gastrostomy tube."

Critical Thinking–Learning Model

A model for teaching adult learners that emphasizes collaboration between teacher and learner was developed by McDonald.[17] The conceptual basis for this model, called the Critical Thinking–Learning Model, is an open system of simultaneous interaction between teacher, learner, and the teaching–learning environment. (See Exhibit 19-2.) The model shows the continual influence of each component on all other components, even when overt interaction is taking place. This model represents a departure from the linear interaction of traditional teaching, in which response from the student occurs as a result of stimulus from the teacher. The Critical Thinking–Learning Model shows a balance of influence from all components, with no single component dominating the exchange. Core elements are considered central to each component and are necessary for the outcome of critical thinking to occur. Each component contains five basic characteristics, as seen in Exhibit 19-3.

EXHIBIT 19-2
Critical Thinking–Learning Interaction

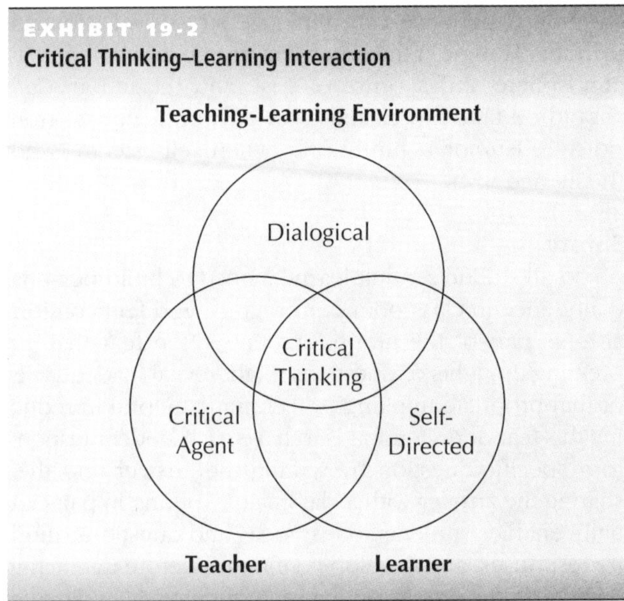

EXHIBIT 19-3
Characteristics of the Components in the Critical Thinking–Learning Model

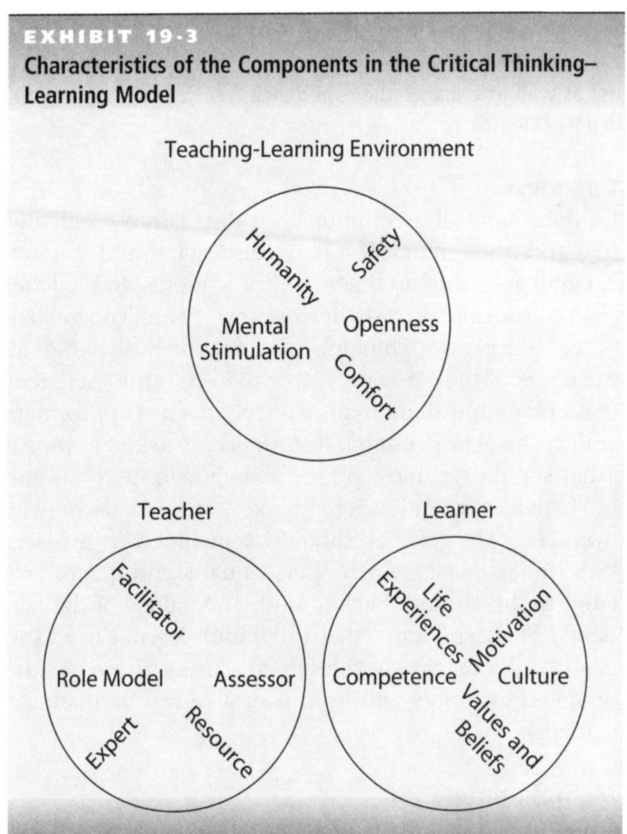

Teaching–Learning Environment

The core element in the teaching–learning environment is dialogical. This concept places the process of dialogue as the central focus in the classroom. (See Exhibit 19-4.) To arrive at the desired outcome of critical thinking, students must be able to relate their new ideas and experiences to previous knowledge. Students must be able to share, justify, and validate their new understanding. Dialogue implies a struggle for insight into possible alternatives and a consideration of new perspectives. The development of critical thinking involves the acting on and sharing of knowledge through discourse. This rational process takes place in the creative and unpredictable environment that occurs with dialogic classes.[18] Five characteristics are necessary for the provision of a teaching–learning environment that supports the process of critical thinking and learning: comfort, openness, mental stimulation, safety, and humanity.

Comfort

When a working adult student arrives at class to participate in learning activities, demanding work schedules and responsibilities already surround the learning experience. The teacher must take into consideration factors such as fatigue and distraction or simply the role change that accompanies adult learners to the classroom. An environment that provides for comfort is a first step in promoting collaboration between teacher and student. Comfortable seating, good lighting, access to beverages, and thermostat control can make a difference between actively attending to learning activities and simply enduring a class session. This attention to environmental factors is particularly applicable in the longer class sessions that are typical of programs structured for adult learners.

EXHIBIT 19-4
Comparison of Traditional, Stimulus–Response Interaction, and Critical Dialogue

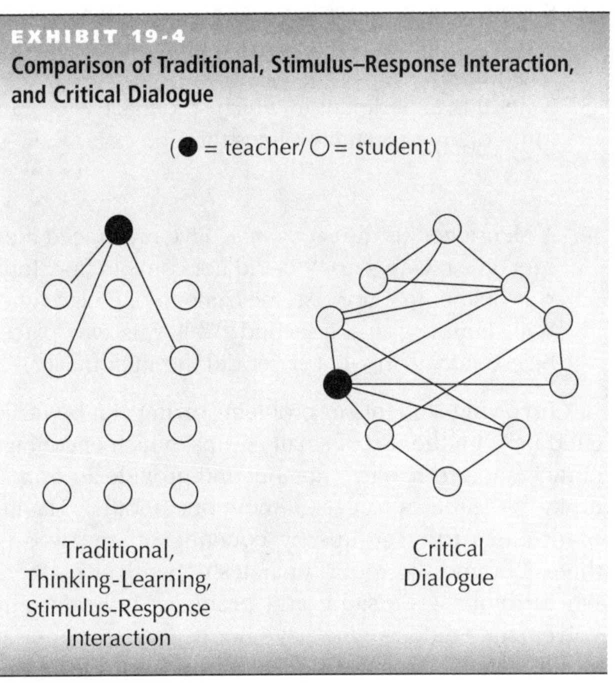

Source: Created by Nancy McDonald for research study, "The Measurement of Selected Aspects of Critical Thinking."

Unique experiences and life skills can contribute to the teaching–learning process as well as enhance the confidence of the participants.

Openness

Establishment of a community in the classroom creates free and open interaction between teacher and student. A circular seating arrangement for students and teacher promotes a nonlinear sharing of power. The dialogue that is central to critical thinking occurs more easily when all members of the class are visible to each other. Activities that encourage sharing among students are appropriate at the initial class session. If students are asked to repeat other students' names and name their favorite foods and fun activities, attention is more likely to be focused away from self. The teacher should be included in this ice-breaking exercise, which offers valuable information related to the culture, background, and values of the students. The experience that each adult learner brings to the classroom can be identified during these get-acquainted exercises and used later as a resource among students.

Mental Stimulation

Classes that begin with a mental warm-up assist with the transition of adults from working professionals to students. The following activities stimulate thinking:

1. Round robin sessions in which students name things involving threes (examples: triangles, butcher–baker–candlestick maker, French hens).
2. Round-robin sessions in which students name things involving time (examples: ETA, timeout, Greenwich mean time).
3. Nine-dots experiment in which students try to draw four continuous straight lines through dots.(• • •)
   (• • •)
   (• • •)
4. A Mensa genius quiz (*example:* Five men raced their cars on a racing strip. Will did not come in first. John was neither first nor last. Joe came in one place after Will. James was not second. Walt was two places below James. In what order did the men finish?)

Involving students in problem solving can be facilitated through the use of small groups, which encourage participation from each member and provide an opportunity for students to get to know one another. Having participants form groups by counting off by twos or threes, around the room separates dependent partners, which minimizes visiting and promotes individual involvement. Students who have not had the opportunity to talk can then engage in dialogue and learn from one another. The infusion of humor and pleasure into the learning experience can minimize stress and stimulate learning. Humor in the classroom promotes a community atmosphere and a sense of ease and relaxation. Care should be taken to establish an environment safe from ridicule. Humor is funny only when self-esteem is not threatened.

Safety

As do all students, adult learners need to build personal confidence in classroom performance and feel comfortable as part of the group. Students often fear that expressing thoughts or questions might reveal inadequacies or inappropriate thinking. A technique helpful in reducing this fear or discomfort is to have each student respond to a specific question by writing the answer and then sharing the answer with a classmate. Working in pairs initially enables students to test ideas and questions, modify responses, and develop confidence before interacting with the larger group. Pairing each student with a different classmate for several of these exercises establishes a known support base and provides a network with other students.

An environment that is safe and nonthreatening is essential to the development of critical thinking. The response of the teacher to each student and to the group must convey respect, caring, and support. A student who fears reprisal, humiliation, or embarrassment will be unlikely to voice opinions or engage in dialogue. Adult learners are often fearful of the unknown and are usually eager to establish credibility and make a good impression.

The learning environment must be supportive of the efforts of adults while providing an atmosphere that supports humor and enjoyment of the learning experience. Strategies such as brainstorming encourage and release the competence for active learning that is in human nature.

Humanity

A person-centered approach to the teaching–learning process means emphasizing the competence of the learners. Teachers who are not afraid to show that they are human value each student's personal choice, responsibility, and contribution to the process of learning. Humanity pervades all interactions within the teaching–learning environment. Human qualities that are essential for the teacher to possess include valuing the student as a fellow human being, regardless of the quality or quantity of class work; trusting the student to engage in self-discovery; being genuine in responses and interactions; and offering empathy.

The Learner

Self-direction is the core element for the learner in the Critical Thinking–Learning Model. The element of self-direction is intimately related to critical thinking and must be present for the student to be a critical thinker. Responsibility for the internal process of cognition rests with the learner and is a precondition for the development of understanding and knowledge. Each learner who participates in the critical thinking–learning process brings life experiences, competence, motivation, culture, and values and beliefs to the educational experience.[19]

Life Experiences

Adult learners are individuals who have accumulated experience, skills, and wisdom through the process of living. These students are not as malleable as are 20-year-olds and may be more resistant to change. In the Critical Thinking–Learning Model, reciprocal interaction occurs in a continuous process in which the teacher learns from the student and vice versa. Life experiences of adult students are a valuable resource for the teaching–learning process. Teachers who recognize and use this resource enrich the process and help build the self-esteem of the learners.

Competence

The educator of adults who subscribes to the concepts of critical thinking and learning must assume that each student is competent to engage in active learning, unless individual performance over time proves otherwise. Creative thinking is an inherent characteristic of human beings, but for a given person it may have been suppressed by rigid and punitive methods encountered in previous educational experiences. Development of competence to assume individual responsibility for learning may be necessary before students can become responsible for personal learning. The teacher should challenge the tendencies toward convergent thinking, give positive feedback for risk taking or creative thinking, and encourage consideration of alternative solutions. Brainstorming is a process that develops competence in self-discovery and critical thinking. No response generated during the exercise of brainstorming can be seen as incorrect, no viewpoint or statement must be justified, and all members of the group are given the opportunity to participate. This process frees students from censoring others' or their own responses. Rewarding uninhibited and outrageous thinking encourages divergent rather than convergent thinking.

Motivation

Adult learners return to the classroom for various reasons. Identifying these motivators can help the learner develop and maintain the initiative needed to engage in critical thinking activities. Insight into intrinsic and extrinsic aspects of motivation to learn can promote integration of new ideas and highlight the approaches best suited for the exploration of these ideas. Understanding individual motivators can enable teacher and student to anticipate and adjust to the stress and anxiety that may accompany new learning experiences. Styles of learning can be diagnosed through tools and measurement scales such as those previously described. Students who can understand personal methods of learning are more able to choose approaches that facilitate critical thinking and learning. Preferences, habits, and aptitudes of each student ideally should be identified to enable teacher and students to select effective strategies for learning.

Culture

Cultural background is the basis for many of the assumptions, values, and beliefs held by an individual. Political stances, life choices, and much of behavior in general are grounded in the time and place of birth and maturation. To become aware of personal choices, students must examine the scripts inherited from acculturation. Students may experience for the first time the basis of personal choices when engaging in critical thinking and learning. In this process, students question and challenge rules that have governed past actions. The disruption and discomfort that result from this process are part of the examination of previously held assumptions. The open interchange of the Critical Thinking–Learning Model indicates that self-directed learning includes the learner's right to challenge both the teacher's assumptions and the learner's personal assumptions. This interchange should never be conducted in an autocratic or intimidating manner by teacher or by student. When familiar assumptions, such as those resulting from cultural influence, are the launching point for the critical thinking–learning process, students are able to respond specifically and with familiarity. Easily identifiable areas of questioning will be more readily broached than will sophisticated or complicated conceptual areas.

Values and Beliefs

Many individuals believe that absolute truths exist, and some individuals are certain of what these truths are. The emotional responses that result from challenging personal values and beliefs may be difficult for individual students, the group, and the facilitator or teacher. An environment of safety, trust, and caring must exist for adult learners to engage in critical thinking—learning related to personal commitments. As with all groups of people, the classroom will have individuals who are more developed or mature and who more readily exhibit skepticism, analysis, and divergent thinking. Those students who have not yet reached this level of self-discovery cannot be forced into using imaginative thought. The teachers of adults can only support, challenge, and offer alternatives to those learners who are resistant to the process. Acceptance of the values and beliefs of others must be role-modeled by the teacher, who continues to offer ways to achieve insight into values and beliefs.

The Teacher

The teacher is the catalyst for the process of critical thinking–learning and must function as a critical agent to provide diversity of thinking, disagreement, and the challenging ideas in the classroom. In leading students toward critical thinking, the teacher must engage in activities that identify and challenge students' assumptions and assist them in imagining and exploring alternatives. Unnecessary criticism and unrealistic utopianism must be avoided.[20]

Facilitator

Effective listening skills are crucial to the collaborative process between student and teacher in the Critical Thinking–Learning Model. Attention to body language and nonverbal communication is as important as is attending to the spoken interchanges among fellow students and between student and teacher. Effective listening assists students in clarifying concepts and problem solving. Responding specifically and thoughtfully to a student's viewpoint indicates that the teacher values that individual, which enhances the individual's self-esteem. Learning can be facilitated through specific classroom activities, such as the use of case studies, team learning, or role playing. Students whose life experiences apply to the concepts being studied can develop case studies. Dialogue then involves the entire class in examining and analyzing the application of the case study to class content. Team learning is a process that uses groups of students who are assigned specific areas of content and then share the concepts with the class. Assignments can be made sufficiently in advance to allow the teams to plan and organize the presentation. All students are given the opportunity to contribute knowledge and expertise. This exercise also develops cooperative work and leadership abilities. Role playing involves assigning a subject or content to be studied and acted out. Several students can participate as a group in the center of a circle of classmates. Observers may chart the interaction of role players, and then participate in an assessment and discussion at the conclusion of the activity to provide learning and feedback.

Role Model

One of the most common means of learning throughout life is by role modeling. Educators of students of all ages are aware of the influence exerted by behavior and of the importance of demonstrating positive qualities in the teaching–learning environment. In the application of critical thinking to role modeling, positive behaviors demonstrated by the teacher include encouraging criticism of one's own actions, refusing to evade difficult questions, and being flexible in changing requirements or behaviors as a result of student input.

Preceptorships encourage extensive role modeling. The preceptor acts as a role model by displaying knowledge of patient care and making critical decisions for implementing quality patient care. The preceptor models technical skills and proper communication with the interdisciplinary team.[21]

Resource

The role of teacher as resource begins with the collaboration process in which learning projects and contracts are identified in the learning environment. Once goals are established, the teacher serves as a resource and then guides the student toward other resources appropriate for achievement of these goals. Student learning styles can be used as a basis for selecting human and other resources as well as methods to promote goal achievement. Emphasis should be placed on adjusting resource selection to meet individual strengths and weaknesses. Resources for personal communication include friends, faculty, other students, and experts in the area to be examined. Professional journals, textbooks, videotapes, and cassettes are also available as resources. Teachers should guide students toward appropriate methods for achievement of goals while individualizing resources for the learning environment. Methods for meeting goals range from random approaches to trial-and-error methods and from sequential to structured approaches. Management plans are often useful in assisting students to map goals, presentations, and resources or for simply organizing time.

Expert

Lecture is rarely used in the Critical Thinking–Learning Model, but if deemed necessary by the teacher, it can be appropriate if limited to time frames of 10 to 20 minutes. Lecturing frees students from active learning and, if lengthy, is not assimilated. Activities that promote student involvement in the learning process are crucial to critical thinking. The teacher as expert in the teaching–learning process uses methods to minimize passivity and promote activity in the learning process.

Assessor

A needs assessment conducted at the first class session provides information related to the classroom. Students are also given the opportunity at this time to recognize and appreciate the knowledge they and their fellow students bring to the learning experience. The teacher in the role of assessor may then explore ways to use student expertise for teaching–learning. The motivation or willingness to learn is an area that the teacher must address in the role of assessor. When the adult learner has already identified the need to learn, goal achievement is more likely to occur. Motivation may be intrinsic or extrinsic. When the student engages in learning for the sake of learning, motivation is intrinsic or occurs for personal motives. Extrinsic motivation is based on external, or social, motives and occurs when the student engages in learning for other personal reasons. During evaluation procedures, the teacher functions as assessor, although the role may be simplified if grade contracts are used. Students and teacher may collaborate to set standards of evaluation or may also evaluate the abilities of students against set criteria. Self-analysis is another method of evaluation that students may use to assess goal achievement. Targeting areas and expertise that need developing or improving should follow assessment by teacher and students.

Teaching Methods

To maximize learning, staff should be aware of three important aspects involved in teaching adult learners.

1. Collaboration between teacher and student is essential for active learning to occur. Learning should be a shared activity in which teacher and students have responsibilities. Learning is more likely to take place when students are active participants. Teaching as a collaborative effort may be viewed as negotiating rather than imparting ready-made knowledge.
2. Critical thinking may be seen as a basic principle of adult education. This process is one of logical reasoning that involves the recognition of assumptions underlying beliefs and behaviors and justification for ideas and actions. Information should be analyzed to make sense of external experiences. Critical thinking demands comprehension. Students are conditioned to be passive when a teacher begins to lecture. Lecture should not be used as a way to challenge students' thinking. The wealth of experience brought to the classroom by adult learners can be incorporated into critical thinking activities that result in greater involvement with the learning experience.
3. Self-directed learning has an important place in the educational activities of adults. Adults have a deep need to be self-directing, which involves being able to make decisions and manage personal experiences. The teacher should determine what the student already knows and must be open about the intent to share responsibility for learning.

Evaluation Procedures

Evaluation is essential to provide staff with information to improve programs or determine whether training programs should be continued. Each course, seminar, class, or workshop is evaluated when it is completed to determine whether the program met the needs for which it was designed. Evaluation includes the learner as well as the program.

Learner Evaluation

Adult learners should have a sense of progress toward their goals and should be involved in evaluating their learning. Teachers should involve learners in developing mutually acceptable criteria and methods for measuring progress toward the learning objectives. When objectives are written in behavioral terms, the standard for evaluation is included in each objective. It can then be observed whether the knowledge, skill, attitude, or practice is accomplished. When measuring learning, a before-and-after approach should be used so that learning can be related to the training program. When possible, learning should be measured objectively, such as by a written test. Also, when practical, a control group should be compared with the experimental group that receives the training.

Three types of techniques can be used to evaluate learning:

1. Observation of skills or behavior is often useful. Observation guides need to be developed, and observers need to be told specifically what they should be scrutinizing. Validity may be a problem if learners perform in a particular way because they are being observed or if the perception of the observer is incorrect.
2. Paper-and-pencil methods, such as true-false, multiple-choice, or fill-in-the-blank tests are frequently used. Pretesting and posttesting should be done so that comparisons can be made. For some students, tests produce anxiety, which may contribute to poor test results.
3. Unobtrusive measures, when used with other evaluation data, can be valuable. Examples of unobtrusive measures are chart reviews, audits, wear of textbook pages, or numbers of staff using self-directed learning modules.

Program Evaluation

The content, process, and method of a program offering should be evaluated. A survey or questionnaire is often used to elicit participants' reaction to the program. The following information can be obtained by a survey:

- What the participants liked or disliked about the program.
- Whether the faculty and speakers were prepared.
- Whether objectives were met.
- How well the program was organized.
- Whether the facilities were adequate.
- Suggestions for improvements.
- Suggestions for future programs.

Problems can arise when questionnaires are too long or unwieldy for the participants to complete or for the person who must tabulate them. The following guides are useful for preparing questionnaires:

- Determine what you want to find out and avoid unnecessary questions.
- Design the form so that a computer can tabulate most reactions.
- Make the form anonymous.
- Give participants the opportunity to make additional comments.
- Perform a pilot-test of the questionnaire on a sample target audience.

Exhibit 19-5 is an example of an evaluation questionnaire.

EXHIBIT 19-5
Evaluation Questionnaire

PURPOSE

To provide feedback to program planners so presentations can be improved. Complete the following anonymously. Evaluation of the Burn Therapy course, August 12. Circle the number that represents your feelings about each statement.

	STRONGLY DISAGREE	DISAGREE	AGREE	STRONGLY AGREE	NO OPINION
1. The content presented is applicable to my work.	1	2	3	4	5
2. The goals of the program were clear to me.	1	2	3	4	5
3. The content presented reflected the goals.	1	2	3	4	5
4. The content presented was what I expected.	1	2	3	4	5
5. The content was valuable to me.	1	2	3	4	5
6. The instructor's presentation was clear and informative.	1	2	3	4	5
7. The instructor made good use of audiovisuals.	1	2	3	4	5
8. The level of presentation was too theoretical.	1	2	3	4	5
9. The level of presentation was not practical.	1	2	3	4	5

Please respond to the following questions:

10. What were the most positive aspects of this presentation?

____

____

11. What did you like best about the presentation?

____

____

12. Please make any other comments or suggestions.

____

____

13. Do you have any suggestions for future presentations?

____

____

Summary

The purposes of staff development include the improvement of care given to clients and of participants' quality of life. Nurse managers who present successful staff development programs understand and apply principles of adult education. Staff members, as adult learners, are self-directed and want to be involved in diagnosing their learning needs, developing objectives, and evaluating their own learning. Adult learners have a wide variety of experiences on which to build new learning and are looking for experiential teaching techniques that allow them to share their knowledge. They want educational programs that are problem-centered and can be applied in their work or life roles. Nurse managers as educators in staff development programs are facilitators of learning. This role is enhanced when the educator possesses attributes such as openness, flexibility, and spontaneity.

APPLICATION EXERCISES

EXERCISE 19-1 Read the job description of the staff development manager. Describe the various roles of the staff development manager.

EXERCISE 19-2 Staff development programs should be aimed at preparing individuals for various life roles and for maintaining competence in those roles. Identify three roles filled by nurses and give examples of staff development programs that will assist them in coping with these social roles and related tasks.

EXERCISE 19-3 Write a philosophy of staff development for your unit or organization.

EXERCISE 19-4 Staff development program planners do careful needs assessments before designing programs. Locate a needs survey done in your organization.

- Is it adequate?
- How has it been used?
- What would you do to improve it?

EXERCISE 19-5 Locate the goals of two staff development programs for your unit or organization. If they are not learner-centered, change them to make them so.

EXERCISE 19-6 Design a questionnaire to evaluate an in-service or continuing education program presented in your workplace. Use it, and analyze the results.

EXERCISE 19-7 Refer to the Critical Thinking–Learning Model in this chapter. Evaluate a staff development program using this model as a standard. Analyze the results and make a management plan to correct any deficiencies.

NOTES

1. Blegen, M., Vaughn, T., & Goode, C. (2001). Nurse experience and education: Effect on quality of care. *Journal of Nursing Administration*, *31*(1), 33–39.
2. Sochalski, J. (2002). Nursing shortage redux: Turning the corner on an enduring problem. *Health Affairs*, *21*(15), 157–164.
3. O'Very, D. I. (1999). Self-Paced: The right pace for staff development. *Journal of Continuing Education in Nursing*, *4*, 182–187.
4. Cross, K. (1982). *Adults as learners*. San Francisco: Jossey-Bass, 16.
5. Knowles, M. (1978). *The adult learner: A neglected species* (2nd ed.). Houston: Gulf Publishing.
6. Wlodkowski, R. J. (1999). *Enhancing adult motivation to learn* (Rev. ed.). San Francisco: Jossey-Bass.
7. Furze, G. & Pearcey, P. (1999). Continuing education in nursing: A review of the literature. *Journal of Advanced Nursing*, *29*(2), 355–363.
8. Letizia, M. & Jennrich, J. (1998). A review of preceptorship in undergraduate nursing education: Implications for staff development. *Journal of Continuing Education in Nursing*, 211–217.
9. Reilly, D. E. & Oermann, M. H. (1992). Clinical teaching in nursing education (2nd ed.). New York: National League for Nursing.
10. Knowles, M. (1984). *Andragogy in action*. San Francisco: Jossey-Bass.
11. Spencer, J. A. & Jordan, K. R. (1999). Learner centered approaches in medical education. *British Medical Journal*, 1280–1283.
12. Cavanagh, S. J. (1990). Educational aspects of cardiopulmonary resuscitation (CPR) training. *Intensive Care Nursing*, *6*, 38–44.
13. Beeler, J. R., Young, P. A., & Dull, S. M. (1990). *Professional development framework. Journal of Nursing Staff Development*, 296–301.
14. Moore, M. & Dutton, P. (1978). Training needs analysis. *Academy of Management Review*, 532–545.
15. Swansburg, R. C. (1995). Nursing staff development: A component of human resource development. Sudbury, MA: Jones and Bartlett.
16. Gould, J. E. & Bevis, E. O. (1992). Here there be dragons. *Nursing and Health Care*, *3*, 126–133.
17. McDonald, N. C. (2002). The nurse manager of staff development. In R. C. Swansburg & R. J. Swansburg (Eds.), *Introduction to management and leadership for nurse managers* (3rd ed.) Sudbury, MA: Jones and Bartlett, 488–501.
18. Brookfield, S. D. (1990). Passion, purity, and pillage: Critical thinking about critical thinking. *Adult Education Research Conference Proceedings*. Athens, GA: The University of Georgia, 25–30.
19. Candy, P. C. (1991). Self-Direction for lifelong learning. San Francisco: Jossey-Bass.
20. Garrison, D. R. (1991). Critical thinking and adult education: A conceptual model for developing critical thinking in adult learners. *International Journal of Lifelong Education*, *5*, 287–303.
21. Gates, G. E. & Cutts, M. (1995). Characteristics of effective preceptors: A review of allied health literature [Electronic version]. *Journal of the American Dietetic Association*, *2*, 225–229.

REFERENCES

Bowen, M., Lyons, K. J., & Young, B. E. (2000). Nursing and health care reform: Implications for curriculum development. *Journal of Nursing Education*, *39*(1), 27–33.

Facione, N. D. & Facione, P. A. (1996). Externalizing the critical thinking in knowledge development and clinical judgment. *Nursing Outlook*, *44*, 129–136.

Fowler, L. P. (1998). Improving critical thinking in nursing practice. *Journal for Nurses in Staff Development*, *14*(4), 183–187.

French, P. & Cross, D. (1992). An interpersonal-epistemological curriculum model for nurse education. *Journal of Advanced Nursing*, *17*, 83–89.

Greenwood, J. (2000). Critical thinking and nursing scripts: The case for the development of both. *Journal of Advanced Nursing*, *31*(2), 428–436.

Hadley, C. S. (1999). Capitalizing on nursing creativity. *AWHONN Lifelines*, 47–49.

Haislett, J., Hughes, R. B., Atkinson, G., & Williams, C. L. (1993). Success in baccalaureate nursing programs: A matter of accommodation? *Journal of Nursing Education*, 64–70.

Kintgen-Andrews, J. (1991). Critical thinking and nursing education: Perplexities and insights. *Journal of Nursing Education*, 152–157.

Lindeman, C. (1996). A vision for nursing education. *Creative Nursing*, *2*(1), 5–12.

Maynard, C. A. (1996). Relationship of critical thinking ability to professional nursing competence. *Journal of Nursing Education*, *35*(1), 12–18.

Morton-Cooper, A. & Palmer, A. (2000). *Mentoring, preceptorship and clinical supervision: A guide to professional roles in clinical practice* (2nd ed.). London: Blackwell Science.

Nielsen, B. B. (1992). Applying andragogy in nursing continuing education. *Journal of Continuing Education in Nursing*, 148–151.

Padberg, R. M. & Padberg, L. F. (1990). Strengthening the effectiveness of patient education: Applying principles of adult education. *Oncology Nursing Forum*, *17*(1), 65–69.

Rew, L. (2000). Acknowledging intuition in clinical decision making. *Journal of Holistic Nursing*, *18*(2), 94–113.

Ward, D. & Berkowitz, B. (2004). Arching the flood: How to bridge the gap between nursing schools and hospitals. *Health Affairs*, *21*(5), 42–52.

Subject Index

E

F

N

O

P

Q

R

S

W

X

Y

Z